Recent Advances in

Histopathology
22

Recent Advances in Histopathology 21
Edited by Massimo Pignatelli & James Underwood

ISBN 1-85315-598-5

ISSN 0-0143 6953

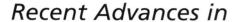

Recent Advances in

Histopathology
22

Edited by

Massimo Pignatelli MD PhD FRCPath

Professor of Histopathology and Head of Department,
Department of Clinical Science South Bristol, University of Bristol, UK

James C. E. Underwood MD FRCP FMedSci FRCPath

Joseph Hunter Professor of Pathology, Academic Unit of Pathology,
University of Sheffield, Sheffield, UK

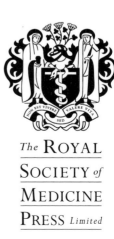

The ROYAL
SOCIETY *of*
MEDICINE
PRESS *Limited*

© 2007 Royal Society of Medicine Press Ltd

Published by the Royal Society of Medicine Press Ltd
1 Wimpole Street, London W1G 0AE, UK
Tel: +44 (0)20 7290 2921
Fax: +44 (0)20 7290 2929
Email: publishing@rsm.ac.uk
Website: www.rsmpress.co.uk

British Library Cataloguing in Publication Data
A catalogue record for this book is available from the British Library
ISBN 978–1-85315-649–6

Distribution in Europe and Rest of World:

Marston Book Services Ltd
PO Box 269, Abingdon
Oxon OX14 4YN, UK
Tel: +44 (0)1235 465500
Fax: +44 (0)1235 465555
Email: direct.order@marston.co.uk

Distribution in the USA and Canada:

Royal Society of Medicine Press Ltd
c/o BookMasters Inc
30 Amberwood Parkway
Ashland, OH 44805, USA
Tel: +1 800 247 6553/+1 800 266 5564
Fax: +1 419 281 6883
Email: order@bookmasters.com

Distribution in Australia and New Zealand:

Elsevier Australia
30-52 Smidmore Street
Marrikville NSW 2204, Australia
Tel: +61 2 9517 8999
Fax: +61 2 9517 2249
Email: service@elsevier.com.au

Editorial services and typesetting by GM & BA Haddock, Ford, Midlothian, UK

Printed in The Netherlands by Krips

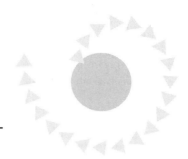

Contents

Contributors

Salim M. Anjarwalla MB ChB MRCPath
Specialist Registrar in Histopathology, Gloucestershire Royal Hospital,
Gloucester, UK

Emyr W. Benbow BSc MB ChB FRCPath
Senior Lecturer in Pathology, University of Manchester and Honorary
Consultant Histopathologist for Central Manchester and Manchester
Children's University Hospitals NHS Trust, Manchester, UK

Fred T. Bosman MD PhD
Professor of Pathology and Director, Institut Universitaire de Pathologie,
Lausanne, Switzerland

Marta C. Cohen MD CCPM
Consultant Paediatric and Perinatal Histopathologist at Sheffield Children's
Foundation Trust and an honorary Senior Lecturer at the University of
Sheffield, UK

Phillip Cox MBBS PhD FRCPath
Consultant Perinatal Pathologist, Birmingham Women's Healthcare NHS
Trust, Birmingham, UK

Karin J. Denton MB ChB FRCPath
Consultant Cytopathologist, Department of Cellular Pathology, Southmead
Hospital, Westbury on Trym, Bristol, UK

Silvana Di Palma MD MRCPath
Senior Fellow, University of Surrey and Consultant Histopathologist, Royal
Surrey County Hospital, Guildford, UK

Paola Domizio BSc MBBS FRCPath FHEA
Professor of Pathology Education, Barts and The Royal London School of
Medicine, Queen Mary College, University of London; and Professor,
Department of Cellular Pathology, The Royal London Hospital, London, UK

Antony J. Freemont MD FRCP FRCPath
Professor, Division of Regenerative Medicine, School of Medicine, The University of Manchester, Manchester, UK

Judith A. Hoyland PhD
Senior Lecturer in Molecular Pathology, Division of Regenerative Medicine, School of Medicine, The University of Manchester, Manchester, UK

Sebastian Lucas BM BCh FRCP FRCPath
Professor, Department of Histopathology, King's College London School of Medicine, St Thomas' Hospital, London, UK

Gillian Murphy BSc PhD FMedSci
Chair of Cancer Cell Biology, Deputy Head of Cancer Research UK, Department of Oncology, University of Cambridge, Cancer Research UK Cambridge Research Institute, Li Ka Shing Centre, Cambridge, UK

Pramila Ramani MB BS PhD FRCPath
Consultant Paediatric Pathologist, Department of Histopathology, Bristol Royal Infirmary, Bristol, UK

Ian S.D. Roberts BSc MB ChB FRCPath
Consultant Pathologist, Oxford Radcliffe Hospitals NHS Trust, Oxford, UK

Neil A. Shepherd DM FRCPath
Consultant Histopathologist and Professor of Gastrointestinal Pathology in the Department of Histopathology, Gloucestershire Royal Hospital, Gloucester, UK

Roderick H.W. Simpson BSc MB ChB MMed(Anat Path) FRCPath
Consultant Histopathologist, Royal Devon and Exeter Hospital, Exeter, UK

David N. Slater BMedSci MB ChB FRCPath
Consultant Dermatopathologist, Department of Histopathology, Royal Hallamshire Hospital, Sheffield, UK

Helen L. Whitwell MBChB FRCPath DMJPath FACBS FFFLM
Professor and Consultant Home Office Accredited Forensic Pathologist, West Midlands Forensic Centre, Sandwell District General Hospital, West Bromwich, UK

Paola Domizio

1

Pathology in the undergraduate curriculum

Five trays of biopsy slides are placed on my desk at the same time as a group of first-year students arrive at my door for their Human Sciences PBL session. I know which task I'd rather be doing but etiquette prevents me from telling the students to go away. No doubt their long-term education will benefit from knowing how social services help Mrs A to get her housework done but there's hardly a mention of her underlying disease. 'What about her breast carcinoma?' I whisper. I have to try really hard to stop myself from teaching them some pathology – one isn't allowed to do that – and have to keep quiet when all they want to do is discuss the nutritional value of meals-on-wheels. Two hours this session is scheduled for! By 45 minutes I'll already be longing to get back to my slides and I'll have to hurry them along. There's no way I'm agreeing to facilitate these PBL tutorials again. If only I could give a few pathology lectures, or even demonstrate an autopsy, I'd be happy to be involved in the teaching. But the way the curriculum is going nowadays I just can't be bothered any more. These students have no idea what a pathologist does – apart from the rubbish they see on television – so how will any of them be stimulated to become the pathologists of the future? It's no good. I'm way too busy to do this again. They'll just have to find somebody else.

Although this scenario is fictional, similar episodes are almost certainly played out by pathologists across the country in response to being involved in medical student teaching. But is this reaction justified? Has pathology teaching been reduced so much that it is virtually extinct? If so, why has this happened? How is pathology represented in modern medical curricula? Is problem-based learning truly the nemesis of pathology teaching? What effect will modern curricula have on pathology recruitment in the future? I shall explore these issues and discuss ways of restoring the profile of pathology teaching.

Paola Domizio BSc MBBS FRCPath FHEA
Professor of Pathology Education, Barts and The Royal London School of Medicine, Queen Mary College, University of London; and Professor, Department of Cellular Pathology, Royal London Hospital, 80 Newark St, London EC1 2ES, UK.   E-mail: p.domizio@qmul.ac.uk

1

WHY TEACH PATHOLOGY?

Pathology bridges the gap between basic sciences and clinical medicine; a proper understanding of pathological processes is vitally important for medical practice. The main goals of undergraduate pathology teaching have always been to provide a language or framework for the description of disease and to provide students with knowledge of the functional and structural changes in disease so that clinical signs and symptoms can be understood and interpreted.

There has been much debate recently in the pathology popular literature about whether medical students should be taught pathology at all. Voluble arguments have been put forward both for and against the motion that 'Doctors don't need to know about the pathological basis of disease'.[1,2] The proponents maintain that 'medicine comprises more than a science and that more attention must be given to the humanist elements of medical practice and medical education' and that 'greater understanding of the pathological basis of disease has not contributed substantially to improved morbidity and mortality rates'. Opponents, on the other hand, respond that proper communication with colleagues and patients depends on a proper understanding of pathological language, that evidence-based practice depends on the scientific basis of medicine and that many advances in public health have been based on understanding of the underlying pathology of a disease.

Most pathologists would undoubtedly oppose the motion, but in which camp do medical students – the current 'consumers' of pathology teaching – lie? A first-year student at one of the new medical schools sides with the opponents,[1] arguing that it is unethical for doctors to treat diseases that they have not been properly taught about: 'Not understanding how these diseases arise, present and are treated would be a criminal flaw. Ignorance is no defence.' Good communication skills are essential for tomorrow's doctors, but they must also have a sufficient knowledge base to communicate about.

IS PATHOLOGY TEACHING EXTINCT?

There is little doubt that, in recent years, the undergraduate medical curriculum has shifted away from didactic, discipline-based teaching towards integrated, systems-based education with an emphasis on self-directed learning.[3] Rightly or wrongly, pathology has been perceived as a fact-based discipline, and so has suffered the same fate as many of the basic science subjects in having its teaching time drastically cut. From the position two decades ago of underpinning much of the medical curriculum, there is increasing concern that pathology as a discipline is largely disappearing from undergraduate curricula, especially those that are centred on problem-based learning.[3]

But does this matter? For several reasons, I would argue that it does. First, medical students may fail to understand the disease mechanisms on which to base their clinical practice. The importance of this is highlighted by a recent study in which graduates of a problem-based course rated themselves as worst in understanding disease mechanisms and poor at making best use of laboratory services.[4] Second, doctors of the future will have poor knowledge of pathology terminology and hence fail to understand pathology reports. Third, the chance will be lost to bring the pathology specialties to the attention of students and junior doctors as they consider their career choices.

WHAT HAVE BEEN THE DRIVERS FOR CURRICULUM CHANGE?

The last 25 years have brought significant changes in patterns of disease and in the way that healthcare is organised and delivered. These changes have fundamentally altered the way that medicine is practiced with redistribution of some tasks and responsibilities away from doctors and towards multidisciplinary teams. This role redesign has been reflected by changes in curriculum content and methods of teaching.

Over the last two decades, the public expectation of doctors has increased, leading to a change in the doctor–patient relationship towards patient-centered medicine. Increasingly, doctors are being faced with difficult ethical and moral issues without sufficient instruction in how to manage these problems. The need for effective communication is greater than ever. It is no longer sufficient for medical students to acquire these skills by observation, so subjects such as ethics and communication skills – which 25 years ago did not feature – now form an increasing part of the undergraduate curriculum at the expense of more traditional science-based disciplines.

Lastly, despite the repeated recognition over many years that curriculum overload is detrimental to medical education, it is only recently that this concept has prompted curricular change. As far back as 1876, Thomas Huxley in an address on university education[5] said: '*The burden we place on a medical student is far too heavy ... a system of medical education that is actually calculated to obstruct the acquisition of knowledge and to heavily favour the crammer and grinder is a disgrace'.*

TOMORROW'S DOCTORS

In response to these drivers for change, the General Medical Council (GMC) began a major review of medical education that culminated in 1993 with the publication of *Tomorrow's Doctors*.[6] Through this document, the GMC set out to 'promote the development of a curriculum which corrects the existing faults of overload and didacticism' and to 'equip the new graduate with the necessary knowledge, skills and attitudes to enable him or her to enter the pre-registration period with confidence and enthusiasm'. In 2003, the guidelines were updated[7] to 'put the principles set out in Good Medical Practice at the centre of undergraduate education' and to 'identify the knowledge, skills, attitudes and behaviour expected of new graduates'.

The main recommendations of *Tomorrow's Doctors* are that the curriculum should be organised around a core of essential knowledge and skills, augmented by a series of options (or selected study modules) that enable students to study more thoroughly areas of particular interest to them. The core curriculum should be based on systems rather than on disciplines, and should be integrated, with loss of the traditional divide between pre-clinical and clinical years. The course should emphasise the development and assessment of clinical, communication and practical skills and the development of professional attitudes and behaviour. More emphasis should be put on the teaching of public health, ethics and law and more of the curriculum should be taught in the community. The burden of factual information on medical students should be substantially reduced and self-directed learning and critical evaluation should be encouraged, thereby preparing the student for life-long learning.

Tomorrow's Doctors has caused a major shift in the objectives of the undergraduate medical curriculum, away from the scientific basis of medicine – a sound knowledge of which had been repeatedly advocated since the early 20th century – towards patient-centred medicine. Newly qualified doctors nowadays have arguably better communication and practical skills, but their knowledge of the basic medical sciences is inevitably much reduced. The effects of this curriculum shift on pathology teaching have been profound.

THE EFFECTS OF *TOMORROW'S DOCTORS* ON PATHOLOGY TEACHING

Since the publication of the first edition of *Tomorrow's Doctors*, there have been major changes in the pathology component of the medical curriculum, not only in the amount of time dedicated to pathology teaching, but also in the content and structure of pathology courses and in the teaching methods used.

In 2001, a survey on pathology teaching on behalf of the Pathological Society was presented at a meeting on the future of academic pathology.[8] This survey showed that, in the preceding decade, 10 of 19 medical schools in the UK (53%) reported a reduction in pathology teaching time, while only one medical school reported an increase. Despite the fact that this study was not peer-reviewed, it does suggest, along with anecdotal evidence from individual lead teachers in pathology, that there has been a real reduction in pathology teaching time in the last 15 years.

The aspects of pathology teaching that have suffered most from this reduction no doubt vary from school to school, but it would seem that the axe has fallen most heavily on histology and general pathology (personal observation). These two subjects were traditionally considered to be basic medical sciences and so were drastically cut in efforts to reduce factual overload. Certainly, medical students no longer spend hours looking down a microscope at the detailed structure of organs and tissues. Systematic pathology has fared somewhat better but, even so, teaching on the morphological changes in disease is often neglected in favour of epidemiology and public health issues. The traditional practice of teaching general pathology in the first two 'pre-clinical years' and systematic pathology in the clinical years has all but disappeared. Instead, pathology teaching is integrated throughout the course. As a consequence, in many medical schools, pathology is no longer recognised as a stand-alone subject.

The change in emphasis from teaching to learning has led to the undergraduate curriculum becoming student-centred rather than teacher-centred.[3] Didactic instruction in the form of pathology lectures and tutor-led pathology tutorials have given way, in varying degree, to self-directed learning and problem-based learning. Pathology is included in PBL case scenarios and pathology tutors have been converted to PBL facilitators.

MODERNISATION OF PATHOLOGY TEACHING

Despite huge advances in pedagogic theory over the past two decades, the question 'What is the best way for students to learn pathology?' has yet to be answered.[9,10] Most pathology teachers would not disagree that students need to assimilate pathology information in two main 'areas' – knowledge and context. The 'knowledge' section comprises understanding of basic disease mechanisms (general pathology) and how diseases present in the patient (systematic pathology). The 'context' section is more of a 'users' guide' in which students learn about use and abuse of laboratories and pathologists, particularly what information doctors can expect from each pathology discipline and the limitations of that information.

The knowledge section is largely based on understanding of pathological mechanisms and pathogenesis but requires factual knowledge to back this up. It can be taught in a variety of settings, including problem-based learning, self-directed learning and web-based tutorials (described below) and, increasingly rarely, dedicated pathology courses.

DEDICATED PATHOLOGY COURSE OR INTEGRATED TEACHING?

The teaching of pathology in dedicated blocks, a common practice until recently, is now limited to only a few traditional medical schools. That does not mean that this method has no advantages. The proponents of course-based teaching argue that it focuses the students' minds and allows them to devote their energies entirely to pathology for the duration of the course. In contrast, the opponents maintain that since pathologists are clinicians, the best way for students to recognise the role and value of pathology is to study it in an integrated setting. Learnt otherwise, it is easy for pathology to become just another science to be forgotten when the examination is over. The teaching of histology, which in many medical schools is now taught alongside pathology by pathologists, has undoubtedly benefited from an integrated approach. Students may no longer know the detailed structure of individual cells, but the relevance of what they do learn is much clearer. Integrated curricula are unquestionably here to stay, so there seems little point in yearning for the traditional, intensive pathology course of yesteryear.

PROBLEM-BASED LEARNING

Problem-based learning (PBL) is a student-centered method that encourages deep learning through the solution of open-ended problems. Students are responsible for solving problems or investigating answers themselves, thereby encouraging active learning. During PBL sessions, the function of the teacher is not to disseminate information, as is the case in a traditional tutorial, but rather to act as a facilitator or learning coach, encouraging student interaction. Consequently, PBL facilitators are not required to be experts in the subject matter of the PBL tutorial they are facilitating.

PBL has many advantages over didactic teaching methods. It encourages a problem-solving approach and reflective practice as well as enhancing communication and team-working skills. It also promotes the skills required for life-long learning, which is now compulsory for doctors throughout postgraduate education and beyond. The main disadvantage of PBL is that it is resource intensive in terms of tutor numbers and time. The maximum number of students for the PBL process to work effectively is 8–10; above that and the interactive process does not work nearly as well. Consequently, the number of tutors needed for a PBL-based curriculum is large. PBL also disadvantages shy students who might feel inhibited in the interactive setting and so are reluctant to engage in the learning process. In the author's experience, tutors have mixed feelings about PBL. Some enjoy witnessing the students' interaction and active learning, while others find it frustrating that they have little control over the content of the session, that they are prevented from 'teaching' the students, and that if they are not experts in the subject of the tutorial they are facilitating, they may lack the specialist knowledge required to correct students if they do go wrong.

Most medical schools have now adopted PBL to a greater or lesser extent, but its effectiveness has recently been called into question by Colliver,[11] who argues that there is 'no convincing evidence that PBL improves knowledge base and clinical performance, at least not of the magnitude expected given the resources required'.

What about PBL and pathology specifically? The fact that pathology bridges the gap between the basic sciences and clinical medicine makes it an ideal subject to be studied in the PBL setting. Anecdotal evidence suggests that interaction between pathology staff and students is enhanced by PBL, which is obviously a positive factor. But the evidence whether PBL influences student awareness of pathology as a career is conflicting. Some authors argue that PBL may improve pathology recruitment by presenting pathology in a more enriching and satisfying context.[12] Most studies, however, claim that PBL will limit students' contact with pathologists, and so recruitment will be threatened.[9,13,14] One recent Canadian study has shown no difference in the number of graduates entering pathology residency programmes from PBL-based medical schools compared to those from non-PBL based schools.[15] There seems little doubt that how pathology fares in an increasingly PBL-based curriculum will depend on the enthusiasm with which pathologists seek to embrace it and take it forward.

COMPUTER-ASSISTED LEARNING

In recent years, there has been an explosive proliferation in computer-assisted resources available for pathology teaching (Fig. 1). These include a multitude of pathology educational websites,[16,17] self-assessment packages,[18] online access to popular textbooks,[19] virtual pathology museums[20] and virtual slide teaching programmes.[21,22] Indeed, so popular has e-learning become that it is now being developed for postgraduate pathology training as well as undergraduate education. Due to the large number of images that most pathology educational material contains, pathology lends itself well to computer-based learning, perhaps more so than many other medical specialties.

The many benefits of computer-assisted learning (CAL) include the use of unlimited images, which can be altered, updated or replaced immediately.

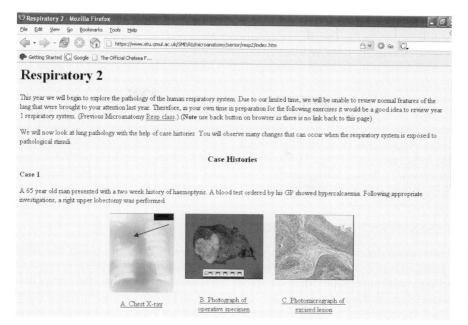

Respiratory 2

This year we will begin to explore the pathology of the human respiratory system. Due to our limited time, we will be unable to review normal features of the lung that were brought to your attention last year. Therefore, in your own time in preparation for the following exercises it would be a good idea to review year 1 respiratory system. (Previous Microanatomy Resp class.) (**Note** use back button on browser as there is no link back to this page)

We will now look at lung pathology with the help of case histories. You will observe many changes that can occur when the respiratory system is exposed to pathological stimuli.

Case Histories

Case 1

A 65 year old man presented with a two week history of haemoptysis. A blood test ordered by his GP showed hypercalcaemia. Following appropriate investigations, a right upper lobectomy was performed.

A. Chest X-ray   B. Photograph of operative specimen   C. Photomicrograph of excised lesion

Fig. 1 Screen capture of a year-2, case-based, pathology tutorial at Barts and the London School of Medicine.

Students can study at their own pace and in their preferred location and can repeat tutorials as many times as they wish. CAL packages often include self-assessment items that give contemporaneous feedback to students in an interactive way. Once set up, CAL requires few or no tutors, and so, particularly given the wide-spread dearth of pathology teachers, it is highly cost effective. Finally, computers never get tired or bored, nor are they judgmental towards below-average students.

CAL has its drawbacks, however. For example, the time and effort required to develop and maintain sites can be problematic for hard-pressed teachers. It goes without saying that a computer is essential for CAL, and one may not always be available. In addition, just as the presence of a tutor may be perceived as threatening to a sensitive student, so may the absence of a teacher be detrimental, as difficult concepts cannot be explained.

INNOVATIVE TEACHING METHODS

The wide-spread loss of dedicated pathology courses has meant that innovative ways of getting pathology into the curriculum are being developed. The new Medical School at the University of East Anglia has formulated a 'casenote-based clinico-pathological conference (CPC)' for third-year students.[23] Small groups of students are given anonymised case-notes from real patients, together with images from the patient's pathology and radiology. They use this material to prepare a CPC, which is subsequently delivered to their peers and teachers. Feedback from this type of teaching has been positive, with students 'relishing the freedom to set their own learning objectives

7

without input from facilitators'.[23] There is also evidence that students emerge from this part of the course understanding the need for, and the context within which, laboratory tests are carried out.[23]

Multidisciplinary team meetings (MDTMs) can also be a useful forum for teaching pathology to medical students. The usual practice of medical students attending MDTMs is to congregate at the back of the room, where they sit silently and rapidly lose interest. If time allows, students can be encouraged to participate actively in the meetings by presenting a patient's history or by answering questions about the patient's pathology. In the author's experience, the initial response of students to this type of teaching is reluctance to become involved, followed by enthusiasm and gratitude once the learning opportunities have been realised.

ASSESSMENT IN PATHOLOGY

There is no doubt that the old-style pathology examination – much like final examinations in the other 'ologies' - has all but disappeared in most medical schools. Although an anathema to most medical educationalists, the adage that 'assessment is the main driver for learning' is as true for pathology as it is for other specialties. Until relatively recently, students would be heard to boast that they 'never knew any pathology until they had to do the exam'. With the integrated assessments now commonplace in most medical schools, this particular driver no longer exists. Indeed, the loss of the monospecialty pathology examination may be perceived by students as an indication that the subject is not important. This effect is compounded by the relative lack of contact that medical students have with pathologists compared to ward-based clinicians. Some might argue that the lack of pathology assessment does not matter, but this would be a short-sighted view. Who could deny the importance of assessing students' knowledge of blood transfusion, infection control and autopsy procedure given the recent media furore surrounding serious transfusion hazards, the spread of MRSA and the 'organ retention scandal'?

It is vitally important, therefore, that pathology teachers are involved in assessment to ensure that pathology subjects are included. Innovative methods of assessment are being developed to fit in with the integrated approach to teaching now widely used. Examples of communication skills OSCE stations that are pathology based include explaining a histopathology report to a patient and seeking consent for autopsy. Similarly, practical skills stations include issuing death certificates after reading an autopsy report. Formative assessments are a good way of assessing students' progress and stimulating learning, albeit to a lesser extent than summative assessments.

WHO SHOULD TEACH PATHOLOGY?

The result of curricular changes in recent years is that, in some medical schools, pathology is no longer taught by pathologists. This has led to understandable anxiety that it is possible for students to complete their undergraduate education without tuition from a pathologist.[9] In such medical schools, what little pathology remains in the curriculum is incorporated into

PBL scenarios and is supervised by PBL tutors. The fundamental principle of PBL-based curricula, namely that students should 'learn' and not 'be taught', could be used to question whether it really matters who facilitates PBL tutorials, even if this involves supervision of pathology learning? There is evidence, however, that students prefer to be taught (or supervised) by experts in the subjects they are learning.[24–28] There is also evidence that student achievement is greater if their PBL learning is facilitated by a subject-matter expert, particularly in their first curriculum year.[24] So, in the ideal world, pathologists should 'teach' pathology, just as surgeons should 'teach' surgery and psychiatrists should 'teach' psychiatry.

In addition, there is evidence that enthusiastic role models and a positive undergraduate experience are more important in encouraging students and junior doctors to enter pathology than they are for other medical careers.[29] While this is not the prime objective of a pathology curriculum, this particular advantage conferred by good pathology teachers should not be forgotten.

SANITISATION OF PATHOLOGY LEARNING

There is little doubt that modern medical curricula have lost much of their 'messiness', becoming sanitised and distilled in the process. Even actors are used instead of real patients in many parts of the curricula. The proliferation in use of CAL packages has occurred at the expense of direct observation of diseased organs during anatomy dissection and post-mortem demonstrations. But can pathology really be learnt from images on a computer screen? Many of the CAL packages available nowadays are very good and as a component of self-directed learning, such material can be very valuable. Virtually all students rate computer-based learning highly,[18,30] but there is no doubt that it has led to sanitisation of pathology learning. It seems obvious that just as clinical and communication skills are better developed on real patients, so the understanding of disease is greater if a student has 'got his or her hands dirty' by studying preserved specimens in a pathology museum or seeing diseased organs fresh at a post-mortem demonstration.

THE DEMISE OF AUTOPSY TEACHING

The organ retention problems at Bristol and Alder Hey have had several deleterious effects on pathology teaching. First, the closure of pathology museums, which were already under threat by lack of funding, has been hastened. Second, the number of consented autopsies, which had been in decline for some time, has fallen even further, so that autopsy demonstrations are now exceedingly rare (Fig. 2). Those that do occur hardly ever attract a student audience. Consequently, the opportunities for today's medical students to observe real-life macroscopic pathology have virtually disappeared.

The advantages of the autopsy as an educational tool have been well documented in the literature[31–34] and students who do have the opportunity to attend post-mortem demonstrations almost always describe the experience as 'positive and valuable', despite the perceived unpleasantness of the post-mortem room environment.[35,36] Unfortunately, however, even coroner's

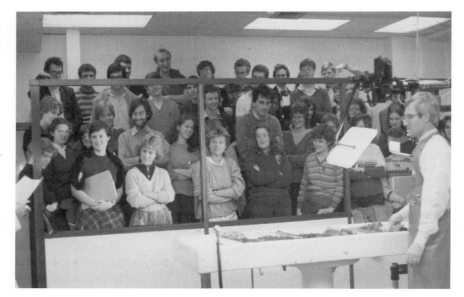

Fig. 2 Autopsy demonstrations such as this (*ca.* 1985) are now exceedingly rare.

autopsies, which have not suffered the same reduction in number as consent autopsies, may no longer be available for teaching due to stringent consent issues following implementation of the *Coroner's (Amendment) Rules 2005.*[37] The time has almost come when the only way for medical students to observe post-mortems is by participating in selected study modules or clinical attachments in pathology. During such attachments, they can claim to be observing routine clinical practice rather than being taught.

THE IMPACT OF CHANGING CURRICULA ON PATHOLOGY RECRUITMENT

The foregoing discussion illustrates how, in the last 20 years, the undergraduate medical curriculum has evolved from being teacher-centred to student-centred, from discipline-based to integrated core and options-based. Passive acquisition of knowledge imparted by real teachers has given way to active problem-based learning with reliance on computers. Pathology learning has changed from seeing preserved specimens in pathology museums and fresh organs at autopsy to looking at images on CDs and websites. No longer is there daily contact with pathologists, instead there is irregular interaction with anonymous computer screens.

In parallel with these changes in medical education, the number of consultant vacancies in all the pathology specialties has risen substantially, resulting in a significant recruitment crisis. In histopathology particularly, the rise in vacancies has been rapid and spectacular, from four in 1992 to a peak of 219 in 2004 (figures supplied by The Royal College of Pathologists). This huge increase in vacancies is partly explained by early retirements but, until recently, it has not been known whether it was also accounted for by a fall in the number of medical graduates entering pathology.

A recent study looking at the career choices of medical graduates showed that the number of newly qualified doctors selecting pathology as their first choice of career halved between 1983 and 1993 and has remained static ever since.[29] The reasons behind this worrying trend were not specifically sought by the study, but there was evidence that 'experience of the subject as a student' and the influence of 'a particular teacher or department' are more important in encouraging students and junior doctors to enter pathology than they are for other medical careers. While the impact of *Tomorrow's Doctors* cannot explain fully the substantial drop in pathology as a career choice, there is no doubt that the current medical curriculum, in which pathology is low profile and there is virtually no exposure to charismatic pathologists acting as role models, will do nothing to remedy the situation.

ACADEMIC PATHOLOGISTS – AN ENDANGERED SPECIES?

Continued funding cuts in higher education in the last few decades have meant that medical schools have struggled to maintain sufficient staffing levels to sustain the major curricular changes adopted. In particular, the savage funding cuts instigated by the last Research Assessment Exercise (RAE) have hit academic pathologists particularly hard. Whole departments have disappeared with individuals retiring early or being re-badged as NHS consultants. Those who have survived the cuts have had the strongest research output but, not surprisingly, their enthusiasm for undergraduate teaching is sometimes poor.

A recent survey by the Council for Heads of Medical Schools (CHMS) has highlighted the dramatic fall in the number of clinical academics in pathology.[38] Between 2003 and 2004, the total number of academic pathologists fell by 40%, leaving only 45% of the numbers that there were in 2000. The situation with clinical lecturers in pathology is even worse. Numbers have dropped by 64% since 2003 and now stand at only 19% of their 2000 numbers. These figures are the worst for any of the medical specialties and prompted CHMS to state in their commentary on the survey that: 'a shortage of academic pathologists at all levels will compromise medical training as well as the UK's medical research capacity'. There is little doubt that the wide-spread dearth of academic pathologists has left pathology teaching in crisis, particularly as NHS consultants have been reluctant to take on the teaching mantle due to their own burgeoning workload and generally low morale.

In contrast to the fall in clinical academic numbers, medical student numbers are continually rising – by 40% since 2000, fuelled by the opening of four new medical schools. More students need more teachers, particularly in PBL-based curricula where the small group nature of the teaching means that the teacher:student ratio has to be high. But where will the teachers needed come from?

Until now, universities have appointed academics on the basis of research profile and have then expected delivery of a significant teaching work-load. In the current educational climate, this practice is no longer acceptable. Many of the skills required for research and teaching are different and very few academics shine in both. To date, universities have not had to face financial consequences as a result of teaching quality assessments, but this is likely to change in the future as students become 'consumers' rather than 'learners' following the introduction of tuition fees. Market forces will then ensure that good teachers attract funding to universities, in the same way that good researchers currently do.

The financial impact of the RAE has placed the diminishing number of research academics under greater pressure than ever. This is particularly true of research-active pathologists, who, due to the applied nature of much of their research, often have to work very hard to secure high-profile grants and publish papers in high-impact journals. It is no great surprise, therefore, that their enthusiasm for teaching is at an all-time low.

Universities must recognise that there are fundamental differences in the research and teaching pathways, and must appoint not just high-profile researchers but specialist teachers as well. Policies should be developed for career enhancement and promotion on the basis of a teaching portfolio alone. Such a strategy, allowing committed teachers the time and resources to develop not only their courses but also their own careers, would have an invigorating effect on the pathology specialties, suffering as they are from chronic staff shortages and an ever-increasing clinical workload.

THE FUTURE FOR PATHOLOGY TEACHING

There is no doubt that if medical graduates of the 21st century are to have an adequate understanding of disease mechanisms and are to be interested in pursuing pathology as a career, pathology teachers of the future must restore the profile of pathology teaching in the undergraduate curriculum. Success in this venture depends on effectively tackling three main issues: (i) the loss of pathology from modern curricula must be corrected; (ii) pathologists must act as role models; and (iii) the pathology teaching workload must be adequately managed.

Managing the teaching work-load will be a particularly difficult challenge and novel solutions will need to be found. Given the savage loss of academic pathologists, unless the trend is reversed, it will be impossible for universities to deliver pathology teaching without the help of NHS colleagues. Academic and NHS pathologists will need to work together to agree a model for delivering teaching. This might involve negotiation of job plans at a departmental level with protected time for teaching. Development of formulae for calculating the time required for teaching and its preparation will be particularly important, as will identifying and obtaining appropriate funding. Other ways of spreading the load include involvement of non-consultant staff in teaching, such as trainees, clinical scientists, postgraduate students or retired pathologists.

Raising the profile of pathology teaching depends on pathologists being actively involved in curriculum design and planning at a local level. It is no longer constructive for pathologists to complain about the demise of pathology teaching or the loss of pathology lectures – instead, they must 'step out of their ivory towers and assume new identities'.[9] Innovative ways of getting pathology into the curriculum have been described above. Other ways of exposing students to pathology include offering selected study modules and research projects or clinical attachments. Intercalated degrees in pathology are one of the best ways of stimulating interested students and, in the author's experience, provide a strong motivation for eventual choice of pathology as a career.

The importance of charismatic role models cannot be overemphasised. One medical student describes her time on a clinical attachment at the Norfolk and Norwich hospital:[39] 'My experience in the pathology department has been wonderful. All staff members are very enthusiastic and keen to teach new students, even when we sometimes ask what might be irrelevant questions.' So, encouraging students and junior doctors to come to the department, being friendly and welcoming, and making time available are vitally important.

The Royal College of Pathologists, in conjunction with other pathology organisations such as the Pathological Society, have been active in trying to re-invigorate pathology teaching. Initiatives include development of a core curriculum in pathology, which is outcomes based, mapped to the objectives in *Tomorrow's Doctors* and encourages analysis and problem solving rather than factual recall. Other projects include a database of e-resources, with images, tutorials and other computer-based teaching materials for use by hard-pressed pathology teachers nation-wide, and specific grants for educational projects, such as that awarded by the Pathological Society for the modernisation of the Crane Pathology Museum at the University of Sheffield.[40] Through these initiatives, it is hoped to keep educational issues high on the pathology agenda well into the future.

PATHOLOGY IN THE FOUNDATION YEAR

Although the Foundation programme for medical graduates in the UK is not strictly part of the undergraduate curriculum, the fact that medical schools are important stakeholders in Foundation Schools means that they will have an influence on the curriculum for the Foundation programme. Several Foundation Schools across the UK have included pathology 'taster' posts, usually of 3 months' duration, in Foundation year 2 (FY2). These posts will include an introduction to autopsy and surgical pathology. Some posts are in academic pathology and will offer exposure to pathology research and teaching in addition to clinical work.

This development is to be welcomed, particularly given the dearth of academic pathologists described above, but there remains concern that it could be a double-edged sword – first because the investment in time and effort involved in supervising FY2 trainees may not be repaid in the number eventually joining the profession and, second, because 3 months may not be long enough to develop a liking for the specialty. It is currently too early to judge whether these posts are a success, but pathology educationalists will follow their progress with interest.

Points for best practice

- Major reforms in medical education have led to a shift away from didactic discipline-based teaching with 'factual overload' towards integrated, systems-based education with an emphasis on self-directed learning.

(continued on next page)

Points for best practice *(continued)*

- Pathology is central to the study of medicine but has, nevertheless, been perceived as a fact-based discipline, and so has suffered the same fate as many of the basic science subjects in having teaching time drastically cut.

- Modern curricula have brought drastic changes to the way pathology is learnt and taught, away from personal contact with a pathologist and experiencing 'real' pathology, towards computer-assisted learning.

- Academic pathology is under threat of extinction, but the danger has been recognised and remedial measures are being implemented.

- Pathology teachers of the future must restore the profile of their subject so that newly qualified doctors will understand the mechanisms of disease, use laboratories properly and be stimulated to become pathologists themselves..

References

1. Jackson M, Arnott B, Benbow EW, Marshall R, Maude P. Doctors don't need to know about the pathological basis of disease. *ACP News* 2003; **Spring**: 33–39.
2. Wright NA. Doctors don't need to know about the pathological basis of disease? Absolute cobblers! *ACP News* 2003; **Summer**: 10–12.
3. Nash JR. Pathology in the new medical curriculum: what has replaced the subject courses? *Pathol Oncol Res* 2000; **6**: 149–154.
4. Jones A, McArdle PJ, O'Neill PA. Perceptions of how well graduates are prepared for the role of pre-registration house officer: a comparison of outcomes from a traditional and an integrated PBL curriculum. *Med Educ* 2002; **36**: 16–25.
5. Huxley TH. Lecture delivered at the opening of Johns Hopkins University, Baltimore, 1876.
6. General Medical Council. *Tomorrow's Doctors: Recommendations on Undergraduate Medical Education*. London: GMC, 1993.
7. General Medical Council. *Tomorrow's Doctors*. London: GMC, 2003.
8. Pathological Society. *Future of Academic Pathology*. Report of the residential meeting held at the Bellhouse Hotel, Beaconsfield, 28–30 March 2001.
9. Marshall R, Cartwright N, Mattick K. Teaching and learning pathology: a critical review of the English literature. *Med Educ* 2004; **38**: 302–313.
10. Mattick K, Marshall R, Bligh J. Tissue pathology in undergraduate medical education: atrophy or evolution? *J Pathol* 2004; **203**: 871–876.
11. Colliver JA. Effectiveness of problem-based learning curricula: research and theory. *Acad Med* 2000; **75**: 259–266.
12. Black WC, Anderson RE. Problem-based teaching of pathology: is it cost-effective? *Hum Pathol* 1990; **21**: 879–880.
13. Herdson PB. Pathology, pathologists and problem-based learning. *Pathology* 1998; **30**: 326–327.
14. Nash JR, West KP, Foster CS. The teaching of anatomic pathology in England and Wales: a transatlantic view. *Hum Pathol* 2001; **32**: 1154–1156.
15. Ford JC. Influence of a problem-based learning curriculum on the selection of pathology as a career: evidence from the Canadian match of 1993–2004. *Hum Pathol* 2005; **36**: 600–604.
16. Florida State University College of Medicine. *The Internet Pathology Laboratory for Medical Education* <http://library.med.utah.edu/WebPath/webpath.html> accessed 10 August 2006.
17. New York University. *Department of Pathology Case Studies* <http://mchip00.med.nyu.edu/path-cases/pathcases.html> accessed 10 August 2006.

18. Velan GM, Kumar RK, Dziegielewski M, Wakefield D. Web-based self-assessments in pathology with Questionmark Perception. *Pathology* 2002; **34**: 282–284.
19. Underwood JCE. *General and Systematic Pathology*. London: Churchill Livingstone, 2006.
20. Monash University. *Museum of Pathology* <http://museum.med.monash.edu.au/index.cfm> accessed 10 August 2006.
21. Kumar RK, Velan GM, Korell SO, Kandara M, Dee FR, Wakefield D. Virtual microscopy for learning and assessment in pathology. *J Pathol* 2004; **204**: 613–618.
22. Kumar RK, Freeman B, Velan GM, De Permentier PJ. Integrating histology and histopathology teaching in practical classes using virtual slides. *Anat Rec B New Anat* 2006; **289**: 128–133.
23. Wilkinson M, Beales I, Jamieson C. Teaching students to use medical notes. *Med Educ* 2005; **39**: 516–517.
24. Schmidt HG, van der Arend A, Moust JH, Kokx I, Boon L. Influence of tutors' subject-matter expertise on student effort and achievement in problem-based learning. *Acad Med* 1993; **68**: 784–791.
25. Kaufman DM, Holmes DB. The relationship of tutors' content expertise to interventions and perceptions in a PBL medical curriculum. *Med Educ* 1998; **32**: 255–261.
26. Bochner D, Badovinac RL, Howell TH, Karimbux NY. Tutoring in a problem-based curriculum: expert versus nonexpert. *J Dent Educ* 2002; **66**: 1246–1251.
27. Gilkison A. Techniques used by 'expert' and 'non-expert' tutors to facilitate problem-based learning tutorials in an undergraduate medical curriculum. *Med Educ* 2003; **37**: 6–14.
28. Groves M, Rego P, O'Rourke P. Tutoring in problem-based learning medical curricula: the influence of tutor background and style on effectiveness. *BMC Med Educ* 2005; **5**: 20.
29. Lambert TW, Goldacre MJ, Turner G, Domizio P, du Boulay C. Career choices for pathology: national surveys of graduates of 1974–2002 from UK medical schools. *J Pathol* 2006; **208**: 446–452.
30. Reid WA, Harvey J, Watson GR, Luqmani R, Harkin PJ, Arends MJ. Medical student appraisal of interactive computer-assisted learning programs embedded in a general pathology course. *J Pathol* 2000; **191**: 462–465.
31. Burton JL. The autopsy in modern undergraduate medical education: a qualitative study of uses and curriculum considerations. *Med Educ* 2003; **37**: 1073–1081.
32. Welsh TS, Kaplan J. The role of postmortem examination in medical education. *Mayo Clin Proc* 1998; **73**: 802–805.
33. Hill RB, Anderson RE. The uses and value of autopsy in medical education as seen by pathology educators. *Acad Med* 1991; **66**: 97–100.
34. Sanchez H, Ursell P. Use of autopsy cases for integrating and applying the first two years of medical education. *Acad Med* 2001; **76**: 530–531.
35. Benbow EW. Medical students' views on necropsies. *J Clin Pathol* 1990; **43**: 969–976.
36. Benbow EW. The attitudes of second- and third-year medical students to the autopsy. A survey by postal questionnaire. *Arch Pathol Lab Med* 1991; **115**: 1171–1176.
37. Statutory Instrument 2005 No. 420. *The Coroners (Amendment) Rules 2005*. London: HMSO, 2005.
38. Council of Heads of Medical Schools and Council of Heads and Deans of Dental Schools. *Clinical Academic Staffing Levels in UK Medical and Dental Schools: data update 2004*. 2005.
39. Nakato H, Tumwebaze F. Learning pathology in a new course in a new medical school: what a great opportunity! *Bull R Coll Pathol* 2003; **124**: 17–18.
40. Bury J, Burton J. *Modernisation of the WAJ Crane Museum of Pathology*. Report on work funded through the 'Open' scheme of the Pathological Society, 2003–2005. 2005.

Roderick H.W. Simpson Silvana Di Palma

2

Primary carcinomas of the salivary glands: selected recent advances

After the major changes of the 1991 WHO Blue Book, the 2005 revised classification of salivary gland tumours includes 15 benign tumours and 23 carcinomas, as well as soft tissue, haematolymphoid and secondary tumours (Table 1).[1] The main changes from 1991 are:

1. Exclusion of non-neoplastic tumour-like lesions.

2. Benign epithelial tumours remain almost the same.

3. Carcinoma categories increased from 18 to 23.

4. Relatively few new entities have been accepted: clear cell carcinoma not otherwise specified (NOS), sialoblastoma and low-grade cribriform cystadenocarcinoma (low-grade salivary duct carcinoma); cribriform adenocarcinoma of the tongue is included as a variant of polymorphous low-grade adenocarcinoma. Several tumour subtypes noted in 1991 are now accorded separate categories. These are carcinoma ex pleomorphic adenoma, carcinosarcoma, metastasising pleomorphic adenoma, sebaceous neoplasms, sebaceous lymphadenoma/carcinoma, lymphoepithelial, small- and large-cell undifferentiated carcinomas.

The classification solved some problems, but not all. Those remaining include the terminology and nature of some of the new entities and their relationship to existing ones, as well as the position of several rare lesions such as sclerosing polycystic adenosis, which may be neoplastic.

Roderick H.W. Simpson BSc MB ChB MMed(Anat Path) FRCPath
Consultant Histopathologist, Royal Devon and Exeter Hospital, Barrack Road, Exeter, Devon EX2 5DW, UK. E-mail: roderick.simpson@virgin.net

Silvana Di Palma MD MRCPath
Senior Fellow, University of Surrey and Consultant Histopathologist, Royal Surrey County Hospital, Guildford, Surrey GU2 7XX, UK
E-mail : silvana.dipalma@royalsurrey.nhs.uk

17

Table 1 WHO histological classification of tumours of the salivary glands[1]

Malignant epithelial tumours	Acinic cell carcinoma
	Mucoepidermoid carcinoma
	Adenoid cystic carcinoma
	Polymorphous low-grade adenocarcinoma
	Epithelial–myoepithelial carcinoma
	Clear cell carcinoma, not otherwise specified (NOS)
	Basal cell adenocarcinoma
	Sebaceous carcinoma
	Cystadenocarcinoma
	Low-grade cribriform cystadenocarcinoma
	Mucinous adenocarcinoma
	Oncocytic carcinoma
	Salivary duct carcinoma
	Adenocarcinoma, not otherwise specified (NOS)
	Myoepithelial carcinoma
	Carcinoma ex pleomorphic adenoma
	Carcinosarcoma
	Metastasising pleomorphic adenoma
	Squamous cell carcinoma
	Small cell carcinoma
	Large cell carcinoma
	Lymphoepithelial carcinoma
	Sialoblastoma
Benign epithelial tumours	Pleomorphic adenoma
	Myoepithelioma
	Basal cell adenoma
	Warthin tumour
	Oncocytoma
	Canalicular adenoma
	Sebaceous adenoma
	Lymphadenoma: sebaceous / non-sebaceous
	Ductal papillomas: inverted ductal papilloma / intraductal papilloma / sialadenoma papilliferum
	Cystadenoma
Soft tissue tumours	Haemangioma
Haematolymphoid tumours	Hodgkin lymphoma
	Diffuse large B-cell lymphoma
	Extranodal marginal zone B-cell lymphoma
Secondary tumours	

The aim of this chapter is to cover the most important recent advances in primary carcinomas, particularly highlighting newly accepted entities. However, there is insufficient space for a comprehensive review of all salivary malignancies, such as can be found elsewhere.[1–5]

ACINIC CELL CARCINOMA

Acinic cell carcinoma is a malignancy in which at least some neoplastic cells demonstrate serous acinar cell differentiation with PAS-diastase positive zymogen granules. Diagnostic difficulties arise from the wide spectrum of growth patterns, including solid, microcystic (microfollicular), follicular and papillary-cystic. The cytomorphology is similarly variable, encompassing acinar (serous; blue dot), intercalated ductal, vacuolated, hobnail, clear and oncocytic cells.[1] Immunohistochemistry is generally unhelpful in its diagnosis.

The clinical course is characterised by local recurrences in 30–50% of patients, metastases in fewer and death from tumour in about 16%. Clinical stage at the time of diagnosis and completeness of excision are the best predictors of outcome.[1] Attempts at histological grading have not been successful, although poor prognostic factors include necrosis, extraglandular extension, increased pleomorphism, high mitotic rate and prominent infiltration of nerves and blood vessels.[1] A particularly aggressive variant is the dedifferentiated form, in which a poorly differentiated adenocarcinoma develops in an ordinary acinic cell carcinoma.[1,2] In contrast, circumscribed well differentiated acinic cell carcinoma with abundant lymphoid stroma has an excellent prognosis.[1,2] It is characterised by a microfollicular growth pattern, MIB1 index < 5% and plentiful stromal lymphocytes with germinal centre formation. All these features must be present, as lymphocytic infiltration by itself is common in acinic cell carcinoma and has no predictive value. One other useful prognostic indicator is the Ki67 (MIB1) proliferative index.[6] In a series of 30 cases, no patient with an index < 5% developed a recurrence or metastasis, in contrast to those with > 5%, most of whom suffered tumour progression.

MUCOEPIDERMOID CARCINOMA

Mucoepidermoid carcinoma is a malignant epithelial neoplasm characterised by mucous, intermediate and epidermoid (keratinisation is exceptional) cells, with additional clear and oncocytic populations. The proportion of the different cell types and their architectural configuration (including cyst formation) varies between tumours and sometimes within an individual neoplasm. Recent developments have mainly concerned predicting clinical outcome from histology.

All mucoepidermoid carcinomas are malignant with metastatic potential, regardless of their microscopic appearance (Fig. 1). Nevertheless, histological features can predict outcome to some degree, and a grading system has been developed based on the extent of the cystic component, neural invasion, necrosis, cytological pleomorphism and mitotic activity.[5] This assessment has considerable prognostic significance, with death rates due to disease of 3.3%, 9.7% and 46.3% for grades 1, 2 and 3, respectively.[5] Recent proposed modifications appear to improve accuracy by adding vascular invasion and pattern of infiltration.[7] Special techniques of value include MIB1 index,[1] and expression of different membrane-bound mucins: MUC4 is related to a much better prognosis than MUC1.[8] Mucoepidermoid carcinoma can be subdivided at the molecular level into two types on the basis of a recurrent t(11;19) (q21; p13) translocation resulting in a MECT1–MAML2 fusion. The median survival of fusion-positive patients was > 10 years compared to 1.6 years for those without it.[9]

ADENOID CYSTIC CARCINOMA

Adenoid cystic carcinoma is a basaloid tumour consisting of epithelial and myoepithelial cells in variable morphological configurations, including tubular, cribriform and solid patterns. It has a relentless clinical course and usually a fatal outcome.[1]

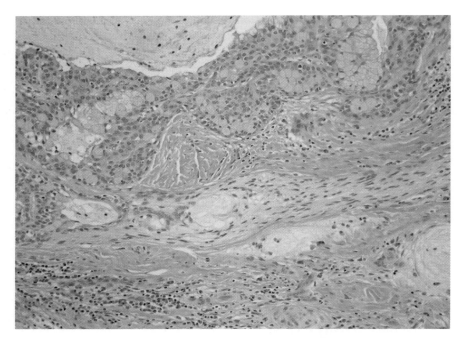

Fig. 1 Mucoepidermoid carcinoma. Although cytologically bland, in this case the nerve invasion suggests a more aggressive tumour, confirmed later by metastases.

Differentiation from less aggressive neoplasms is important, and whilst this is done mainly on haematoxylin and eosin stained sections, immunohistochemistry has some value. Pleomorphic adenoma may contain adenoid cystic-like areas, but myxochondroid matrix and plasmacytoid or spindle-shaped myoepithelial cells are usually present.[10] Both adenoid cystic and polymorphous low-grade adenocarcinomas are diffusely infiltrating neoplasms displaying morphological diversity, but can be distinguished cytologically: the former typically have closely packed dark, angular, atypical nuclei and frequent mitotic figures, in contrast to the uniform, bland nuclei of the latter. There are some immunohistochemical guides but, with one exception, no absolute discriminants. For example, S100 staining is usually more diffuse and stronger in polymorphous low-grade adenocarcinoma, and p63 typically reacts with cells at the periphery of the islands in adenoid cystic carcinoma. CD117 is of uncertain significance and diagnostic usefulness. Much more reliable is the MIB1 index, which is usually < 5% in polymorphous low-grade adenocarcinoma (and pleomorphic adenoma) and > 10% in adenoid cystic carcinoma.[11] Basal cell adenoma and adenocarcinoma resemble the solid pattern of adenoid cystic carcinoma, but mitotic and MIB1 indices are much lower. Basaloid squamous cell carcinoma also simulates solid pattern adenoid cystic carcinoma, but lacks any small epithelial-lined spaces; furthermore, the diagnosis requires the presence of a malignant squamous component.

The average 5- and 10-year survival rates are about 60% and 40%, respectively, but most patients eventually die of, or with, their disease. Overall, the main prognostic factors are site (*e.g.* submandibular worse than parotid), clinical stage and histological pattern. Predominantly tubular and cribriform adenoid cystic carcinomas have a better outcome than tumours with a solid component, especially if this exceeds 30% of the total volume. Another unfavourable feature is the frequent involvement of resection margins, particularly as the result of extensive perineural infiltration. Metastases occur in 40–60% of patients but, unlike other salivary malignancies, adenoid cystic carcinoma metastases tend to involve distant organs (lung, bone and liver) rather than local lymph nodes.[1]

POLYMORPHOUS LOW-GRADE ADENOCARCINOMA

Polymorphous low-grade adenocarcinoma is a malignant epithelial tumour characterised by cytological uniformity, morphological diversity, an infiltrative growth pattern and low metastatic potential.[1] It is the second commonest intra-oral salivary carcinoma, more frequent in women and with a wide age range.[5] Most arise in minor salivary glands, particularly the palate, with only rare examples in the parotid.

Cytologically, there is a uniform population of small to medium-sized cells with bland, round or oval nuclei, sometimes with intranuclear vacuoles[12] and absent or small nucleoli. In contrast, any tumour can encompass several architectural patterns, including ducts, fascicles, micropapillary, cribriform and solid structures. Diffuse infiltration of tumour cells in single file and concentric growth around nerves is reminiscent of lobular breast carcinoma. Mitotic figures are scanty and never atypical. The stroma varies from fibromyxoid to densely hyaline, but the chondroid matrix of pleomorphic adenoma is not seen. The most useful immunohistochemical markers are cytokeratins (broad spectrum, cytokeratin 7) and S100 protein. Positivity is also seen with EMA, vimentin, bcl-2 and sometimes with CEA, αSMA and GFAP; MIB1 proliferation is low – mean 2.4% (range, 0.2–6.4%) in one study.[11]

The most important histopathological differential diagnosis is the much more aggressive adenoid cystic carcinoma (see above). Other potential mimics include pleomorphic adenoma, often less well circumscribed in minor glands than in the parotid. Any chondroid matrix or circumscription favours pleomorphic adenoma, but it is sometimes impossible to distinguish these tumours on a small biopsy, though both should be excised.

Polymorphous low-grade adenocarcinoma behaves as a low-grade malignancy, with recurrence rates of about 20%, nodal metastases in < 10%, distant metastases in < 2%, and death due to disease in < 1%.[12] Long-term studies suggest late recurrences and metastases may be more frequent,[13] perhaps due to incompleteness of excision at original surgery.

Papillary structures form part of the spectrum of growth patterns seen in polymorphous low-grade adenocarcinoma; when extensive, such tumours have slightly more frequent nodal metastases,[13] although the same long-term outlook. Genuine, high-grade malignancy occurs rarely, as either a poorly differentiated version of the low-grade carcinoma or salivary duct carcinoma.[14]

CRIBRIFORM ADENOCARCINOMA OF THE TONGUE

A newly described tumour so far reported only in the tongue has a characteristic morphology, thus suggesting origin from remnants of lingual thyroid tissue. Nevertheless, it shares some histological features with

2A

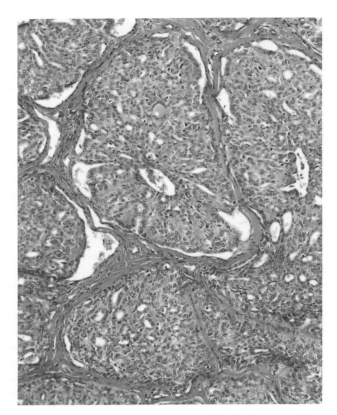

Fig. 2 Cribriform adenocarcinoma of the tongue. (A) Cribriform and glomeruloid architecture. (B) Papillary thyroid carcinoma-like nuclei.

polymorphous low-grade adenocarcinoma, to which it may be related, and thus, it was not accepted in the WHO classification as a separate entity.[1] Cribriform adenocarcinoma of the tongue usually arises in adults with a mean age of 50 years (range, 25–70 years) and equal sex incidence in the root of the tongue. Generally, there are cervical nodal metastases at the time of diagnosis, either unilaterally or bilaterally, but distant spread has not been described.

Microscopy shows lobules composed of solid and microcystic growth patterns, separated by fibrous septa. In the solid areas, tumour nests often display a well-developed peripheral layer which detaches, leaving papillae or glomeruloid structures surrounded by apparent clefts (Fig. 2A). In the microcystic areas, the lobules comprise intermingled cribriform and tubular structures; typically, the tubules are approximately the same size and consist of one cell layer. The tumour is composed of one cell type with pale and vacuolated nuclei, sometimes containing up to three small nucleoli. The nuclei often overlap one another, thus resembling papillary thyroid carcinoma (Fig. 2B), but psammoma bodies were identified in only one case. Mitotic figures are sparse. Immunohistochemically, a strong or patchy reaction is seen with staining for cytokeratins and S100 protein, but actin, calponin and smooth muscle myosin heavy chain (SMMHC) are evident in only a few areas. Thyroglobulin and TTF-1 are completely negative.

2B

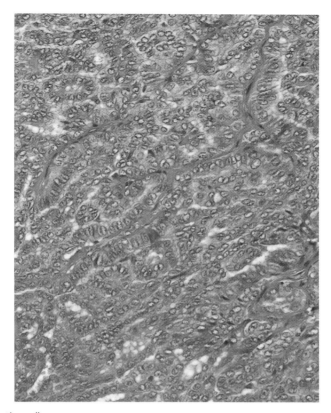

Fig. 2 (Continued)

Patients treated with surgical excision and neck node dissection, possibly with radiotherapy, have a good chance of prolonged survival.[1]

EPITHELIAL–MYOEPITHELIAL CARCINOMA

Epithelial–myoepithelial carcinoma is rare with a wide age range (8–103 years; mean, 60 years). It occurs in any salivary gland, predominantly the parotid;[5] analogous neoplasms have been described in the bronchus, breast and biliary tract.

It is composed throughout of lumina lined by an inner layer of small epithelial cells, surrounded by an outer layer of often clear myoepithelial cells, beyond which is a periodic acid–Schiff (PAS)-positive basement membrane of variable thickness. Cytological pleomorphism is usually mild. The inner cells express cytokeratin and the outer actin, SMMHC, calponin and p63. S100 and cytokeratin 14 immunostains are less specific and sometimes react with both layers.

The differential diagnosis depends on the predominant component, *e.g.* other tumours composed of clear cells (Table 2),[2,15] or pleomorphic adenoma if the stroma is abundant and bi-layered ducts inconspicuous; any invasiveness indicates carcinoma. Areas resembling epithelial–myoepithelial carcinoma can be seen in more aggressive neoplasms such as myoepithelial carcinoma

3A

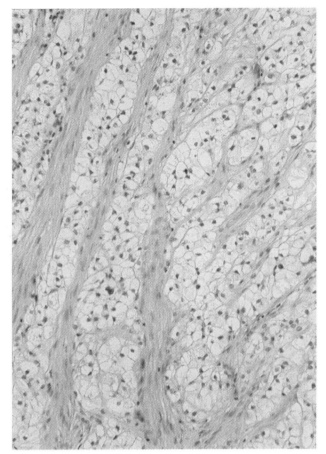

Fig. 3 Clear cell carcinoma, NOS. (A) A monomorphic population of clear cells. (B) Perineural invasion, but no staining of the carcinoma itself with myoepithelial markers such as S100 protein.

Table 2 Classification of clear cell tumours involving the salivary glands

Benign
  Pleomorphic adenoma, myoepithelioma, sebaceous adenoma, oncocytoma and oncocytic hyperplasia (MNOH)

Malignant, primary
  Carcinomas not usually characterised by clear cells, but with rare clear cell variants, *e.g.* mucoepidermoid and acinic cell carcinomas

  Carcinomas usually characterised by clear cells:
    (i)   Dimorphic – epithelial–myoepithelial carcinoma
    (ii) Monomorphic – hyalinising clear cell carcinoma; clear cell myoepithelial carcinoma (malignant myoepithelioma)
    (iii) Sebaceous carcinoma

Malignant, metastatic
  Carcinomas, especially kidney, thyroid. Also melanoma

Miscellaneous
  Some odontogenic neoplasms

3B

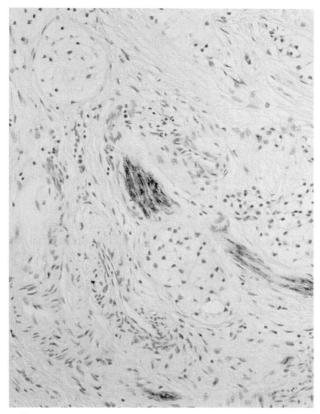

Fig. 3 *(Continued)*

(particularly the clear cell variant) and adenoid cystic carcinoma; therefore, any tumour with epithelial–myoepithelial growth must be sampled widely.

Cases of epithelial–myoepithelial carcinoma have been associated with multiple nodules of intercalated duct hyperplasia in the surrounding parotid gland.[16,17] This suggests a ductal origin, and also why in hybrid tumours of the salivary glands (themselves very rare), the most frequent combination is that of epithelial–myoepithelial and adenoid cystic carcinomas.[17]

The behaviour of epithelial–myoepithelial carcinoma in most series is low grade, typically with recurrences in 31%, cervical node metastases in 18%, distant metastases in 7%, and death due to tumour in 7%.[2] Higher rates of recurrence (50%) and death (40%) in a series from a large referral centre in Portugal probably reflect a patient population with advanced disease.[18] The only morphological feature found to correlate with a poor prognosis was nuclear atypia in more than 20% of tumour cells. Epithelial–myoepithelial carcinoma can occasionally dedifferentiate as a high-grade myoepithelial or glandular malignancy.[2]

CLEAR CELL CARCINOMA, NOT OTHERWISE SPECIFIED (NOS)

Monomorphic, clear cell carcinomas are either epithelial or myoepithelial (clear cell variant of myoepithelial carcinoma). The former is included in the

2005 WHO classification as clear cell carcinoma, not otherwise specified (NOS), a malignant epithelial neoplasm composed of a single population of cells having optically clear cytoplasm on H&E stained sections. The diagnosis requires the exclusion of other salivary tumours with a clear cell component.[1]

The sex incidence is equal, and the age range wide (1–86 years; mean, 52 years).[5,15] Most arise in minor salivary glands, mainly in the palate,[1,5,15] and less frequently elsewhere such as the parotid.[15] Patients typically present with a long-standing, painless mass, usually < 30 mm in diameter. Exceptionally, cervical lymph node metastases are seen at initial presentation.

Microscopy shows invasive nests, sheets and trabeculae of polygonal glycogen-rich cells separated by dense collagen bands or thin fibrous septa (Fig. 3B).[1] The nuclei display usually mild pleomorphism and inconspicuous nucleoli; mitotic figures are rare. In some cells, particularly in deeper parts of the tumours, the cytoplasm appears weakly eosinophilic rather than clear. Occasional tumours demonstrate squamous or ductal differentiation, with rare intracellular mucin droplets. Otherwise, mucin stains are negative. Clear cell carcinomas express epithelial markers, including cytokeratin 7 (but not cytokeratin 20) and epithelial membrane antigen (EMA); myoepithelial markers (e.g. S100 protein, actin) are consistently negative (Fig. 3B).[2] Ultrastructural studies have demonstrated epithelial, but not myoepithelial, features.[15]

Clear cell carcinoma, NOS is one of several salivary tumours composed of clear cells (Table 2).[2,15] They are either benign or malignant, the latter subdivided into those carcinomas usually characterised by clear cells and those in which clear cells constitute an unusual variant; metastases are an additional category. Benign clear cell oncocytoma and multifocal nodular oncocytic hyperplasia usually include admixed typical eosinophilic granular cells and show strong staining with antimitochondrial antibody. Scattered clear cells are not uncommon in benign myoepithelioma, but the pure clear cell variant is very rare. It is well circumscribed, comprising a population of relatively bland cells, positive for some myoepithelial markers. Acinic cell and, in particular, mucoepidermoid carcinomas can have clear cell areas, on occasions extensive, but careful sampling shows scattered cells with the characteristic features (e.g. PAS-diastase positive zymogen granules, mucinous goblet cells and squamous-like foci) of either neoplasm. Primary carcinomas typically composed of clear cells are either dimorphic or monomorphic. The former is epithelial–myoepithelial carcinoma, with a biphasic cell population (see above). A monomorphic proliferation characterises clear cell carcinoma and clear cell predominant myoepithelial carcinoma.[2] The latter is more aggressive, usually occurs in major glands, shows areas of necrosis and expresses myoepithelial markers. Neoplastic sebaceous cells have foamy, vacuolated cytoplasm (often indenting the nucleus), compared to the completely clear cytoplasm of clear cell carcinoma. Metastatic clear cell renal carcinoma can present as a parotid mass. This tumour has a prominent vascular background and usually some nuclear atypia, and expresses broad-spectrum cytokeratins, vimentin and CD10, but not cytokeratin 7, keratin 903 or CEA.[19] Imaging of the kidneys also identifies any primary with metastatic potential. Other metastases sometimes composed of clear cells include melanoma, positive for S100 protein, HMB45 and other markers.

The treatment of clear cell carcinoma is surgical excision. The prognosis of this low-grade malignancy is generally good; a few patients have developed metastases in the neck nodes and rarely the lungs, but no deaths have been reported.[1,15]

BASAL CELL ADENOCARCINOMA

Basal cell adenocarcinoma is rare and arises mainly in the parotid, but also elsewhere.[1] Microscopically, it has the architecture of basal cell adenoma, but displays infiltrative growth. Four architectural patterns are recognised: solid (composed of variably sized nests), tubular (contains luminal spaces), trabecular and membranous. In all patterns, there is a mixture of small basal-type and large pale cells; nuclei are often palisaded at the periphery of tumour islands; focal squamous eddies are seen in some tumours. Nuclear pleomorphism and mitotic activity are usually minimal. Hyalinised eosinophilic basal lamina material is present in variable amounts, but is abundant in the membranous subtype, together with hyaline intercellular droplets.

The most important differential diagnosis is the solid variant of adenoid cystic carcinoma which, as described above, shows nuclear pleomorphism and mitotic activity. Also, it is much commoner in the submandibular and minor glands, in contrast to the usual parotid location of basal cell adenocarcinoma.

Basal cell adenocarcinoma is a low-grade malignancy with local recurrences in 37%, nodal and distant metastases in 8% and 4%, respectively.

SALIVARY DUCT CARCINOMA AND VARIANTS

Salivary duct carcinoma is an aggressive malignancy of major glands, most often found in men over 50 years old. Histologically, it resembles high-grade breast ductal carcinoma.[1] Recent developments include new immunohisto-chemical findings and the recognition of morphological variants.

Most cases show positive distinct membrane staining for HER-2/neu protein, although there is some variation depending which antibody is used;[20] in some cases amplification of the HER-2 gene can be demonstrated by FISH analysis. Unlike breast cancer, there is no significant oestrogen or progesterone receptor expression.[21] In contrast, > 90% (in both sexes) express androgen receptors.[21–23] Staining with prostatic markers has been found in some studies,[22] but not others.[21]

In addition to the usual type of salivary duct carcinoma, a few, rare, morphological variants have been reported: micropapillary, sarcomatoid, mucin-rich and oncocytic, as well as pure *in situ* cases. In the micropapillary variant, clusters of cells without fibrovascular cores are each surrounded by a clear space, and there is an 'inside-out' pattern of EMA staining.[24] The mucin-rich variant includes areas of typical salivary duct carcinoma and mucin lakes containing malignant cells (Fig. 4A,B).[25] The sarcomatoid type is a composite of usual salivary duct and spindle cell sarcomatoid carcinomas.[1] It may account for some tumours previously classified as carcinosarcoma ('true malignant mixed tumour'). A few cells with oncocytic features can be seen in any salivary duct carcinoma, but a genuine oncocytic variant has been described only in outline. Most tumour cells should show evidence of

4A

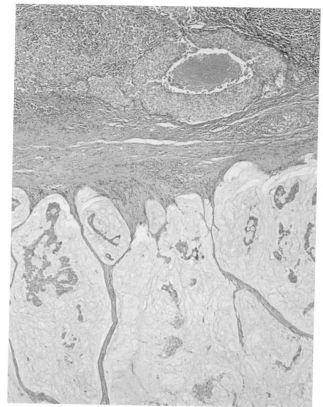

Fig. 4 Salivary duct carcinoma, mucin-rich variant. (A) usual type salivary duct carcinoma and mucin lakes containing tumour cells. (B) Nuclear positivity for androgen receptors.

oncocytic differentiation in a neoplasm with morphological and immuno-histochemical features of salivary duct carcinoma (Fig. 5).[26] Occasional examples of purely *in situ* salivary duct carcinoma have been described in both major and minor glands; they differ from low-grade cribriform cystadenocarcinoma[27,28] by displaying nuclear atypia and the same immunoprofile as their invasive counterparts, *i.e.* S100 negative, androgen receptor positive, gross cystic disease fluid protein (GCDFP)-15 positive.

At present, the preferred treatment of salivary duct carcinoma is complete surgical excision with neck dissection followed by radio- and chemotherapy. Future patients may benefit from anti-androgen therapy[22] or Herceptin.[20] Peroxisome proliferator-activated receptor gamma (PPAR-γ) is often strongly expressed in the cytoplasm, and is a possible molecular target for drugs that specifically bind to and activate this receptor.[29]

ONCOCYTIC CARCINOMA

Only a few dozen cases of oncocytic carcinoma have been reported, mostly in the parotid glands of patients with an average age of 63 years (range, 29–91 years) and male predominance.[5] A few cases have arisen in Warthin tumours.

4B

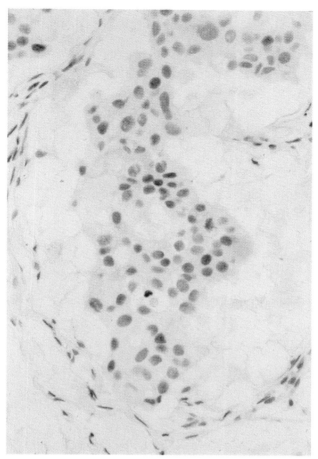

Fig. 4 *(Continued)*

The diagnosis requires evidence of oncocytic differentiation (by phospho-tungstate acid and haematoxylin [PTAH] staining, immunohistochemistry or electron microscopy) and demonstration of malignant behaviour. The literature is limited, but the consensus is that oncocytic carcinoma is an aggressive tumour with over half of reported patients either dying of disease or suffering recurrences.[5]

The authors' view is that it is probably not a single entity but a mixture of several carcinomas showing oncocytic differentiation, most often salivary duct carcinoma.[26]

MUCINOUS ADENOCARCINOMA

Mucinous (colloid) adenocarcinoma is composed of round and irregularly shaped clusters of epithelial cells floating in mucus-filled cysts, themselves separated by fibrous strands. The cells are cuboidal, columnar or irregular in shape, usually possessing clear cytoplasm and small dark nuclei; signet ring cells may be present. Mitotic figures are sparse. The mucus is PASD and mucicarmine positive.[1]

5A

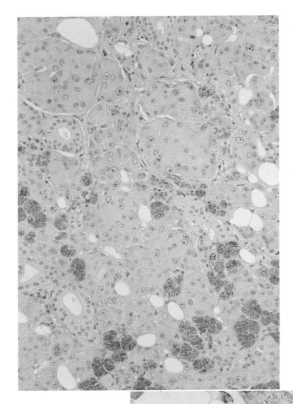

5B

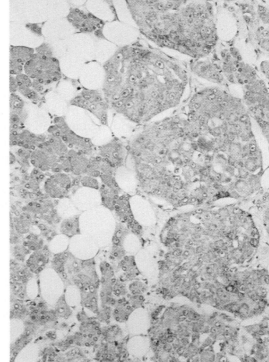

Fig. 5 Salivary duct carcinoma, oncocytic variant; invading normal gland.
(A) H&E; (B) anti-mitochondrial antibody; (C) androgen receptors; (D) invasive and *in situ* lesions, cytokeratin 14.

5C

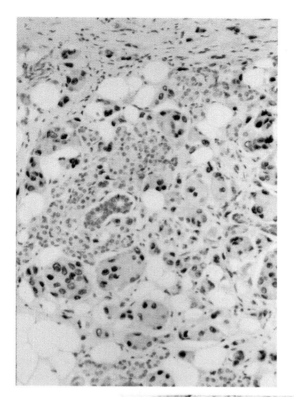

5D

Fig. 5 *(Continued)*

The carcinoma cells express epithelial markers, but not high molecular weight cytokeratins, actin, HER2/neu protein, oestrogen or progesterone receptors.

The differential diagnosis includes mucoepidermoid carcinoma, in which there are also squamous-like and intermediate cells. Mucin-rich salivary duct carcinoma includes areas of the usual type, and expresses GCDFP-15 and androgen receptors.[25]

It is unclear whether low-grade signet ring cell (mucin-producing) adenocarcinomas of minor salivary gland are related, as they lack mucus pools.[30]

From the relatively few published cases, mucinous adenocarcinoma has a propensity for local recurrence and lymph node metastases. Four of the 11 cases described by Gnepp *et al.*[4] died of disease.

LOW-GRADE CRIBRIFORM CYSTADENOCARCINOMA

Low-grade cribriform cystadenocarcinoma is defined as: 'a rare, cystic, proliferative carcinoma that resembles the spectrum of breast lesions from atypical ductal hyperplasia to micropapillary and cribriform low-grade ductal carcinoma *in situ*'.[1] It was previously named 'low-grade salivary duct carcinoma'.

The average age of patients is 64 years (range, 32–93 years), with an equal sex incidence. All but one case arose in the parotid glands, the other in the submandibular.

Microscopically, this tumour is unencapsulated and generally displaces rather than truly invades salivary tissue. Multiple cysts and solid structures of varying sizes (Fig. 6A) are composed of small, bland ductal cells with regular nuclei and clear to eosinophilic cytoplasm (Fig. 6B). They proliferate to form papillae or cribriform structures, but no necrosis or comedocarcinoma are seen. Mitotic figures are sparse. Very occasional cells contain lipofuscin pigment. At the periphery of the tumour islands, there is often a population of flattened myoepithelial cells. The stroma is partly sclerotic with occasional microcalcifications. Moderate amounts of extracellular mucus are found, but goblet cells only rarely. The predominant cells express cytokeratins 7, 8, 18, 19, EMA and S100 protein (Fig. 6C), and the peripheral cells react with myoepithelial markers (Fig. 6D). Cytokeratin 14 immunocytochemistry shows strong staining at the periphery, but also in some inner cells. The MIB1 proliferation index is usually < 1%. No significant staining is seen with antibodies to CEA, GCDFP-15 or HER2/neu protein, and variable results have been found with androgen receptors.[31,32] Occasional tumours have demonstrated foci of stromal invasion, and three neoplasms have shown transition from low to intermediate or high-grade cytology, with scattered mitotic figures and focal necrosis.

The main differential diagnosis is salivary duct carcinoma of usual type, particularly purely *in situ* lesions. They display nuclear atypia and the same immunoprofile as their invasive counterparts, *i.e.* S100 negative, expression of androgen receptor, GCDFP-15. Ductal proliferation is the sole feature common to both tumours, which otherwise are two different entities. Occasional reports of low-grade cribriform cystadenocarcinoma with high-grade elements were relatively solid, not resembling usual type salivary duct carcinoma. The papillary cystic variant of acinic cell carcinoma includes at least some cells

6A

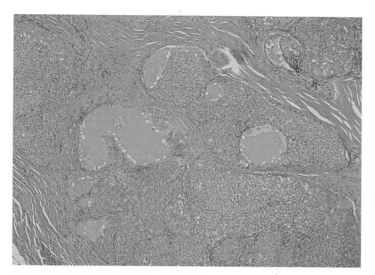

6B

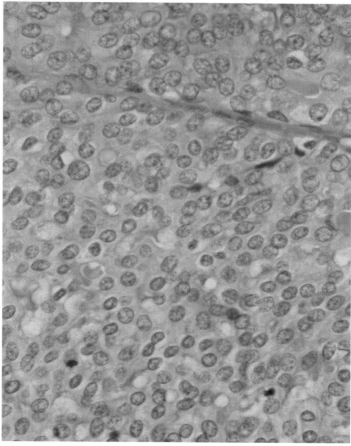

Fig. 6 Low-grade cribriform cystadenocarcinoma. (A) Architecture. (B) No cytological atypia. (C) Tumour cells are S100 positive. (D) Myoepithelial cell rim (smooth muscle myosin heavy chain).

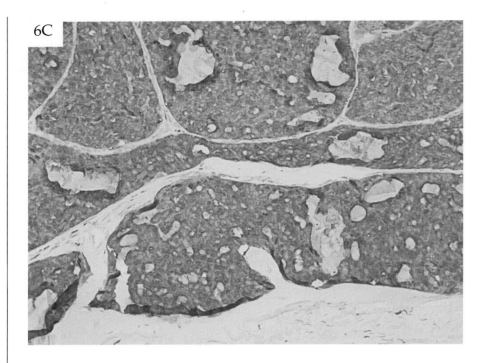

Fig. 6 *(continued)* Low-grade cribriform cystadenocarcinoma. (A) Architecture. (B) No cytological atypia. (C) Tumour cells are S100 positive. (D) Myoepithelial cell rim (smooth muscle myosin heavy chain).

with PASD-positive granules and is usually S100 negative. Other variants of cystadenocarcinoma lack the resemblance to atypical ductal hyperplasia or carcinoma-*in-situ* of the breast.[27]

Generally low-grade cribriform cystadenocarcinoma follows a non-aggressive clinical course; all but one patient were recurrence-free after 6–144 months (median, 32 months).[31] One recent case transformed to a higher grade neoplasm and developed cervical nodal metastases.[32] Thus, conservative resection of the involved gland, without neck dissection or adjuvant radiotherapy is adequate treatment, unless there is histological evidence of high-grade disease.

OTHER FORMS OF CYSTADENOCARCINOMA

The WHO fascicle defines cystadenocarcinoma as:[1] 'a rare malignant tumour characterised by predominantly cystic growth that often exhibits intraluminal papillary growth. It lacks any additional specific histopathological features that characterise the other types of salivary carcinomas showing cystic growth. It is conceptually the malignant counterpart of benign cystadenoma.' However, it is not universally accepted as a specific entity.[33]

Microscopically, there are numerous cysts of different sizes, some of which contain mucin, separated by fibrous connective tissue. The cell types include small and large, cuboidal and columnar, but mucous, clear and oncocytic cells are rare. The nuclei are typically bland and mitotic figures few.

Cystadenocarcinoma is a low-grade malignancy, and no deaths have been reported, although a few patients have developed regional nodal metastases.

MYOEPITHELIAL CARCINOMA

Myoepithelial carcinoma (malignant myoepithelioma) is an infiltrative neoplasm with potential for metastasis, composed almost exclusively of tumour cells with myoepithelial differentiation.[1]

The average age of patients is 55 years (range, 14–86 years), with an equal sex incidence. They arise at any site (mostly the parotid), sometimes *de novo*, but at least 50% develop in pre-existing pleomorphic adenomas or benign myoepitheliomas.[34]

Myoepithelial carcinomas often form multiple cellular nodules containing plentiful myxoid or hyaline material, and central necrosis (Fig. 7). Small cysts and cleft-like spaces are frequent, and some authors allow a few small true lumina. The cells can be monomorphic or a mixture of epithelioid (the most frequent), clear, vacuolated (resembling lipoblasts), hyaline (plasmacytoid), spindle to stellate, or occasionally oncocytic. The nuclei vary from small and bland to large and pleomorphic. Mitotic figures may be plentiful, including atypical forms. Metaplastic changes are frequent, most often squamous with keratinisation.[5]

All cases stain to some degree for S100, vimentin and broad-spectrum cytokeratins. Myoepithelial markers such as CK14, αSMA, SMMHC, calponin and p63 are positive in most, but by no means all, cases. The mean MIB1 index is high, with any count above 10% said to be diagnostic of malignancy in a myoepithelial neoplasm.[35] It has recently been shown that myoepithelial

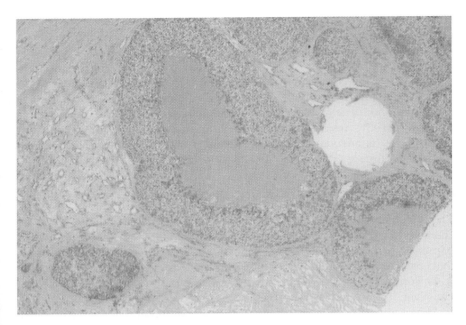

Fig. 7 Myoepithelial carcinoma is typically composed of multiple nodules, some of which have necrotic centres.

carcinomas secrete compounds with anti-invasive properties; although as yet poorly understood, they could affect the biological aggressiveness of any particular tumour.[36]

The variable appearance leads to a wide differential diagnosis, including other salivary carcinomas. The spindle cell type mimics soft tissue sarcomas and the plasmacytoid cell type must be distinguished from melanoma. The clear cell variant resembles the many other salivary tumours composed of clear cells (Table 2).[2] Extensive squamous metaplasia suggests mucoepidermoid or metastatic squamous carcinoma.

The prognosis of myoepithelial carcinoma is variable, but about one-third of patients die of disease, another third have residual tumour or recurrences (often multiple) and the remaining third are disease-free.[5,34,35] There is only a weak statistical correlation for outcome with cytological atypia (high grade), but other parameters (tumour size, site, cell type, mitotic rate, presence of a benign tumour, necrosis, perineural and vascular invasion) are not helpful. Tumours arising in ordinary pleomorphic adenomas behave the same as *de novo* carcinomas,[34] but those developing in recurrent pleomorphic adenomas may pursue a prolonged course.[2,36]

MALIGNANCY IN PLEOMORPHIC ADENOMA

Malignancy in pleomorphic adenoma encompasses three entities – carcinoma ex pleomorphic adenoma, carcinosarcoma and metastasising pleomorphic adenoma. The latter two are exceedingly rare. Published figures for incidence vary considerably from series to series: those quoted in the 2005 WHO fascicle are 3.6% of all salivary gland tumours (range, 0.9–14%) and 12% of malignancies (range, 2.8–42.4%). Malignancy develops in 6.2% of all pleomorphic adenomas (range, 1.9–23.3%), and the incidence increases with the length of history, but can still be short.[1]

CARCINOMA EX PLEOMORPHIC ADENOMA

The malignancy in carcinoma ex pleomorphic adenoma is restricted to the epithelial or myoepithelial component, and metastases are composed solely of carcinoma.

It occurs over a wide age range, with the majority of cases in the sixth to eighth decades, about 10 years later than uncomplicated pleomorphic adenoma; most series report a slight female predominance. Any gland can be involved, though the parotid is most common. The tumour typically presents with a long history (usually > 3 years) of a nodule that suddenly increases in size.

The main histological requirement for the diagnosis is the presence of a benign pleomorphic adenoma and a carcinoma. The former is often largely hyalinised and/or calcified, and may require extensive sampling to detect it; sometimes, the origin can only be inferred from the history. Most types of carcinoma have been described, the commonest being poorly differentiated adenocarcinoma and undifferentiated carcinoma. There is evidence that many of the former are salivary duct carcinoma and the latter myoepithelial.[1,2]

The most important feature to assess is whether the carcinoma has breached the capsule; it is thus classified as non-invasive, minimally invasive (< 1.5 mm penetration beyond the capsule) or invasive (> 1.5 mm).[1] Non-invasive carcinoma (the terminology preferred to 'intracapsular carcinoma' and 'carcinoma *in situ*') is defined as 'pleomorphic adenoma with multifocal areas containing carcinoma' (Fig. 8A). Despite its malignant microscopic appearance, it generally behaves indolently,[37] with only one report of a patient developing lymph node metastases.[38] In invasive carcinomas, the extent is important: one study[39] found that no patient whose tumour penetrated < 6 mm beyond the capsule died of disease, whereas all patients with invasion of > 8 mm succumbed.

Immunohistochemical and molecular studies of HER-2/neu proto-oncogene have shown protein overexpression and gene amplification in all high-grade invasive carcinoma ex pleomorphic adenoma.[20] Similar findings have been demonstrated in the malignant component of non-invasive carcinomas (protein overexpression in 55%, gene amplification in 37%).[37] In these studies, benign areas of the original tumour were constantly negative. Thus, staining for HER-2/neu can be used to detect early carcinoma in a pleomorphic adenoma (Fig. 8B).

The main practical difficulties with carcinoma ex pleomorphic adenoma are:

1. Its rarity, which makes it an unfamiliar feature for most pathologists.

2. If the capsule of the pleomorphic adenoma is ill-defined, assessment of the extent of invasion becomes less reliable.

3. Sampling of the capsule must be extensive to ensure identification of maximum invasion.

4. It can be difficult to separate non-invasive carcinoma from a pleomorphic adenoma with atypical histological features. Focal nuclear atypia in oncocytic and myoepithelial cells is seen occasionally and is probably not of clinical significance. Necrosis, squamous metaplasia and epithelial atypia may follow fine-

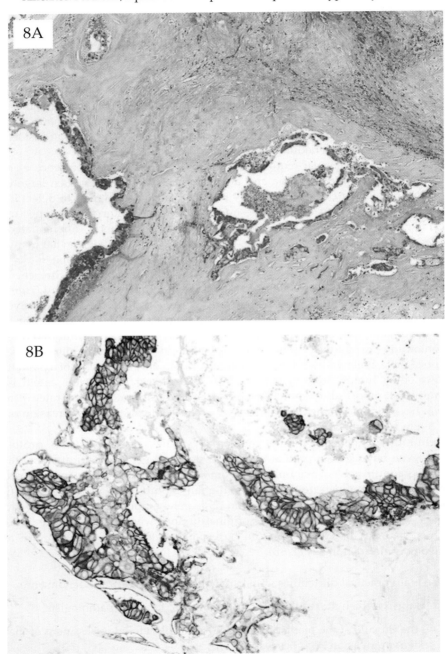

Fig. 8 Non-invasive carcinoma in a densely fibrotic pleomorphic adenoma. (A) H&E and (B) HER2/neu oncoprotein.

needle aspiration of a benign tumour, as perhaps can focal vascular permeation. Immunohistochemical staining for MIB1 and HER-2/neu can differentiate true malignant cells from bizarre nuclear changes in benign cells.[37]

5. The differential diagnosis includes a wide range of other salivary carcinomas, and the main problem results from the under-recognition of the pre-existent pleomorphic adenoma.

The treatment is radical surgery and neck dissection, perhaps with radiotherapy. The prognosis for widely invasive carcinoma ex pleomorphic adenoma is poor, with a 5-year survival of about 50%. Regional and distant metastases are frequent.

CARCINOSARCOMA IN A PLEOMORPHIC ADENOMA (TRUE MALIGNANT MIXED TUMOUR)

Carcinosarcoma is an exceedingly rare malignant tumour composed of a mixture of carcinomatous and sarcomatous elements,[1] with either component capable of metastasis. The mean age at presentation is 58 years (range, 14–87 years), and most cases are found in the parotid gland. It may arise in a pre-existing pleomorphic adenoma, or de novo.

Microscopy shows a biphasic tumour in which the epithelial component is generally a poorly differentiated adenocarcinoma. The mesenchymal element is usually chondrosarcoma, but osteosarcoma and other differentiation have been described. Epithelial markers are detected in the epithelial component and sometimes the mesenchymal; both elements have similar p53 and genetic profiles. In a subset with osteoclast-type giant cells, the same mutation was found of the same allele on chromosome 17p13, a known mutation of salivary duct carcinoma.[40] This suggests that carcinosarcomas are metaplastic carcinomas, possibly sarcomatoid salivary duct carcinomas.[1]

The differential diagnosis includes spindle cell squamous carcinoma, primary salivary sarcomas and carcinoma ex pleomorphic adenoma. The first arises from the mucosal surface and may simulate carcinosarcoma of minor salivary glands. Its epithelial component is epidermoid, not glandular; dysplasia of the surface squamous epithelium is diagnostic. Primary salivary sarcomas are exceptionally rare and must be well sampled to identify any minor carcinomatous component.

The outcome of carcinosarcoma is usually poor with 60% of patients dying of disease.

METASTASISING PLEOMORPHIC ADENOMA

Metastasising pleomorphic adenoma is defined as a histologically benign pleomorphic adenoma that manifests local or distant metastasis.[1] Common factors in most reported cases were long intervals (up to 50 years) between the primary tumour and metastases, and simultaneous occurrence of distant metastases and local recurrences, usually multiple. This suggests that surgical manipulation of recurrences could cause vascular implantation but, in many cases that later metastasised, it was not possible histologically to demonstrate actual vascular permeation. The microscopic picture is that of the usual mixture of mesenchyme, epithelial and myoepithelial cells of any pleomorphic adenoma, and there are no predictive histological features. Metastases can be found in bone, lung, lymph nodes and, rarely, other sites such as kidney. They are generally indolent tumours, and patients may survive for extended periods with metastatic disease. Recommended therapy is wide local excision for both primary and metastases.

UNDIFFERENTIATED CARCINOMA

Undifferentiated carcinomas of the salivary glands are uncommon malignant epithelial neoplasms that are too poorly differentiated by their light microscopic features to be placed into a specific category. They are generally subclassified into three groups – lymphoepithelial, small cell and large cell carcinomas. Almost all small cell and some large cell carcinomas exhibit neuroendocrine differentiation.[1]

LYMPHOEPITHELIAL CARCINOMA

Lymphoepithelial carcinoma is exceptionally rare, except for a high incidence among Eskimos and Chinese, in whom it is consistently linked with EBV infection.[1] There is no clinical association with Sjögren's syndrome.

Histologically, it closely resembles analogous nasopharyngeal neoplasms; syncytial nests of carcinoma cells infiltrate the surrounding salivary tissue accompanied by lymphoid stroma. The cells are anaplastic, large and polygonal or sometimes spindled with a vesicular nucleus and prominent eosinophilic nucleoli. In non-Caucasian patients, EBV-encoded small RNA (EBER) is generally detected in the tumour cells by *in situ* hybridisation.[1]

The 5-year survival rate is 75–86%,[1] even though nodal and distant metastases are common.

SMALL CELL CARCINOMA

Small cell carcinoma of the salivary glands is a very rare malignant epithelial tumour characterised by proliferation of small anaplastic cells with scanty cytoplasm, fine nuclear chromatin, and inconspicuous nucleoli.[1] Most are positive for cytokeratin, sometimes showing a paranuclear dot-like pattern, and also react with neuroendocrine markers. All are negative for S100, HMB45, myoepithelial and lymphoid markers. In addition, about three-quarters of cases express cytokeratin 20; on this basis, salivary small cell carcinoma may be subdivided into Merkel cell and pulmonary varieties.

The 2- and 5-year survival rates are 38–70% and 13–46%, respectively, although patients with the Merkel cell subtype (*i.e.* cytokeratin 20 positive) have a better prognosis than cytokeratin 20 negative cases.

LARGE CELL CARCINOMA

Large cell carcinoma is exceptionally rare and composed of invasive sheets of large pleomorphic cells (> 30 μm in diameter), with abundant eosinophilic or clear cytoplasm. They usually express cytokeratins (not cytokeratin 20) and EMA, but never lymphoid, melanoma or myoepithelial markers. About one in five cases exhibits neuroendocrine differentiation, *i.e.* large-cell neuroendocrine carcinoma.[1]

It is aggressive with frequent local recurrences, nodal and distant metastases. The 2-year survival rate is 36%.[1]

SIALOBLASTOMA

Most sialoblastomas are identified in the perinatal period or first year of life.[5] The male:female ratio is 2:1; three-quarters of tumours arise in the parotid glands, the remainder in the submandibular. Tumours are well circumscribed, up to 150 mm in diameter and composed of numerous solid hypercellular islands of primitive basaloid cells, some with peripheral palisading, and often with small central ducts, bud-like structures and solid organoid nests. The tumour cells have large, round-to-oval, vesicular nuclei and variable amounts of eosinophilic cytoplasm. Immunohistochemistry and electron microscopy show both epithelial and myoepithelial cells.[1,5] There is diffuse expression of S100 protein and vimentin, with cytokeratin highlighting any ducts. Mitotic figures may be numerous (especially in recurrences[1]), but none is atypical. The intervening stroma appears loose and immature. Criteria for malignancy include invasion of nerves or vascular spaces, necrosis and marked cytological atypia.[1] Of fifteen reported cases, four recurred and another metastases to regional lymph nodes. One death has been recorded, but most cases are cured by excision.[1]

MISCELLANEOUS OTHER CARCINOMAS[1,5]

Sebaceous carcinoma and lymphadenocarcinoma are both very rare and high grade. Primary squamous cell carcinoma must be distinguished from metastases, which are far commoner.

Points for best practice

- The new WHO classification is a reasonably up-to-date summary of our current knowledge, and is readily usable in practice, but does leave some issues unresolved.

- Newly accepted entities include clear cell carcinoma NOS, sialoblastoma and low-grade cribriform cystadenocarcinoma.

- Whilst morphology remains the mainstay in the diagnosis of salivary tumours, immunohistochemistry is valuable in, for example, the differential diagnosis of clear cell lesions.

- MIB1 index gives important prognostic information in acinic cell carcinoma and is useful in the differential diagnosis between adenoid cystic and polymorphous low-grade adenocarcinoma.

- Salivary duct carcinoma includes several newly-described histological variants. Androgen receptor expression and positive HER2/neu status may become therapeutically important.

- The most useful prognostic indicator in carcinoma ex pleomorphic adenoma is the extent of invasion beyond the original benign tumour. Identification of early malignant change can be aided by HER2/neu immunostaining.

References

1. Barnes EL, Eveson JW, Reichart P, Sidransky D. Tumours of the salivary glands. In: *World Health Organization Classification of Tumours: Pathology and Genetics of Head and Neck Tumours*. Lyon: IARC, 2005; 209–281.

2. Di Palma S, Simpson RHW, Skálová A, Leivo I. Major and minor salivary glands. In: Cardesa A, Slootweg PJ. (eds) *Pathology of the Head and Neck Pathology*. Berlin: Springer, 2006; 131–170.

3. Dardick I, Kini S, Bradley G *et al*. *Atlas of Salivary Gland Tumor Cytopathology, Oral and Surgical Pathology*. Pathology Images Inc., 2006.

4. Gnepp DR, Brandwein MS, Henley JD. Salivary and lacrimal glands. In: Gnepp DR (ed) *Diagnostic surgical pathology of the head and neck*. Philadelphia, PA: WB Saunders, 2001; 325–430.

5. Ellis GL, Auclair PL. *Atlas of Tumor Pathology: Tumors of the Salivary Glands*. Washington, DC: Armed Forces Institute of Pathology, 1996.

6. Skálová A, Leivo I, von Boguslawsky K, Saksela E. Cell proliferation correlates with prognosis in acinic cell carcinomas of salivary gland origin. Immunohistochemical study of 30 cases using the MIB1 antibody in formalin-fixed paraffin sections. *J Pathol* 1994; **173**: 13–21.

7. Brandwein MS, Ivanov K, Wallace DI *et al*. Mucoepidermoid carcinoma: a clinicopathologic study of 80 patients with special reference to histological grading. *Am J Surg Pathol* 2001; **25**: 835–845.

8. Alos L, Lujan B, Castillo M *et al*. Expression of membrane-bound mucins (MUC1 and MUC4) and secreted mucins (MUC2, MUC5AC, MUC5B, MUC6 and MUC7) in mucoepidermoid carcinomas of salivary glands. *Am J Surg Pathol* 2005; **29**: 806–813.

9. Behboudi A, Enlund F, Winnes M *et al*. Molecular classification of mucoepidermoid carcinomas – prognostic significance of the MECT1–MAML 'fusion oncogene'. *Genes Chromosomes Cancer* 2006; **45**: 470–481.

10. Ogawa I, Miyauchi M, Matsuura H *et al*. Pleomorphic adenoma with extensive adenoid cystic carcinoma-like cribriform areas of parotid gland. *Pathol Int* 2003; **53**: 30–34.

11. Skálová A, Simpson RHW, Lehtonen H, Leivo I. Assessment of proliferative activity using the MIB1 antibody helps to distinguish polymorphous low grade adenocarcinoma from adenoid cystic carcinoma of salivary glands. *Pathol Res Pract* 1997; **193**: 695–703.

12. Castle JT, Thompson LDR, Frommelt RA, Wenig BM, Kessler HP. Polymorphous low-grade adenocarcinoma: a clinicopathologic study of 164 cases. *Cancer* 1999; **86**; 207–219.

13. Evans HL, Luna MA. Polymorphous low-grade adenocarcinoma: a study of 40 cases with long-term follow up and evaluation of the importance of papillary areas. *Am J Surg Pathol* 2000; **24**: 1319–1328.

14. Simpson RHW, Reis-Filho JS, Pereira EM, Ribeiro AC, Abdulkadir A. Polymorphous low grade adenocarcinoma of the salivary glands with transformation to high grade carcinoma. *Histopathology* 2002; **41**: 250–259.

15. Wang B, Brandwein MS, Gordon R *et al*. Primary salivary clear cell tumors – a diagnostic approach: a clinicopathologic and immunohistochemical study of 20 patients with clear cell carcinoma, clear cell myoepithelial carcinoma, and epithelial–myoepithelial carcinoma. *Arch Pathol Lab Med* 2002; **126**: 676–685.

16. Di Palma S. Epithelial–myoepithelial carcinoma with co-existing multifocal intercalated duct hyperplasia of the parotid gland. *Histopathology* 1994; **25**: 494–496.

17. Chetty R. Intercalated duct hyperplasia: possible relationship to epithelial–myoepithelial carcinoma and hybrid tumours of salivary gland. *Histopathology* 2000; **37**: 260–263.

18. Fonseca I, Soares J. Epithelial–myoepithelial carcinoma of the salivary glands. A study of 22 cases. *Virchows Archiv A Pathol Anat* 1993; **422**: 389–396.

19. Rezende RB, Drachenberg CB, Kumar D *et al*. Differential diagnosis between monomorphic clear cell adenocarcinoma of salivary glands and renal (clear) cell carcinoma. *Am J Surg Pathol* 1999; **23**: 1532–1538.

20. Skálová A, Stárek I, Vanecek T *et al*. Expression of HER-2/neu gene and protein in salivary duct carcinoma of parotid gland as revealed by fluorescence *in-situ* hybridization and immunohistochemistry. *Histopathology* 2003; **42**: 348–356.

21. Kay PA, Roche PC, Olsen KD, Lewis JE. Salivary duct carcinoma: immunohistochemical

analysis of androgen receptor, prostate markers and HER-2/neu oncoprotein in 40 cases [Abstract]. *Mod Pathol* 2001; **14**: 150A.

22. Fan C-Y, Wang J, Barnes EL. Expression of androgen receptor and prostatic specific markers in salivary duct carcinoma: an immunohistochemical analysis of 13 cases and review of the literature. *Am J Surg Pathol* 2000; **24**: 579–586.

23. Moriki T, Ueta S, Takahashi T, Mitani M, Ichien M. Salivary duct carcinoma: cytologic characteristics and application of androgen receptor immunostaining for diagnosis. *Cancer (Cancer Cytopathol)* 2001; **93**: 344–350.

24. Nagao T, Gaffey TA, Visscher DW *et al.* Invasive micropapillary salivary duct carcinoma: a distinct histologic variant with biologic significance. *Am J Surg Pathol* 2004; **28**: 319–326.

25. Simpson RHW, Prasad A, Lewis JE, Skálová A, David L. Mucin-rich variant of salivary duct carcinoma: a clinicopathological and immunohistochemical study of four cases. *Am J Surg Pathol* 2003; **27**: 1070–1079.

26. Simpson RHW. Salivary duct carcinoma. In: Bedossa P. (ed) *20th European Congress of Pathology: Update in Pathology*, 2005; 240–243.

27. Cheuk W, Miliauskas JR, Chan JKC. Intraductal carcinoma of the oral cavity: a case report and a reappraisal of the concept of pure ductal carcinoma *in situ* in salivary duct carcinoma. *Am J Surg Pathol* 2004; **28**: 266–270.

28. Anderson C, Muller R, Piorkowski R, Knibbs DR, Vignoti P. Intraductal carcinoma of major salivary gland. *Cancer* 1992; **69**: 609–614.

29. Mukunyadzi P, Ai L, Portilla D, Barnes EL, Fan C-Y. Expression of peroxisome proliferators-activated receptor gamma in salivary duct carcinoma: immunohistochemical analysis of 15 cases. *Mod Pathol* 2003; **16**: 1218–1223.

30. Ghannoum JE, Freedman PD. Signet ring cell (mucin-producing) adenocarcinomas of minor salivary gland. *Am J Surg Pathol* 2004; **28**: 89–93.

31. Brandwein-Gensler M, Hille J, Wang BY *et al.* Low-grade salivary duct carcinoma: description of 16 cases. *Am J Surg Pathol* 2004; **28**: 1040–1044.

32. Weinreb I, Perez-Ordonez B. Low-grade cribriform cystadenocarcinoma of salivary gland is a low-grade intraductal carcinoma not a variant of cystadenocarcinoma. [Abstract]. *Mod Pathol* 2006; **19 (Suppl 1)**: 212A.

33. Batsakis JG. Cystadenocarcinoma: a specific diagnosis or just another adenocarcinoma NOS? *Adv Anat Pathol* 1997; **4**: 252–255.

34. Savera AT, Sloman A, Huvos AG, Klimstra DS. Myoepithelial carcinoma of the salivary glands: a clinicopathologic study of 25 patients. *Am J Surg Pathol* 2000; **24**: 761–774.

35. Nagao T, Sugano I, Ishida Y *et al.* Salivary gland malignant myoepithelioma: a clinicopathologic and immunohistochemical study of ten cases. *Cancer* 1998; **83**: 1292–1299.

36. Simpson RHW. Myoepithelial tumours of the salivary glands. *Curr Diagn Pathol* 2002; **8**: 328–337.

37. Di Palma S, Skálová A, Vanecek T *et al.* Non-invasive (intracapsular) carcinoma ex pleomorphic adenoma: recognition of focal carcinoma by HER-2/neu and MIB1 immunohistochemistry. *Histopathology* 2005; **46**: 144–152.

38. Félix A, Rosa-Santos J, Mendoca ME, Torrina F, Soares J. Intracapsular carcinoma ex pleomorphic adenoma: report of a case with unusual metastatic behaviour. *Oral Oncol* 2002; **38**: 107–110.

39. Tortoledo ME, Luna MA, Batsakis JG. Carcinomas ex pleomorphic adenoma and malignant mixed tumors: histomorphologic indexes. *Arch Otolaryngol* 1984; **110**: 172–176.

40. Tse LLY, Finkelstein SD, Siegler RW, Barnes EL. Osteoclast-type giant cell neoplasm of salivary gland. A microdissection-based comparative genotyping assay and literature review. *Am J Surg Pathol* 2004; **28**: 953–961.

Salim M. Anjarwalla Neil A. Shepherd

3

Barrett's oesophagus for the practising histopathologist

Barrett's oesophagus (columnar-lined oesophagus, CLO) is defined as the replacement of the lower oesophageal squamous mucosa by metaplastic glandular mucosa as a result of gastro-oesophageal reflux disease (GORD). Over recent decades, there has been a rapid rise in the incidence of CLO in the UK, as in other Western populations.[1–4] Although increased detection by endoscopy may be partly responsible for this, there is also a true increase in its prevalence. The escalating incidence of CLO is coupled with a marked increase in the incidence of its malignant complication. At one time, in Western populations, squamous cell carcinoma was the predominant type of oesophageal cancer but the ratio has been reversed; there has been an 8-fold increase in adenocarcinoma over the past 30 years.[5] The estimated incidence of oesophageal adenocarcinoma in the UK is in the order of 10 cases per 100,000 population. Overall, oesophageal cancer is now the ninth most common cancer and the fifth most common cause of cancer death in the UK. However, there have been, some believe controversial, claims that the rise in adenocarcinoma has been exaggerated[6] and some evidence has been advanced that cancer is, in fact, a rare cause of death in CLO.[7,8] This 'epidemic' of adenocarcinoma of the oesophagus seems to be confined to Western Europe and North America. Other parts of the world appear to remain relatively unaffected. Even in Japan, which has a much higher rate of oesophageal carcinoma than that in Western countries, adenocarcinoma of the oesophagus accounts only for about 2% of primary oesophageal cancers and it has not been convincingly shown to have increased in the last 30 years despite the trend towards a more Westernised diet.[9]

Salim M. Anjarwalla MB ChB MRCPath
Specialist Registrar in Histopathology, Gloucestershire Royal Hospital, Great Western Road, Gloucester GL1 3NN, UK
E-mail: salim.anjarwalla@glos.nhs.uk

Neil A. Shepherd DM FRCPath (for correspondence)
Consultant Histopathologist and Professor of Gastrointestinal Pathology in the Department of Histopathology, Gloucestershire Royal Hospital, Great Western Road, Gloucester GL1 3NN, UK
E-mail: neil.shepherd@glos.nhs.uk

The rising incidence of CLO in the West can be attributed to the same risk factors as those for GORD (male, middle-age, Caucasian, overweight, alcohol, smoking and family history). One retrospective review has demonstrated dramatically that an overweight male with a long-term history of reflux disease has a greatly increased (up to 180-fold) risk of oesophageal adenocarcinoma compared to a lean subject without a history of reflux disease.[10] The role of acid reflux has long been known, but in the 1990s it became apparent that the reflux of bile and alkali from the duodenum also had an important part to play, particularly with regard to the development of neoplasia.[11] Another factor, believed to be protective against CLO is *Helicobacter pylori* infection of the stomach. The lack of *H. pylori* infection in Western populations is thought to encourage a higher stomach acid level and, therefore, promote the development of CLO if there are other predisposing factors to reflux disease.[12]

Despite all the advances in our understanding of CLO and the factors leading to its development, there remain many unresolved issues. The 'cell of origin', for instance, is not yet known. Candidates include multipotential stem cells at the basal aspect of the squamous mucosa of the oesophagus and the cells lining oesophageal gland ducts.[13] The varying terminology and classification of the condition causes considerable confusion. Owing to the natural variation of up to 2 cm between the oesophagogastric junction and the squamocolumnar junction, the disease was originally diagnosed only when at least 3 cm of columnar-lined epithelium was present in the lower oesophagus. 'Short segment CLO' (SSCLO) was then used to describe those cases in which less than 3 cm of columnar-lined epithelium was present in the lower oesophagus. To make matters more confusing, the term 'ultrashort segment CLO' (USSCLO) was introduced for cases where there was essentially intestinal metaplasia at the cardia. Furthermore, others use this term to mean true CLO that is effectively microscopic and not demonstrable at endoscopy.

Notwithstanding the controversies over the epidemiology of CLO and its adenocarcinoma, pathologists in the UK, North America and Western Europe are in no doubt that they are seeing a massive increase in the number of biopsies of CLO and resections for oesophageal adenocarcinoma. This is despite continuing doubts over their role in the diagnosis of Barrett's oesophagus. Furthermore, the diagnosis of the neoplastic complications of CLO, very much the endeavour of pathologists, is also not without controversy. In this review, we will address some of these issues and discuss the impact on pathology of emerging modern methods of surveillance and treatment.

PATHOLOGY AND DIAGNOSIS OF CLO

Classical or long-segment CLO is essentially an endoscopic diagnosis,[14] with pathological corroboration necessary in some 30% of the cases. There are infrequent cases where pathology may be diagnostic and endoscopy is not, especially when there is stricturing or peptic ulceration. The diagnosis of SSCLO requires more pathological corroboration.[13,15] On the other hand, USSCLO is an entirely pathological diagnosis. As we will discuss later, this is best regarded as a gastric disease rather than part of the spectrum of CLO and

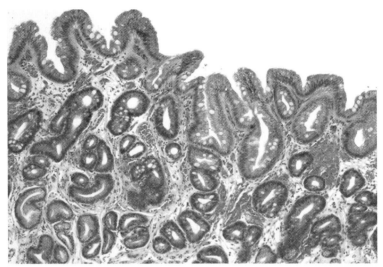

Fig. 1 A 'typical' CLO biopsy. There is a patchwork of cardiac and incomplete intestinal glands.

is better termed 'cardia intestinal metaplasia' (CIM). Thus, the role of the pathologist in the diagnosis of classical and short segment CLO is to corroborate the endoscopic diagnosis. At the current time, we believe that a definitive diagnosis can only be made on the grounds of histopathology alone when glandular metaplasia is seen associated with native oesophageal structures, such as oesophageal gland ducts or submucosal glands, indicating that the glandular metaplasia is unequivocally in the oesophagus.[13,14]

Three main types of epithelium are recognised in CLO – cardiac, fundic and intestinal phenotypes. The intestinal epithelium is usually of the incomplete type although the complete type is occasionally seen.[16] A characteristic histopathological feature of the disease is the presence of a 'patchwork' of these different types (Fig. 1). The intestinal metaplasia (IM) in CLO has been termed 'specialised', implying that it is unique to CLO and differs from that seen in the stomach. Many attempts have been made to confirm or refute this. Basic mucin histochemical stains have proved unhelpful. Various immunohistochemical mucin stains have also been tried, including cdx2,[17] but again none have been convincingly shown to be specific for IM in CLO. Perhaps the most encouraging results have been seen with MUC-1 and MUC-6. One study showed that these markers were 90% specific for goblet cells in CLO compared to those in the stomach, but their use in routine practice is limited by poor sensitivity of the markers.[18]

In recent years, there has been much debate concerning the value of differential cytokeratin immunohistochemistry to distinguish between CLO and gastric IM. Some studies have claimed that a specific pattern of staining can be seen with CLO, namely diffuse staining of the glandular epithelium with cytokeratin 7 and staining of the surface epithelium with cytokeratin 20.[19–21] However, a similar pattern has since been observed in gastric IM, especially immature IM, as well as in biopsies from the gastro-oesophageal junction (GOJ).[22–25] The use of differential cytokeratin staining in practice is further complicated by evidence that staining patterns may differ because of technical variations in the methods and the types of fixative used: observer variation in the interpretation of staining patterns has also been demonstrated.[26–28] At present, we firmly believe that these methodologies cannot be advocated for routinely distinguishing true intestinal-type glandular metaplasia in the oesophagus from that occurring in the stomach, whether at the cardia or elsewhere.

The association of hiatus hernia with CLO presents a potential minefield for both pathologists and endoscopists. The two conditions often co-exist[29] and distinguishing between the two at endoscopy is frequently difficult. Pathologists, on the other hand, know little about the mucosal histological appearances of hiatus hernia, in particular the prevalence of IM. Accurate endoscopic and pathological correlation is, therefore, essential in these cases.[13]

The importance of IM in the neoplastic sequence of CLO cannot be disputed. However, the role of IM demonstration in the diagnosis of the disease is much more controversial.[13] In North America, the histopathological demonstration of IM remains an absolute diagnostic requirement.[30–32] However, North American pathologists accept the argument that the demonstration of IM should not be a *sine qua non* for the diagnosis and the requirement for the demonstration of IM is shortly to be revised there (Odze R.D., personal communication). This is because the demonstration of IM depends critically on the number of biopsies taken.[13] Since, in the UK, the median number of biopsies taken at the diagnostic endoscopy is just three, a requirement for the demonstration of IM would mean that many patients would not be diagnosed with CLO at that time, even with diagnostic endoscopic features.[13] The British Society of Gastroenterology (BSG) guidelines for the management of CLO indicate that the diagnosis should be endoscopic, with pathology only corroborating the diagnosis and with no requirement for the identification of intestinalisation at the initial endoscopy.[14]

It has been suggested that IM in CLO is preceded by the development of an 'intermediate' or 'transitional' type of epithelium. A seemingly unique type of multilayered epithelium (ME) has been demonstrated at the squamocolumnar junction and within the columnar mucosa in patients with CLO (Fig.2).[33] The morphological, ultrastructural and immunohistochemical features of this epithelium are intermediate between those of squamous epithelium and columnar epithelium, suggesting that this may represent a precursor stage in the development of CLO.[33] One study has also shown that ME is strongly associated with reflux-associated carditis, when compared to *H. pylori*-induced carditis.[34] This not only indicates that it may be useful in this, often difficult, differential diagnosis, but lends further support to the theory that ME may be a precursor of CLO. It remains to be proven definitely that ME is specific to reflux-related disease and CLO but tantalising new studies have suggested that, apart from the demonstration of native oesophageal structures and ME, there may be other morphological features which aid the pathologist in the distinction of CLO from cardia IM. These include squamous epithelium overlying crypts with IM and hybrid glands (Fig. 3).[35] The latter are glands with a bimodal composition of intestinal crypts in the superficial portions and cardiac-type glands towards the base. More studies are required to test the specificity of these changes for CLO but it may well be that routine morpho-logical assessment can enhance the pathologist's role in the diagnosis of CLO.

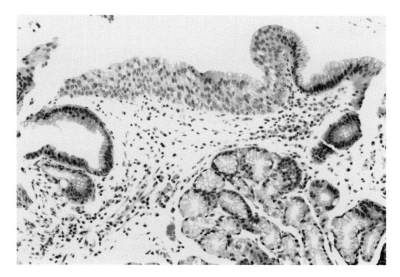

Fig. 2 Multilayered epithelium in CLO. The ME has an appearance very similar to that of immature squamous metaplasia in the endocervix. There are cardiac-type glands below.

A feature commonly seen in intestinalised CLO mucosa, alongside goblet cells, is the presence of non-goblet columnar cells that also stain with Alcian blue. There is some evidence to suggest that these 'blue cells' may be more prevalent than goblet cells[36] and, as such, may be markers of IM. There is also an apparent association with ME, suggesting that they may represent 'early' goblet cells.[37] Whether an intermediate phase of IM exists is debatable, but in any case it will have no bearing on UK pathological opinion: that is, not to rely on the presence of IM for the diagnosis of CLO.

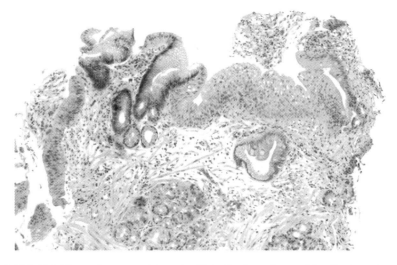

Fig. 3 This CLO biopsy shows a patchwork of intestinal, cardiac and fundic phenotypes. There is a focus of ME on the surface and, below the ME, is a hybrid gland with well-defined and discrete intestinal and cardiac phenotypes.

Table 1 The pathological reporting strategy for CLO (British Society of Gastro-enterology, 2005)[14]

Category	Reporting strategy	Pathological features	Observations
1	Biopsies diagnostic for CLO	Native oesophageal structures with juxta-position to glandular mucosa	–
2	Biopsies corrob-rative of an endo-scopic diagnosis of CLO	Intestinalised metaplastic glandular mucosa with or without non-organised arrangement, villous architecture, patchwork of different glandular types	Could yet repre-sent incomplete IM in the stomach, especially hiatus hernia or USSCLO
3	Biopsies in keeping with, but not specific for, CLO	Gastric type mucosa without intestinal metaplasia, non-organised arrangement, patchwork appearance	Could yet repre-sent the GOJ or the stomach, with or without hiatus hernia
4	Biopsies without evidence of CLO	Oesophageal type squamous epithelium with no evidence of glandular epithelium	–

In summary, the pathological diagnosis of CLO is critically dependent on the endoscopic information provided, especially the site of biopsies and the presence or absence of a hiatus hernia. Adequacy of the size and number of biopsies is also important. To aid the pathologist in the reporting of CLO, the BSG guidelines have introduced four reporting categories (Table 1).[14] This reporting system should prevent unhelpful or misleading pathological reports and provide pathologists with a better understanding of what they can and cannot infer from biopsies of putative CLO.

CYTOLOGY AND CLO

Cytology has no generally accepted role in establishing the diagnosis of CLO.[14] There may be a role in surveillance of patients but this is controversial. Some success has been obtained with balloon abrasion techniques as a non-endoscopic means of surveillance, but they have not gained wide acceptance.[38,39] Cytology has proven useful, in some centres, for the diagnosis of neoplastic complications,[40,41] especially in corroborating a histological diagnosis. The limitations of cytology lie in its inability to distinguish reliably between dysplasia and invasive carcinoma[42] and the difficulty with differentiating low grade dysplasia from inflammatory changes.[43]

SHORT SEGMENT CLO

Short segment CLO is used to describe glandular metaplasia in the lower oesophagus less than 3 cm in length, including non-circumferential metaplasia and tongues of columnar epithelium extending from the squamocolumnar junction. SSCLO is much commoner, affecting 8–17% of the endoscopic population, compared with 1–2% for classical CLO.[5,44] The disease may be more difficult to diagnose endoscopically, due to its smaller size, particularly when there is associated stricturing, ulceration or a hiatus hernia. Hence, corroboration by histology is of more importance than with classical CLO.[14] SSCLO is thought to have significant neoplastic potential, but there is some evidence that the length of the segment is directly proportional to the neoplastic risk. There is also some evidence to suggest that SSCLO is more likely to regress than classical disease.[45] For these reasons, there remains much uncertainty regarding surveillance strategies for SSCLO.[15,46]

ULTRASHORT SEGMENT CLO

Ultrashort segment CLO is controversial. Some use this term to imply true glandular metaplasia in the oesophagus that is scarcely or not visible at endoscopy. Most believe that this term refers to IM in the gastric cardia. It is now believed that such cardia IM is a gastric disease and is better served by the term cardia intestinal metaplasia (CIM). There is considerable evidence that gastric *H. pylori* infection has a role in its development but reflux disease may also possibly play a part.[26] CIM is a common finding in biopsies from the normal GOJ, being present in 16–35% of an endoscopic population (Fig. 4). Since little is known about its significance or neoplastic potential, current guidelines, including those of the BSG, recommend that the normal GOJ should not be biopsied – and CIM not be diagnosed – in routine practice, mainly because we have no idea how to manage the condition once it has been demonstrated.[13,14] This is not to deny the

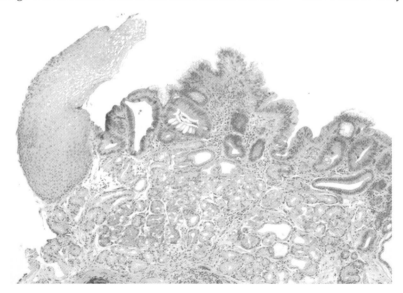

Fig. 4 A biopsy from the endoscopically normal oesophagogastric junction. There is intestinalisation indicating CIM. Some of the intestinal glands, especially those immediately adjacent to the squamocolumnar junction, show dysmaturation: a diagnosis of 'mucosa indefinite for dysplasia' was made. It would seem likely that this CIM may account for many of the junctional cancers that occur without evidence of CLO.

importance of research into a condition likely to have a considerable bearing on the incidence of junctional adenocarcinoma.

PATHOLOGY AND TREATMENT OF CLO

The practising pathologist should be aware of modern trends in the treatment of CLO and the resulting pathological changes encountered, as there is an increasing need for the histological assessment of treatment response. Acid-suppressive therapy is the mainstay of treatment of reflux disease. H2-receptor antagonists can be used to provide symptomatic relief, especially with mild reflux, but their efficacy may decrease over time. Proton pump inhibitors (PPIs) are widely acclaimed as the agents of choice. They are more effective both in providing symptomatic relief and in healing erosive GORD. Consequently, there has been much interest in their potential role in inducing regression of CLO. The evidence so far is conflicting. Partial regression can certainly occur, and one double-blind, controlled trial convincingly demonstrated a decrease in both the length and the area of the Barrett's segment.[47] Several other studies, however, have shown no regression.[48]

Surgical correction of reflux, typically performed laparoscopically and usually using Nissen fundoplication, is aimed at improving the competency of the gastro-oesophageal junction through plication of the gastric fundus. The success of acid-suppressive therapy in the management of GORD has lessened the need for surgical intervention.[49] However, studies have indicated that anti-reflux surgery is an effective approach, with overall outcomes equal to and possibly superior to those achieved with medication.[50] There has been increasing interest in various methods of ablation of CLO, being especially suitable for patients unfit for major surgery. Techniques include laser,

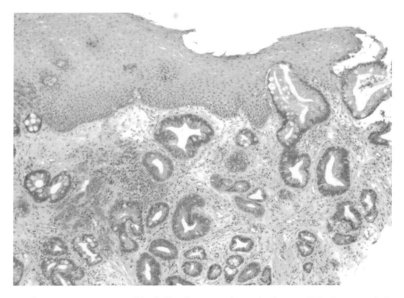

Fig. 5 Surface squamous re-epithelialisation over intestinal-type CLO. Because it is not possible to assess surface maturation, the appearance of the intestinal-type crypts may trap the unwary into making a diagnosis of dysplasia.

photodynamic therapy (PDT), and argon beam plasma coagulation (ABC). PDT and ABC have gained some popularity over recent years. A recent, randomised, prospective trial comparing the two methods showed that they are equally effective in eradicating Barrett's mucosa, although PDT appears to be more effective in eradicating dysplasia.[51]

The pathological response to ablation therapy can be dramatic, with extensive necrosis and florid reactive changes that may be difficult to distinguish from residual dysplasia. The characteristic, and most important, response to treatment is squamous re-epithelialisation of the Barrett's segment (Fig. 5). This can occur both as endoscopically visible squamous islands as well as microscopic foci.[48] Such squamous re-epithelialisation can occur following treatment with PPIs alone, or in combination with anti-reflux surgery, laser ablation and PDT.[52] It seems, therefore, that acid-suppressing therapy is necessary for squamous re-epithelialisation to occur. The squamous regeneration shows three differing patterns. The first is encroachment of adjacent squamous epithelium at the squamocolumnar junction. The second pattern, seen particularly following long-term PPI treatment,[48] is extension of squamous epithelium from the superficial portion of the submucosal gland duct, leading to defined squamous islands. Finally, squamous metaplasia of the Barrett's columnar mucosa itself has been recognised, following laser therapy and PDT, and provides evidence of the existence of multipotential stem cells within Barrett's mucosa.[48]

A potentially problematic pathological finding is the demonstration of residual CLO glands lying 'hidden' beneath the neosquamous epithelium. Such glandular epithelium may tempt the pathologist into an erroneous diagnosis of dysplasia as the cells of the crypts of intestinalised epithelium appear hyperchromatic and maturation to the surface cannot be seen because

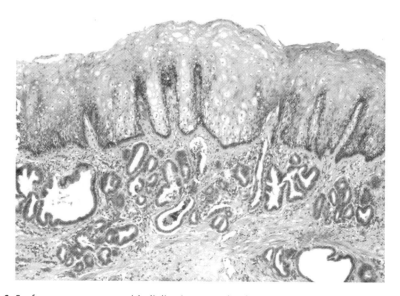

Fig. 6 Surface squamous re-epithelialisation over dysplastic CLO in a patient known to have HGD, treated with PDT. Such changes should not be interpreted as representing adenocarcinoma beneath native squamous mucosa of the oesophagus.

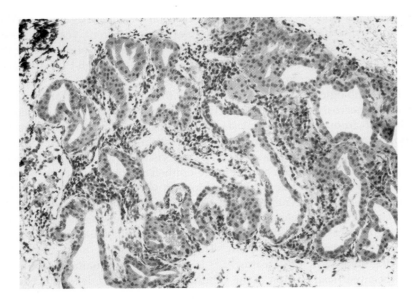

Fig. 7 Apocrine change in an oesophageal submucosal gland in CLO patient treated with PDT. This is a distinctive response of this native oesophageal structure to such ablative therapy.

of the overlying squamous mucosa. When such glands are truly dysplastic, the unwary pathologist may be tempted to interpret this as adenocarcinoma infiltrating beneath native squamous epithelium (Fig. 6). Whether dysplastic or not, there is obvious concern regarding the neoplastic potential of the residual glands, emphasising the need for histological assessment of endoscopically suspected squamous re-epithelialisation with deep biopsies. Some re-assurance can be gained from the fact that squamous metaplasia of these buried glands too has been demonstrated, particularly following PDT. Complete squamous re-epithelialisation of the Barrett's segment, and a plausible reduction in neoplastic potential, is therefore a distinct possibility after ablation therapy.[52,53]

Increasingly, pathologists recognise seemingly unique changes caused by the effects of treatment, especially ablation therapy. We have seen occasional cases where the entire oesophageal gland duct has become lined by squamous epithelium and, very rarely, when the submucosal gland has also undergone complete squamous metaplasia. One increasingly recognised feature of ablation therapy, especially PDT, is focal apocrine change in the submucosal gland (Fig. 7).

PATHOLOGY AND NEOPLASIA IN CLO

There is now general consensus that dysplasia in CLO should be categorised according to a Riddell-type classification originally introduced for dysplasia in ulcerative colitis (Table 2).[54,55] Such a classification has been recommended for use in CLO for 15 years and more. Even so, one of us (NAS) still observes pathologists regularly using the mild, moderate and severe dysplasia

Table 2 The recommended neoplasia classification of CLO in Western countries (after Riddell *et al.* 1983)[55]

•   Negative for dysplasia
•   Indefinite for dysplasia
•   Low-grade dysplasia
•   High-grade dysplasia
•   Intramucosal carcinoma
•   Invasive adenocarcinoma

classification. As there are well-established guidelines for the management of indefinite for dysplasia, low grade dysplasia and high grade dysplasia,[54] there can be no excuse for using older, outmoded and unacceptable classifications.

A major problem for pathologists is the lack of definitive criteria for the diagnosis of dysplasia and even more so for the separation of the various categories. The cytological features of dysplasia have been well described: nuclear enlargement, nuclear pleomorphism, nuclear hyperchromasia, prominent nucleoli, nuclear stratification, increased mitotic activity and atypical mitotic figures are all commonly cited. Although these changes are important, architectural changes are usually more useful. We believe that a lack of maturation toward the surface is the single most useful criterion for the diagnosis of dysplasia. Villous configuration is also frequently associated with dysplasia, although it is not entirely specific.

Strict criteria cannot be defined for the distinction of low grade dysplasia from high grade dysplasia. Tables 3 and 4 give practical guides to aid in this differentiation. However, there is variation even amongst experts and low

Table 3 Useful pathological criteria for the diagnosis of low grade and high grade dysplasia in Barrett's oesophagus[13]

Low grade
- Cytology approximates to that of mild and moderate adenomatous dysplasia
- Nuclei are enlarged, crowded, hyperchromatic and ovoid (Fig. 9)
- Mitotic activity may be substantial and atypical mitoses may be present
- Stratification is often present
- Architectural change, including villosity, may be present but in the appropriate cytological setting
- There is loss of the basal-luminal maturation/differentiation axis

High-grade
- Cytology approximates to that of severe adenomatous dysplasia
- Nuclei are enlarged, usually spheroidal, and have an open chromatin pattern with nucleoli (Fig. 10)
- Mitotic activity may be substantial and atypical mitoses are usually present
- Stratification may be present but there is usually pronounced cellular disorganisation
- Architectural change, including villosity, glandular budding and complex glandular structures, is often present
- There is loss of the basal-luminal maturation/differentiation axis

Table 4 Cytological and architectural features of low- and high grade dysplasia in CLO (Odze, 2006)[56]

Feature	Low-grade	High-grade
Cytology		
Increased N/C ratio	+	++
Loss of cell polarity	−	+
Mitosis	+	++
Atypical mitosis	±	+
Full-thickness nuclear stratification	−	+
Decreased goblet cells (± dystrophic)	+	++
Hyperchromasia	+	++
Multiple nucleoli	±	±
Large irregular (prominent) nucleoli	−	±
Irregular nuclear contour	+	++
Nuclear pleomorphism	−	+
Architecture		
Villiform change	−	±
Crypt budding/branching	±	++
Crowded (back-to-back) crypts	±	++
Irregular crypt shapes	±	+
Intraluminal papilla/ridges	−	±
Lamina propria between glands	+	±

N/C, nuclear/cytoplasmic ratio; −, absent; ±, may be present; +, usually present.

grade dysplasia and the indefinite category tend to be associated with poorer levels of interobserver agreement. The distinction between dysplasia and carcinoma is also not clear cut and there are differences in opinion between Eastern and Western pathologists. In Japan, in particular, emphasis is placed on cytological changes rather than the architecture and definitive invasion through the basement membrane is not a requirement to diagnose carcinoma. These differences have prompted the introduction of the Vienna system of classification of dysplasia in CLO (Table 5).[57] Currently used in most Far Eastern and some European countries, it differs from the IBD-based system in that the term 'non-invasive neoplasia' is used in place of 'low grade' or 'high

Table 5 The Vienna classification for gastrointestinal neoplasia (after Schlemper *et al.* 2000)[57]

Category 1	Negative for neoplasia/dysplasia
Category 2	Indefinite for neoplasia/dysplasia
Category 3	Non-invasive low grade neoplasia (low grade adenoma/dysplasia)
Category 4	Non-invasive high grade neoplasia
	4.1 High-grade adenoma/dysplasia
	4.2 Non-invasive carcinoma (carcinoma *in situ*)
	4.3 Suspicion of invasive carcinoma
Category 5	Invasive neoplasia
	5.1 Intramucosal carcinoma
	5.2 Submucosal carcinoma or beyond

Table 6 Common causes for error in the pathological diagnosis of dysplasia in CLO

Inflammation and regenerative change
- Expansion of proliferative compartment
- Hyperproliferation
- Nuclear activity
- Villous/papillary architecture

Polymorphism of cell types
- Differences in position of proliferative compartments in different CLO epithelial types
- Morphological changes in mucin
- Juxtaposition of intestinal mucosa to other blander-appearing cell types

Artefact
- Biopsy technique, especially crush artefact (Fig. 8)
- Tangential sectioning
- Staining variation

Squamous re-epithelialisation
- Overlying squamous mucosa obscures evidence of maturation
- Only prominent intestinal crypt bases seen

grade' dysplasia and an additional subcategory of 'suspicious for invasive carcinoma' has been included.[57]

The category 'indefinite for dysplasia' should be used, and pathologists are encouraged to do so, when it is not possible to exclude dysplasia confidently (Figs 4 and 8).[54] It should be understood that there are many situations, especially those highlighted in Table 6, in which a definitive diagnosis of dysplasia cannot and

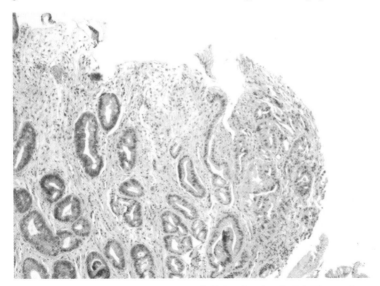

Fig. 8 A CLO biopsy reported as 'mucosa indefinite for dysplasia'. The patient was known to have dysplasia. Crush artefact of these crowded and somewhat concerning glands renders a definitive diagnosis of dysplasia unwise.

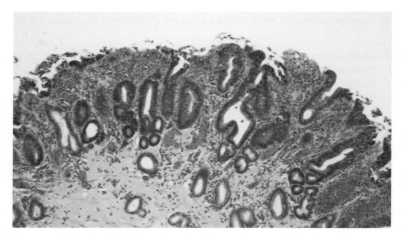

Fig. 9 Low-grade dysplasia in CLO. There is failure of maturation toward the surface and the dysplastic glands show diffuse abnormality with oval, hyperchromatic and stratified nuclei.

should not be made and yet it is important to identify the concern for dysplasia to the clinician. Failure to recognise the pathologist's limitations in many of these situations can lead to the dangerous overcalling of dysplasia. One of the commonest of these occurs because of the 'patchwork' of the different CLO phenotypes. The intestinal mucosa in CLO has a prominent proliferative zone showing nuclear enlargement and mitotic activity. This can give worrying appearances when seen juxtaposed to relatively bland-appearing cardia-type mucosa. Tangential sectioning can make this assessment even more difficult.

What then are the features that can help one distinguish between true dysplasia and reactive changes? Epithelial changes due to inflammation are usually most prominent in the inflamed foci, and there is a gradual reduction

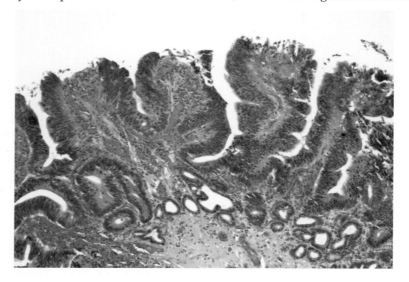

Fig. 10 High-grade dysplasia in CLO. There is a villous architecture with pronounced cytological abnormality. Nuclear stratification is especially prominent.

in the degree of cytological change towards the non-inflamed areas. In contrast, abrupt transition between normal and abnormal epithelium favours true dysplasia. The most useful feature, and one that argues strongly against dysplasia, is the presence of surface maturation. However, the findings of a recent study challenge this long-held theory.[58] 'Basal crypt dysplasia-like atypia' (BCDA), with surface maturation in a group of patients with long-standing CLO, has been proposed as representing a rare sub-type of true dysplasia. The assessment of surface maturation can also not be applied to post-treatment specimens where there is squamous re-epithelialisation of the surface. In all such difficult cases, the category 'indefinite for dysplasia' is entirely appropriate.

The poorer interobserver reproducibility of 'indefinite for dysplasia' and low grade dysplasia is well documented.[59] The interobserver agreement for high grade dysplasia is much better[59] and this is important because many of these cases will have co-existent adenocarcinoma, especially if ulceration is present.[59] The pathologist should be aware of the implications of the various diagnostic categories for management. 'Indefinite for dysplasia' is managed by early repeat endoscopy and multiple biopsies, often after treatment of inflammation with a course of PPI therapy.[54] The management of low grade dysplasia is similar, with close (6-monthly) endoscopic surveillance as long as the disease remains stable.[54] In Europe and North America, high grade dysplasia remains an indication for oesophagectomy, an operation that carries very significant morbidity and mortality risks, because of the strong association between biopsy-diagnosed high grade dysplasia and (presumed contemporaneous) adenocarcinoma.[53,54,60] Endoscopic ablation or mucosal resection are indicated for cases of low- and high grade dysplasia in patients unfit for surgery. Because of the implications of a diagnosis of high grade dysplasia, management guidelines recommend that such a diagnosis is confirmed by a second, preferably expert, specialist gastrointestinal pathologist.[61]

Comprehensive sampling of the Barrett's segment is of paramount importance. The established Seattle biopsy protocol employs quadrantic and segmental (every 2 cm) biopsies of the Barrett's segment, preferably using Jumbo-type biopsy forceps, in addition to sampling of any visible lesion.[62] This is because endoscopic appearances do not correlate well with the histological diagnosis of dysplasia. High-grade dysplasia, and even adenocarcinoma, has been detected in biopsies from macroscopically unremarkable, or minimally affected, Barrett's areas.[63] Dysplasia can also be multifocal and extensive. Current imaging techniques, such as endoluminal ultrasound, are poor at detecting early malignancy in CLO and, therefore, histological evaluation remains the principal means of assessing dysplasia.

MOLECULAR MARKERS OF NEOPLASIA

In view of the difficulties encountered in the management of CLO, it is not surprising that there has been much interest in the search for molecular markers to aid in the diagnosis and grading of dysplasia. Immuno-histochemical detection of p53 protein overexpression and of proliferation markers such as Ki-67 has been extensively assessed.[64,65] Whilst there is no doubt that expression of these markers correlates with increasing grade of dysplasia, it is uncertain whether they add any real diagnostic value in practice. One potential hope for the future is the antibody α-methylacyl-CoA racemase (AMACR). This has been shown to be useful in distinguishing between reactive and dysplastic epithelium.[66] Even so, all such 'biomarkers' are still regarded as experimental currently and their routine use, outside the research setting, cannot yet be recommended.

SURVEILLANCE

Surveillance of CLO is now recommended if the patient wishes it and if they are fit for the treatment that the diagnosis of dysplasia and malignancy implies. Some have suggested that surveillance should be concentrated in those with particular risk factors, such as long-segment disease, associated ulceration and stricturing and previously diagnosed dysplasia. Pathologists are increasingly seeing a large number of such surveillance biopsies and these are likely to increase and comprise a high proportion of the gastrointestinal workload in histopathology departments. It is of critical importance that pathologists do not overcall dysplasia and are aware of the management implications of their diagnoses. Furthermore, we believe that all diagnoses of CLO dysplasia demand full discussion in a multidisciplinary team meeting as the treatment options are so varied. We also agree with the recommendation that all such diagnoses should be double reported.

In recent years, advanced endoscopic techniques have been applied to CLO surveillance, including magnification endoscopy, high-resolution endoscopy and chromoscopy.[67] Whilst these methods offer advantages over standard endoscopy in terms of visualisation of early neoplastic lesions, they ultimately rely on the pathological demonstration of dysplasia on biopsy – the current 'gold standard'.[67] There is, therefore, much interest in the development of techniques which allow the accurate *in situ* detection of dysplasia. This involves the combination of endoscopy with microscopic tools, such as confocal microscopy, molecular tools, such as fluorescence *in situ* hybridisation (FISH) and spectroscopic analytical techniques. In our view, Raman spectroscopy offers some hope for the development of such a 'smart endoscope'. This technique is based on the detection of inelastically scattered light from molecules and can be used to map out a specific molecular fingerprint. The major advantages are that it is non-invasive, can be used for real-time analysis and is compatible with current endoscope technology. Our recent study showed rates of sensitivity and specificity for neoplastic change in CLO well above 90% and overall Raman achieved a better performance than an independent pathologist.[68]

CONCLUSIONS

Although pathologists have a role in the diagnosis of CLO, it is important that they understand the limitations of histopathology and that they are critically reliant on clinical and endoscopic correlation to make an accurate histological assessment. We commend to all pathologists the four-category reporting strategy of the British Society of Gastroenterology, especially when insufficient clinical and endoscopic information is provided or biopsy sampling is suboptimal.

Intestinal metaplasia is certainly important in the neoplastic progression of CLO but its demonstration is dependent on the number of biopsies taken. For this reason, UK pathological consensus is that it should not be used as a defining factor and that its demonstration is not essential for the diagnosis of CLO.

There has been considerable effort in the attempts to demonstrate a phenotype specific for CLO. The efficacy of cytokeratin subset immuno-histochemistry is highly controversial in this regard. On the other hand, newer data suggest that morphological features, such as native oesophageal structures, multilayered epithelium and hybrid glands, may be very helpful to the pathologist in the attempt to make a definitive diagnosis of CLO. The need for the pathological assessment of response to treatment, especially ablation therapy, is increasing. The principal change is that of squamous re-epithelialisation, although residual glands remain buried underneath in many cases, causing pathological diagnostic difficulties and considerable concern for its neoplastic potential.

The diagnosis and management of short segment CLO and so-called ultrashort segment CLO (cardia intestinal metaplasia, CIM) remain problematic. The recommendation is that the normal oesophagogastric junction should not be biopsied as, in about one-third of all endoscopies, in the UK at least, CIM will be seen and little is known about the significance or neoplastic potential of this condition.

Pathology is central to the diagnosis of dysplasia but the difficulties faced are exemplified by poor interobserver agreement, particularly for the indefinite category and low grade dysplasia. The search for molecular markers to aid in the diagnosis of dysplasia continues but none has been shown to be useful in the routine clinical setting so far. There is also considerable interest in the development of a 'smart endoscope', which would allow the *in situ* detection of dysplasia and early cancer. Surveillance for Barrett's oesophagus is now widely undertaken in Europe and North America and is recommended in the UK BSG management guidelines. However, it is likely that such surveillance will have little effect on the alarming increase in adenocarcinoma of the oesophagus. This is because the great majority of patients still present clinically not with Barrett's oesophagus, but with the adenocarcinoma that complicates it.[69,70]

Points for best practice

- Barrett's oesophagus, generally, is an endoscopic diagnosis corroborated by histology.

- There are characteristic histopathological features of Barrett's oesophagus including the 'patchwork' of cardiac, fundic and intestinal epithelial types, hybrid glands, multilayered epithelium and the association with native oesophageal structures.

- The importance of the role of intestinal metaplasia in the neoplastic sequence of Barrett's oesophagus is undeniable. However, the importance of observing intestinal metaplasia in biopsies for the diagnosis of the disease is much more controversial.

(continued on next page)

Points for best practice *(continued)*

- Treatment of Barrett's oesophagus by acid-suppressing drugs and ablative therapy causes squamous re-epithelialisation and this may cause confounding biopsy appearances.

- Pathologists must now use the low- and high grade categories for reporting definitive dysplasia in Barrett's oesophagus. There are well-established management guidelines for these categories; there are none for the former mild, moderate and severe categorisation.

- Pathologists are encouraged to use the category 'indefinite for dysplasia' when the pathological features are equivocal, either due to inflammation or because of other confounding features.

- Endoscopic appearances do not correlate well with the histological diagnosis of dysplasia, emphasising the need for comprehensive sampling of the Barrett's segment.

- The literature would suggest that 25–50% of high grade dysplasia cases have co-existent adenocarcinoma.

- Management guidelines recommend that a diagnosis of high grade dysplasia is confirmed by a second, preferably expert, specialist gastrointestinal pathologist.

References

1. Wild CP, Hardie LJ. Reflux, Barrett's oesophagus and adenocarcinoma: burning questions. *Nat Rev Cancer* 2003; **3**: 676–684.
2. van Soest EM, Dieleman JP, Siersema PD, Sturkenboom MC, Kuipers EJ. Increasing incidence of Barrett's oesophagus in the general population. *Gut* 2005; **54**: 1062–1066.
3. Shaheen NJ. Advances in Barrett's esophagus and esophageal adenocarcinoma. *Gastroenterology* 2005; **128**: 1554–1566.
4. Prach AT, MacDonald TA, Hopwood DA, Johnston DA. Increasing incidence of Barrett's oesophagus: education, enthusiasm, or epidemiology? *Lancet* 1997; **350**: 933.
5. Watson A. Barrett's oesophagus – 50 years on. *Br J Surg* 2000; **87**: 529–531.
6. Shaheen NJ, Crosby MA, Bozymski EM, Sandler RS. Is there publication bias in the reporting of cancer risk in Barrett's esophagus? *Gastroenterology* 2000; **119**: 333–338.
7. Hage M, Siersema PD, van Dekken H *et al*. Oesophageal cancer incidence and mortality in patients with long-segment Barrett's oesophagus after a mean follow-up of 12.7 years. *Scand J Gastroenterol* 2004; **39**: 1175–1179.
8. van der Burgh A, Dees J, Hop WC, van Blankenstein M. Oesophageal cancer is an uncommon cause of death in patients with Barrett's oesophagus. *Gut* 1996; **39**: 5–8.
9. Tachimori Y. Clinical strategies for adenocarcinoma of the esophagus at the National Cancer Centre, Japan. In: Imamura M. (ed) *Superficial Esophageal Neoplasm: Pathology, Diagnosis and Therapy*. Tokyo: Springer, 2002; 66–74.
10. Lagergren J, Bergstrom R, Lindgren A, Nyren O. Symptomatic gastroesophageal reflux as a risk factor for esophageal adenocarcinoma. *N Engl J Med* 1999; **340**: 825–831.
11. Owen WJ, Warren BF. Pathogenesis and pathophysiology of columnar-lined oesophagus. In: Watson A, Heading RC, Shepherd NA. (eds) *Guidelines for the diagnosis and management of Barrett's columnar-lined oesophagus*. London: British Society of Gastroenterology, 2005.
12. Blaser MJ. *Helicobacter pylori* and gastric diseases. *BMJ* 1998; **316**: 1507–1510.

13. Coad RA, Shepherd NA. Barrett's oesophagus: definition, diagnosis and pathogenesis. *Curr Diagn Pathol* 2003; **9**: 218–227.

14. Hellier MD, Shepherd NA. Diagnosis of columnar-lined oesophagus. In: Watson A, Heading RC, Shepherd NA. (eds) *Guidelines for the diagnosis and management of Barrett's columnar-lined oesophagus*. London: British Society of Gastroenterology, 2005.

15. Sampliner RE, Sharma P. Short-segment Barrett's esophagus. *J Clin Gastroenterol* 1998; **26**: 357–358.

16. Jass JR. Histopathology of early neoplasia in Barrett's esophagus. In: Imamura M. (ed) *Superficial Esophageal Neoplasm: Pathology, Diagnosis and Therapy*. Tokyo: Springer, 2002; 13–21.

17. Phillips RW, Frierson Jr HF, Moskaluk CA. Cdx2 as a marker of epithelial intestinal differentiation in the esophagus. *Am J Surg Pathol* 2003; **27**: 1442–1447.

18. Glickman JN, Shahsafaei A, Odze RD. Mucin core peptide expression can help differentiate Barrett's esophagus from intestinal metaplasia of the stomach. *Am J Surg Pathol* 2003; **27**: 1357–1365.

19. Ormsby AH, Goldblum JR, Rice TW *et al*. Cytokeratin subsets can reliably distinguish Barrett's esophagus from intestinal metaplasia of the stomach. *Hum Pathol* 1999; **30**: 288–294.

20. Ormsby AH, Vaezi MF, Richter JE *et al*. Cytokeratin immunoreactivity patterns in the diagnosis of short-segment Barrett's esophagus. *Gastroenterology* 2000; **119**: 683–690.

21. Couvelard A, Cauvin JM, Goldfain D *et al*. Cytokeratin immunoreactivity of intestinal metaplasia at normal oesophagogastric junction indicates its aetiology. *Gut* 2001; **49**: 761–766.

22. El-Zimaity HM, Graham DY. Cytokeratin subsets for distinguishing Barrett's esophagus from intestinal metaplasia in the cardia using endoscopic biopsy specimens. *Am J Gastroenterol* 2001; **96**: 1378–1382.

23. Glickman JN, Wang H, Das KM *et al*. Phenotype of Barrett's esophagus and intestinal metaplasia of the distal esophagus and gastroesophageal junction: an immunohisto-chemical study of cytokeratins 7 and 20, Das-1 and 45 MI. *Am J Surg Pathol* 2001; **25**: 87–94.

24. DeMeester SR, Wickramasinghe KS, Lord RV *et al*. Cytokeratin and DAS-1 immunostaining reveal similarities among cardiac mucosa, CIM, and Barrett's esophagus. *Am J Gastroenterol* 2002; **97**: 2514–2523.

25. Mohammed IA, Streutker CJ, Riddell RH. Utilization of cytokeratins 7 and 20 does not differentiate between Barrett's esophagus and gastric cardiac intestinal metaplasia. *Mod Pathol* 2002; **15**: 611–616.

26. Goldblum JR. Ultra-short segment Barrett's oesophagus, carditis and intestinal metaplasia at the oesophago-gastric junction: pathology, causation and implications. *Curr Diagn Pathol* 2003; **9**: 228–234.

27. Odze R. Cytokeratin 7/20 immunostaining: Barrett's oesophagus or gastric intestinal metaplasia? *Lancet* 2002; **359**: 1711–1713.

28. Glickman JN, Ormsby AH, Gramlich TL, Goldblum JR, Odze RD. Interinstitutional variability and effect of tissue fixative on the interpretation of a Barrett cytokeratin 7/20 immunoreactivity pattern in Barrett esophagus. *Hum Pathol* 2005; **36**: 58–65.

29. Cameron AJ. Barrett's esophagus: prevalence and size of hiatal hernia. *Am J Gastroenterol* 1999; **94**: 2054–2059.

30. Rice TW, Mendelin JE, Goldblum JR. Barrett's esophagus: pathologic considerations and implications for treatment. *Semin Thorac Cardiovasc Surg* 2005; **17**: 292–300.

31. Spechler SJ. Barrett's esophagus. *Semin Gastrointest Dis* 1996; **7**: 51–60.

32. Riddell RH. The biopsy diagnosis of gastroesophageal reflux disease, 'carditis', and Barrett's esophagus, and sequelae of therapy. *Am J Surg Pathol* 1996; **20 (Suppl 1)**: S31–S50.

33. Glickman JN, Chen YY, Wang HH, Antonioli DA, Odze RD. Phenotypic characteristics of a distinctive multilayered epithelium suggests that it is a precursor in the development of Barrett's esophagus. *Am J Surg Pathol* 2001; **25**: 569–578.

34. Wieczorek TJ, Wang HH, Antonioli DA, Glickman JN, Odze RD. Pathologic features of reflux and *Helicobacter pylori*-associated carditis: a comparative study. *Am J Surg Pathol* 2003; **27**: 960–968.

35. Srivastava A, Glickman JN, Odze RD. Morphological parameters are useful in distinguishing Barrett's esophagus from carditis with intestinal metaplasia. *Mod Pathol* 2005; **18 (Suppl 1)**: 119A.

36. Offner FA, Lewin KJ, Weinstein WM. Metaplastic columnar cells in Barrett's esophagus: a common and neglected cell type. *Hum Pathol* 1996; **27**: 885–889.

37. Chen YY, Wang HH, Antonioli DA *et al.* Significance of acid-mucin-positive non-goblet columnar cells in the distal esophagus and gastroesophageal junction. *Hum Pathol* 1999; **30**: 1488–1495.

38. Falk GW, Chittajallu R, Goldblum JR *et al.* Surveillance of patients with Barrett's esophagus for dysplasia and cancer with balloon cytology. *Gastroenterology* 1997; **112**: 1787–1797.

39. Fennerty MB, Ditomasso J, Morales TG *et al.* Screening for Barrett's esophagus by balloon cytology. *Am J Gastroenterol* 1995; **90**: 1230–1232.

40. Wang HH, Doria Jr MI, Purohit-Buch S *et al.* Barrett's esophagus. The cytology of dysplasia in comparison to benign and malignant lesions. *Acta Cytol* 1992; **36**: 60–64.

41. Saad RS, Mahood LK, Clary KM *et al.* Role of cytology in the diagnosis of Barrett's esophagus and associated neoplasia. *Diagn Cytopathol* 2003; **29**: 130–135.

42. Hardwick RH, Morgan RJ, Warren BF, Lott M, Alderson D. Brush cytology in the diagnosis of neoplasia in Barrett's esophagus. *Dis Esophagus* 1997; **10**: 233–237.

43. Falk GW. Cytology in Barrett's esophagus. *Gastrointest Endosc Clin North Am* 2003; **13**: 335–348.

44. Spechler SJ. The columnar-lined esophagus. History, terminology, and clinical issues. *Gastroenterol Clin North Am* 1997; **26**: 455–466.

45. Weston AP, Badr AS, Hassanein RS. Prospective multivariate analysis of factors predictive of complete regression of Barrett's esophagus. *Am J Gastroenterol* 1999; **94**: 3420–3426.

46. Richter JE. Short segment Barrett's esophagus: ignorance may be bliss. *Am J Gastroenterol* 2006; **101**: 1183–1185.

47. Peters FT, Ganesh S, Kuipers EJ *et al.* Endoscopic regression of Barrett's oesophagus during omeprazole treatment; a randomised double blind study. *Gut* 1999; **45**: 489–494.

48. Shepherd NA. Barrett's oesophagus and proton pump inhibitors: a pathological perspective. *Gut* 2000; **46**: 147–149.

49. Scarpignato C, Pelosini I, Di Mario F. Acid suppression therapy: where do we go from here? *Dig Dis* 2006; **24**: 11–46.

50. Moayyedi P, Talley NJ. Gastro-oesophageal reflux disease. *Lancet* 2006; **367**: 2086–2100.

51. Ragunath K, Krasner N, Raman VS *et al.* Endoscopic ablation of dysplastic Barrett's oesophagus comparing argon plasma coagulation and photodynamic therapy: a randomized prospective trial assessing efficacy and cost-effectiveness. *Scand J Gastroenterol* 2005; **40**: 750–758.

52. Biddlestone LR, Barham CP, Wilkinson SP, Barr H, Shepherd NA. The histopathology of treated Barrett's esophagus: squamous re-epithelialization after acid suppression and laser and photodynamic therapy. *Am J Surg Pathol* 1998; **22**: 239–245.

53. Barr H. The pathological implications of surveillance, treatment and surgery for Barrett's oesophagus. *Curr Diagn Pathol* 2003; **9**: 242–251.

54. Barr H, Shepherd NA. The management of dysplasia. In: Watson A, Heading RC, Shepherd NA. (eds) *Guidelines for the diagnosis and management of Barrett's columnar-lined oesophagus*. London: British Society of Gastroenterology, 2005.

55. Riddell RH, Goldman H, Ransohoff DF *et al.* Dysplasia in inflammatory bowel disease: standardized classification with provisional clinical applications. *Hum Pathol* 1983; **14**: 931–968.

56. Odze RD. Diagnosis and grading of dysplasia in Barrett's oesophagus. *J Clin Pathol* 2006; **59**: 1029–1038.

57. Schlemper RJ, Riddell RH, Kato Y *et al.* The Vienna classification of gastrointestinal epithelial neoplasia. *Gut* 2000; **47**: 251–255.

58. Lomo LC, Blount PL, Sanchez CA *et al.* Crypt dysplasia with surface maturation: a clinical, pathologic and molecular study of a Barrett's esophagus cohort. *Am J Surg Pathol* 2006; **30**: 423–435.

59. Montgomery E, Bronner MP, Goldblum JR *et al.* Reproducibility of the diagnosis of

dysplasia in Barrett esophagus: a reaffirmation. *Hum Pathol* 2001; **32**: 368–378.

60. Sampliner RE. Updated guidelines for the diagnosis, surveillance, and therapy of Barrett's esophagus. *Am J Gastroenterol* 2002; **97**: 1888–1895.

61. Loft DE, Alderson D, Heading RC. Screening and surveillance in columnar-lined oesophagus. In: Watson A, Heading RC, Shepherd NA. (eds) *Guidelines for the diagnosis and management of Barrett's columnar-lined oesophagus*. London: British Society of Gastroenterology, 2005.

62. Levine DS, Haggitt RC, Blount PL *et al.* An endoscopic biopsy protocol can differentiate high-grade dysplasia from early adenocarcinoma in Barrett's esophagus. *Gastroenterology* 1993; **105**: 40–50.

63. Levine DS. Management of dysplasia in the columnar-lined esophagus. *Gastroenterol Clin North Am* 1997; **26**: 613–634.

64. Reid BJ, Blount PL, Rabinovitch PS. Biomarkers in Barrett's esophagus. *Gastrointest Endosc Clin N Am* 2003; **13**: 369–397.

65. Hong MK, Laskin WB, Herman BE *et al.* Expansion of the Ki-67 proliferative compartment correlates with degree of dysplasia in Barrett's esophagus. *Cancer* 1995; **75**: 423–429.

66. Dorer R, Odze RD. AMACR immunostaining is useful in detecting dysplastic epithelium in Barrett's esophagus, ulcerative colitis and Crohn's disease. *Am J Surg Pathol* 2006; **30**: 871–7.

67. van Dam J. Novel methods of enhanced endoscopic imaging. *Gut* 2003; **52 (Suppl 4)**: iv12–iv16.

68. Kendall C, Stone N, Shepherd NA *et al.* Raman spectroscopy, a potential tool for the objective identification and classification of neoplasia in Barrett's oesophagus. *J Pathol* 2003; **200**: 602–609.

69. Brown CM, Jones R, Shirazi T, Codling BW, Valori RM. Prior diagnosis of Barrett's oesophagus is rare in patients with oesophageal carcinoma. *Gut* 1996; **38**: A23.

70. Cameron AJ. Epidemiology of Barrett's esophagus and adenocarcinoma. *Dis Esophagus* 2002; **15**: 106–108.

Fred T. Bosman

4

Cancer invasion and metastasis: the concept of epithelial–mesenchymal transition

Invasion and metastasis constitute important hallmarks of malignant neoplasia. It is in most cases not the primary tumour that makes the outlook of malignant disease so bleak for the patient; metastases are what eventually kills. In the last decade, intense research efforts have focused on the mechanisms involved in these processes. It has become clear that in order to invade, cancer cells must detach from their neighbouring cells, migrate into the surrounding tissue, pass through vessel walls and enter into the bloodstream, exit the bloodstream at the metastatic site and reconstitute a tissue environment which resembles that of the primary site. In order to develop this migratory behaviour, epithelial cancer cells acquire properties that come close to those of mesenchymal cells. Consequently, this phenomenon has been called epithelial–mesenchymal transition (EMT). In establishing a metastasis, the cells that grow out to become the metastatic tumour, go through the inverse process of mesenchymal–epithelial transition. This plasticity resembles that of various cell types during embryonic development. In this review, I shall discuss in some detail the process of EMT, the molecular pathways involved, the on-going debate as to the validity of the concept and its implications for the diagnosis and treatment of cancer.

BACKGROUND

In spite of the remarkable progress that has been made in the last decade regarding our understanding of the biology of cancer, it remains a devastating disease. In general terms, many molecular (genetic) mechanisms involved in carcinogenesis have been unravelled. For more and more specific types of cancer, we know how they develop and which molecular pathways are involved. Progress in the use of this knowledge for the development of new

Fred T. Bosman MD PhD
Professor of Pathology and Director, Institut Universitaire de Pathologie, Rue du Bugnon 25, 1011 Lausanne, Switzerland. E-mail: fred.bosman@chuv.ch

treatment modalities has been slow but, in the last few years, a steady flow of new drugs has become available, allowing what is fashionably called 'targeted' therapy – interference of the drug with a specific molecular pathway involved in the development of the cancer.

For a long period of time, the main research emphasis was on the cancer cell itself and on the mechanisms involved in its transformation – conversion from a regulated normal cell to an autonomously proliferating cell, no longer responding to the micro-environmental cues that regulate its growth and differentiation. The last decade much additional emphasis has been on the processes involved in the interaction between the developing cancer and the host in the process of invasive growth. These allow the cancer cells their migratory behaviour and ultimately the development of metastases. The latter field is in explosive development as our understanding of how cancer cells manage to do this is still incomplete and the importance is paramount: for most cancer types the presence or absence of metastases will ultimately determine the outcome of the disease.

CHARACTERISTICS OF EPITHELIAL AND MESENCHYMAL CELLS

EPITHELIAL CELLS

Normal epithelial cells are characterised by strong intercellular adhesive interactions, structurally reflected in the existence of adherence junctions. These play a role in the maintenance of continuous cell layers, as a single layer or as a multilayered structure. Single cell layers are mostly glandular in nature as in the digestive or respiratory tract. In these tissues epithelial cells are characterised by specialised membrane domains:

1. The **basal domain** interacting with the basement membrane.

2. The **lateral domains** which form the adherence junctions but also the tight junctions which are, more than the adherence junctions, responsible for keeping the epithelial cell layer impenetrable.

3. The **apical domain** of which the characteristics depend on the functional needs of the cell.

A characteristic example is the enterocyte with its brush border, essential for the resorptive activity of the cell. The basal domain shows specific interaction with a specialised compartment of the extracellular matrix – the basement membrane. This is morphologically reflected in the hemidesmosomes that form between the basal domain of the cell membrane and the adjacent basement membrane. Laminin-5 is an important molecule here, mediating adhesion to the basement membrane through interaction with ($\alpha_6\beta_1$ and $\alpha_6\beta_4$) integrins, which also provide signalling cues from the extracellular environment.

In the lateral domain of the plasma membrane, junctional complexes are the characterising element. In the intercellular adherence junctions, E-cadherin plays a dominant role as organising principle. Furthermore, the E-cadherin–catenin complex links the cell membrane and its junctions to the cytoskeleton. The tight junctions seal the intercellular connections through transmembrane proteins such as claudins and occludins. In addition, the lateral domain contains desmosomes and gap junctions. The cytoplasm tends to be polarised as well with secretory organelles; for example, concentrated in the apical part of the cell. All these attributes limit the mobility of the cell: as a rule, epithelial cells do not move around. It is only when the surface epithelial cells are traumatised, for example on the cornea or in the epidermis, that the remaining adjacent epithelial cells start to migrate. The resident character of the cells is reflected in a cytoskeleton mostly composed of cytokeratins. Epithelial cells do have a cortical actin filament network adjacent to the plasma membrane but only epithelial cells with contractile functions also contain smooth muscle actin microfilaments.

MESENCHYMAL CELLS

The mesenchymal compartment is remarkably different. The cells do not form continuous sheets but do make connections and may form a loose network which they fill with extracellular matrix. There is no particular spatial arrangement of the cells and they do not dispose of specific membrane domains. There is no cytoplasmic polarity. The secretory activity is targeted towards the production of extracellular matrix components. The cells are potentially mobile with a cytoskeleton composed of vimentin, in the case of myofibroblasts completed by smooth muscle cell actin. When mobile, the cells develop cytoplasmic extensions, the so-called filopodia, which contain an active cytoskeleton and on the plasma membrane expression of matrix adhesion proteins as well as matrix metalloproteinases. The latter reflects the fact that migration is the result of interaction between the migrating cells and the extracellular matrix. Proteases loosen up the matrix and liberate migration activating molecules whereas the focal adhesion contacts that develop between membrane domains and collagen fibres permit anchoring of the cells for traction.[1]

EPITHELIAL CELL PLASTICITY UNDER PATHOLOGICAL CONDITIONS

It has become clear that, under pathological conditions, epithelial cells can dramatically change the morphology and behaviour described above. This is notably the case in wound healing and fibrosis as well as in cancer. In this context it is worthwhile to be reminded of Dvorak's metaphor of 'cancer as wounds that do not heal'. What happens to epithelial cells under these very different pathological conditions is in many ways quite similar.[2] This striking epithelial plasticity is now called epithelial–mesenchymal transition (EMT).

WOUND HEALING

Epithelial cell plasticity has been studied extensively in the process of wound healing, notably in the skin and the cornea.[3,4] Ultimately, in the re-establishment of a competent covering epithelial layer, epithelial cell proliferation and differentiation will be essential. But these take time to develop. A more rapid recovery is favoured by migratory behaviour of resident epithelial cells and this is what happens in the skin and the cornea when damaged. Rapidly after wounding of the epidermis, the adherence junctions disassemble and E-cadherin expression is down-regulated, vimentin expression is up-regulated, the cytoskeleton is activated and the cells start to migrate.[5] They do not do this as individual cells but as sheets, which, therefore, to some extent maintain epithelial cell characteristics. It has been shown that the transcription factor SNAI2, member of a family which will be discussed later in more detail, plays an important orchestrating role in this process.[6] When the cornea is wounded, epithelial stem cells residing in the limbus are activated.[7] They show the phenomena described for keratinocytes above but in addition show β-catenin expression shifting from a cell membrane associated pattern to the nucleus.

CHRONIC INFLAMMATORY CONDITIONS

In chronic inflammatory conditions leading to fibrosis, epithelial cell plasticity has been demonstrated, notably in chronic kidney disease.[8] Many chronic kidney diseases end up with diffuse fibrosis of the parenchyma. This is essentially caused by the emergence of myofibroblasts, that deposit the extracellular matrix proteins making up the fibrotic tissue. It is now believed that these myofibroblasts, at least partly, derive from kidney tubular epithelial cells. In chronic inflammatory processes leading to renal fibrosis, the inflammatory response induces the presence in the micro-environment of growth factors such as TGF-β, EGF and FGF-2.[9] These are all capable of inducing EMT. Studies on experimental mouse models of interstitial kidney disease have shown that part of the interstitial fibroblasts are derived from tubular epithelial cells. In human tubulo-interstitial renal disease, there is also compelling evidence in favour of such a mechanism. Even in liver fibrosis, conversion of epithelial cells into mesenchymal cells has been proposed as a mechanism for the recruitment of (myo)fibroblasts.[10]

CANCER

Extensive attention has been paid to the modifications in morphology and behaviour of epithelial cells in invasive cancer.[11-13] Transformed epithelial cells in a carcinoma maintain, to a certain extent, their social behaviour in keeping up a multicellular organisation. Cohesive cell masses constitute one of the morphological hallmarks of epithelial differentiation in a malignant tumour. The morphology and expression of various markers in the invasion front of an adenocarcinoma and a squamous cell carcinoma are illustrated in Figures 1 and 2. In adenocarcinomas, often the characteristic polarity of glandular epithelial cells has disappeared (Fig. 1A). There might still be glandular formations but the lining epithelium becomes pseudostratified and the ordered domains of the plasma membrane disappear, along with a decrease in density of adherence junctions. Especially in the invasive front, E-cadherin expression decreases (Fig. 1D), N-cadherin expression may increase and the pattern of integrin expression changes to allow interaction with interstitial

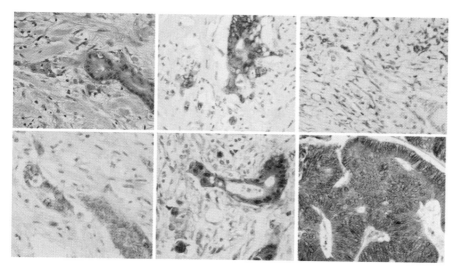

Fig. 1 Invasion front of a colorectal carcinoma (all micrographs original magnification x400). (A) Invasive tumour cells 'budding' off a glandular structure (HE). (B) Invasive (partly individuals) carcinoma cells express cytokeratins. (C) Carcinoma cells do not express vimentin. (D) Carcinoma cells irregularly express E-cadherin in a membranous pattern; individual invasive cells show cytoplasmic E-cadherin immunoreactivity. (E) nuclear and cytoplasmic β-catenin staining at the invasion front. (F) Well-differentiated glands in the tumour centre predominantly express β-catenin in a membranous pattern; no nuclear immunoreactivity.

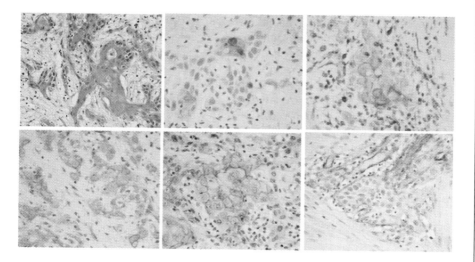

Fig. 2 Invasion front of an oral squamous cell carcinoma (all micrographs original magnification x400). (A) Individual invasive carcinoma cells assume a spindle shape and blend in with the surrounding tumour stroma. (B) Significant loss of cytokeratin immunoreactivity. (C) Some carcinoma cells express vimentin. (D) Even in areas with high invasive activity, many cells retain significant membranous E-cadherin immunoreactivity. (E) Likewise β-catenin immunoreactivity remains largely membranous. Note total absence of nuclear staining. (F) Irregular type IV collagen deposition around nests of carcinoma cells in the invasion front.

matrix collagens and fibronectin rather than with the basement membrane. The cytoskeleton might change with emergence, in certain types of carcinoma, of vimentin intermediate filaments (Fig. 2B,C) and a more active actin microfilament network. The tendency to deposit a basement membrane is decreased (Fig. 2F) and may disappear completely once the cells become invasive. Laminin-5 is no longer deposited extracellularly but is retained in the cytoplasm. This goes along with the expression of proteinases involved in the dissolution of the extracellular matrix (notably matrix metalloproteinases, MMPs), essential for the invasive cells to migrate through the matrix. MMPs also liberate activating factors such as FGF-2 from the extracellular matrix.

EPITHELIAL PLASTICITY IS BI-DIRECTIONAL

It is important to note that the altered behaviour and morphology of epithelial cells under pathological conditions, notably also in invasive cancer, are reversible. Once an invasive and metastatic cell has reached its target site, tissue infrastructure needs to be re-established. Morphologically, this is reflected in the re-emergence of the histological characteristics of the primary tumour. One might call this mesenchymal–epithelial transition (MET). At a molecular level, E-cadherin expression is up-regulated, adherence junctions re-establish, the cytoskeleton changes into a resting state, basal integrin expression again allows interaction with a basement membrane, that is (often in a lacunary fashion) deposited in close apposition to the epithelial cell, including the formation of hemidesmosomes.

These observations indicate that epithelial cell behaviour in wound healing, fibrosis or invasive cancer mimics that of mesenchymal cells. It usually does so, however, in a transient fashion and in a very dynamic way, the cell adapting to the requirements dictated by its micro-environment. Only in a limited number of carcinoma types is E-cadherin expression permanently incapacitated as, for example, in diffuse gastric cancer or in lobular breast cancer. In these cancer types, the constitutive loss of E-cadherin expression, due to a mutation in the coding gene, goes along with stable incompetence of the cells to form cohesive multicellular aggregates that infiltrate diffusely. It is important to emphasise that neither does loss of E-cadherin always induce 'mesenchymal' behaviour nor does activation of SNAI1 or SNAI2 always induce a mesenchymal phenotype.[14,15]

EPITHELIAL–MESENCHYMAL TRANSITION

For what has been reviewed above (epithelial cell plasticity in response to pathological cues from the tissue micro-environment), the term epithelial–mesenchymal transition (EMT) has become rather commonplace. The reverse phenomenon, back to the epithelial phenotype, is called mesenchymal–epithelial transition (MET). This terminology was established in developmental biology and was, by analogy, subsequently proposed also for the modified morphology and behaviour of epithelial cells in pathological conditions as described above (see review by Thiery and Sleeman[16]). During embryogenesis, a variety of extracellular signals appear capable of triggering the conversion of epithelial into mesenchymal cells. Clearly, in the developing embryo, mesenchymal cells do not only derive from the mesoderm but epithelial cells derived from the ectoderm or from the endoderm are also capable of delivering mesenchymal cells. This process of EMT is quite important in the early stages of development of the embryo and experimental interference with this process yields embryos that do not proceed beyond the stage of a blastula. Also, MET is an essential mechanism in embryogenesis, where it plays a role in the development of the somites, in the morphogenesis of the kidney and in the formation of the coelomic cavities. The discussion around EMT and MET has been complicated by the misconception that a lineage switch is involved, which is clearly not necessarily the case. Neither in developmental processes nor under pathological conditions do all the cellular and molecular changes that have been associated with EMT obligatorily occur.

In the debates[17,18] relating to the validity of EMT in a cancer context, the question as to whether or not the epithelial–mesenchymal transition is complete in cancer is probably irrelevant and evidently a derivative of rigid thinking along classical concepts of cell lineages. As we have seen, there is no doubt that human epithelial cancer cells, in culture or in human cancer tissues, can assume properties that are strikingly similar to those of mesenchymal cells. Classical morphological examples are squamous cell carcinomas with a sarcomatous spindle cell component and mixed Müllerian tumours of the female genital tract. Biphasic neoplasms, such as mesothelioma and synovial sarcoma, are examples of morphological plasticity in cancer of mesenchyme-derived 'epithelial' cells (re)assuming mesenchymal characteristics. These examples illustrate the limitations of the cell-lineage concepts when applied in the context of cancer cell differentiation. Tumours break rules: what looks

Table 1 Cellular modifications associated with EMT

In vitro morphology and function	
	Stellate or spindle shape
	Resistance to anoikis
	Increased migration
	Invasion into collagen matrix
Down-regulated proteins	
	E-cadherin
	Cytokeratin
	Occludin
	Claudin
Up-regulated proteins	
	N-cadherin
	Vimentin SNAI1
	Snail2
	Twist
	MMPs (2, 3, 9)
	Integrin $\alpha_v\beta_6$
Activated proteins	
	ILK
	GSK-3β
	Rho
Nuclear expression of proteins	
	β-Catenin
	Smad (2, 3)
	Snail1
	Snail2
	Twist

epithelial is not necessarily derived from an ectodermal or an endodermal cell nor is what looks mesenchymal necessarily derived from mesoderm.

Against this background, the whole question of the validity of the EMT concept is rather semantic. There is no doubt that invasive cancer cells assume morphological, functional and molecular properties (listed in Table 1) that are quite characteristic of mesenchymal cells; however, usually, not all.[12] In studying invasion in colorectal cancer,[19,20] for example, we noticed that the invasive cells have a strikingly different morphology, which has led to the term 'budding' in this purportedly early phase in the process of invasion. Budding cells escape the control of adjacent epithelial cells and take off into the stroma. In human colon cancer tissues, as well as in colon cancer cell line derived xenograft cancers in mice, we have found these cells to change the pattern of expression of E-cadherin (Fig. 1D) while no longer depositing a regular basement membrane on the face exposed to the extracellular matrix. These cells did not loose the expression of cytokeratins nor did they start to express vimentin (Fig. 1B,C). Remarkably, they retained deficient laminin-5 in the cytoplasm (comprising a β3 and a γ2 chain but not α3). Also, the pattern of integrin expression was different from that of non-invasive adenoma cells. Interestingly, in xenograft experiments of human colorectal carcinoma cells in nude mice, it became clear that in orchestrating the 'budding' phenomenon, interaction between the cancer cells and the host stromal cells plays an important role. Subcutaneous xenografts of human colorectal cancer cells did not show any budding, no cytoplasmic retention of laminin-5 but extensive E-cadherin staining. In contrast, orthotopic xenografting of the same cells in the wall of the caecum led to extensive transmural infiltration of the bowel wall and a budding-type spreading of the cancer cells, which had retained laminin-5 together with decreased E-cadherin expression. Vimentin expression, however, was not induced. It is likely that, in this interaction, TGF-β plays an important role.[21]

SIGNALLING PATHWAYS IN EMT

The question as to whether or not the modifications in morphology and behaviour displayed by invasive cancer cells constitute 'genuine' EMT might be addressed by comparing signalling and effector pathways in physiological and pathological EMT. Significant molecular homology would lend support to the validity of the concept of EMT as a leading force in cancer cell invasion. Crucial differences, however, would point towards intrinsically different biological processes. It is beyond the purpose of this brief review to describe in detail the signalling pathways involved in EMT; the reader is referred to excellent recent reviews for the details.[11,12,16] The key pathways and their role in EMT are summarised in Table 2.

MICRO-ENVIRONMENTAL CUES INDUCE EMT

In general terms, EMT is induced by stimulating factors in the micro-environment, for which the responding cells express receptors. These factors include extracellular matrix molecules (such as collagens, hyaluronic acid and

Table 2 Pathways involved in the regulation of EMT

Receptor	Ligand	Signalling molecules	Intermediate signalling end-point	Effect
TGF-β receptor	TGF-β	RhoA Smad family		Stress fibres Migration
Receptor tyrosine kinase	FGF	Sarc	SNAI2	Cytoskeleton activation
	HGF EGF	Ras, MAPK		Migration Focal adhesion re-arrangement
Integrins	Collagens Fibronectin	FAK, Paxillin, Rac	SNAI2	Increased migration
Frizzled	Wnt	APC, axin, GSK3β, β-catenin	SNAI1	E-cadherin down-regulation Reduced cell adhesion

fibronectin), growth factors (such as members of the TGF, the FGF and the EGF families and scatter factor, also known as hepatic growth factor or HGF) and ligands of the Wnt, Notch and AKT pathways.[22,23] These act through their cognate receptors, the integrins, the TGFR, the receptor tyrosine kinases (RTK) and Frizzled, the Wnt receptor. Constitutively activating mutations in the receptors or in downstream signalling molecules are involved in EMT in some cancers.[22] The pathways that have been identified as essential in EMT in development have also been implicated in cancer cell invasion.[11,24]

THE ROLE OF TGF-β

A key role for TGF-β is suggested by a variety of studies showing that inhibitors of TGF-β or TGF-β receptors attenuate invasive and metastatic capability, presumably through inhibition of EMT.[24] Members of the TGF-β family are also involved in EMT in developmental processes, partly in interaction with the Wnt pathway. TGF-β induces EMT in a variety of epithelial cell types *in vitro* and TGF-β1 is expressed in sites of fibrosis and in cancer stroma,[21] underlining the important role of TGF-β signalling in a pathological context. One of the key molecules involved in EMT downstream of TGF-β is Twist, a transcription factor which regulates cell movement and tissue re-organisation during early embryogenesis.[25]

SNAI1 AND SNAI2 ARE CENTRAL REGULATORS

Interaction of FGF, EGF or HGF with their respective RTKs activates members of the small GTPase family (Ras, Rho and Rac) and Sarc and, subsequently, key transcription factors such as SNAI1 (formerly known as Snail) and SNAI2 (formerly known as Slug). An essential role is played by SNAI1 in the regulation of EMT. Activation of RTKs and signalling of the Wnt, TGF-β and Notch pathways all pass through SNAI1. A central element in the Wnt-pathway

GSK3β, for example, phosphorylates SNAI1, which allows its translocation to the nucleus to down-regulate E-cadherin expression.[26] SNAI1 and SNAI2, furthermore, orchestrate the modifications in the pattern of genes expressed responsible for remodelling the cytoskeleton, including up-regulation of vimentin expression and activation of the contractile apparatus, modification of the integrin expression, ultimately responsible for the characteristic changes in the morphology and behaviour of invasive cells.[27]

THE ROLE OF E-CADHERIN

Complex interactions between the signalling pathways during EMT all seem to gravitate towards down-regulation of E-cadherin expression, leading to disassembly of junctional complexes. This liberates β-catenin from the cadherin–catenin complexes into the cytoplasm, allowing it to translocate into the nucleus and to activate the Wnt pathway through LEF/TCF4. Disassembly of junctional complexes signals directly to integrins: E-cadherin is endocytosed, which activates Rap1 (a small GTPase protein), responsible for cytoplasmic activation of integrins,[28] an example of the intensive cross-talk between the different signalling pathways. TGF-β induced signalling, for example, requires co-signalling through β_1-integrins. Conversely, TGF-β induces the expression of adapter molecules (such as DAB-2) essential for β_1-integrin activation,[29] which induces formation of focal adhesions and prevents the cells from going into anoikis. Signalling through collagens and FGF receptors also requires $\alpha_2\beta_1$-integrins. ECM-induced signalling through β_1- and β_3-integrins activates integrin-linked kinase (ILK) which down-regulates E-cadherin expression. ILK is also necessary for TGF-β signalling. In addition, β_1-integrin signalling activates RhoA and Rac1, which constitutes one of the mechanisms involved in adhesion complex disassembly.[30] Integrin signalling, furthermore, contributes to the activation of focal adhesion kinase (FAK).

In summary, therefore, in different tissues and under different morpho-genetic or pathological conditions, the molecular pathways that regulate physiological EMT or epithelial cell adaptation to pathological conditions do show differences in detail. However, the molecular pathways that govern epithelial cell plasticity in invasion and those responsible for EMT in a developmental context are sufficiently homologous to warrant the use of EMT as a metaphor for what happens to the invasive carcinoma cell. The use of the term EMT should not be taken as suggestive of a cell lineage shift: the transition in an invasive cell is usually incomplete and reversible. Furthermore, cancer cell invasion might include molecular events that are not connected with EMT.[12]

DO EMT CELLS HAVE TUMOUR STEM CELL PROPERTIES?

An interesting concept has emerged from a series of studies conducted on colorectal cancer. These have shown that the changes in growth pattern observed at the invasion front of the tumour, described earlier as 'budding', go along with striking alterations in the pattern of β-catenin expression. While in the centre of a colorectal cancer the tumour cells may grow in tubules composed of polarised cells held together by E cadherin in adherence junctions, in the invasion front, the cells lose polarity along with loss of E-cadherin expression, and dissociate. In the centre, β-catenin expression is membranous; in the invasion front, this becomes cytoplasmic and nuclear (Fig. 2E,F). This is, however, not a universal rule for all types of cancer (Fig. 2D,E). This finding underlines the importance of Wnt signalling in EMT. Kirchner and co-workers[31–33] associated the nuclear expression of β-catenin with the acquisition of stem cell properties by the cancer cells. Even though the concept of stem cells in cancer is not yet firmly established and a consensus definition of tumour stem cells has not been reached, the idea makes sense. These cells have invasive properties and they will circulate and metastasise; only those cells that have clonogenic potential, tumour stem cells, would be capable of giving rise to sustained cell proliferation in a metastatic site. At least a fraction of the cells capable of EMT, therefore, must have tumour stem cell properties.

WHAT IS THE IMPORTANCE OF THE EMT CONCEPT IN THE DIAGNOSIS AND TREATMENT OF CANCER?

Although invasion and metastasis are the most important characteristics of malignant cells, they remain relatively poorly understood in terms of molecular mechanisms involved. We have argued that EMT is a concept that explains some of the characteristics of invasive cells. It is crucial that further research uncovers additional essential aspects of the process of invasion and metastasis. In that sense, the EMT hypothesis is serving an important conceptual purpose: generating discussion, stimulating original ideas and the exploration of new avenues in metastasis research. It is likely that, in coming years, basic research will provide essential new insight.

The available knowledge, however, is already applied in diagnostic practice and drug developers are using this knowledge in exploring new avenues in targeted therapy. In terms of diagnostic pathology, two important problems might find solutions in the application of new knowledge or of the tools developed – the borderline between non-invasive and invasive neoplasia and prediction of tumour cell behaviour. Immunohistochemistry might be used to detect expression of molecular markers of invasion. A multitude of papers in the histopathological literature, describing the use of extracellular matrix molecules such as collagen IV and laminin, integrins, E-cadherin or β-catenin, underline the potential of these molecular markers for diagnostic purposes. Gontero et al.[34] have recently reviewed this for bladder cancer, but this is just one example. Immunohistochemical staining of EMT involved molecules might also be used to predict metastatic behaviour.[35,36]

Drug developers are using the new knowledge to develop specific (ant)agonists for key molecules in the process of invasion and metastasis. An example is the use of cystatin C to inhibit EMT in breast cancer.[37] This might also become important for the diagnostic histopathologist, as sensitivity to these new agents might be predicted through the immunohistochemical detection of the expression of involved molecules as, for example, sensitivity for the EGF inhibitors in lung cancer patients.[38,39]

Points for best practice

- Under physiological conditions, epithelial cells are characterised by their organisation in multicellular masses, immobility, a cytoskeleton mostly composed of cytokeratin intermediate filaments, specialised plasma-membrane domains and a polarised cytoplasm.

- Under pathological conditions such as healing wounds, chronic inflammation and cancer cell invasion, epithelial cells may assume characteristics of mesenchymal cells.

- Epithelial cell plasticity in pathological conditions implies dissolution of adhesion junctions with down-regulation of E-cadherin expression, migrating behaviour, vimentin intermediate filaments and cytoskeletal activation.

- EMT and MET are essential processes in organogenesis. They do not necessarily represent a lineage shift.

- EMT can be used as a metaphor for cell epithelial plasticity under pathological conditions. EMT is usually reversible (MET) and does not imply a lineage shift.

- Cancer cells in the invasion front of a carcinoma that have undergone EMT may express β-catenin in the nucleus. This might be a hallmark of their tumour stem cell properties.

- EMT-associated molecules will increase in importance as markers for prediction of prognosis and response to targeted therapy.

References

1. Yamaguchi H, Wyckoff J, Condeelis J. Cell migration in tumors. *Curr Opin Cell Biol* 2005; **17**: 559–564.
2. Dvorak HF. Tumors: wounds that do not heal. Similarities between tumor stroma generation and wound healing. *N Engl J Med* 1986; **315**: 1650–1659.
3. SundarRaj N, Rizzo JD, Anderson SC, Gesiotto JP. Expression of vimentin by rabbit corneal epithelial cells during wound repair. *Cell Tissue Res* 1992; **267**: 347–356.
4. Midwood KS, Mao Y, Hsia HC, Valenick LV, Schwarzbauer JE. Modulation of cell–fibronectin matrix interactions during tissue repair. *J Invest Dermatol* 2006; **126 (Suppl)**: 73–78.
5. Martin P. Wound healing – aiming for perfect skin regeneration. *Science* 1997; **276**: 75–81.
6. Savagner P, Kusewitt DF, Carver EA *et al.* Developmental transcription factor Slug is required for effective re-epithelialization by adult keratinocytes. *J Cell Physiol* 2005; **202**: 858–866.
7. Kawakita T, Espana EM, He H *et al.* Intrastromal invasion by limbal epithelial cells is mediated by epithelial-mesenchymal transition activated by air exposure. *Am J Pathol* 2005; **167**: 381–393.
8. Hay ED, Zuk A. Transformations between epithelium and mesenchyme: normal, pathological, and experimentally induced. *Am J Kidney Dis* 1995; **26**: 678–690.
9. Liu Y. Epithelial to mesenchymal transition in renal fibrogenesis: pathologic significance, molecular mechanism, and therapeutic intervention. *J Am Soc Nephrol* 2004; **15**: 1–12.

10. Sicklick JK, Choi SS, Bustamante M *et al*. Evidence for epithelial–mesenchymal transitions in adult liver cells. *Am J Physiol* 2006; **291**: G575–G583.

11. Thiery JP. Epithelial–mesenchymal transitions in tumour progression. *Nat Rev Cancer* 2002; **2**: 442–454.

12. Christiansen JJ, Rajasekaran AK. Reassessing epithelial to mesenchymal transition as a prerequisite for carcinoma invasion and metastasis. *Cancer Res* 2006; **66**: 8319–8326.

13. Lee JM, Dedhar S, Kalluri R, Thompson EW. The epithelial–mesenchymal transition: new insights in signaling, development, and disease. *J Cell Biol* 2006; **172**: 973–981.

14. Rosivatz E, Becker I, Specht K *et al*. Differential expression of the epithelial–mesenchymal transition regulators Snail, SIP1, and twist in gastric cancer. *Am J Pathol* 2002; **161**: 1881–1891.

15. Come C, Magnino F, Bibeau F *et al*. Snail and Slug play distinct roles during breast carcinoma progression. *Clin Cancer Res* 2006; **12**: 5395–5402.

16. Thiery JP, Sleeman JP. Complex networks orchestrate epithelial–mesenchymal transitions. *Nat Rev Mol Cell Biol* 2006; **7**: 131–142.

17. Tarin D. The fallacy of epithelial mesenchymal transition in neoplasia. *Cancer Res* 2005; **65**: 5996–6000.

18. Thompson EW, Newgreen DF. Carcinoma invasion and metastasis: a role for epithelial–mesenchymal transition? *Cancer Res* 2005; **65**: 5991–5995.

19. Sordat I, Bosman FT, Dorta G *et al*. Differential expression of laminin-5 subunits and integrin receptors in human colorectal neoplasia. *J Pathol* 1998; **185**: 44–52.

20. Sordat I, Rousselle P, Chaubert P *et al*. Tumor cell budding and laminin-5 expression in colorectal carcinoma can be modulated by the tissue micro-environment. *Int J Cancer* 2000; **88**: 708–717.

21. De Wever O, Mareel M. Role of tissue stroma in cancer cell invasion. *J Pathol* 2003; **200**: 429–447.

22. Larue L, Bellacosa A. Epithelial–mesenchymal transition in development and cancer: role of phosphatidylinositol 3′-kinase/AKT pathways. *Oncogene* 2005; **24**: 7443–7454.

23. Leong KG, Karsan A. Recent insights into the role of Notch signaling in tumorigenesis. *Blood* 2006; **107**: 2223–2233.

24. Zavadil J, Böttinger EP. TGF-beta and epithelial-to-mesenchymal transitions. *Oncogene* 2005; **24**: 5764–5774.

25. Yang J, Mani SA, Weinberg RA. Exploring a new twist on tumor metastasis. *Cancer Res* 2006; **66**: 4549–4552.

26. Zhou BP, Deng J, Xia W *et al*. Dual regulation of Snail by GSK-3beta-mediated phosphorylation in control of epithelial-mesenchymal transition. *Nat Cell Biol* 2004; **6**: 931–940.

27. Barrallo-Gimeno A, Nieto MA. The Snail genes as inducers of cell movement and survival: implications in development and cancer. *Development* 2005; **132**: 3151–3161.

28. Balzac F, Avolio M, Degani S *et al*. E-cadherin endocytosis regulates the activity of Rap1: a traffic light GTPase at the crossroads between cadherin and integrin function. *J Cell Sci* 2005; **118**: 4765–4783.

29. Prunier C, Howe PH. Disabled-2 (Dab2) is required for transforming growth factor beta-induced epithelial to mesenchymal transition (EMT). *J Biol Chem* 2005; **280**: 17540–17548.

30. Gimond C, van der Flier A, van Delft S *et al*. Induction of cell scattering by expression of beta1 integrins in beta1-deficient epithelial cells requires activation of members of the rho family of GTPases and downregulation of cadherin and catenin function. *J Cell Biol* 1999; **147**: 1325–1340.

31. Kirchner T, Brabletz T. Patterning and nuclear beta-catenin expression in the colonic adenoma-carcinoma sequence. Analogies with embryonic gastrulation. *Am J Pathol* 2000; **157**: 1113–1121.

32. Brabletz T, Hlubek F, Spaderna S *et al*. Invasion and metastasis in colorectal cancer: epithelial–mesenchymal transition, mesenchymal-epithelial transition, stem cells and beta-catenin. *Cells Tissues Organs* 2005; **179**: 56–65.

33. Brabletz T, Jung A, Spaderna S, Hlubek F, Kirchner T. Opinion: migrating cancer stem cells – an integrated concept of malignant tumour progression. *Nat Rev Cancer* 2005; **5**: 744–749.

34. Gontero P, Banisadr S, Frea B, Brausi M. Metastasis markers in bladder cancer: a review of the literature and clinical considerations. *Eur Urol* 2004; **46**: 296–311.

35. Yang MH, Chang SY, Chiou SH *et al.* Overexpression of NBS1 induces epithelial-mesenchymal transition and co-expression of NBS1 and Snail predicts metastasis of head and neck cancer. *Oncogene* 2006; Epub ahead of print.

36. Shioiri M, Shida T, Koda K *et al.* Slug expression is an independent prognostic parameter for poor survival in colorectal carcinoma patients. *Br J Cancer* 2006; **94**: 1816–1822.

37. Sokol JP, Neil JR, Schiemann BJ, Schiemann WP. The use of cystatin C to inhibit epithelial–mesenchymal transition and morphological transformation stimulated by transforming growth factor-beta. *Breast Cancer Res* 2005; **7**: R844–R853.

38. Thomson S, Buck E, Petti F *et al.* Epithelial to mesenchymal transition is a determinant of sensitivity of non-small-cell lung carcinoma cell lines and xenografts to epidermal growth factor receptor inhibition. *Cancer Res* 2005; **65**: 9455–9462.

39. Yauch RL, Januario T, Eberhard DA *et al.* Epithelial versus mesenchymal phenotype determines *in vitro* sensitivity and predicts clinical activity of erlotinib in lung cancer patients. *Clin Cancer Res* 2005; **11**: 8686–8698.

Gillian Murphy

5

Matrix metalloproteinases in neoplastic progression: where are we now?

Matrix metalloproteinases (MMPs) have been recognised as important components of tumourigenesis for decades, charged with the role of regulators of the extracellular matrix (ECM) environment of cancer cells and mediating their invasion and metastasis. Their considerable up-regulation in malignant tissues made them promising drug targets, but the resulting early generations of synthetic inhibitors, although effective in several animal models of cancer, were extremely disappointing in clinical trials.[1,2] In the meantime, we have learnt a great deal more about these enzymes and can now rethink their roles in neoplastic progression and the potential for their therapeutic regulation.[3,4] This short review will present the methodologies that have been used to study the expression of MMPs and tissue inhibitors of metalloproteinases (TIMPs) in tumours, with some examples of the interpretation of the data.

MMPs AND CANCER

In the human, there are 23 MMPs, many of which are up-regulated in tumour systems. Six of these enzymes are membrane anchored, the membrane-type MT-MMPs, and the remainder are ostensibly secreted, but may have strong associations with cell-surface molecules or the extracellular matrix.[5] Interestingly, most MMP activity (detected at the mRNA, protein or enzyme activity level) is associated with the stromal, 'host'-derived component of carcinomas, including fibroblasts and myofibroblasts, endothelial cells and inflammatory cells.[4] Studies in cells and in mice deficient in individual MMPs have shown that they not only play roles in tumour cell invasion and metastasis, due to their combined ability to degrade all major components of the ECM, but also in cell–cell communication, such as the activity of growth

Gillian Murphy BSc PhD FMedSci
Chair of Cancer Cell Biology, Deputy Head of Cancer Research UK.
Department of Oncology, University of Cambridge, Cancer Research UK Cambridge Research Institute, Li Ka Shing Centre, Robinson Way, Cambridge CB2 0RE, UK. E-mail: gm290@cam.ac.uk

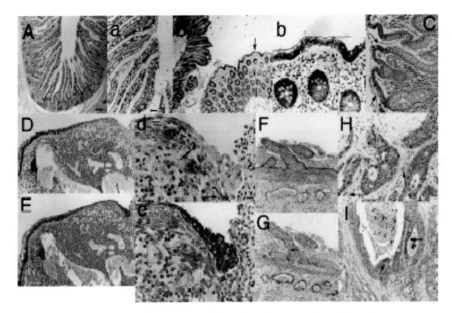

Fig. 1 MMP-19 is expressed in the normal gut but down-regulated in colon cancer. (A) MMP-19 protein in the epithelium of the ileal villi; (a) higher magnification of (A). (B) Positive immunostaining for MMP-19 in normal colon; (b) higher magnification of the area shown by the arrow in (B). (C) MMP-19 protein is evident in the shedding epithelium in ulcerative colitis. (D) MMP-19 is not expressed by migrating cells in an ulcer associated with inflammatory bowel disease; (d) higher magnification of the epithelial tip in (D). Arrows mark stromal macrophage/activated fibroblast-like MMP-19 positive cells. (E) Serial section stained for laminin-5; (e) higher magnification of the migrating epithelial tip in (E). (F) MMP-19 staining in an ulcer caused by ischaemic colitis. (G) A serial section stained for type IV collagen. (H) The invasive front of a Duke's C colon tumour is devoid of MMP-1 protein, which is only detected in occasional fibroblasts (arrows). (I) A Duke's A colon cancer displaying MMP-19 only sporadically in cancer cells (arrow). Scale bars: 50 μm (A); 25 μm (a,B,G,J); 12.5 μm (b,H); 6.3 μm (d,e). Figure from Bister VO et al.[6] by agreement with Plenum Publishing Corporation.

factors, chemokines and their receptors and adhesion molecules (Table 1). The MMPs can be involved in the regulation of tumour growth and metastasis, apoptosis, angiogenesis and aspects of innate immunity and may have protective functions in some cases. In general, few MMPs are expressed in normal tissues and are up-regulated in response to injury and other stimuli, notably during tumourigenesis. However, Bister and colleagues[6] have shown that MMP-19, MMP-26 and MMP-28 are exceptions to these rules and are expressed in normal intestine. Using immunohistochemistry, MMP-19 was shown to be expressed in the apical regions of human colonic villi and in the crypts in normal colon surface epithelium (Fig. 1). MMP-19 was up-regulated in inflammatory conditions and could be detected in fibroblasts, macrophages and shedding epithelium in inflammatory bowel disease and colonic ischaemia. However, it was not detected in ulcerated areas in migrating enterocytes, as assessed by laminin-5 staining. MMP-19 was detected in areas where type IV collagen was absent. Unlike many previously characterised MMPs, MMP-19 was not present in the invasive front of colon cancers, was

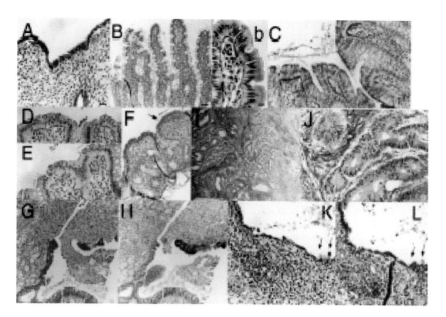

Fig. 2 MMP-26 protein localises to the basement membrane in normal and diseased colon and is absent from cancer epithelium. (A) Positive cytoplasmic staining for MMP-26 in the endometrial epithelium. (B) MMP-26 protein is detected in a linear pattern in the basement membrane zone at the villus tips of the ileum; (b) higher magnification of (B). (C) MMP-26 is detected in a linear pattern in the basement membrane zone in a sample representing inflamed colitis ulcerosa. (E) Negative control stained with MMP-26 pre-immune serum. (F) Ischaemic colitis representing diminished MMP-26 staining in a more inflamed area (arrow). (G) A Duke's B colon cancer stained for MMP-26. The direction for invasion to the right and the fairly well differentiated tumour surface area is seen at the left. (H) Higher magnification of cells. (J) Serial section stained for laminin-5. Cytoplasmic staining in migrating enterocytes co-localises for MMP-26 (K) and MMP-7 (L) in a sample of ulcerative colitis. Scale bars: 25 μm (B,F,I); 12.5 μm (A,C,D,E,G,H,J,K,L); 6.3 μm (b). Figure from Bister VO et al.[6] by agreement with Plenum Publishing Corporation.

down-regulated in the cancer epithelium and could only occasionally be detected in fibroblasts (Fig. 1). In normal ileum, MMP-26 protein was detected in the basement membrane zone (Fig. 2). In colon, MMP-26 was also in the basement membrane area and associated with epithelia. MMP-26 was also found at the edges of gut wounds in ulcerative colitis in cells with migratory potential, as suggested by the cytoplasmic staining for laminin-5. In colon carcinomas, however, MMP-26 was located around cancer cell islets in the matrix as a thread-like meshwork and appeared to be down-regulated in areas of histologically more aggressive and de-differentiated cancer.[6]

The tumour phenotype of MMP-2, MMP-7, MMP-9, MMP-11 and MMP-19 null mice generally reflects decreased tumour growth and/or metastases, whereas MMP-3, MMP-8 and MMP-12 null mice show increased tumour growth, progression or metastases.[7]

It is, therefore, clear that we need to have a very detailed understanding of the precise action of MMPs in different tumour cell types and at different disease stages. This must be coupled with an ability to design inhibitors that specifically target the correct enzymes if useful therapeutic agents are to emerge.

Table 1 Novel substrates of matrix metalloproteinases

Matrix metallo-proteinase	Substrate
MMP-1	proIL-1β, proTNF-α, insulin-like growth factor-binding protein (IGFBP)-2, -3, -5, stromal derived factor (SDF)-1, MCP-1, -2, -3, L-selectin, α_1-proteinase inhibitor, α_1-antichymotrypsin, α_2-macroglobulin
MMP-2	proIL-1β proTNF-α, proTNF-β, IGFBP-3, -5, FGFR-1, SDF-1, MCP-3, α_1-proteinase inhibitor, α_2-macroglobulin, metastin, endothelin-1
MMP-3	proIL-1β, proTNF-α, proHB-EGF, IGFBP-3, SDF-1, MCP-1, -2, -3, -4, E-cadherin, L-selectin, endostatin, plasminogen, α_1-proteinase inhibitor, α_1-antichymotrypsin, α_2-macroglobulin, antithrombin III
MMP-7	proTNF-α, pro-α-defensin, proHB-EGF, Fas ligand (FasL), RANK ligand, E-cadherin, β_4-integrin, endostatin, plasminogen, syndecan, α_1-proteinase inhibitor, α_2-macroglobulin
MMP-8	proTNF-α, IGFBP, MCP-1, IP-10, MIG, GCP-2, LIX, L-selectin, α_1-proteinase inhibitor, α_2-macroglobulin, α_2-antiplasmin
MMP-9	proIL-1β, IL-2Rα, proIL-8, proTNF-α, proTGF-β, IFN-β, FGFR-1, SDF-1, GROα, CTAP-III, IP-10, MIG, GCP-2, ENA-78, Kit ligand, tumstatin, plasminogen, α_1-proteinase inhibitor, α_2-macroglobulin, metastin
MMP-11	IGFPB-1, α_1-antitrypsin, α_1-proteinase inhibitor, α_2-macroglobulin
MMP-12	proTNF-α, endostatin, plasminogen, α_1-proteinase inhibitor
MMP-13	proTNF-α, SDF-1, MCP-3, Endostatin, α_1-antichymotrypsin, α_2-macroglobulin
MMP-14	proTNF-α, CTGF, IL-8, GROα, GROγ, SDF-1, WISP-2, PDGFR, $\alpha_v\beta_3$-integrin, CD44, tissue transglutaminase, syndecan, α_1-proteinase inhibitor, α_2-macroglobulin, metastin
MMP-15	proTNF-α, tissue transglutaminase
MMP-16	proTNF-α, syndecan, tissue transglutaminase, metastin
MMP-17	proTNF-α
MMP-24	metastin
MMP-25	α_1-proteinase inhibitor
MMP-26	IGFBP-1, α_1-proteinase inhibitor
MMP-28	TGF-β

The majority of these substrates have been identified in *in vitro* or cell-based studies and have not been yet verified *in vivo*.

The MMPs are usually expressed in low amounts, and their transcription is tightly regulated. Activation of secreted MMPs occurs by removal of the prodomain by proteolytic mechanisms that are not well understood.[5] MMPs that contain a furin-like recognition domain in their propeptide (MMP-11, MMP-28, and the MT-MMPs) are activated intracellularly. Many MMPs are activated at the cell surface by the action of plasmin or MMPs. MMP-2, which is constitutively produced, is activated on the cell surface by MT1-MMP and this may act as the start of a cascade of pro-MMP activation events. Once activated, MMPs are further regulated by endogenous inhibitors, notably the tissue inhibitors of metalloproteinases (TIMPs), autodegradation, and selective endocytosis. Most cells secrete both MMPs and TIMPs, as well as activators of

MMPs. Hence, the function of activated MMPs tends to be limited to short bursts of time in the pericellular micro-environment. MMPs bound to the cell surface are thought to be partially protected from inhibition.

The TIMPs, of which there are four, are the most important physiological inhibitors[8] and have a wide capability to inhibit all the MMP family members. There are, however, variations in their efficiency; for instance, TIMP-1 is a rather poor inhibitor of a number of the transmembrane sub-group of MMPs, the MT-MMPs and of MMP-19. Some TIMPs have activity against other families of metzincins, notably against the disintegrin metalloproteinases, ADAMs and the related ADAM-TS, disintegrin metalloproteases with thrombospondin repeats. TIMP-3 is the most promiscuous in this respect, although TIMP-1 may also have some activity.[8] One other major potential regulator is the general proteinase inhibitor of serum, α_2-macroglobulin, which is involved in MMP endocytosis through a scavenger–receptor mechanism. It is thought that the balance between the proteinases and their inhibitors is critical for levels of proteolysis and due attention needs to be paid to their level of expression and regulation during tumourigenesis.[5] It is also thought that some TIMPs may have other cellular roles that may be independent of their MMP inhibitory activity.[9,10] Once again, studies of the effect of ablation or overexpression of individual TIMP genes in animal models of cancer have been useful in determining their role.[11–14]

The identification of the many biological functions of MMPs and the re-evaluation of their relevance in cancer has led to the recognition of their importance in the early stages of disease. As well as remodelling or degrading the ECM, the processing of bioactive molecules contributes to the formation of a complex micro-environment that promotes malignant transformation. Additionally, activation or release of growth factors from the ECM stimulates proliferation and suppresses apoptosis.

CURRENT EVALUATION TECHNIQUES FOR MMPs

The biggest challenge for MMP researchers at this stage is to accumulate the appropriate data from human cancers which give information not only of levels of expression relative to the disease state, but of the localisation of individual enzymes with respect to different sites. Correlation between tissue levels of MMPs and the levels in serum, *etc.*, relative to other markers, is also essential and may go some way, alongside laboratory studies, to evaluate the role of individual MMPs. We also need to assess whether the activities MMPs and TIMPs in cancer patients are prognostic markers for disease. To evaluate newer generations of therapeutic inhibitors, it would be advantageous to monitor loss of enzyme activity either directly or by the use of surrogate markers in relation to clinical functionality. Clinically relevant animal models are also essential to this process.

mRNA STUDIES OF MMPs

The larger scale evaluation of MMP expression at the mRNA level in tumours is proceeding efficiently since the advent of microarray and automated, real-time polymerase chain reaction (RT-PCR) techniques. A customised Affymetrix protease microarray (Hu/Mu ProtIn chip[15]) was recently developed and has been used to identify genes transcribed by human tumour xenografts in the mouse, as well as in the host cells.[16] Using an orthotopic lung cancer model, it was shown that murine matrix metalloproteinases MMP-12 and MMP-13 were up-regulated in tumour tissue compared with normal mouse lung. To determine the relevance of stromal proteases detected using this model system, the results were compared to an analysis of human lung adenocarcinoma specimens using an Affymetrix microarray. MMP-12 and MMP-13 showed an increase in expression in human tumours compared with normal lung similar to that seen in the orthotopic model. Overall and Dean[17] described the development of a dedicated and complete human protease and inhibitor microarray named the CLIP-CHIP. Oligonucleotides (70-mers) identifying all 715 human proteases, inactive homologues and inhibitors were spotted onto glass slides with a dedicated subarray containing oligonucleotides for specific human breast carcinoma genes. Initial analyses revealed that MMPs showed a restricted expression pattern in both normal and cancerous breast tissues, with most expressed at low levels. However, of the several MMPs expressed in significant quantities (with the exception of MMP-28 which was strongly elevated), the carcinoma samples showed only slightly increased levels. RT-PCR has been used in a large number of studies and is particularly powerful when coupled with laser dissection techniques, generating more data on spatial details, such as cell-type specificity of expression. RNA from normal bladder and urothelial carcinoma specimens was profiled for each of the 23 human MMPs, the four endogenous TIMPs and several key growth factors and their receptors using quantitative RT-PCR.[18] Laser capture microdissection of RNA from 22 tumour and 11 normal frozen sections was performed allowing accurate RNA extraction from either stromal or epithelial compartments. MMP-2, MT1-MMP and MMP-28 were very highly expressed in tumour samples while MMPs 1, 7, 9, 11, 15, 19 and 23 were highly expressed. There was a significant positive correlation between transcript expression and tumour grade for MMPs 1, 2, 8, 10, 11, 12, 13, 14, 15 and 28 ($P < 0.001$). At the same confidence interval, TIMP-1 and TIMP-3 also correlated with increasing tumour grade. Laser capture microdissection revealed that most highly expressed MMPs are located primarily within the stromal compartment, except MMP-13 which localised to the epithelial compartment.[18] Pedersen and colleagues[19] used laser capture microdissection and RT-PCR to quantify the mRNA expression of components of matrix-degrading proteolytic systems in cancer and stromal areas of mouse mammary tumours genetically induced by the polyoma virus middle T (PyMT) antigen. They examined the mRNA levels of MMPs 2, 3, 11, 13 and 14, and found that all seven genes are predominantly expressed by stromal cells. The results were qualitatively supported by *in situ* hybridisation analysis of the expression of mRNAs for MMP-2, MMP-3 and MMP-13 in the PyMT tumours. Statistical analyses indicated that the quantitative expression patterns observed in cancer and stromal cells isolated from individual tumours from different PyMT mice are quite reproducible. The use of *in situ* hybridisation to study MMP mRNA *in situ* is clearly important, as shown by the extensive works of Saarialho-Kere and colleagues. In a recent study,[20] they showed that during oesophageal tumourigenesis, MMP-21 and MMP-26 have different, unique expression patterns both being tightly regulated and induced in the vicinity of inflammation. They propose that MMP-21 may provide a marker for differentiating tumour areas.[20] It is difficult to quantify this technique, particularly in a high-throughput format, but it has yielded important clues to both spatial and temporal MMP expression in tumour and host tissues, alongside appropriate cell markers.

PROTEIN AND ENZYME ACTIVITY

Some data on protein expression within tumour tissues have always been available from immunohistochemistry. This continues to be the most powerful technique to identify MMP localisation at the protein level, in conjunction with suitable markers and, where possible, *in situ* hybridisation assessment of the same genes. There are still some concerns about antibody specificity, as even some monoclonal antibodies that have been raised to peptides may not be yielding an accurate picture. Hence, the use of tissue array technology requires very careful validation. In such cases, adequate controls and the validation of the antibody by immunoblotting of tumour extracts relative to purified protein is recommended. Emphasis has been placed on the importance of active, rather than total, MMP levels in tumours. However, technical problems in the identification of activated MMPs in tissues have limited this assessment. The fact that activated MMPs have not been detected in the blood of cancer patients suggests that endogenous inhibitors rapidly bind and inactivate mature proteases in tissues and blood.[21] The high ratio of MMPs to TIMPs in cancer tissue specimens has been proposed to reflect dominant proteolytic activity and has been correlated with poor prognosis (reviewed by Overall and Lopez-Otin[22]). MMP activity can be detected either using tissue extracts or by *in situ* zymography.[23–25] Techniques are being developed to quantify MMP activity levels, which has proved difficult. Fluorimetric and colorimetric peptide substrates have been developed as activity-based probes for tissue slices, or in an attempt to measure MMP activities directly in tissue extracts. To date, these have not been highly selective and have been inadequate in reporting low levels of activity since the MMPs turn over peptides rather poorly. The most innovative way around this problem is the use of a specific antibody to isolate the MMP of interest (immunocapture), followed by the use of a general MMP assay.[26] Such assays for MMPs and ELISA techniques for the quantitation of a limited number of MMP protein levels are also available commercially. Hesek and colleagues[27] have reported a resin-immobilised, potent, broad-spectrum, synthetic MMP inhibitor for the selective detection of active forms of MMPs in experimental samples. Only the free, active MMPs, and not the zymogens or MMP/TIMP complexes, were bound specifically to the resin. On examination of human tissue, active (free) MMP-2 and MMP-14 were detected in cancerous, but not in benign, human tissue extracts. The authors propose that the identification of the active MMP profile for individual cancer types will help to target specific MMPs on an individual basis, hence encouraging future development of specific/selective inhibitory drugs for treatment of cancer. Based on the data presented, it would appear that a fluorescent, immobilised resin approach might also be applicable for *in situ* detection of active MMPs in living tissue. A variety of factors, including tissue extraction procedure and sample storage, will affect detection of active MMPs in tissue samples which may limit the use of this technique for the examination of clinical tissues for diagnosis, staging, and prognosis of cancer. An alternative is the development of techniques to identify the cleavage products released following activation of a proMMP. These neo-markers remaining after MMP activation include the N-terminal and C-terminal activation products released from MMPs themselves[28] or fragments cleaved from extracellular matrix proteins.

It is advisable to assess the MMP expression by a range of techniques if at all possible. Yokoyama and colleagues[29] compared gastric carcinomas of the scirrhous (SC) and non-scirrhous (NSC) type. SC are characterised by diffuse invasive growth patterns with marked fibrosis, frequent peritoneal dissemination and lymph-node metastases and poor prognosis, while NSC show medullary growth patterns and common haematogeneous metastases. To study the differences in local expression levels of MMPs and TIMPs between SC and NSC, several methods were used including sandwich-enzyme immunoassay systems, gelatin zymography, real-time quantitative PCR, immunoblotting, immunohistochemistry and *in situ* zymography. Of the seven MMPs and two TIMPs tested, only proMMP-2 levels were remarkably higher in SC than in NSC, and proMMP-2 activation ratio was significantly lower in SC than in NSC. TIMP-3 mRNA levels were remarkably about 2-fold higher in SC than in NSC tissues. TIMP-3 production in SC was confirmed by immunoblotting and TIMP-3 was immunolocalised to stromal fibroblasts in SC. TIMP-3 mRNA levels inversely correlated with proMMP-2 activation ratios, although the expression levels of MT1-MMP and MT2-MMP were not different in SC and NSC. By *in situ* zymography, gelatinolytic activity appeared to be weaker in SC than in NSC. All these data suggest that proMMP-2 activation is down-regulated by TIMP-3 in SC, which may explain the differences in clinical behaviours of SC and NSC. The early detection of both primary tumours and metastatic disease continue to be significant challenges in the diagnosis and staging of cancer. The development of therapeutic strategies using proteinase inhibitors, has necessitated methods to detect tumour-associated proteolytic activities. Non-invasive imaging techniques with enhanced sensitivity can be obtained by enzymatic amplification to increase the efficacy of imaging contrast agents. Some studies have already established MMP activity probes for *in vivo* detection of their activity. Bremer and colleagues[30] showed that novel, biocompatible, near-infrared, fluorigenic MMP substrates could be used as activatable reporter probes to sense MMP activity in intact tumours in nude mice. Moreover, the effect of MMP inhibition could be directly imaged using this approach within hours after initiation of treatment using the synthetic MMP active site inhibitor, prinomastat (AG3340). The development of further probes, together with novel near-infrared, fluorescence imaging technology, will enable the detailed analysis of a number of proteinases, albeit relatively non-specific for MMPs. McIntyre and colleagues[31] have described a novel, polymer-based, fluorigenic substrate with some specificity for MMP7 which has been tested in a mouse xenograft model. The current status of imaging MMP expression, including the types of tracers being developed and the types of imaging modalities available has been reviewed by Li and Anderson.[32]

ASSESSMENT OF TIMP LEVELS

The balance between MMPs and their major physiological inhibitors, the TIMPs clearly plays a role in the regulation of tumourigenesis. The evaluation of TIMP levels can be achieved by techniques such as quantitative RT-PCR, *in situ* hybridisation, immunohistochemistry as discussed for the MMPs. Free, active TIMPs can be measured more quantitatively using ELISA techniques in tissue extracts,[33] or in plasma.[34] Extreme care is needed in the latter case since circulating platelets have very high levels of stored TIMP-1, as well as some TIMP-2 and TIMP-4. Hoikkala and colleagues[35] investigated the tumour immunoreactive protein of MMP-2, MMP-9 and TIMP-1, as well as the levels of circulating total TIMP-1 and MMP-2/TIMP-2-complex, as prognostic factors in stage I–III lung carcinoma. Serum levels were measured by ELISA assay and the protein expression in primary tumours was analysed by streptavidin–biotin immunohistochemical staining using specific monoclonal antibodies. High levels of MMP-2 or MMP-9 in tumours predicted a poor prognosis. The 5-year survival rates were 83 or 85% in patients negative for MMP-2 or MMP-9, respectively. Tissue MMP-2 correlated with high expression of MMP-9, but the serum levels of MMP-2/TIMP-2-complex or TIMP-1 did not correlate with the immunostaining of the corresponding tumours. The authors concluded that, in lung carcinoma, the best prognostic value is achieved by using immunohistochemistry for MMP-2 and MMP-9. In early disease, however, serum TIMP-1 or MMP-2/TIMP-2-complex could offer some further prognostic value.

CONCLUSIONS

The need to understand fully the roles of MMPs in individual cancer settings has fuelled the development of techniques to analyse their expression, localisation and activity in human disease. A particular focus on preclinical studies to determine the specific roles in different stages of tumour progression and the development of appropriate animal models are key components of these efforts. Such activities will allow the evaluation of new generations of more appropriate inhibitors. However, the validation of techniques for the monitoring of molecularly targeted anti-tumour agents such as MMP inhibitors is required prior to any large-scale trials. The assessment of MMP inhibition therapies has relied on indirect evidence of efficacy such as tumour markers, size, histological changes and the measurement of MMPs in blood or tissue which do not provide a reliable end point for assessing inhibition of MMP activity *in vivo*. More direct methods of molecular target assessment are, therefore, being developed and such novel reporters of enzyme activity are making it possible to visualise enzyme function *in vivo*. Imaging probes that can be used in non-invasive optical imaging have the potential to make a significant impact. Already, positron emission tomography and magnetic resonances imaging using probes to detect gene expression and molecular interactions are making an increasing contribution in clinical development of such therapeutic approaches.[35]

Points for best practice

- Matrix metalloproteinases (MMPs) have roles in the turnover of cellular receptors, growth factors, cytokines and chemokines, as well as extracellular matrix.

- MMPs are made by tumour cells and the associated tumour stromal cells.

- To target MMPs effectively in therapeutic strategies, we need to understand the role of individual MMPs in cancers, requiring detailed studies in human cancers and animal models.

- The expression patterns and activities of the major natural inhibitor family, the tissue inhibitors of metalloproteinases (TIMPs), is also necessary.

- Studies at the level of mRNA and protein are being substantiated by the use of novel techniques to assess enzyme activity.

- Recent developments include non-invasive imaging techniques..

ACKOWLEDGEMENTS

I am indebted to Dr Ulpu Saarialho-Kere for permission to reproduce her data. Our work is supported by Cancer Research UK and the European Union Framework Programme 6.

References

1. Coussens LM, Fingleton B, Matrisian LM. Matrix metalloproteinase inhibitors and cancer: trials and tribulations. *Science* 2002; **295**: 2387–2392.
2. Pavlaki M, Zucker S. Matrix metalloproteinase inhibitors (MMPIs): the beginning of phase I or the termination of phase III clinical trials. *Cancer Metastasis Rev* 2003; **22**: 177–203.
3. Overall CM, Kleifeld O. Tumour microenvironment – opinion: validating matrix metalloproteinases as drug targets and anti-targets for cancer therapy. *Rev Cancer* 2006; **6**: 227–239.
4. Jodele S, Blavier L, Yoon JM, DeClerck YA. Modifying the soil to affect the seed: role of stromal-derived matrix metalloproteinases in cancer progression. *Metastasis Rev* 2006; **25**: 35–43.
5. Egeblad M, Werb Z. New functions for the matrix metalloproteinases in cancer progression. *Nat Rev Cancer* 2002; **2**: 161–174.
6. Bister VO, Salmela MT, Karjalainen-Lindsberg ML *et al.* Differential expression of three matrix metalloproteinases, MMP-19, MMP-26, and MMP-28, in normal and inflamed intestine and colon cancer. *Dig Dis Sci* 2004; **49**: 653–661.
7. Fingleton B. Matrix metalloproteinases: roles in cancer and metastasis. *Bioscience* 2006; **11**: 479–491.
8. Baker AH, Edwards DR, Murphy G. Metalloproteinase inhibitors: biological actions and therapeutic opportunities. *J Cell Sci* 2002; **115**: 3719–3727.
9. Lambert E, Dasse E, Haye B, Petitfrere E. TIMPs as multifacial proteins. *Crit Rev Oncol Hematol* 2004; **49**: 187–198.
10. Chirco R, Liu XW, Jung KK, Kim HR. Novel functions of TIMPs in cell signaling. *Metastasis Rev* 2006; **25**: 99–113.

11. Soloway PD, Alexander CM, Werb Z, Jaenisch R. Targeted mutagenesis of Timp-1 reveals that lung tumor invasion is influenced by Timp-1 genotype of the tumor but not by that of the host. *Oncogene* 1996; **13**: 2307–2314.

12. Ikenaka Y, Yoshiji H, Kuriyama S et al. Tissue inhibitor of metalloproteinases-1 (TIMP-1) inhibits tumor growth and angiogenesis in the TIMP-1 transgenic mouse model. *Int J Cancer* 2003; **105**: 340–346.

13. Cruz-Munoz W, Sanchez OH, Di Grappa M, English JL, Hill RP, Khokha R. Enhanced metastatic dissemination to multiple organs by melanoma and lymphoma cells in TIMP-3(−/−) mice. *Oncogene* 2006; **25**: 6489–6496.

14. Cruz-Munoz W, Kim I, Khokha R. TIMP-3 deficiency in the host, but not in the tumor, enhances tumor growth and angiogenesis. *Oncogene* 2006; **25**: 650–655.

15. Chen X, Su Y, Fingleton B et al. Increased plasma MMP9 in integrin alpha$_1$-null mice enhances lung metastasis of colon carcinoma cells. *Int J Cancer* 2005; **116**: 52–61.

16. Acuff HB, Sinnamon M, Fingleton B et al. Analysis of host- and tumor-derived proteinases using a custom dual species microarray reveals a protective role for stromal matrix metalloproteinase-12 in non-small cell lung cancer. *Cancer Res* 2006; **66**: 7968–7975.

17. Overall CM, Dean RA. Degradomics: systems biology of the protease web. Pleiotropic roles of MMPs in cancer. *Cancer Metastasis Rev* 2006; **25**: 69–75.

18. Wallard MJ, Pennington CJ, Veerakumarasivam A et al. Comprehensive profiling and localisation of the matrix metalloproteinases in urothelial carcinoma. *Br J Cancer* 2006; **94**: 569–577.

19. Pedersen TX, Pennington CJ, Almholt K et al. Extracellular protease mRNAs are predominantly expressed in the stromal areas of microdissected mouse breast carcinomas. *Oncogene* 2005; **24**: 1233–1240.

20. Ahokas K, Karjalainen-Lindsberg ML, Sihvo E, Isaka K, Salo J, Saarialho-Kere U. Matrix metalloproteinases 21 and 26 are differentially expressed in esophageal squamous cell cancer. *Tumour Biol.* 2006; **27**: 133–141.

21. Zucker S, Doshi K, Cao J. Measurement of matrix metalloproteinases (MMPs) and tissue inhibitors of metalloproteinases (TIMP) in blood and urine: potential clinical applications. *Adv Clin Chem* 2004; **38**: 37–85.

22. Overall CM, Lopez-Otin C. Strategies for MMP inhibition in cancer: innovations for the post-trial era. *Nat Rev Cancer* 2002; **2**: 657–672.

23. Snoek-van Buerden PA, Von den Hoff JW. Zymographic techniques for the analysis of matrix metalloproteinases and their inhibitors. *Biotechniques* 2005; **38**: 73–83.

24. Nemori R, Yamamoto M, Kataoka F et al. Development of *in situ* zymography to localize active matrix metalloproteinase-7 (matrilysin-1). *J Histochem Cytochem* 2005; **53**: 1227–1234.

25. Fujiwara A, Shibata E, Terashima H et al. Evaluation of matrix metalloproteinase-2 (MMP-2) activity with film *in situ* zymography for improved cytological diagnosis of breast tumors. *Breast Cancer* 2006; **13**: 272–278.

26. Hanemaaijer R, Visser H, Konttinen YT, Koolwijk P, Verheijen JH. A novel and simple immunocapture assay for determination of gelatinase-B (MMP-9) activities in biological fluids: saliva from patients with Sjogren's syndrome contain increased latent and active gelatinase-B levels. *Matrix Biol* 1998; **17**: 657–665.

27. Hesek D, Toth M, Meroueh SO et al. Design and characterization of a metalloproteinase inhibitor-tethered resin for the detection of active MMPs in biological samples. *Chem Biol* 2006; **13**: 379–386.

28. Osenkowski P, Toth M, Fridman R. Processing, shedding, and endocytosis of membrane type 1-matrix metalloproteinase (MT1-MMP). *J Cell Physiol* 2004; **200**: 2–10.

29. Yokoyama T, Nakamura H, Otani Y et al. Differences between scirrhous and non-scirrhous human gastric carcinomas from the aspect of proMMP-2 activation regulated by TIMP-3. *Clin Exp Metastasis* 2004; **21**: 223–233.

30. Bremer C, Bredow S, Mahmood U, Weissleder R, Tung CH. Optical imaging of matrix metalloproteinase-2 activity in tumors: feasibility study in a mouse model. *Radiology* 2001; **221**: 523–529.

31. McIntyre JO, Fingleton B, Wells KS et al. Development of a novel fluorogenic proteolytic beacon for *in vivo* detection and imaging of tumour-associated matrix metalloproteinase-7 activity. *Biochem J* 2004; **377**: 617–628.

32. Li WP, Anderson CJ. Imaging matrix metalloproteinase expression in tumors. *Q J Nucl Med* 2003; **47**: 201–208.
33. Schrohl AS, Christensen IJ, Pedersen AN *et al.* Tumor tissue concentrations of the proteinase inhibitors tissue inhibitor of metalloproteinases-1 (TIMP-1) and plasminogen activator inhibitor type 1 (PAI-1) are complementary in determining prognosis in primary breast cancer. *Mol Cell Proteomics* 2003; **2**: 164–172.
34. Holten-Andersen MN, Murphy G, Nielsen HJ *et al.* Quantitation of TIMP-1 in plasma of healthy blood donors and patients with advanced cancer. *Br J Cancer* 1999; **80**: 495–503.
35. Hoikkala S, Paakko P, Soini Y, Makitaro R, Kinnula V, Turpeenniemi-Hujanen T. Tissue MMP-2/TIMP-2-complex are better prognostic factors than serum MMP-2, MMP-9 or TIMP-1 in stage I–III lung carcinoma. *Cancer Lett* 2006; **236**: 125–132.
36. Rudin M, Weissleder R. Molecular imaging in drug discovery and development. *Nat Rev Drug Discov* 2003; **2**: 123–131.

Antony J. Freemont Judith A. Hoyland

6

Osteoarthritis: new concepts

Osteoarthrosis or osteoarthritis is a very common disorder of synovial joints[1] that has long been regarded as 'degenerative' and either part of the ageing process, or found in those who have 'abused' their joints through repeated trauma and/or obesity.

It was considered that the only treatments for osteoarthritis were either symptomatic or replacement of the joint with prosthetic implants. To researchers, this disorder appeared to offer little. However, there has been a recent explosion of interest in osteoarthritis, triggered by a realisation that far from being 'degenerative', it is a very active disorder characterised by imbalanced catabolic and anabolic processes affecting a number of different tissues in and around the joint. Furthermore, the disease processes of osteoarthritis are now recognised as being driven by complex molecular events from which it is hoped putative molecular therapeutic targets will be identified. In the dawning age of regenerative and molecular medicine, osteoarthritis has suddenly become a potentially treatable disorder, and molecular pathology holds all the clues to the new generation of therapeutics that could relieve this significant source of pain and disability.

NORMAL ANATOMY AND PHYSIOLOGY OF SYNOVIAL JOINTS

STRUCTURE AND STABILITY

The structure of synovial joints allows complex movements. The smooth surface of the articular cartilage that covers and separates the bone ends, and

Antony J. Freemont MD FRCP FRCPath (for correspondence)
Professor, Division of Regenerative Medicine, School of Medicine, Stopford Building, The University of Manchester, Oxford Road, Manchester M13 9PT, UK
E-mail: tonyfreemont@hotmail.com

Judith A. Hoyland PhD
Senior Lecturer in Molecular Pathology, Division of Regenerative Medicine, School of Medicine, Stopford Building, The University of Manchester, Oxford Road, Manchester M13 9PT, UK
E-mail: judith.hoyland@manchester.ac.uk

the lubricating action of synovial fluid facilitate these movements. The wide range of movements of synovial joints comes at a cost. The bone ends are not tethered together as they are in fibrous or cartilaginous joints, making the joint inherently unstable. Stability in synovial joints comes from the capsule/ligament/muscle/articular cartilage complex. Put very simply, the two opposing forces of the cartilage trying to push the bone apart and the capsule, ligaments and muscle preventing it, maintains stability. It follows that should there be a reduction in the thickness of the cartilage, or should the capsule, ligaments or muscles become lax or weakened, the joint will become unstable. Instability *per se* may lead to an increased risk of osteoarthritis or be a consequence of it.

SYNOVIUM AND SYNOVIAL FLUID

This space enclosed by the capsule is lined over the bone ends by cartilage and elsewhere by synovium. Synovium consists of:

1. An incomplete surface cell layer of synoviocytes made up of two cell populations, macrophages and fibroblast-derived cells, specialised to produce hyaluronans.

2. The subintima consisting of the fat and/or fibrous tissue that supports the synoviocyte layer. It contains the only blood vessels and nerves within the lining tissues of the joint.

Synovial fluid is a unique body fluid consisting of a transudate of plasma supplemented by hyaluronans.[2]

ARTICULAR CARTILAGE

Articular cartilage lies on, and is bound to, a surface consisting of a thin plate of bone (bone end plate [BEP]). Blood vessels in the bone marrow and penetrating into the BEP provide nutrients to the adjacent cartilage. Cartilage consists predominantly of extracellular matrix (ECM) in which are scattered chondrocytes. The ECM has two major components – type II collagen and proteoglycans.

The collagen bundles are arranged in loops with their free ends embedded in either the subchondral bone or the layer of calcified cartilage (Fig. 1) and their looped end close to, or at the surface of, the cartilage. These loops effectively tether the cartilage to the bone.

The main proteoglycan is aggrecan. This molecule is heavily sulphated, by virtue of the large number of chondroitin sulphate molecules attached to its core protein, and hydrophilic. By imbibing water, it swells, generating a high swelling pressure. The swelling pressure is resisted by the tethering effect of the collagen loops and, when the two forces are in equilibrium, cartilage becomes hard enough to withstand considerable loads.

Recently, Scott[3] has elucidated the role of different types of proteoglycan in cartilage morphology and function. He has shown that the collagen fibres are bound together by proteoglycan 'shape modules' which gives the cartilage strength and elasticity. The hydrophilic aggrecan is not uniformly distributed,

Function 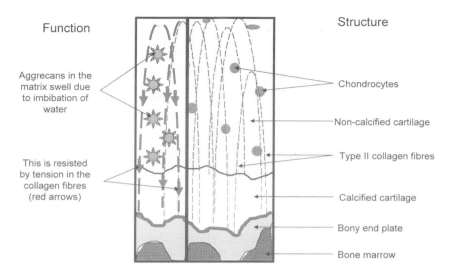 Structure

Aggrecans in the matrix swell due to imbibation of water

This is resisted by tension in the collagen fibres (red arrows)

Chondrocytes

Non-calcified cartilage

Type II collagen fibres

Calcified cartilage

Bony end plate

Bone marrow

Fig. 1 A diagram showing the structure of cartilage and its relationship to subchondral bone on the right and how the opposing forces of aggrecan swelling pressure and tension in the collagen fibres are balanced.

but instead has a predominantly pericellular distribution. This distribution means the cells are surrounded by a water-rich zone, which protects them and also acts as water 'sumps'.[4] Under load, water is forced out of the cartilage absorbing energy and allowing movement of nutrients in and out of the cartilage.

The chondrocytes lie in lacunae in the centre of the sumps (Fig. 2). Each lacune consists of a sphere of matrix rich in type VI collagen, which also protects the cell from damage during loading. The cell is attached to the inside of the sphere by cell adhesion molecules, it is thought predominantly $\alpha_4\beta_1$

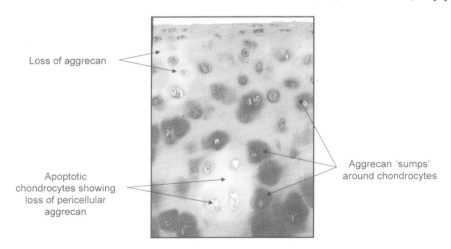

Loss of aggrecan

Apoptotic chondrocytes showing loss of pericellular aggrecan

Aggrecan 'sumps' around chondrocytes

Fig. 2 The superficial region of cartilage in early osteoarthritis. Shown is the normal distribution of aggrecan (purple staining) in pericellular 'sumps' and also loss of aggrecan in the superficial layers and around apoptotic chondrocytes.

integrin.[5] Although resistant to complete compression, the sphere is distensible. Through its attachments, the chondrocyte 'senses' the altered shape of the sphere and reacts by gene transcription. This process is known as mechanotransduction. Regular, cyclical loading is necessary for normal chondrocyte function.

It used to be thought that chondrocytes in adult cartilage were an unreplenishable population. It is now recognised that there is a 'stem cell' pool in the superficial layers of the cartilage.[6]

Molecular regulation of normal chondrocyte function is largely unknown, but *in vitro* studies suggest that extracellular matrix synthesis is regulated through the growth hormone/insulin-like growth factor axis, by IGF-1, IGF-2 and IGF-1-binding proteins (IGFBPs).[7] TGF-β1 can also stimulate proteoglycan core protein synthesis *in vitro* and levels are responsive to load which is significant in an habitually loaded tissue.

Much more is known about the regulation of chondrocyte biology during cartilage development, particularly as the precursor structure of long bones. For instance, in the embryo, chondrogenesis starts from mesenchymal precursor cells under the influence of extracellular growth and differentiation factors, which include bone morphogenic proteins, fibroblast growth factors (FGFs), parathyroid-hormone-related peptide (PTHrP), and members of the hedgehog and Wnt families. Members of the Sox family play a leading role in the process. Some of these genes are believed to play a part in the homeostasis of articular cartilage. Two members of the Sox family, L-Sox5 and Sox6, are linked to chondrocyte maturation and matrix formation[8] and Sox9 plays a role in the prevention of chondrocyte apoptosis. Fibroblast growth factor and PTHrP formed in peri-articular perichondrium and Indian hedgehog co-operate to retain a chondroid phenotype, preventing articular chondrocytes progressing to hypertrophy and apoptosis. The major difference between articular and growth plate cartilage is this failure of chondrocytes to undergo 'full maturation' to the hypertrophic phenotype in the former. The reasons for this are not well understood.

PATHOLOGY OF OSTEOARTHRITIS

All the tissues in the joint, cartilage, bone, synovium and synovial fluid, are affected in osteoarthritis.[9] The most recent advances in understanding osteoarthritis come from new knowledge of its molecular pathology, but, this is only meaningful when related to the 'conventional' macroscopic and microscopic pathology. Whilst the ideal would be to correlate molecular and morphological changes in tissue biology in human tissue, this is not possible because human osteoarthritis tissue is difficult to obtain during the progression of the disorder, most coming to the pathologists only as part of the treatment of end-stage disease. Such is the nature of human biopsy pathology that, even when tissue is obtained with different morphological characteristics, the progression of the disease can only be assumed by extrapolation. To understand fully the morphological and molecular events during the progression of osteoarthritis, particularly in its earliest stages, requires the use of animal models.

ANIMAL MODELS

The most widely used model is the Pond–Nuki[10] cruciate ligament transection model in the dog, which has become a gold standard for exploring the mechanisms of osteoarthritis and its treatment. Spontaneous forms of osteoarthritis in rats, guinea pigs, dogs, horses, monkeys and other species have also been studied; some, such as the STR/ort mouse, have reached the same status as the dog model.

Novel gene manipulation models including those with targeted deletions directed at components of the matrix, degradative enzymes and other molecules have also given interesting insights into potential disease mechanisms.[11]

These models offer new ways for: (i) studying the initial (and later) stages of the molecular pathology of osteoarthritis process; (ii) identifying candidate genes; (iii) biomarker identification; and (iv) investigating therapeutic interventions.

ARTICULAR CARTILAGE

The initial changes in the cartilage are focal loss of proteoglycan from the superficial layers. The reduction in proteoglycan disturbs the balance between the swelling pressure of the proteoglycan and the tension of the type II collagen fibres, making the cartilage softer and more susceptible to load-induced changes, including damage to the collagen fibre arrays (Fig. 3). Damage to the collagen fibres leads to the development of superficial splits (fissures) that propagate both parallel with, and at right angles to, the surface. Ultimately, this results in an area from which articular cartilage is completely lost and bone/calcified cartilage exposed. This area is surrounded by a region of damaged cartilage, often containing clusters of calcium crystals (notably calcium pyrophosphate). The exposed bone becomes worn smooth (eburnation), the articular surface develops an abnormal shape, and the joint becomes unstable.

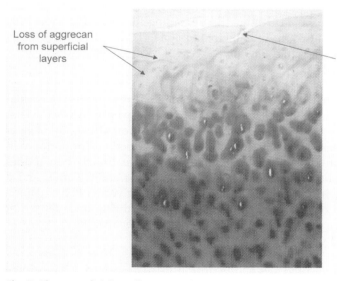

Loss of aggrecan from superficial layers

Reduced swelling pressure leads to 'softening' of superficial cartilage and damage under load

Fig. 3 The superficial cartilage in early osteoarthritis. Loss of aggrecan has lead to softening of the superficial layers and the early development of trauma-induced slits.

During this process, there is a general loss of chondrocytes from the cartilage, initially leaving empty chondrocyte lacunae, but residual chondrocytes, particularly those deep in the cartilage undergo division to form clusters. Radiotracer studies have shown that the residual chondrocytes are hypermetabolic.

Matrix degradation

The loss/change of matrix molecules in osteoarthritis has been a driver to investigate the mechanisms by which the matrix turns over normally and how that changes in osteoarthritis. Cartilage matrix turnover requires matrix degradation as well as synthesis. Degradation is a key element in both normal matrix regulation and the excessive breakdown that characterises osteoarthritis.

Aggrecan has an average turnover in adult cartilage of a few years, compared to several decades for collagen II. Aggrecan loss is an early event in osteoarthritis. *In vitro*, matrix metalloproteinases (MMPs) and particularly the related ADAMTS (a disintegrin and metalloprotease with thrombospondin motifs), have aggrecansase activity but are active at different sites. Thus MMP-13 degrades aggrecan core protein at the Asn341–Phe342 whereas ADAMTS 4 and 5 cleave the molecule at the Glu373–Ala374.[12] Because they are the most active aggrecan degrading enzymes ADAMTS 4 and ADAMTS 5 are known as 'aggrecanase'. ADAMTS synthesis is stimulated by interleukin-1 (IL-1) and retinoids and inhibited by tissue inhibitor of matrix metalloproteinases 3 (TIMP-3).[13] Overexpression occurs in osteoarthritis and synthetic inhibitors will protect cartilage from breakdown *in vitro*.[14] The thrombospondin motif is essential for enzyme function by binding to the GAG chains of aggrecan.

MMPs are involved in matrix turnover and in osteoarthritis. Many MMPs are up-regulated in osteoarthritis but the key MMPs are the collagenases, particularly MMP-13 which is the most active type II collagenase.[15] Different MMPs are, in part, found in different zones of the cartilage, indicating different roles. The membrane-bound proteases, TM-MMPs, participate in activation of MMPs but may also have a direct matrix-degrading function. The same cells that produce MMPs also produce their inhibitors, TIMPs. In osteoarthritis there is an imbalance, leading to relative excess of MMPs over TIMPs.

Matrix proteins

One matrix protein that is the source of considerable current interest in normal and osteoarthritis joints is cartilage oligomeric matrix protein (COMP). First described in 1992, COMP is a highly anionic protein found in a number of tissues, but particularly cartilage. It is of paramount functional importance in regulating the structure of embryonic and adult cartilage. Exactly how it does this is unknown, but it is a member of the thrombospondin family and a pentamer allowing it to bind to several glycosaminoglycans. It has gained particular attention as an investigative tool in osteoarthritis since its serum concentration relates to development of progressive osteoarthritis.[16]

Cytokines

As understanding of the processes of osteoarthritis have developed, it has become clear that so called 'pro-inflammatory mediators' including cytokines (IL-1, IL-8, TGF-β, CSF, PAF, TNF, VEGF) and other mediators (NO, eicosanoids, PTH) play a fundamental role in the initiation and progression of osteoarthritis[17] and are being increasingly identified as therapeutic targets in osteoarthritis.[18]

IL-1 and TNF-α play key roles in altering cartilage extracellular matrix turnover. *In vitro*, IL-1 will stimulate MMP-3 mRNA synthesis and suppress TIMP, increase expression of the enzyme plasminogen activator (PA) and reduce its inhibitor. Active IL-1 has been found in osteoarthritis synovial membrane suggesting that activated synoviocytes are responsible for producing the IL-1 in osteoarthritis.

Other cytokines produced during flares of osteoarthritis (IL-6, IL-8, IL-17) can supplement IL-1 activity and others are inhibitory (IL-4, IL-10, IL-13, interferon-γ).[19] A unifying hypothesis[20] states that soluble mediators characteristic of inflammation pathways lead to chondrocyte and synoviocyte activation that, in turn, initiate and cause progression of osteoarthritis. It follows that, if this hypothesis is correct, effective therapies for osteoarthritis would be targeted at these molecules. Trials of IL-1 inhibitors (IL-1 receptor antagonist and the soluble decoy type II receptor) support this hypothesis.[21]

TNF-α has similar effects to IL-1[19,22] and two TNF-α blocking agents have been shown to suppress some of the mechanisms active in A-cartilage degradation. Taken together, these results suggest that cytokine networks involving IL-1 and TNF-α, working individually or synergistically, amplify cartilage tissue injury responses in osteoarthritis.

Nitric oxide

One mechanism by which IL-1 and TNF-α are believed to work in osteoarthritis is through production of NO by activating the inducible synthase, iNOS. Human chondrocytes obtained from osteoarthritis cartilage express iNOS and produce micromolar amounts of NO in culture whereas iNOS is not expressed by normal chondrocytes. The mechanism of action of NO is not clear. Current data suggest that it is multifactorial, inhibiting matrix synthesis and promoting chondrocyte apoptosis affecting chondrocyte adhesion and cell-surface signalling pathways and through COX-2 mediated production of prostaglandin E_2. Whatever the mechanism of action, selective inhibition of iNOS with *N*-iminoethyl-L-lysine (L-NIL) reduces matrix damage in the Pond–Nuki model.[23]

Apoptosis and cartilage regeneration

The longevity of chondrocytes in normal articular cartilage is a testament to their having inherent resistance to apoptosis. Evidence from *in vitro* studies suggests that chondrocytes require an intact 3-D matrix to resist apoptosis which may partly explain the increased apoptosis in a disorder characterised by matrix degradation. Recent observations that cartilage contains a stem-cell population may indicate that cell turnover (presumably through apoptosis) is occurring in normal cartilage.[6]

In osteoarthritis, apoptosis is increased and the cells are not replaced, as shown by a high proportion of empty lacunae on microscopy (Fig. 4). As discussed above, local NO production is believed to be a key mediator of apoptosis in osteoarthritis.[24]

Tissue repair does occur in osteoarthritis but it is not known whether the new chondrocytes are formed from the cartilage stem-cell pool. Once the

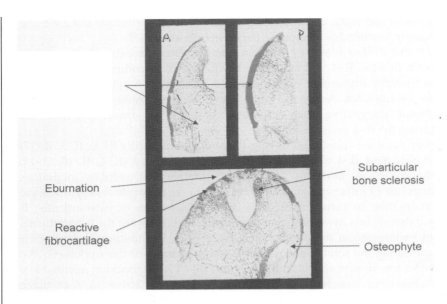

Eburnation

Subarticular
bone sclerosis

Reactive
fibrocartilage

Osteophyte

Fig. 4 Sections through a femoral head in end-stage osteoarthritis to show eburnation, bione sclerosis, osteophytes and an intra-osseous cyst (geode)

collagen network has been damaged, it is not possible to repair the cartilage as such. Instead, there is a cellular repair response which starts at the periphery of the joint. Cellular cartilage extends over, and sometimes dissects into, the damaged cartilage. This repair cartilage is usually much more cellular than the pre-existing articular cartilage and the matrix is fibrocartilage. Small islands of fibrocartilage may also form within, and extend up to the surface of, the eburnated bone. In this setting, chondrocytes are thought to form from mesenchymal stem cells (MSCs) within the marrow. Dependent upon the load environment, the fibrocartilage can (but rarely does) grow over the eburnated surface.

Crystal deposition

Deposition of calcium pyrophosphate dehydrate (CPPD) crystals is a common finding in osteoarthritis cartilage, synovium and fibrocartilage and basic calcium phosphate and calcium hydroxyapatite are also commonly seen.[25] CPPD is easily detected radiographically. In several studies, the prevalence of crystal occurrence relates to duration and severity of osteoarthritis, particularly in less commonly involved joints such as shoulder, elbows and wrists. Perhaps surprisingly, the incidence of pseudogout is not much higher in these patients. Injection of CPPD into joints affected by osteoarthritis accelerates the progression of disease[26] but injection into normal joints does not induce osteoarthritis. Calcium crystals exert their effects by up-regulating eicosanoids and MMPs and through inducing altered signal transduction through calcium-dependent protein and MAP kinases. Basic calcium phosphate can induce MMP production synergistically with IL-1 and TNF-α and can even lead to production of these cytokines.

OTHER STRUCTURES WITHIN THE JOINT

The changes within the osteoarthritic joint are not restricted to the articular cartilage. The disease process also affects the subchondral and marginal bone and the synovium and synovial fluid.

Subchondral bone

There is a view[27] that the first detectable changes in joints that will go on to become osteoarthritic are thickening and increased density of the subchondral bone plate, raising the suggestion that the initiating event in osteoarthritis is an alteration of the flow of nutrients into the articular cartilage from the adjacent bone marrow. How this reconciles with the pathology of avascular bone necrosis, in which the only part of the tissue not to be affected by profound ischaemia at bone ends is the articular cartilage, is just one element in an on-going debate. Other contributions include: (i) in the Pond–Nuki osteoarthritis model, disturbed proteoglycan metabolism are the initial events, and only later do subchondral and other bone changes occur; and (ii) by contrast, in a spontaneous form of osteoarthritis in the macaque, the earliest changes were seen in bone rather than cartilage.[28] A further view has been developed from studies of subchondral bone thickness and density in human knee joint preparations using high-resolution radiography. Cartilage damage in the tibial or femoral region did not correlate with subchondral bone thickness or quality, perhaps indicating that the subchondral bone changes observed in osteoarthritis may be more related to age than to osteoarthritis.[29]

There is, however, no doubt that in most cases of osteoarthritis there is a generalised anabolic effect in bone. This causes increased cell activity generally, but with an excess of osteoblastic bone deposition leading to subchondral bone sclerosis and osteophyte formation.

Osteophytes

It is believed that instability causes osteophyte formation but the mechanism(s) is/are still unknown. The net effect of osteophyte formation is to increase the area of the articulating surface. Some osteophytes form because of a change in phenotype of mid-zone chondrocytes near the edge of the cartilage. These develop behaviour similar to that of fetal growth plate chondrocytes, becoming hypertrophic and leading to new bone formation through endochondral ossification.[30] Other osteophytes form by endochondral ossification from foci of chondroid metaplasia at the enthesis (the junction of capsular and ligamentous insertions into bone) at the joint margins. They are almost certainly the result of traction injuries secondary to joint instability.

Bone cysts

Bone cysts or geodes are a feature of advanced osteoarthritis. They form as a consequence of synovial fluid entering the bone marrow. Unlike cartilage, bone is naturally permeated by narrow channels, either in the form of Haversian systems or the canaliculi linking osteocyte lacunae, making convenient routes for synovial fluid to be forced under pressure through the bone. Once in the marrow, the synovial fluid elicits a bipolar reaction with osteoclastic bone destruction and osteoblastic bone deposition, ultimately causing the formation of bone cysts containing fibrous or myxoid tissue, and lined by sclerotic bone and fibrous tissue.

Synovium

In osteoarthritis, the synovium is thrown into finger-like folds or villi. There is an increase in the number and size of synoviocytes in the synovial membrane. As many of these cells are effectively activated macrophages, it is not surprising that the milieu of the osteoarthritis joint is one rich in cytokines and inflammatory mediators.

In many cases, particularly early in the course of the disease, the synovium appears inflamed to the naked eye. This is due to increased blood flow through the subintima and perivascular oedema associated with a mast cell infiltrate.[31] As disease advances, there is progressive synovial fibrosis. Whilst there is never the florid accumulation of lymphocytes and plasma cells in the villi and synovial subintima that is seen in the inflammatory arthropathies, frequently, particularly in advanced osteoarthritis, perivascular aggregates of lymphocytes are seen in the synovium and, more rarely, occasional plasma cells. Occasionally, bone and cartilage debris enter the synovium and elicit a macrophage response. Aggregates of calcium pyrophosphate crystals are also sometimes seen in the synovium.

In the Pond–Nuki model, synovitis is common. Similarly, there may be classical, low-grade chronic inflammation with increased numbers of NK cells even in early osteoarthritis.[32] In the STR/ORT spontaneous mouse model of osteoarthritis, cellular inflammation is also a feature, which is different to the pathology in humans.

Synovial fluid

In osteoarthritis, the synovial fluid often increases in volume, particularly during the acute 'flares' that characterise the clinical course of osteoarthritis. The fluid remains viscid but contains debris (*e.g.* articular cartilage, pyrophosphate and hydroxyapatite crystals, bone, and fragments of synovial villi) shed into the fluid from the deteriorating articular surfaces and joint lining. The cell count is always low, never exceeding 1000 cells/mm^3.[2]

LOAD AND OSTEOARTHRITIS

In vitro studies have established that normal chondrocyte function is dependent on intermittent loading, without which matrix synthesis stops. By extrapolation, cartilage health should be dependent upon repetitive low-impact exercises and the available data support this view. There is, however, an association between osteoarthritis and abnormal patterns of load in some clinical or life-style settings,[33] particularly those associated with repetitive, high-impact movements. Gait analysis has also shown a correlation between loading and imaging evidence of osteoarthritis.

During normal movement, articulating surfaces are exposed to very high loads (*e.g.* several times body weight in the hip and knees). Chondrocytes within their lacunae undergo deformation when cartilage is compressed initiating mechanotransductive events. At the same time, water and solutes such as cytokines move in and out of the cartilage. These fluxes in regulatory molecules and nutrients critically influence chondrocyte biology. Studies using explants from normal joints have shown that cyclical loading stimulates whereas constant load inhibits matrix synthesis, supporting the view that chondrocyte phenotype is load-dependent. Within acceptable limits, strenuous exercise in dogs causes increased cartilage proteoglycan content and tri-athletes evolve larger weight-bearing joint surfaces in the knee, indicating two adaptive mechanisms to prolonged increased mechanical stress.[34]

Exploring the mechanisms behind the mechanotransductive events leading to cartilage changes following loading Salter's group has shown that load causes its effects through an integrin-dependent IL-4 autocrine/paracrine loop.[5,35] Osteoarthritis chondrocytes do not show this anabolic type of response. The integrin $\alpha_5\beta_1$ serves as the mechanoreceptor in both osteoarthritis and normal chondrocytes but downstream signalling appears abnormal in osteoarthritis.

FUTURE ROLE OF THE PATHOLOGIST IN THE MANAGEMENT OF OSTEOARTHRITIS

The pathogenesis of osteoarthritis is becoming better understood as a consequence of the application of new techniques (particularly those of molecular pathology) to its study. These data are already yielding new therapeutic targets. More targets will evolve as the complex interactions between chondrocytes and their environment (humoral, cartilage matrix and load) begin to be unravelled. It has already been shown that: (i) at the molecular level (or the morphological), osteoarthritis is not the same disease in all joints;[36] (ii) distinct genetic risk factors may predispose different joint sites to osteoarthritis; and (iii) different joints show differences in resistance to the development of osteoarthritis.[37] Improved experimental models, in part based on gene manipulation, and expanding knowledge of the cell biology of joint tissue will bring new insights to disease processes and, in turn, novel methods of repairing osteoarthritis joints and in prevention of progression of joint damage.[38]

That individual patients might have different patterns of molecular disturbances in what at first sight appears to be a single disease is very reminiscent of the emerging understanding of cancer. Is it possible, therefore, that just as the molecular pathologist is becoming increasingly involved in identifying diagnostic and prognostic features in individuals with cancer, so he or she will come to play a pivotal role in tailoring treatment to the needs of individual patients with osteoarthritis?

Points for best practice

- The point prevalence of osteoarthritis is the highest of any disease on earth.
- Although the cartilage changes may be the same in different joints affected by osteoarthritis, the underlying molecular mechanisms are different.

(continued on next page)

Points for best practice (continued)

- The synovium in osteoarthritis might well show evidence of inflammation in the absences of an underlying inflammatory arthropathy.

- In established osteoarthritis there may be large numbers of lymphocytes and occasional plasma cells in fibrotic synovium. This is a normal accompaniment of osteoarthritis.

- Osteoarthritis can present as a single 'red and hot' and surgeons often describe the synovium of osteoarthritic joints as 'inflamed' at arthroscopy.

- Calcium pyrophosphate crystals in the synovium or synovial fluid are a common feature of osteoarthritis and do not indicate pseudogout unless there is associated acute inflammation.

- The presence of calcium crystals in the synovium of an osteoarthritic joint is a poor prognostic sign, usually indicating a faster decline to end-stage osteoarthritis.

- In the future, the pathologist will be called upon to determine the molecular pathways leading to osteoarthritis changes in particular joints in order to direct targeted therapy.

References

1. Sharma L, Kapoor D, Issa S. Epidemiology of osteoarthritis: an update. *Curr Opin Rheumatol* 2006; **18**: 147–156.
2. Freemont AJ, Denton J. *Atlas of Synovial Fluid Cytopathology*. Dordrecht: Kluwer, 1991.
3. Scott JE. Elasticity in extracellular matrix 'shape modules' of tendon, cartilage, *etc*. A sliding proteoglycan-filament model. *J Physiol* 2003; **553**: 335–343.
4. Scott JE, Stockwell RA. Cartilage elasticity resides in shape module decoran and aggrecan sumps of damping fluid: implications in osteoarthrosis. *J Physiol* 2006; **574**: 643–650.
5. Salter DM, Millward-Sadler SJ, Nuki G, Wright MO. Integrin–interleukin-4 mechano-transduction pathways in human chondrocytes. *Clin Orthop* 2001; **391 (Suppl)**: S49–S60.
6. Dowthwaite GP, Bishop JC, Redman SN *et al*. The surface of articular cartilage contains a progenitor cell population. *J Cell Sci* 2004; **117**: 889–897.
7. Middleton J, Manthey A, Tyler J. Insulin-like growth factor (IGF) receptor, IGF-I, interleukin-1β (IL-1β), and IL-6 mRNA expression in osteoarthritic and normal human cartilage. *J Histochem Cytochem* 1996; **44**: 133–141.
8. Ikeda T, Kawaguchi H, Kamekura S *et al*. Distinct roles of Sox5, Sox6, and Sox9 in different stages of chondrogenic differentiation. *J Bone Miner Metab* 2005; **23**: 337–340.
9. Martel-Pelletier J, Pelletier JP. New insights into the major pathophysiological processes responsible for the development of osteoarthritis. *Semin Arthritis Rheum* 2005; **34 (Suppl 2)**: 6–8.
10. Pond MJ, Nuki G. Experimentally-induced osteoarthritis in the dog. *Ann Rheum Dis* 1973; **32**: 387–388.
11. Salminen H, Vuorio E, Samaanen AH. Expression of Sox9 and type IIA procollagen during attempted repair of articular cartilage damage in a transgenic mouse model of osteoarthritis. *Arthritis Rheum* 2001; **44**: 947–955.
12. Struglics A, Larsson S, Pratta MA *et al*. Human osteoarthritis synovial fluid and joint cartilage contain both aggrecanase- and matrix metalloproteinase-generated aggrecan fragments. *Osteoarthritis Cartilage* 2006; **14**: 101–113.

13. Kevorkian L, Young DA, Darrah C *et al.* Expression profiling of metalloproteinases and their inhibitors in cartilage. *Arthritis Rheum* 2004; **50**: 131–141.
14. Malfait AM, Liu RQ, Ijiri K *et al.* Inhibition of ADAM-TS4 and ADAM-TS5 prevents aggrecan degradation in osteoarthritic cartilage. *J Biol Chem* 2002; **277**: 22201–22208.
15. Freemont AJ, Byers RJ, Taiwo YO, Hoyland JA. *In situ* zymographic localisation of type II collagen degrading activity in osteoarthritic human articular cartilage. *Ann Rheum Dis* 1999; **58**: 357–365.
16. Punzi L, Oliviero F, Plebani M. New biochemical insights into the pathogenesis of osteoarthritis and the role of laboratory investigations in clinical assessment. *Crit Rev Clin Lab Sci* 2005; **42**: 279–309.
17. Goldring SR, Goldring MB. The role of cytokines in cartilage matrix degeneration in osteoarthritis. *Clin Orthop* 2004; **427 (Suppl)**: S27–S36.
18. Malemud CJ. Cytokines as therapeutic targets for osteoarthritis. *BioDrugs* 2004; **8**: 23–35.
19. Goldring MB. The role of cytokines as inflammatory mediators in osteoarthritis: lessons from animal models. *Connect Tissue Res* 1999; **40**: 1–11.
20. Pelletier J-P, Martel-Pelletier J, Abramson SB. Osteoarthritis, an inflammatory disease. Potential implication for the selection of new therapeutic targets. *Arthritis Rheum* 2001; **44**: 1237–1247.
21. Evans CH, Gouze JN, Gouze E, Robbins PD, Ghivizzani SC. Osteoarthritis gene therapy. *Gene Ther* 2004; **11**: 379–389.
22. Westacott CI, Baraket AF, Wood L *et al.* Tumor necrosis factor alpha can contribute to focal loss of cartilage in osteoarthritis. *Osteoarthritis Cartilage* 2000; **8**: 213–221.
23. Pelletier JP, Jovanovic DV, Lascau-Coman V *et al.* Selective inhibition of inducible nitric oxide synthase reduces progression of experimental osteoarthritis *in vivo*: possible link with the reduction in chondrocyte apoptosis and caspase 3 level. *Arthritis Rheum* 2000; **43**: 1290–1299.
24. Aigner T, Kim HA, Roach HI. Apoptosis in osteoarthritis. *Rheum Dis Clin North Am* 2004; **30**: 639–653.
25. Olmez N, Schumacher Jr HR. Crystal deposition and osteoarthritis. *Curr Rheumatol Report* 1999; **1**: 107–111.
26. Fam AG, Morava-Protzner I, Purcell C *et al.* Acceleration of experimental lapine osteoarthritis by calcium pyrophosphate microcrystalline synovitis. *Arthritis Rheum* 1995; **38**: 201–210.
27. Hunter DJ, Spector TD. The role of bone metabolism in osteoarthritis. *Curr Rheumatol Report* 2003; **5**: 15–19.
28. Carlson CS, Loeser RF, Purser CB *et al.* Osteoarthritis in cynomolgus macaques. III: Effects of age, gender, and subchondral bone thickness on the severity of disease. *J Bone Miner Res* 1996; **11**: 1209–1217.
29. Yamada K, Healey R, Amiel D *et al.* Subchondral bone of the human knee joint in aging and osteoarthritis. *Osteoarthritis Cartilage* 2002; **10**: 360–369.
30. Hoyland JA, Thomas JT, Donn R *et al.* Distribution of type X collagen in normal and osteoarthritis human cartilage. *Bone Miner* 1991; **15**: 151–164.
31. Dean G, Hoyland JA, Denton J *et al.* Mast cells in the synovium and synovial fluid in osteoarthritis. *Br J Rheum* 1993; **32**: 671–675.
32. Smith MD, Triantafillou S, Parker A *et al.* Synovial membrane inflammation and cytokine production in patients with early osteoarthritis. *J Rheumatol* 1997; **24**: 365–371.
33. Kurz B, Lemke AK, Fay J, Pufe T, Grodzinsky AJ, Schunke M. Pathomechanisms of cartilage destruction by mechanical injury. *Ann Anat* 2005; **187**: 473–485.
34. Eckstein F, Faber S, Muhlbauer R *et al.* Functional adaptation of human joints to mechanical stimuli. *Osteoarthritis Cartilage* 2002; **10**: 44–50.
35. Chowdhury TT, Appleby RN, Salter DM, Bader DA, Lee DA. Integrin-mediated mechanotransduction in IL-1 beta stimulated chondrocytes. *Biomech Model Mechanobiol* 2006; **5**: 192–201.
36. Kuettner KE, Cole AA. Cartilage degeneration in different human joints. *Osteoarthritis Cartilage* 2005; **13**: 93–103.
37. Cole AA, Kuettner KE. Molecular basis for differences between human joints. *Cell Mol Life Sci* 2002; **59**: 19–26.
38. Ge Z, Hu Y, Heng BC *et al.* Osteoarthritis and therapy. *Arthritis Rheum* 2006; **55**: 493–500.

David N. Slater

7

Cutaneous pseudolymphoma

Pseudolymphoma is a term which, over the years, has met variable acceptability. In particular, there was a dip in credibility in the 1990s, with the discovery that many historical pseudolymphomas were examples of mucosa-associated lymphoid tissue (MALT) lymphoma. Despite this, however, the term has remained in frequent use. Dermatologists, in particular, support the term and include it in a long list of so-called pseudodermatoses.

Histopathologically, the diagnosis of cutaneous pseudolymphoma is now used either in the context of specific disease entities which incorporate the term or when an exogenous cause for the reactive cellular response can be identified. In other instances, especially when the cause is not known, the term cutaneous lymphoid hyperplasia is favoured.

The term cutaneous pseudolymphoma now enjoys unreserved acceptance following the recent World Health Organization (WHO) publication on skin tumours.[1] One chapter is specifically titled 'Lymphoid infiltrates of the skin mimicking lymphoma (cutaneous pseudolymphoma)'. Cutaneous pseudolymphoma is defined by the WHO as a reactive polyclonal benign lymphoproliferative disease, predominantly composed of either B-cells or T-cells, localised or disseminated. It heals spontaneously after cessation of the causative factor (*e.g.* drugs) or after non-aggressive treatment.

CLINICAL ASPECTS OF CUTANEOUS PSEUDOLYMPHOMA

Clinical manifestations of cutaneous pseudolymphoma are frequently not diagnostic and overlap with lymphoma. Two main problems exist:

1. Lesional regression is common in cutaneous lymphoma and, accordingly, regression does not necessarily indicate that the lesion is pseudolymphoma.

David N. Slater BMedSci MB ChB FRCPath
Department of Histopathology, Royal Hallamshire Hospital, Glossop Road, Sheffield S10 2JF, UK
E-mail: david.slater@sth.nhs.uk

2. Occasional cases of initial cutaneous pseudolymphoma can evolve into lymphoma (so-called 'pseudo-pseudolymphoma').

In general, pseudolymphoma is rare on the scalp and never displays clinical poikiloderma. In addition, lesions showing variability in size, shape and colour and occurring in non-sun-exposed skin (such as the buttocks) should be regarded as cutaneous T-cell lymphoma (CTCL) until proved otherwise.

In practice, however, cutaneous lymphoma remains a rare disease and is numerically overshadowed by cases of cutaneous pseudolymphoma. Although diagnostically important not to miss cutaneous lymphoma, it is equally important that lymphoma is not overdiagnosed. As many cutaneous lymphomas are of low-grade biological type, there should be a low clinicopathological threshold for adopting a follow-up and re-biopsy approach in difficult and uncertain cases. All of the latter should receive detailed immunohistochemical and genotypic investigations and be discussed in a multidisciplinary team setting. Clinico-pathological correlation remains paramount and distinction between cutaneous lymphoma and pseudolymphoma should rely on a constellation of criteria and not on a solitary feature.

SPECIFIC DISEASES THAT CAN MIMIC CUTANEOUS LYMPHOMA

EPITHELIAL NEOPLASMS

Neoplastic epithelial cells in tumours such as neuroendocrine carcinoma (Merkel cell tumour), neuroblastoma and primitive neuro-ectodermal tumour can mimic cutaneous lymphoma. Epidermal involvement in Merkel cell tumour can result in intra-epidermal collections of cells that mimic Pautrier micro-abscesses in CTCL and distinction from lymphoma may depend on immunohistochemistry.

LYMPHOCYTE-RICH EPITHELIAL NEOPLASMS

Some epithelial neoplasms can, at times, contain sufficient numbers of lymphocytes to mimic cutaneous lymphoma. Classically, these include eccrine spiradenoma and lympho-epithelioma-like carcinoma of the skin. A more recent entity is cutaneous lympho-adenoma, although increasingly this is regarded as a trichoblastoma with adamantinoid features (Fig. 1).[2] Immunohistochemistry may be necessary to reveal the underlying epithelial component.

IMMUNE RESPONSE TO EPITHELIAL DYSPLASIA OR MALIGNANCY AND OTHER NEOPLASMS

Cutaneous neoplasms such a basal cell carcinoma, malignant melanoma and dermatofibroma can elicit extremely strong lymphocytic stromal responses, in which the underlying neoplasm can be difficult to identify. Indeed, complete regression of the neoplasm can result in a residual dense lymphoid infiltrate and no evidence of the original tumour.

Lymphomatoid variants of actinic keratosis and benign lichenoid keratosis (lichen planus-like keratosis) exist.[3] Some cases of the latter probably reflect

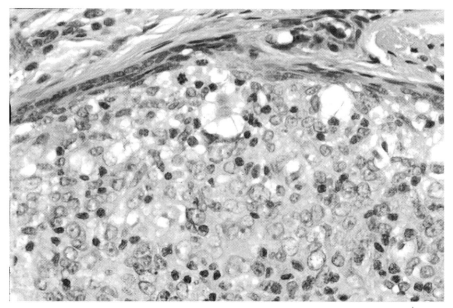

Fig. 1 Cutaneous lymphadenoma characterised by small lymphocytes and larger epithelial cells of adnexal origin.

end-stage regression of an original lesion that may, for example, have been a seborrhoeic keratosis or melanocytic abnormality.[4] In an attempt to identify an underlying lesion, there should be a low threshold for requesting step sections and immunohistochemistry. In this situation, many histopathologists use the melanocytic antibody Melan A to exclude partially regressed melanoma.

DISEASES SEEN UNCOMMONLY IN THE SKIN

The list of diseases seen infrequently in the skin, but which can mimic lymphoma, include extramedullary haemopoiesis, malakoplakia, Whipple's disease ectopic thymus, Rosai–Dorfman disease, inflammatory pseudotumour, Castleman's disease and Kikuchi's disease.

Rosai–Dorfman disease in the skin can herald, co-exist with or follow nodal or systemic disease.[5] Its histological appearance is usefully remembered by the alternative term of histiocytic lymphophagocytic panniculitis. The large cells present are positive for S100 and display emperipolesis (Fig. 2). Moderate numbers of plasma cells are usually present and the stroma can appear sclerotic or storiform.

Inflammatory pseudotumours probably represent a spectrum of disease that incorporates plasma cell granuloma and inflammatory myofibroblastic tumour.[6] The former can display germinal centres, plasma cells and fibrosis. The latter displays myofibroblastic proliferation and 2p23 re-arrangement.

Castleman's disease, especially the plasma cell variant, can present in the skin and in particular the vulva.[7] In difficult cases, the identification of human herpes virus type 8 can be helpful.

Kikuchi's disease can exist in the skin and display the characteristic features of necrosis, karyorrhexis, apoptosis, immunoblasts and plasma cells.[8] All

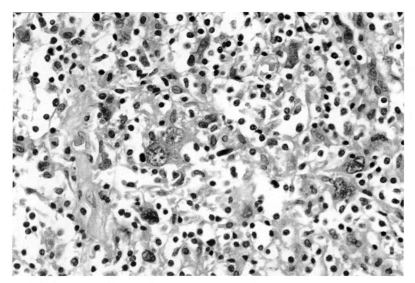

Fig. 2 Cutaneous Rosai–Dorfman disease displaying large atypical histiocytes.

potential cases should be accompanied by investigations to exclude the possibility of lupus erythematosus.

CLASSICAL DERMATOSES

Many classical dermatoses can, at times, mimic lymphoma and this is particularly frequent with autoimmune and connective tissue disorders.

Lupus erythematosus

Lupus erythematosus profundus is now more frequently referred to as lupus erythematosus panniculitis and characteristic features include epidermal involvement, germinal centre formation, plasma cells and hyaline necrosis. Cases may be extremely difficult to distinguish from subcutaneous panniculitis-like T-cell lymphoma and there has been debate whether a spectrum of disease between the two can exist. This has resulted in some acceptance of an intermediary entity within the broad diagnostic group of lymphocytic lobular panniculitis. This has been variably described as indeterminate lymphocytic lobular panniculitis or more recently atypical lymphocytic lobular panniculitis.[9] As well as atypical cells, T-cell monoclones may be identified on gamma T-cell receptor (TCR) gene re-arrangement analysis.

Occasionally, lupus erythematosus can display localisation on hair follicles mimicking the folliculotropic variant of mycosis fungoides. This mimicry can be further intensified by the presence of follicular mucinosis.

The nosological status of tumid lupus erythematosus remains uncertain but a useful histopathological feature is the presence of copious dermal mucin.

Lichen sclerosus

The interface dermatosis present in lichen sclerosus can closely mimic cutaneous CTCL and especially so in early stages.[10] In addition, some cases of lichen sclerosus can display florid, small-to-medium blood vessel lymphocytic vasculitis which closely resembles angiocentric variants of cutaneous lymphoma.[11]

Pigmented purpuric dermatosis and lichen aureus
Some cases of pigmented purpuric dermatosis and lichen aureus can evolve into CTCL.[12] Suspicion is particularly raised in cases which are persistent or contain atypical cells. In these cases, however, consideration should also be given a possible drug-related aetiology.[13]

Lymphomatoid dermatitis/eczema
Although classically described in association with external sensitisation, it is now recognised to occur in occasional cases of atopic dermatitis and, in particular, those with high IgE levels.

Lymphomatoid folliculitis
This entity occurs predominantly in patients under 50 years of age and immunohistochemistry reveals mixed populations of B- and T-cells.[14] In addition, the most characteristic diagnostic feature is the presence of moderate numbers of perifollicular antigen-presenting cells which are CD1a and S100 positive. Another feature is the tendency towards spontaneous regression. Some reported cases may have represented primary cutaneous CD4-positive small/medium-sized pleomorphic T-cell lymphoma.

Acne rosacea
Although poorly described in the dermatological and histopathological literature, acne rosacea can be characterised by follicular interface changes which, together with a paucity of granulomas, can mimic early stages of follicular CTCL.

Angiolymphoid hyperplasia and Kimura's disease
Both can be characterised by large numbers of lymphocytes and/or eosinophils. Prominent hob-nail endothelial cells with vacuoles in small-to-medium sized vessels, and germinal centres are the main diagnostic clues to angiolymphoid hyperplasia. In patients from outside the UK, Kimura's disease can mimic human T-cell lymphotropic lymphoma.

Chronic photodermatoses
Chronic actinic dermatitis (including actinic reticuloid) and polymorphous light eruption are classical mimics of cutaneous lymphoma. Histological clues in chronic actinic dermatitis include dermal fibrosis and multinucleate stromal giant cells. Polymorphous light eruption is often associated with oedema of the papillary dermis. Actinic prurigo has more recently been added to this group and can cause diagnostic problems by a high density of B-cells.

Photodermatoses can display increases in CD8 T-cells but this phenotype can also be present in some variants of CTCL.

Perniosis (chilblains)
Perniosis is an abnormal inflammatory response to cold, seen most frequently in acral locations, but it can occur on the thighs of horse-riders. It can be

mimicked by variants of lupus erythematosus termed chilblain lupus. Both perniosis and chilblain lupus can resemble lymphoma because of dense perivascular collections of lymphocytes.

Annular erythemas

Annular erythemas and especially erythema annulare centrifugum can mimic lymphoma with dense perivascular collection of lymphocytes.

Traumatic ulcerative granuloma (eosinophilic ulcer/granuloma of the tongue)

Located on the tongue, this entity can contain eosinophils and blast cells mimicking lymphoma.

Jessner and Kanof's lymphocytic infiltration of the skin

This entity is loved by many dermatologists but sadly is often diagnosed with suboptimal clinical insight.

Problems surrounding the entity are complicated by the index description being restricted to an unpublished Kodachrome presentation to the Bronx Dermatological Society in 1953.[15] On that basis, the exact nature of the disease has to be extrapolated from other publications, which record comments made by Jessner and Kanof to scientific audiences, on other workers' cases.

Using this approach, the entity appears to exist although it should be restricted to a specific clinicopathological situation. Clinically, the lesions are usually on the face and are discoid in nature. Papules expand peripherally but clear in the centre and give rise to a circinate appearance. Spontaneous remission can occur but with recurrence in weeks, months, or longer. Histologically, there is only a mild perivascular and peri-adnexal lymphocytic infiltrate. There should be no involvement of the epidermis and oedema of the papillary dermis appears frequent. More recently, immunohistology has suggested increased dermal CD8 lymphocytes but no HLA–DR expression. This contrasts with lupus erythematosus which has fewer CD8 lymphocytes and greater HLA–DR expression. Some studies have highlighted the presence of so-called plasmacytoid monocytes. There have been suggestions that the entity may overlap with polymorphous light eruption or lupus erythematosus and, on balance, a light sensitivity association would appear likely. In addition, the entity has been described in human immunodeficiency virus (HIV) positive patients and, occasionally, as a drug-reaction. Direct immunofluorescence for lupus erythematosus must be negative. There is overlap with the palpable arciform migratory erythema described by Clark.

SPECIFICALLY NAMED CUTANEOUS PSEUDOLYMPHOMAS

Acral pseudolymphomatus angiokeratoma of children

For ease, acral pseudolymphomatus angiokeratoma of children is often referred to as APACHE.[16] This was first described in children on the extremities of arms and legs and often multiple and unilateral. Histologically, it is characterised by prominent postcapillary venules and a moderately dense lymphocytic infiltrate. The diagnostic vascular features of angiolymphoid hyperplasia are always absent. The cellular infiltrate may show interface changes with the epidermis and immunohistochemistry reveals mixed populations of B- and T-cells. Linear variants of the disease have been described. More recently, there has been increasing recognition of cases with a solitary lesion and/or in adults.

There appears to be overlap with the entity of papular angiolymphoid proliferation with epithelioid features (referred to as PALEFACE).

Solitary pseudo T-cell lymphoma

Although often accepted as a specific entity, there appears to be some overlap with lymphomatoid benign lichenoid keratosis. The entity is characterised by mixed populations of B- and T-cells, an increase in CD8 T-cells and the presence of histiocytes. Some reported cases may have represented primary cutaneous CD4 positive small/medium pleomorphic T-cell lymphoma. One case of solitary pseudo T-cell lymphoma resolved following treatment for *Helicobacter pylori.*

Pseudolymphoma of haematological disease (insect-bite-like reaction or eosinophilic eruption of haematological disease)

Treatment for haematological disease can be associated with various cutaneous pseudolymphomatus reactions. In particular, this relates to drug eruptions and these are covered below.

Haematological disease, however, can be associated with a specific pseudolymphomatus reaction termed insect-bite-like reaction.[17] It was initially recognised that mosquito bites in patients with chronic lymphocytic leukaemia could be associated with florid cutaneous responses. This was followed by reports of insect-bite-like reactions in patients with chronic lymphocytic leukaemia but no apparent history of insect bites. More recently, this pseudolymphomatus reaction has been reported in patients with mantle zone lymphoma and in association with HIV infection. The entity is generally considered to have an association with altered immunity.

EXOGENOUS CAUSES OF CUTANEOUS PSEUDOLYMPHOMATUS REACTIONS

DRUGS

The list of drugs causing cutaneous pseudolymphomatus reactions is extensive and can be usefully remembered by the prefix 'anti-'. This includes anti-depressants, anticonvulsants, antihypertensives, antibiotics, anti-inflammatory and antihistamines. To this can be added calcium-channel blockers, lipid lowering drugs, colony stimulating factors, interleukins and inhibitors against tyrosinase and tumour necrosis factors. In essence, drugs can be associated with all of the morphological, cytological and immunophenotypic patterns described below.

VIRAL INFECTIONS

Cutaneous pseudolymphomatus reactions are well described in association with molluscum contagiosum, herpes simplex and varicella-zoster virus, parapox, cowpox, Epstein–Barr virus, human T-cell lymphotropic virus and HIV.[18] Molluscum contagiosum and herpes viruses appear to show a specific tendency for follicular reactions. HIV can manifest with a pseudo-lymphomatous interface dermatosis which is CD8 prominent and improves after anti-retroviral therapy.

BACTERIAL INFECTIONS

Cutaneous pseudolymphomatous reactions are classically associated with infections by spirochaetes including *Borrelia burgdorferi* and *Treponema pallidum*.[19]

The cutaneous reaction to borrelia is often specifically termed borrelia lymphocytoma and characteristically occurs in younger patients with frequent involvement of earlobes, nipple or genitals. The histological reaction usually has a pronounced B-cell component, which can mimic marginal zone or follicular centre lymphoma. Germinal centres can appear enlarged, irregular and have no mantle zone. Blast-cell numbers can be increased significantly but there is often a retention of tingible body macrophages. Histiocytes and granulomas can be present and, at times, the infiltrate can be of so-called 'bottom heavy' distribution.

PARASITES AND OTHER EXTERNAL ORGANISMS

This includes scabies and bites from many organisms, including scorpions, spiders and leeches. They all tend to initiate a reaction which is eosinophil-rich with both B- and T-cells (Fig. 3). A similar reaction can occur following external irritation or trauma from coral.

ANTIGEN INJECTIONS

This occurs most frequently with vaccinations containing aluminium hydroxide.[20] The histiocytes display a characteristic purple-grey cytoplasm and particulate aluminium can be identified in some cells at high power

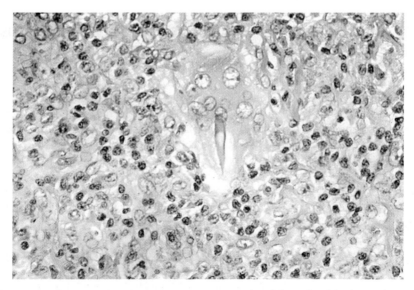

Fig. 3 Insect-bite reaction displaying numerous eosinophils and residual mouth parts.

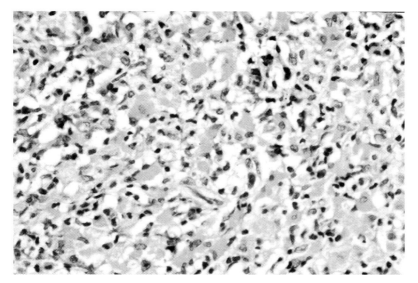

Fig. 4 Aluminium-containing histiocytes in an aluminium hydroxide-related granuloma following vaccination.

magnification (Fig. 4). Histochemical stains for aluminium are positive and aluminium can be identified on X-ray micro-analysis. The histological appearance can be variable and display patterns mimicking marginal zone lymphoma, granuloma annulare, lupus erythematosus or fat necrosis. Pseudolymphomatous reactions have also been reported following desensitising procedures for pollen, dust and house mites.

METALS AND PIGMENT

Cutaneous pseudolymphomatous reactions have been reported most commonly against metal-based pigment in tattoos and the metals in earrings and acupuncture.[21]

ETHNIC SCARIFICATION/FEMALE GENITAL MUTILATION

Cutaneous pseudolymphomatus reactions can follow this procedure. It is believed to represent a reaction to a component part of the applied dressings.

SILICONE

The entry of silicone into soft tissue and skin can be associated with a pseudolymphomatus reaction. It has been described following silicone injection for both breast and genital enlargement.

OTHER CELL TYPES THAT CAN MIMIC CUTANEOUS LYMPHOMA

As well as lymphocytes, other haematological cells, together with histiocytes and antigen-presenting cells can mimic cutaneous lymphoma.

115

PLASMA CELLS

Plasma cells can be sufficiently prominent in certain infective and autoimmune/connective tissue disorders, to mimic cutaneous lymphoma. This applies particularly to spirochaete and *Leishmania* spp. infections and connective tissue disorders such as lupus erythematosus, morphoea and necrobiosis lipoidica.

Plasma cells can be prominent in cutaneous manifestations of Castleman's disease and represent a significant cellular component in the stromal response to epidermal dysplasia and malignancy. Furthermore, as will be discussed later, the occasional presence of a plasma cell monoclone can make distinction between a reactive and neoplastic state difficult.

Cutaneous plasmacytosis and cutaneous angioplasmocellular hyperplasia are two examples of reactive plasma cell proliferation.[22] Distinction from a neoplastic proliferation depends largely on the absence of a monoclone on immunohistochemistry and also preferably genotypic analysis. Patients with cutaneous plasmacytosis should also be screened for potential systemic involvement.

Cutaneous plasmablastic infiltrates in association with HIV infection can be monoclonal in nature but self-healing and a definitive distinction between reactive and neoplastic states can again be difficult.

HISTIOCYTES

Interstitial granulomatous disease is characterised by the presence of palisaded neutrophilic and granulomatous infiltrates with focal collagen degeneration. This disease can present as either a drug eruption or in association with autoimmune/connective tissue diseases, such as rheumatoid arthritis or lupus erythematosus.[23] It can closely mimic granulomatous or interstitial variants of CTCL, but is characterised by a greater population and histiocytes compared to T-cells.

ANTIGEN-PRESENTING CELLS

Reactive Langerhans' cells can show prominence in numerous classical dermatoses. For example, they can become prominent within the epidermis in eczema/dermatitis and mimic Pautrier abscesses as in CTCL. In addition, intra-epidermal Langerhans' cells can become so prominent in CTCL that they can mimic Langerhans cell histiocytosis.

HISTOLOGICAL PATTERNS OF CUTANEOUS PSEUDOLYMPHO-MATOUS REACTIONS

Histological cutaneous pseudolymphomatus patterns can be divided into those of morphological, cellular and cytological type and those revealed by immunohistochemistry. Although some types of cutaneous pseudolymphoma are more frequently associated with certain patterns, there is considerable overlap in the appearances observed.

SCANNING MAGNIFICATION MORPHOLOGICAL PATTERNS

The main types described are those involving the epidermis (epidermo-trophic), dermis (non-epidermotropic), follicular (with or without follicular mucinosis), subcutaneous and vascular. In general, an epidermotropic infiltrate will have a significant T-cell component, whereas other patterns can be of T-cell, B-cell or mixed type. The pattern focused on blood vessels is specifically termed a lymphomatoid vascular reaction and is particularly associated with drug reactions, lupus erythematosus and varicella-zoster virus infection.

CELLULAR AND CYTOLOGICAL PATTERNS

Lymphomatoid
The term lymphomatoid is applied when cellular density and/or nuclear atypia is pronounced or when features of mycosis fungoides (such as Pautrier abscesses or interface changes) are present. Entities receiving this designation include lymphomatoid dermatitis and lymphomatoid actinic and benign lichenoid keratoses.

Pseudo-Pautrier abscesses
Classical Pautrier abscesses represent an intimate association between T-cell lymphocytes and antigen-presenting cells. Pseudo-Pautrier abscesses represent situations where the number of antigen-presenting cells is substantially in excess of lymphocytes present (Fig. 5).[24] They are also termed Langerhans' cell microgranulomas. They can be seen in common dermatoses such as eczema/dermatitis and their presence should not be used as a solitary feature to make an erroneous diagnosis of CTCL.

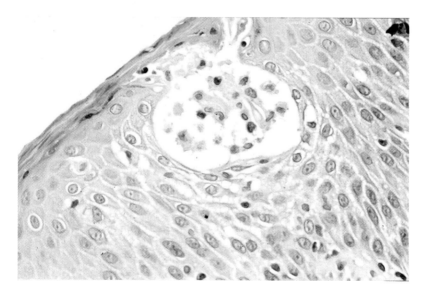

Fig. 5 An intra-epidermal pseudo-Pautrier abscess characterised by numerous antigen-presenting cells rather than lymphocytes.

Adipocyte rimming

The rimming of adipocytes by lymphocytes in subcutaneous fat was initially regarded as a diagnostic feature of subcutaneous panniculitis-like T-cell lymphoma. It is now appreciated, however, not to be specific and can be seen in other examples of lymphocytic lobular panniculitis and especially lupus erythematosus panniculitis.[25] The nuclear proliferation rate, however, of rimming lymphocytes in lymphoma is substantially greater than in reactive disorders.

IMMUNOPHENOTYPIC PROFILES

Pan or subset T-cell antigen loss can be a feature of CTCL but this is recognised to lack specificity and can be seen in reactive T-cell disorders.

CD56 is a relatively new antigen and is used to identify CD56-positive natural killer/T-cell lymphomas. The antigen can, however, be expressed in various pseudolymphomatus situations and, in particular, in relation to herpes simplex and varicella-zoster virus infections.

The CD15 antigen was initially associated with descriptions of Hodgkin's lymphoma. It is now recognised that treatment with, for example, colony stimulating factors can be associated with a cutaneous pseudolymphomatus reaction with CD15 positivity that mimics Hodgkin cells.

CD30-positive pseudolymphomas

As with CD15, CD30 was associated with early immunophenotypic developments in Hodgkin's lymphoma. This was quickly extended into the area of cutaneous CD30-positive T-cell lymphoproliferative disorders including lymphomatoid papulosis and anaplastic large cell lymphoma. It is now appreciated, however, that CD30 positivity can be associated with activation of other cell types including those of B-cell, natural killer cell and myeloid lineage. In addition, normal tissue such as decidua and some non-lymphoid mesenchymal and epithelial tumours can be CD30 positive. Accordingly, the interpretation of CD30 positivity in cutaneous infiltrates should be undertaken with great care.[26] In general, there is a tendency for CD30-positive cells in true primary cutaneous CD30-positive T-cell lymphoproliferative disorders to occur in substantial numbers and in clusters. In addition, they are more frequently associated with larger and atypical nuclei and show T-cell monoclones on genotypic analysis. Nothing, however, is absolute and there is a considerable overlap between reactive and neoplastic processes. Reactive CD30-positive T-cells can occur, in particular, in drug eruptions, viral infections, tuberculosis and scabies (Fig. 6). Furthermore, in some viral infections and scabies, the CD30-positive cells can be large, atypical, clustered and represent over 75% of the cell population. In practice, therefore, CD30-positive T-cells should be regarded as potentially occurring in any cutaneous inflammatory condition and their final interpretation based on the overall histological appearance and clinical setting. CD30-positive decidua can mimic CD30-positive anaplastic large cell lymphoma and CD30-positive cells amongst neutrophils, as in ruptured follicular cysts and hidradenitis suppurativa, can mimic the neutrophil-rich variant of CD30-positive anaplastic large cell lymphomas. The cells in the eruption of lymphocyte recovery following haematological treatment may be CD30 positive, as can the

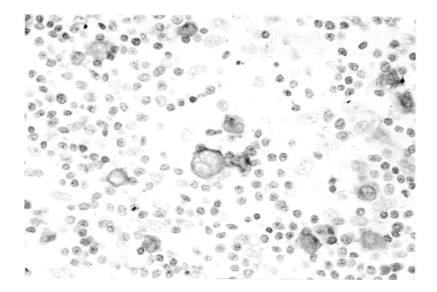

Fig. 6 CD30-positive lymphocytes in a cutaneous drug eruption.

lymphocytes in cutaneous lymphadenoma, traumatic ulcerative granuloma (eosinophil-rich CD30 lymphoproliferative disorder of the oral mucosa) and lymphomatoid benign lichenoid keratosis. Chemotherapy for leukaemia and lymphoma can be associated with cutaneous atypical CD30-positive T-cell reactions, which can be misdiagnosed as recurrent disease.[27]

THE EVOLUTION OF HISTORICAL CUTANEOUS PSEUDOLYMPHOMA INTO LYMPHOMA OR LYMPHOID HYPERPLASIA

HISTORICAL PERSPECTIVE OF CUTANEOUS PSEUDOLYMPHOMA

Over a century ago, Kaposi and Spiegler published independently on cutaneous lymphoid infiltrates. Their descriptions were those of either single or multiple sarcomatous-like skin lesions, referred to as sarcoids. Some cases regressed and were associated with a good prognosis, whereas others spread and caused death. Credit for these observations was given by Darier, who included these diseases in his discourse on sarcoids. For uncertain reasons, however, Darier highlighted the later work of Fendt and designated the group, Spiegler–Fendt rather than Kaposi–Spiegler sarcoid.

Although Kaposi and Spiegler described both fatal and non-fatal cases, authors over the next 70 years focused on the latter. Although meaning the same disease, this resulted in copious different terminology, including lymphocytoma, lymphadenosis benigna cutis, cutaneous lymphoplasia, cutaneous lymphoid hyperplasia, large-cell lymphocytoma and reactive pseudolymphoma. The term 'pseudolymphoma of Spiegler–Fendt', advocated by Lever, erroneously applied the rubber stamp of benign to this group of disorders.[28]

119

In parallel with these historical views on cutaneous pseudolymphoma, the status of primary cutaneous B-cell lymphoma (CBCL) remained uncertain. Clark, as late as 1974, stated that primary CBCL should not be diagnosed by skin biopsy alone.[29] Furthermore, other authors excluded the diagnosis of primary CBCL if there had been no systemic spread after 5 years. This arbitrary definition of CBCL was widely used in many studies which analysed histopathological features believed to be useful in the distinction between benign and malignant cutaneous lymphoid infiltrates.[30] It is, therefore, not surprising that these features were unreliable in practice and that many diagnostic and prognostic difficulties were encountered.

THE ADVENT OF CUTANEOUS MARGINAL ZONE LYMPHOMA

Primary cutaneous marginal zone and follicular centre lymphoma are now recognised in international lymphoma classifications. The existence, however, of primary cutaneous marginal zone lymphoma was not widely accepted for many years and the current consensus classifications were only achieved after prolonged debate.[31]

The advances facilitating the recognition of primary cutaneous marginal zone lymphoma included immunohistochemistry which identified lymphocyte subtypes, immunohistochemical and genotypic methods to assess clonality and finally the recognition of MALT lymphoma in the gastointestinal tract. Many apparent gastric pseudolymphomas were then found to represent MALT lymphoma and the antigenic aetiological role of *H. pylori* in the disease is now legend.

This was followed by recognition that MALT lymphoma also existed in the skin and that some cases could also be linked to antigen presentation, including *B. burgdorferi*, tattoos, vaccination, drugs and more recently, in the ocular area, *Chlamydia psittaci*. It readily became apparent that many cases, which historically would have been regarded as cutaneous pseudolymphoma, were actually examples of lymphoma. Finally, developments in lymphoma classification saw the term MALT lymphoma replaced by marginal zone lymphoma. During this time, several cutaneous entities, such as large cell lymphocytoma and Crosti's reticulohistiocytoma, were recognised to be cutaneous lymphoma.

CUTANEOUS LYMPHOID HYPERPLASIA

Although many cases which historically would have been called cutaneous pseudolymphoma are now regarded as cutaneous lymphoma, there still remain cases which appear reactive. Therefore, to avoid confusion with the term pseudolymphoma, it is now common practice for these cases to be termed cutaneous lymphoid hyperplasia, especially when no aetiological cause is apparent.[32] In addition, based on the presence or absence of epidermal involvement and the phenotypic cell content, they are referred to as either cutaneous T-cell or B-cell predominant lymphoid hyperplasia.

Cutaneous B-cell predominant lymphoid hyperplasia is notoriously difficult to distinguish from cutaneous lymphoma, because reactive germinal centres and tingible body macrophages can also be seen in primary cutaneous marginal zone lymphoma. Furthermore, in both reactive and neoplastic conditions, lymphoid follicles and germinal centres can show similar disturbing morphological changes, including increased size, asymmetry, loss of polarity, confluence, increased blast-cell numbers and increased mitotic activity. In addition, for uncertain reasons, lympho-epithelial lesions are seen rarely in CBCL. Accordingly, as morphological appearances can be unhelpful in the distinction between reactive and neoplastic conditions, detailed immunohistochemistry should always be undertaken. The presence of light chain restriction is invaluable in the diagnosis of lymphoma but immuno-architecture can also be of significant help and attention should be paid to B-cell distribution, nuclear proliferation rate and bcl-2, bcl-6 and CD10 status. In practice, the immunohistochemical demonstration of light chain restriction can be technically difficult and genotypic analysis is often more revealing.

CLONAL DERMATITIS AND CLONAL CUTANEOUS LYMPHOID HYPERPLASIA

Studies into CTCL, using TCR gene re-arrangement analysis, identified a small number of cases of eczema/dermatitis, in the control population, with T-cell monoclones. This observation formed the basis of a new disease entity called clonal dermatitis.

Similar findings were then made in some cases of cutaneous lymphoid hyper-plasia and this led to the equivalent term of clonal cutaneous lymphoid hyperplasia. Although less common than TCR gene re-arrangement, monoclonal B-cell populations have also seen in some cases by immunoglobulin heavy chain gene re-arrangement analysis.

The diagnostic and clinical relevance of these T- and B-cell monoclonal populations has been subject to considerable investigation. Results from different workers have been variable; however, in general, the presence of a monoclone is regarded as clinicopathologically significant, especially in the absence of an aetiological factor for the lymphoid hyperplasia. Most studies have shown that a small percentage of these cases can transform over time into clinically overt cutaneous CTCL or CBCL. On this basis, it is desirable for these patients to be followed up clinically, with a low threshold for re-biopsy, disease staging or both.

Although the aetiological factor may not be apparent, the known existence of antigen-driven primary cutaneous CBCL, lends support to the view that such cases probably lie on a spectrum between reactive and neoplastic. This group of disorders has been usefully described as a lymphoproliferative continuum with lymphomatous potential,[33] although the specific application of the term reactive/benign or neoplastic/malignant to an individual case can be difficult. For example, a B-cell monoclone can be identified in some infiltrates in association with basal or squamous cell carcinoma. It is unresolved whether this represents a reactive monoclonal response to antigens within the tumour or alternatively represents occult neoplasia that is antigenically driven.

As well as in cutaneous lymphoid hyperplasia, the presence of monoclonal populations has been described in a small number of specifically named dermatoses and cutaneous reactions to known external aetiological factors. Excluding variants of pityriasis lichenoides, which probably lie more on the true lymphoproliferative T-cell spectrum, T-cell monoclones have been described in some cases of lichen planus, lichen sclerosus and pigmented purpuric dermatosis.[34] Whereas in lichen planus and lichen sclerosus they are considered to have no known clinical significance, some cases of pigmented purpuric dermatosis may evolve into CTCL. Exogenous aetiological factors that can be associated with a T-cell monoclone include drug reactions and viral infections.[35,36] The latter, in particular, applies to varicella-zoster virus and HIV infections.

The existence of solitary T-cell pseudolymphoma has been contentious and publications have described the variable presence or absence of T-cell monoclones.[37] Although their presence should be regarded with clinical caution, interpretation is difficult as T-cell monoclones have also been described in benign lichenoid keratosis.

A similar debate also exists with respect to lupus erythematosus panniculitis and distinction from subcutaneous panniculitis-like T-cell lymphoma. In general, however, there appears to be increasing agreement that caution should be applied to the diagnosis of lupus erythematosus panniculitis, if a T-cell monoclone is present.[38]

In general, B-cell monoclones are less frequent than T-monoclones in reactive cutaneous dermatoses. They have, however, been described in association with borrelia lymphocytoma, herpes varicella-zoster virus and necrobiosis lipoidica.[39]

The investigation of clonality is also complicated by methodologies that may not always correlate. For example, immunohistochemical light chain restriction may not be accompanied by B-cell monoclonality on genotypic analysis. Similarly, it is recognised that monoclonality in some malignancies may not be demonstrable and that some cases of polyclonal cutaneous lymphoid hyperplasia can transform into lymphoma. Certainly, monoclonality must not be used as the single criterion on which to diagnose malignancy. Different molecular technologies, such as Southern blot analysis and those based on the polymerase chain reaction (PCR), have different degrees of sensitivity and specificity and PCR amplification can be associated with so-called pseudoclones. To avoid false positive or false negative genotypic results, it is imperative that the laboratories undertaking molecular investigations participate in quality assurance schemes.

CONCLUSIONS

In the future, molecular abnormalities specific to the diagnosis of primary cutaneous lymphoma may be identified and new methodologies, such as gene expression profiling, will be useful in this extremely difficult area. At the moment, the co-existence of genotypic and cytogenetic abnormalities should heighten the degree of suspicion for lymphoma, as should the presence of monoclones that are persistent, reproducible and of significant size. Reversible clones have sometimes been used to define the term T-cell or B-cell dyscrasia, but as the term has also been used variably with pre-lymphomatous conditions, it is probably best avoided.[40]

Points for best practice

- Cutaneous pseudolymphoma is an entity now recognised by the World Health Organization.

- Cutaneous pseudolymphoma occurs more frequently clinically and pathologically that cutaneous lymphoma.

- Historical reports of cutaneous pseudolymphoma are now known to have incorporated examples of cutaneous lymphoma.

- Cutaneous pseudolymphoma should only be diagnosed with full clinicopathological correlation.

- The diagnosis should be limited to either specific diseases that incorporate the term or when the exogenous cause of the cellular response is known (such as drugs and infections).

- Numerous diseases, including many classical dermatoses, can mimic cutaneous lymphoma.

- Some cases of cutaneous pseudolymphoma can transform into lymphoma.

- Lesional regression does not automatically imply pseudolymphoma, as it can also be seen in cutaneous lymphoma.

- Cutaneous lymphoid hyperplasia is the preferred term for reactive/benign lymphoproliferative disorders, where no aetiological agent is apparent.

- Clonal dermatitis/clonal cutaneous lymphoid hyperplasia has a low but significant risk of transformation into lymphoma and requires multidisciplinary team discussion, possible staging and follow up with re-biopsy if necessary.

References

1. Burg G, Kempf W, Burg G et al. Lymphoid infiltrates of the skin mimicking lymphoma (cutaneous pseudolymphoma). In: LeBoit PE, Burg G, Weedon D, Sarasin A. (eds) Pathology & Genetics Skin Tumours. Lyon: IARC Press, 2006; 212–214.
2. Santa Cruz DJ, Barr RJ, Headington TJ. Cutaneous lymphadenoma. Am J Surg Pathol 1991; **15**: 101–110.
3. Al-Hoqail IR, Crawford RI. Benign lichenoid keratoses with histologic features of mycosis fungoides: clinicopathologic description of a clinically significant histologic pattern. J Cutan Pathol 2002; **29**: 291–294.
4. Menasce LP, Shanks JH, Howarth VS, Banerjee SS. Regressed cutaneous malignant melanoma mimicking lymphoma: a potential diagnostic pitfall. Int J Surg Pathol 2006; **13**: 281–284.
5. Brenn T, Calonje E, Granter SR et al. Cutaneous Rosai–Dorfman disease is a distinct clinical entity. Am J Dermatopathol 2002; **24**: 385–391.
6. El Shabrawi-Caelen L, Kerl K, Cerroni L, Soyer HP, Kerl H. Cutaneous inflammatory pseudotumour – a spectrum of various disease? J Cutan Pathol 2004; **31**: 605–611.
7. Klein WM, Rencic A, Munshi NC, Nousari CH. Multicentric plasma cell variant of Castleman's disease with cutaneous involvement. J Cutan Pathol 2004; **31**: 448–452.

8. Yen HR, Lin PY, Chuang WY, Chang ML, Chiu CH. Skin manifestations of Kikuchi–Fujimoto disease: case report and review. *Eur J Pediatr* 2004; **163**: 210–213.

9. Magro CM, Crowson AN, Byrd JC, Soleymani AD, Shendrik I. Atypical lymphocytic lobular panniculitis. *J Cutan Pathol* 2004; **31**: 300–306.

10. Citarella L, Massone C, Kerl H, Cerroni L. Lichen sclerosus with histopathologic features simulating early mycosis fungoides. *Am J Dermatopathol* 2003; **25**: 463–465.

11. Regauer S, Liegl B, Reich O, Beham-Schmid C. Vasculitis in lichen sclerosus: an under recognized feature? *Histopathology* 2004; **45**: 237–244.

12. Toro JR, Sander CA, LeBoit PE. Persistent pigmented purpuric dermatitis and mycosis fungoides: simulant, precursor, or both? A study by light microscopy and molecular methods. *Am J Dermatopathol* 1997; **19**: 108–118.

13. Crowson AN, Magro CM, Zahorchak R. Atypical pigmentary purpura: a clinical, histopathologic, and genotypic study. *Hum Pathol* 1999; **30**: 1004–1012.

14. Arai E, Okubo H, Tsuchida T, Kitamura K, Katayama Y. Pseudolymphomatous folliculitis: a clinicopathologic study of 15 cases of cutaneous pseudolymphoma with follicular invasion. *Am J Surg Pathol* 1999; **23**: 1313–1319.

15. Jessner M, Kanof NB, Lymphocytic infiltration of the skin. *Arch Dermatol* 1953; **68**: 447–499.

16. Ramsay B, Dahl MC, Malcolm AJ, Wilson-Jones E. Acral pseudolymphomatous angiokeratoma of children. *Arch Dermatol* 1990; **126**: 1524–1525.

17. Khamaysi Z, Dodiuk-Gad RP, Weltfrient S *et al*. Insect bite-like reaction associated with mantle cell lymphoma: clinicopathological, immunopathological, and molecular studies. *Am J Dermatopathol* 2005; **27**: 290–295.

18. Leinweber B, Kerl H, Cerroni L. Histopathologic features of cutaneous herpes virus infections (herpes simplex, herpes varicella/zoster) a broad spectrum of presentations with common pseudolymphomatous aspects. *Am J Surg Pathol* 2006; **30**: 50–58.

19. Colli C, Leinweber B, Mullegger R *et al*. *Borrelia burgdorferi*-associated lymphocytoma cutis: clinicopathologic, immunophenotypic, and molecular study of 106 cases. *J Cutan Pathol* 2004; **31**: 232–240.

20. Slater DN, Underwood JCE, Durrant TE, Gray T, Hooper IP. Aluminium hydroxide granulomas: light and electron microscopic studies and X-ray microanalysis. *Br J Dermatol* 1982; **107**: 103–108.

21. Slater DN, Durrant TE. Tattoos: a light and electron microscopy study with X-ray microanalysis. *Clin Exp Dermatol* 1984; **9**: 167–173.

22. Gonzalez S, Molgo M. Primary cutaneous angioplasmocellular hyperplasia. *Am J Dermatopathol* 1995; **17**: 307–311.

23. Perrin C, Lacour J-P, Castanet J, Michiels JF. Interstitial granulomatous drug reaction with a histological pattern of interstitial granulomatous dermatitis. *Am J Dermatopathol* 2001; **23**: 295–298.

24. Candiago E, Marocolo D, Manganoni MA, Leali C, Facchetti F. Nonlymphoid intraepidermal mononuclear cell collections (pseudo-Pautrier abscesses). *Am J Dermatopathol* 2000; **22**: 1–6.

25. Lozzi GP, Massone C, Citarella L, Kerl H, Cerroni L. Rimming of adipocytes by neoplastic lymphocytes: a histopathological feature not restricted to subcutaneous T-cell lymphoma. *Am J Dermatopathol* 2006; **28**: 9–12.

26. Cepeda LT, Pieretti M, Chapman SF, Horenstein MG. CD30-positive atypical lymphoid cells in common non-neoplastic cutaneous infiltrates rich in neutrophils and eosinophils. *Am J Surg Pathol* 2003; **23**: 912–918.

27. Su LD, Duncan LM. Lymphoma- and leukaemia-associated cutaneous atypical CD30+ T-cell reactions. *J Cutan Pathol* 2000; **27**: 249–254.

28. Lever WF, Schaumburg-Lever G. *Histopathology of the Skin*, 4th edn. Philadelphia, PA: Lippincott, Williams and Wilkins, 1967; 1–647.

29. Clark WH, Mihm Jr MC, Reed RJ, Ainsworth AM. The lymphocytic infiltrates of the skin. *Hum Pathol* 1974; **5**: 25–43.

30. Evans HL, Winkelmann RK, Banks, PM. Differential diagnosis of malignant and benign cutaneous lymphoid infiltrates. A study of 57 cases in which malignant lymphoma had been diagnosed or suspected in the skin. *Cancer* 1979; **44**: 699–717.

31. Slater DN. MALT and SALT: the clue to cutaneous B-cell lymphoproliferative disease. *Br*

J Dermatol 1994; **131**: 557–561.

32. Caro WA, Helwig EB. Cutaneous lymphoid hyperplasia. *Cancer* 1969; **24**: 487–502.

33. Nihal M, Mikkola D, Horvath N *et al*. Cutaneous lymphoid hyperplasia: a lymphoproliferative continuum with lymphomatous potential. *Hum Pathol* 2003; **34**: 617–622.

34. Cerroni L, Kerl H. Monoclonally rearranged gamma T-cell receptor in lichen sclerosus – a finding of clinical significance? *Am J Dermatopathol* 2004; **26**: 350–351.

35. Brady SP, Magro CM, Diaz-Cano SJ, Wolfe HJ. Analysis of clonality of atypical cutaneous lymphoid infiltrates associated with drug therapy by PCR/DGGE. *Hum Pathol* 1999; **30**: 130–136.

36. Aram G, Rohwedder A, Nazeer T *et al*. Varicella-zoster-virus folliculitis promoted clonal cutaneous lymphoid hyperplasia. *Am J Dermatopathol* 2005; **27**: 411–417.

37. Bakels V, van Oostven JW, van der Putte SCJ *et al*. Immunophenotyping and gene rearrangement analysis provide additional criteria to differentiate between cutaneous T-cell lymphomas and pseudo-T-cell lymphomas. *Am J Pathol* 1997; **150**: 1941–1949.

38. Massone C, Kodama K, Salmhofer W *et al*. Lupus erythematosus panniculitis (lupus profundus): clinical, histopathological, and molecular analysis of nine cases. *J Cutan Pathol* 2005; **32**: 396–404.

39. Cioc AM, Frambach GE, Magro M. Light-chain-restricted plasmacellular infiltrates in necrobiosis lipoidica – a clue to an underlying monoclonal gammopathy. *J Cutan Pathol* 2005; **32**: 263–267.

40. Magro CM, Crowson AN, Kovatich AJ, Burns F. Drug-induced reversible lymphoid dyscrasia: a clonal lymphomatoid dermatitis of memory and activated T cells. *Hum Pathol* 2003; **34**: 119–129.

Karin J. Denton

8

Liquid-based cytology for cervical screening

The cervical smear was pioneered by Dr George Papanicolaou starting in the 1920s, and first used for diagnosis of neoplastic processes in 1928. The technique of removing cells from the surface of the cervix by scraping with a wooden spatula, smearing onto a glass slide, staining and examining them microscopically remained unchanged until the late 1990s.

In the UK, cervical cytology started to be used sporadically in the 1950s, but became more organised over the years. A national programme of computerised call and recall was established in 1987, supported by a series of policy documents, intensively trained staff and robust quality assurance. This

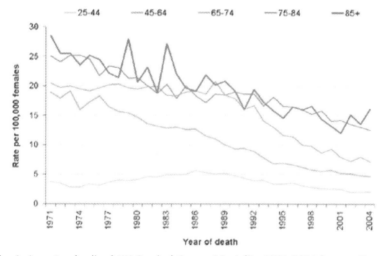

Fig. 1 Age-standardised UK Cervical Cancer Mortality 1971–2004 (source Cancer Screening UK).

Karin J. Denton MB ChB FRCPath
Consultant Cytopathologist, Department of Cellular Pathology, Southmead Hospital, Bristol BS10 5NB, UK
E-mail: karin.denton@nbt.nhs.uk

programme, the National Health Service Cervical Screening Programme (NHS CSP), has been very successful. Incidence and mortality from cervical cancer have fallen consistently (Fig. 1). It is estimated that 80% of all cases of cervical cancer are prevented by the cervical screening programme.[1]

Yet, despite this success, there have been problems. The vast majority of smear tests in England and Wales are carried out by the NHS, and capacity is limited. This issue is less familiar to those working in private healthcare settings but, in the NHS, there has been a limited number of trained staff and financial restrictions on provider organisations with, until recently, little opportunity to generate income. This has, in some cases, contributed to long back-logs for reporting cervical cytology. The national standard is that all women should receive their result in writing within 6 weeks,[2] yet many laboratories working with conventional smears have experienced back-logs of several months. A method which improved screening productivity would have a big impact on this problem, which is viewed as extremely important by women.[3]

A second challenge was the high percentage of inadequate smears – up to 15% in some centres, but generally 9–10%.[4] A smear reported as inadequate generates severe anxiety in women[5] and burdens the system by requiring a repeat. If inadequate smears could be reduced, this would improve the patient experience and improve turn-around time provided, of course, that no abnormalities were missed by inappropriately reporting an inadequate sample as negative.

A further concern was the occurrence of truly negative smears in women who were subsequently found to have had abnormalities at the time. One Possible explanations for this are non-random sampling of the cervix and, even if it is fully sampled, non-random transfer of cells from the sampling device to the glass slide (Fig. 2).[6]

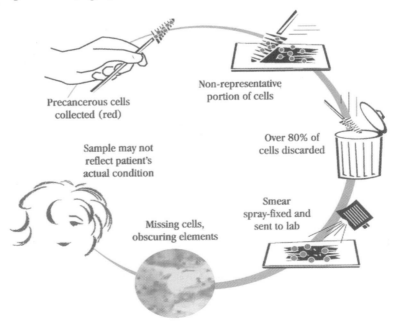

Fig. 2 Non-random sampling in a conventional smear is a potential cause of negative cytology in the presence of a lesion (image courtesy of Cytyc).

LIQUID-BASED CYTOLOGY

The idea for liquid-based cytology (LBC) started to be developed on the 1970s; at that time, it was part of a desire to automate the process of cervical cytology. The automation aspect was unsuccessful at that time, largely because of the inadequate processing power of contemporary computers; however, the idea for LBC continued to be developed. LBC could produce a sample which was fully representative of the material removed, and potentially easier to screen.

SYSTEMS FOR LBC

Two systems for LBC were evaluated in the English, Scottish and Welsh pilots – SurePath® (TriPath imaging) and ThinPrep® (Cytyc). There are other systems under development but these have not been evaluated in the UK and cannot be implemented at this time, so have not been considered further.

The two systems have entirely different theory and methods yet produce similar results. Both use the same collection device, currently the Cervex Broom, though other plastic devices can be used. For ThinPrep®, the broom is rinsed thoroughly in the vial, for SurePath® the broom head is snapped off and retained in the vial.

ThinPrep®

Figure 3 summarises the ThinPrep® process. The vial is received and processed in one of two ways. There is a semi-automated method, the T2000 processor, or the fully automated T3000. In either case, the method is the same. The vial is agitated and then fluid is sucked up through a micropore filter. Neutrophils and red blood cells pass through the filter but epithelial cells do not and they obstruct the pores. Heavily blood-stained or mucoid samples can be treated at this stage to improve cell yield. Obstruction of the pores leads to a pressure differential across the filter which is detected by the machine and used to determine when sufficient cells have become stuck on the filter. The filter is

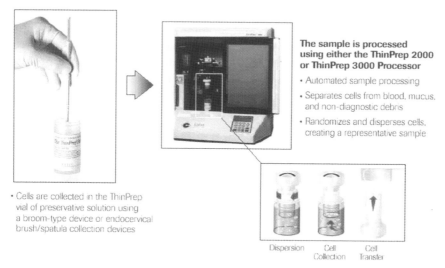

The sample is processed using either the ThinPrep 2000 or ThinPrep 3000 Processor

- Automated sample processing
- Separates cells from blood, mucus, and non-diagnostic debris
- Randomizes and disperses cells, creating a representative sample

- Cells are collected in the ThinPrep vial of preservative solution using a broom-type device or endocervical brush/spatula collection devices

Dispersion   Cell Collection   Cell Transfer

Fig. 3 The ThinPrep® process (image courtesy of Cytyc).

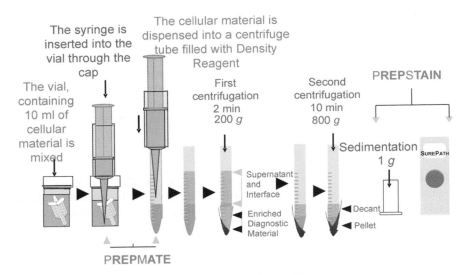

The syringe is inserted into the vial through the cap

The cellular material is dispensed into a centrifuge tube filled with Density Reagent

The vial, containing 10 ml of cellular material is mixed

First centrifugation 2 min 200 g

Second centrifugation 10 min 800 g

PREPSTAIN

Sedimentation 1 g

SUREPATH

Supernatant and Interface

Enriched Diagnostic Material

Decant

Pellet

PREPMATE

Fig. 4 The PrepStain® process (image courtesy of Tripath).

then removed and dabbed onto an electrically charged slide, causing the cells to transfer onto the glass slide. This is then stained in a separate process, using the same staining machine as is used for conventional samples. The T3000 is heavily automated and converts vials into slides ready for staining with no intervention. A single T3000 can handle over 70,000 samples/year, depending on the working day of staff to load and unload it.

SurePath®

The SurePath® process is shown in Figure 4. This system works on the principle of a density gradient. On receipt in the laboratory, vials are vortex mixed to re-suspend cells. An aliquot is then placed into a centrifuge vial and treated through a density gradient centrifugation process. This has the effect of removing unwanted cells and material and produces a concentrated pellet of cells. This is then resuspended, and an aliquot is transferred to a settling chamber mounted on a microscope slide. Cells sediment to form a thin layer and excess fluid is discarded. Staining is an integrated part of the process. The PrepStain™ processor has a higher capacity than the ThinPrep T3000, (48 slides per hour) but is not fully automated and requires more skilled manual operation.

STAINING

The two systems of LBC take a slightly different approach to staining. With ThinPrep®, the slide preparation is automated and yields an unstained slide which can then be inserted into a range of automated staining machines. Protocols for staining will probably not have to be altered from those used for conventional smears. For SurePath®, staining is an integral part of the process, and the results are slightly different to those for conventional cytology in many laboratories, in particular with regard to cytoplasmic staining. This has implications for the cytological appearances of keratinised cells. In the UK, there is a technical external quality assurance scheme (TEQA),[7] which assesses all samples against agreed standards. Both methods perform adequately on TEQA though, because of the cytoplasmic staining, SurePath does not currently achieve high scores.

THE LBC PILOT STUDIES

LBC was the subject of a technology appraisal by the National Institute for Clinical Excellence (NICE) in 2000.[8] This concluded that LBC was safe on the basis of published evidence, but required a pilot of implementation to examine further LBC in a UK setting. LBC was piloted separately in England,[9] Scotland[10] and Wales.[11] The English pilot was the largest in terms of number of samples studied, and it was also the only pilot to study the effects of complete conversion to LBC for the screening population served by a laboratory. This was a pilot of implementation and, therefore, was not designed to address every issue; specifically, it was not designed to look for differences in effectiveness of the two systems. Three pilot sites in England were selected, two larger centres, including one site hosting a cytology training centre, and one district general hospital. Two centres used ThinPrep®, whilst the other used SurePath®. All three sites carried out a pilot of reflex testing for human papilloma virus (HPV) in addition to that for LBC. The results have been reported in the pilot evaluation document.[9] The pilot study showed a decrease in the number of inadequate samples from 9.1% to a mean of 1.6%. Sensitivity of screening was not measured in the pilot; indeed, it is very difficult to measure this directly. A proxy for sensitivity is high-grade dyskaryosis detection rate, provided that coverage remains constant and that there no great change in the population being served. These two features, amongst others, were selection criteria for pilot sites. The high-grade detection rate increased overall in the pilot sites, and this was accompanied by an increase in specificity, measured by the positive predictive value (PPV). Although it is tempting to accept this as evidence that LBC is more sensitive than conventional cytology, there was insufficient evidence to support this conclusion. Therefore, the sensitivity of LBC is accepted as being at least equal to conventional cytology in a UK setting. A concern was also raised that this sensitivity outcome could be due to other factors, including training of smear takers and cytologists and changes in sampling device and technique, rather than to LBC itself. However, as the pilot study was one of implementation into a UK setting, it could be argued that this is irrelevant and if, as seems likely to be the case, this higher detection rate is reproduced in other laboratories, a claim for increased sensitivity may be substantiated. The experience, to date, of the pilot sites is of generally increased detection rates and PPV maintained over several years,[4] and this has also been witnessed in Scotland.[12]

An area of concern raised by the pilot studies was the decrease in detection rate for glandular abnormality. However, the histological detection rate remained unchanged and the conclusion was that LBC is at least as good at detecting glandular lesions.

The pilot study looked at screener productivity and concluded that there was an increase of 9%. However, most laboratories working with LBC now feel this was an underestimate. Productivity is difficult to measure accurately as staff perform varying amounts of screening and other activities, and the results

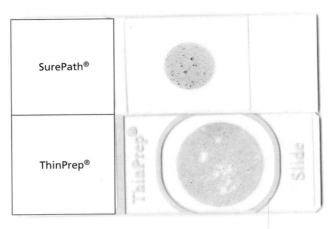

Fig. 5 Macroscopic appearance of ThinPrep® and SurePath® slides.

can easily be skewed by sickness absence, *etc.* The NHS CSP guideline for conventional smears is that all staff should screen a minimum of 3000 samples/year. Many screeners experience difficulty in reaching this target with conventional samples. With LBC, the experience in Bristol is that virtually all staff can attain 4500–5000 samples/year and some can comfortably do many more (up to 8000), with no decline in effectiveness. Speed increases with experience and this continues for months and years after LBC conversion.

SCREENING METHODS FOR LBC

Using LBC, modifications must be made to the conventional screening technique. The area to be screened is smaller (Fig. 5) and circular. Abnormal cells may be located anywhere, will not be confined to streaks of similar cells and may be very sparse, though usually they are not. A screening technique must cover 100% of the deposit and allow for overlap. (Trainee screeners are usually taught to overlap fields by 50%, dropping to 30% when experienced.) Screening should be performed with the x10 objective and screeners are taught that they will frequently need to use a higher power frequently (x40 lens) to examine individual cells.

Cells of interest, including abnormal cells, are often found in the spaces between clumps of normal cells. Screeners need to be taught specifically to look for these cells.

At primary screening, the two methods do have a different appearance. The cells on ThinPrep® are more widely spaced and there is less depth to the field (Fig. 6).

Screening LBC samples is intensive. There are no breaks in the sample, as there are in conventional smears, meaning that the screener must concentrate throughout the process. There has been some concern that this is a risk but no evidence of this has been found. Nonetheless it is recommended that screeners pay attention to usual advice for maintaining concentration, *i.e.* taking short breaks, regular proper breaks, and not exceeding 5 hours per day screening time.[13]

There has been debate in the UK about the necessity of screening SurePath® samples twice, the second screen being at 90° to the first. The rationale for this appears to have been concern that perception of cells altered depending on the direction of approach. However, there is no evidence to support this practice,

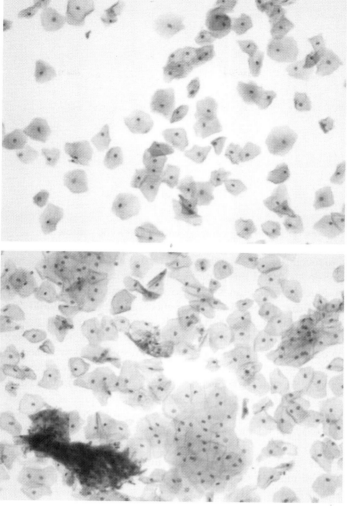

Fig. 6 ThinPrep® (top) and SurePath® (bottom) slides have a different appearance at screening magnification.

which would adversely impact productivity and it is not endorsed by the manufacturer for routine practice, though it may be useful in training.

After primary screening, all negative and inadequate LBC samples are submitted to rapid review. This can be with a variety of screening patterns according to local practice but should take less than 90 seconds. A full rapid review is not widely practiced outside the UK and detailed studies of its effectiveness in LBC are awaited.

MORPHOLOGY

Once the differences in location of the abnormal cells have been accounted for, there are fewer morphological differences between LBC and conventional cytology than might be expected.

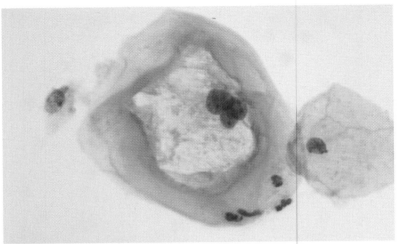

Fig. 7 Borderline nuclear change in a cell with a koilocytic vacuole.

There are several subtle general effects. The prompt fixation of LBC samples leads to good preservation and this is particularly seen in the clarity of presentation of chromatin. Nuclear membranes are also well visualised. In general, cells appear slightly smaller, due to the rounding-up effect of fixation in a liquid. The clarity of nuclear features is helpful in diagnosing dyskaryosis but training needs to address the tendency to overcall dyskaryosis, because subtle variations in chromatin and membrane pattern, invisible on conventional smears, can now be seen. Policies for grading dyskaryosis in the BSCC classification are based on nuclear–cytoplasmic ratio, and this is the same in conventional preparations and LBC.[14] However, other classifications depend on nuclear size and these may require adjustment.[15]

Cells showing low-grade dyskaryosis, especially those with koilocytosis, are usually very easy to find and look identical to similar cells in a conventional smear (Fig. 7).

High-grade dyskaryosis (moderate and severe dyskaryosis) sometimes appears very similar to that seen in conventional smears (Fig. 8). Experience

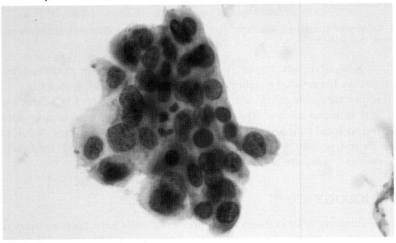

Fig. 8 Severe squamous dyskaryosis.

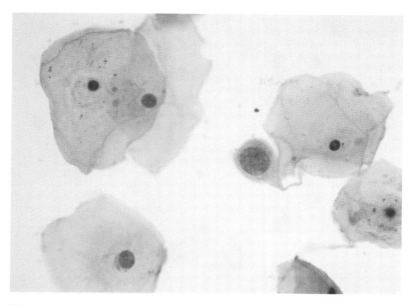

Fig. 9 Severe squamous dyskaryosis in a single cell. These cells may be widely dispersed on the sample.

suggests it is particularly difficult to differentiate the two diagnoses on LBC and this is one of the drivers towards a proposed revision of UK terminology. In LBC, severe dyskaryosis often presents as dispersed single cells, a recognised but less frequent feature on conventional smears (Fig. 9).

Hyperchromatic crowded cell groups (HCCGs) are a problem in conventional and LBC cytology, though the reduced size of the groups and improved nuclear clarity does aid differentiation of benign and abnormal conditions (Fig. 10).

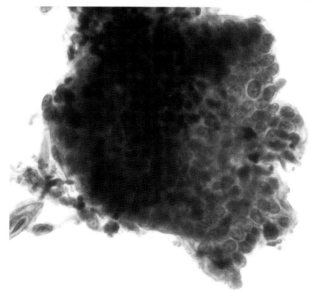

Fig. 10 Severe dyskaryosis in a hyperchromatic crowded cell group. Note that although part of the group is too dense to assess nuclear features, cells on the edge are fully assessable.

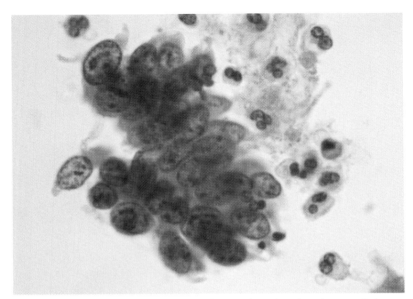

Fig. 11 Nuclei of cells showing '?glandular abnormality' showing characteristic coarse, clumped chromatin.

Concern has focused on the identification of abnormalities in glandular cells on LBC, partly because of the outcome in the English pilot, which found that the incidence of a cytology diagnosis of '?glandular abnormality' decreased in all three sites. However, there is no evidence that histologically diagnosed cervical glandular intra-epithelial neoplasia (CGIN) and adenocarcinoma decreased; indeed, it dramatically increased at one of the sites. The likely explanation for this is that glandular abnormalities were misclassified,

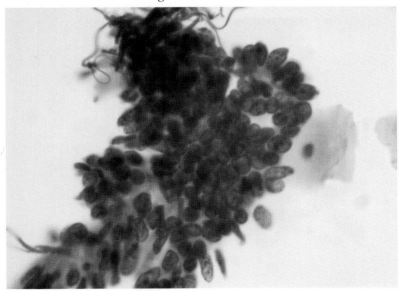

Fig. 12 A group of cells showing '?glandular abnormality' on a ThinPrep® sample. Note the visible micro-acinar structure and the radial discohesion of cells at the periphery of the group.

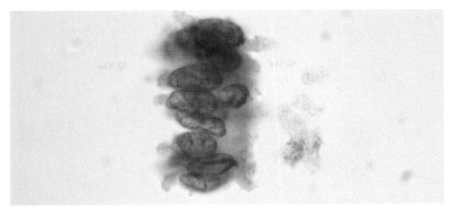

Fig. 13 A strip of cells with raised nuclear/cytoplasmic ratio and nuclear multilayering, diagnostic of '?glandular abnormality' (ThinPrep®).

probably as severe squamous dyskaryosis, with minimal effects on diagnosis and treatment.[10] Glandular abnormalities show similar nuclear features (Fig. 11) on both LBC systems, but architecture and distribution exhibit significant differences. In ThinPrep®, the characteristic appearances are of groups of cells, smaller than in conventional cytology, and showing radial alignment of cells, with occasional feathering (Fig. 12). Feathering, however, is not as prominent as in conventional samples. Palisaded strips with nuclei at multiple levels are seen (Fig. 13) and also, occasionally, micro-acinar structures such as rosettes. Single cells are rarely seen without groups. On SurePath®, groups of cells are seen, but single abnormal glandular cells are also common. Cells show abnormal nuclei distending the cytoplasm (Fig. 14). These cells may be arranged in strips, which often show a shared or community border (Fig. 15). Nuclear features are as for ThinPrep®.

'Severe dyskaryosis ?invasion' also appears to have dropped in frequency with LBC; however, since the specificity of this diagnosis for invasion has always been

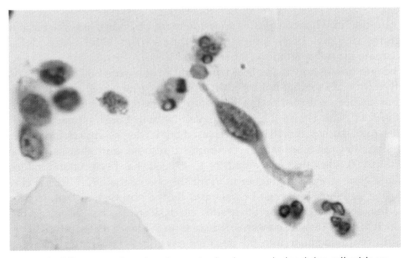

Fig. 14 SurePath® preparation showing a single abnormal glandular cell with an enlarged nucleus which distends the cytoplasm. This has been called the 'snake-and-egg' appearance (image courtesy of Dr D. Rana).

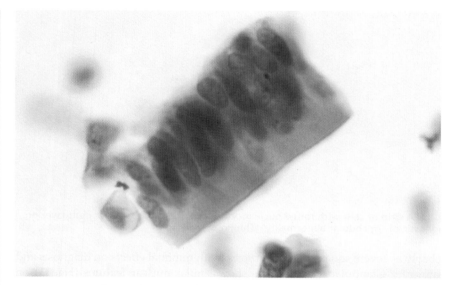

Fig. 15 Surepath® preparation showing a multilayered strip of abnormal endocervical cells showing a shared or community boarder (image courtesy of Dr D. Rana).

low, this is not perceived as a problem. A diathesis can be recognised on LBC but has a different appearance to conventional smears, and nuclear features of poorly differentiated, non-keratinising tumours, are also well seen.

Dyskaryosis in LBC samples may be scanty, though usually it is not. The work of Mitchell and Medley[16] defining the minimum number of abnormal cells on a conventional smear required for diagnosis has not yet been fully repeated for LBC.

ADEQUACY

The question of what constitutes an inadequate LBC sample is the basis for an on-going debate. There are certain appearances which are definitely inadequate for interpretation (Table 1).

The question of how many cells constitute an adequate LBC sample is not yet resolved. In a US setting, Bollick[17] has argued for a threshold of 20,000 cells but this has not been accepted by the Bethesda classification,[18] which has an advisory limit of 5000. This is also the figure quoted by both LBC manufacturers. In the English pilot studies, no cell count was used but it was the impression of the pilot sites that they all used about the same threshold and that it represented 10,000–12,000 cells. In Wales, a limit of 15,000 cells has been set and inadequate rates are correspondingly higher than for the rest of the UK.[19] This is clearly a confusing situation but must be balanced by the observation that, in the pilot sites, the detection rate for all grades of dyskaryosis has risen, as has the specificity (PPV). Despite concerns,[20] there is no evidence that samples have been moved from inadequate into the negative category – rather they seem to have moved proportionately into all other categories.[21] The NHS Health Technology Assessment Programme has commissioned a large multicentre study which aims to resolve the issue in a UK setting.[22]

Table 1 Appearances considered inadequate for interpretation

Before the laboratory	Cervix not fully visualised and sampled (360° x5) Vial broken or leaked No brush in vial (SurePath®) Brush left in vial (ThinPrep®)
No endocervical cells	Only a cause of inadequacy in women after treatment of CGIN, or CIN3 with endocervical margin involved
Obscured by blood or polymorphs	Extremely rare occurrence on LBC
Contamination	Use of inappropriate lubricant (Aquagel with ThinPrep®)
Inadequate cellularity	Thresholds not yet established

IMPLEMENTATION

The English LBC pilot studies commenced in 2001 and were reported in late 2002. The decision to implement LBC was taken in 2003,[8] following on from the same decision already made on Scotland.[10] There was a requirement that LBC in England should be fully implemented by 2008. Initially, apart from the pilot sites, progress was slow in England. Wales and Scotland completed their implementation by 2005, Scotland using ThinPrep® and Wales using SurePath®. Decisions on which system to use were the first hurdle for English laboratories where there was no national requirement for one system or the other. For many areas, this procurement decision constituted the first delay. A second major issue was funding. Although the pilot evaluation claimed that conversion to LBC was cost neutral, this proved in practice not to be the case as some of the savings were impossible to realise, such as a reduction in the time taken by a nurse in general practice to prepare the specimen. Commissioners and purchasers, therefore, have had to identify funding for start-up costs, including alterations to buildings, laboratory staff training and backfill during training, and smear-taker training, as well as the on-going cost of consumables required for LBC. Some of the savings, particularly the reduction in repeat samples required, are not realised for at least 6 months after implementation.

Reviewing the world literature on LBC implementation, it is clear that the results in many countries have not been as good as in the UK.[23] Much of this difference is possibly attributable to differences in training protocols. Although both manufacturers insist on training, this has in many countries been provided in-house to most staff, by non-qualified trainers, after they have attended a manufacturer's course. In the UK, good laboratory staff training was regarded as essential; an in-depth protocol was devised by the NHS CSP[24] and used in the pilot study and subsequently. This involves attendance at a 3-day course in a NHS CSP approved cytology training centre, followed by a consolidation set of 200 slides which are heavily weighted with abnormal cases, then an interim test. Staff who do primary screening then go on to a performance review set of a further 200 slides. Sensitivity targets must be met at all stages, with additional training for those who fail to complete any stage. Since 2001, it has been possible for staff training for the Certificate in Cervical Cytology to do all their training in LBC and the Royal College of Pathologists also allows training and examination in LBC for all MRCPath candidates. All these cytology qualifications are now system specific (conventional, SurePath® and ThinPrep®) and conversion courses exist for those who want or need to change.

There has also been an issue of space. Conventional cervical cytology requires very little laboratory space for preparation, but with both methods of LBC there are increased requirements. Many cytology departments are located in old, cramped buildings which have been difficult to modify. In addition, automated processing machines have a larger capacity than required by many small and average sized laboratories. This has been a driver to centralisation of processing services, which has added a further layer of complexity to the commissioning process.

At the time of writing, it seems likely that the vast majority of British women will be offered LBC screening by late 2008.

PRACTICAL CONSIDERATIONS IN IMPLEMENTING LBC

Converting to LBC is a complex process for laboratories, with numerous processes to review and, in some cases, re-design. The NHS CSP has published guidance derived from the experience of the pilot sites.[25]

SPECIMEN COLLECTION/DELIVERY

Most samples are taken in GP surgeries and collected by hospital transport. Vials take up a lot more space than slides but, in most instances, this has not been a problem. LBC vials can be sent in the post but, being flammable, require special packaging compliant with UN3373.

RECEPTION/NUMBERING

Conventional cervical smears are always received with the patient's identification written on the slide. For LBC there is a potential error because the sample from the labelled vial must be transferred onto a slide, and it is imperative that the correct label accompanies this process. One of the advantages of the T3000 is that it automatically prints a bar code onto the slide, giving a very secure process. With SurePath®, protocols must ensure that the samples are labelled correctly throughout all parts of the process. Staff receiving specimens must ensure the correct vial and form are matched, a process analogous to histology specimen reception.

STOCK CONTROL

LBC vials have a shelf-life which, although long, is limited. Also, unlike glass slides and wooden spatulas, vials have a significant monetary value. Smear-takers, therefore, need to rotate their stock. In some cases, laboratories control the delivery of consumables and have developed methods to control the stock.

STORAGE

Vials take up a lot of space both before and after use. Regular deliveries are needed for unused vials and a racking system for vials after the sample has been prepared are needed. All vials must be kept at least until the specimen in reported. If teaching material is being collected, or research or HPV testing is being performed, vials will need to be kept for longer.

DISPOSAL

Both techniques leave residual material which must be disposed of. This is handled by the manufacturers.

STAINING AND COVER-SLIPPING

Staining techniques have been described above. Both methods are compatible with automated cover-slipping devices. These do not work well with conventional smears because of the variable thickness of the sample; however, LBC is perfect for this process which can save technical time and also laboratory space.

FUTURE ADVANCES

HPV TESTING

The LBC pilot study in England was combined with a pilot of reflex testing of low-grade samples for human papilloma virus (HPV) using Hybrid Capture II, a test which detects a cocktail of high-risk HPV types.[26] Numerous other studies of HPV testing have been carried out[27,28] and interest in HPV testing continues to grow. A large UK trial of HPV as primary screening (ARTISTIC) will report in 2009.[29] One of the great advantages of LBC is that an HPV test can be performed on the same sample. Use of LBC will allow integration of a combination of cervical cytology and HPV testing into cervical cancer prevention; in the longer term, this is probably the most likely outcome.

The next big step forward enabled by LBC will, however, be the development of automation.

AUTOMATION

The desire to automate cervical screening was, as described above, the driver for initial development of LBC. It was probably initially hoped by some that the subjective nature of morphological interpretation could be replaced by a numerical, quantitative process which was not open to any ambiguity. However, the human skills of interpretation have proved to be extremely complex and cannot be entirely replicated. Both LBC manufacturers have developed systems which are effective, though they still require human intervention at some points in the process. There are similarities and differences between the two systems. Both use complex algorithms for the identification of cells which may be abnormal and these are commercially sensitive and have not been published.

TriPath Imaging, the owner of the SurePath® technique, has developed the FocalPoint and FocalPoint GS systems. FocalPoint scans slides prepared by the SurePath® technique and can also be used on conventional smears. It identifies cells which are potentially abnormal then ranks the whole sample on its likelihood of being abnormal. The lowest 25% can then be reported as negative without human intervention. This is the only application of computerised slide reading so far developed which is entirely automated. It has Food and Drug Administration (FDA) approval and is in routine use in the United States of America. The next development is the FocalPoint GS system which captures images, records the location of potentially abnormal cells then, via an automated microscope stage, guides the screener to 10 locations, though the screener must screen the whole slide. This development has not yet received FDA approval.

The Cytyc ThinPrep® Imaging System (TIS) works somewhat differently. Slides are placed in a scanner and the 20 worst cells and two worst groups of cells are identified. The technique of identifying these cells is partly stoichiometric, and a specific staining technique must be used for the TIS. The images are not stored, only the locations, an elegant solution which uses little processing power. Again, an automated stage is used to take the screener to the identified fields. If these are negative, the slide can be classified as negative without full re-screening.

Currently, there is no evidence in the UK literature of the clinical or cost-effectiveness of automated systems. A large trial to address these questions and funded by the HTA is underway in Manchester (MAVARIC).[30] Both systems have FDA approval, backed up by a number of studies in the American and, more recently the European, literature; both claim big increases in productivity with detection equal or superior to manual screening of LBC. Recent experience in Australia comparing conventional, manual screening to automation using the ThinPrep imaging system shows a striking increase in detection rates. The reason for the HTA study is that, once again, international experience is not necessarily applicable to the UK screening programmes, where detection rates are higher than elsewhere in the world[27] and quality assurance and training are far more robust.

However, the existing evidence shows that these systems are practical and this is an exciting development for cervical cytology, long regarded as a technological backwater amongst other pathology specialities. The current impossibility of fully automating the process also demonstrates that cervical cytology interpretation is truly a highly skilled job.

CONCLUSIONS

The implementation of LBC into the NHS CSP is probably the biggest change ever seen in cervical screening and is already resulting in big advantages for women, who now have a reduced chance of an inadequate result, at least as good a chance of any abnormalities being detected, and in most cases a shorter wait for their result. Indeed, the speeding up of reporting has lead to consideration of a much tighter deadline for issuing cervical screening reports.

LBC implementation is also the first example of universal implementation, in a controlled fashion, of an entirely new process in UK cellular pathology, with lessons learned about the procedural and commissioning challenges this involves.

The final message though must be that the UK cervical screening programmes using conventional cytology were amongst the best in the world and prevented the majority of cases of cervical cancer. The very thorough evaluation and controlled implementation of LBC into the UK has ensured that future outcomes will be at least as good and hopefully better.

Key points for clinical practice

- Liquid-based cytology represents the first major technological change in cervical cytology.
- The UK cervical screening programmes are highly effective.
- Liquid-based cytology has been shown to be at least as effective as conventional cytology for the detection of high-grade abnormalities, and offers improvements by decreasing rates of inadequacy and improving screener productivity.
- Two systems have been approved for use in the UK.
- Many lessons have been learnt in implementing this entirely new process.
- Liquid-based cytology provides the platform for future advances in cervical screening which may include human papilloma virus testing and automation of morphological interpretation.

References

1. Peto J, Gilham C, Fletcher O, Matthews FE. The cervical cancer epidemic that screening has prevented. *Lancet* 2004; **364**: 249–256.
2. NHS CSP. *Quality Assurance Guidelines for the Cervical Screening Programme.* NHS CSP publication no. 3. London: Department of Health, 1996.
3. Marteau TM. Psychological costs of screening. *BMJ* 1989; **299**, 527.
4. Department of Health. *Cervical Screening Programme Annual Statistics Bulletin.* London: Department of Health.
5. French DP, Maissi E, Marteau TM. Psychological costs of inadequate smear test results. *Br J Cancer* 2004; **91**: 1887–18-92.
6. Hutchinson ML, Isenstein L, Goodman A *et al.* Homogeneous sampling accounts for the increased diagnostic accuracy using the ThinPrep processor. *Am J Clin Pathol* 1994; **101**: 215–219.
7. NHS CSP. *External Quality Assessment Scheme for the Evaluation of Papanicolaou Staining in Cervical Cytology.* NHS CSP publication 19. London: Department of Health, 2004.
8. NICE. *Guidance on the use of Liquid Based Cytology for Cervical Screening.* NICE Technology Appraisal 69. London: NICE, 2003.
9. Moss S, Gray A, Legood R, Henstock E. *Evaluation of HPV/LBC cervical screening pilot studies. First report to the Department of Health on evaluation of LBC.* London: Department of Health, 2002.
10. Scottish Executive. *Cervical Screening Programme – Liquid Based Cytology (LBC).* Edinburgh: Scottish Executive, 2002.
11. Cervical Screening Wales. *Liquid Based Cytology Pilot Project Report.* Cardiff: Cervical Screening Wales 2003.
12. Williams A. Liquid based cytology and conventional smears compared over two 12 month periods. *Cytopathology* 2006; **17**: 82–85.
13. BSCC. *Codes of Practice for Gynaecological Cytology.* London: BSCC, 1997.
14. Slater DN, Rice S, Stewart R, Melling S, Hewer E, Smith JH. Proposed Sheffield quantitative criteria in cervical cytology to assist the grading of squamous cell dyskaryosis as the BSCC definitions require amendment. *Cytopathology* 2005; **16**: 179–192.

15. Slater DN, Rice S, Stewart R, Melling S, Hewer E, Smith JH. Proposed Sheffield quantitative criteria in cervical cytology to assist the grading of squamous intraepithelial lesions as some Bethesda system definitions require amendment. *Cytopathology* 2005; **16**: 168–178.
16. Mitchell H, Medley G. Differences between Papanicolaou smears with correct and incorrect diagnoses. *Cytopathology* 1996; **7**: 422–424.
17. Bolick DR. Personal communication.
18. Solomon D, Nayar R. *The Bethesda system for reporting cervical cytology: definitions, criteria and explanatory notes*, 2nd edn. New York: Springer, 2003.
19. Cervical Screening Wales. *KC 53/61/65 Statistical report 2005–6*. Cardiff: Cervical Screening Wales 2006.
20. Herbert A, Johnson J. Personal view. Is it reality or an illusion that liquid-based cytology is better than conventional cervical smears? *Cytopathology* 2001; **12**: 383–389.
21. Imrie J, Gardiner DS, Willson A. Is it reality or an illusion that liquid-based cytology is better than conventional cervical smears? *Cytopathology* 2002; **13**: 133.
22. NHS. *Adequacy of LBC cytology specimens for cervical screening*. NHS Health Technology Assessment Programme. London, Department of Health.
23. Davey E, Barrett A, Irwig L et al. Effect of study design and quality on unsatisfactory rates, cytology classification and accuracy in liquid based versus conventional cytology: a systematic review. *Lancet* 2006; **367**: 122–132.
24. NHS CSP. *Training requirements for medical staff working in cervical cytopathology*. LBC Implementation Guide No. 3. London: Department of Health, 2004.
25. NHS CSP. *Advice for cytopathology laboratories on the implementation of liquid based cytology for cervical screening*. LBC Implementation Guide No 2. London: Department of Health, 2004.
26. Legood R, Gray A, Wolstenhome J, Moss S. Lifetime effects, costs and cost effectiveness of testing for HPV to manage low grade cytological abnormalities: results of NHS pilot studies. *BMJ* 2006; **332**: 79–85.
27. Cuzick J, Szarewski A, Cubie H et al. Management of women who test positive for high risk types of HPV: the HART study. *Lancet* 2003; **362**: 1871–1876.
28. ASCUS – LSIL Triage study (ALTS) group. A randomised trial on the management of low grade SIL cytology interpretation. *Am J Obstet Gynecol* 2003; **188**: 1393–1400.
29. NHS. *A randomised trial of HPV virus testing in primary cervical screening (ARTISTIC)*. NHS Health Technology Assessment Programme. London: Department of Health.
30. NHS. MAVARIC. Manual assessment versus automated reading in cytology. NHS Health Technology Assessment Programme. London: Department of Health.

Pramila Ramani

9

Pitfalls in the diagnosis of soft tissue tumours of childhood

Childhood cancer is rare, accounting for less than 1% of all cancers seen in industrialised countries. Nonetheless, it is one of the principal causes of mortality in childhood, resulting in over 20% of deaths in children between 1 and 15 years.

Tumours in children and adolescents differ from those found in adults in several ways. Most malignant neoplasms occurring in adults are carcinomas, and are classified according to their site of origin. Childhood tumours are histologically diverse, and the same tumour can occur at a variety of sites. They are classified into 12 main diagnostic groups,[1] and the age–incidence distribution varies considerably between these groups.[2]

The outcome for most types of childhood cancers has improved dramatically over the last 20 years, in contrast to the very small improvement in survival rates for the common adult cancers. It is estimated that by the year 2010, 1 in every 250 adults will be a survivor of childhood cancer. The most important, long-term, serious, side-effects of therapy are growth failure, reduced fertility, major organ damage, and an approximately 3-fold increase in the risk of secondary cancer in adulthood.[3,4] With that in mind, more attention is now being focused on minimising the toxic effects of therapy while maintaining or improving survival rates.

In the light of increased awareness of the clinical implications of misdiagnosis in paediatric oncology, this review provides a summary of the potential pitfalls encountered in soft tissue tumour pathology. The most helpful features are discussed, together with the main differential diagnoses, where confident diagnosis can sometimes prove problematic, and how best to resolve potential difficulties. The detailed pathology of soft tissue tumours is described in several textbooks;[5–7] in this chapter, only the key diagnostic

Pramila Ramani MB BS PhD FRCPath
Consultant Paediatric Pathologist, Department of Histopathology, Bristol Royal Infirmary, Marlborough Street, Bristol BS2 8HW, UK
E-mail: pramila.ramani@bristol.ac.uk

features will be re-iterated, plus those which differ from adults or pose dilemmas.

Although there is some overlap with adult tumours, paediatric soft tissue tumours present unique challenges. In an ideal situation, the clinician provides the pathologist with full information, including the clinical history and differential diagnosis, before the biopsy arrives in the laboratory. This allows for the planning of laboratory handling and distribution of fresh tissue, which must be dealt with soon after the receipt of the specimen in order to preserve the morphology and the viability of cellular antigens and nucleic acids, particularly RNA.

A wide variety of problems arise in diagnosis, many originating in the interpretation of small or crushed biopsies, or poorly-fixed tissue. Well-prepared sections remain the gold standard for diagnosis. So, the priority for triaging is fixation in 10% neutral-buffered formalin. As there is an overlap in the histology and immunohistoprofile of many tumours, cytogenetic or molecular genetic confirmation of the characteristic translocations is very valuable.[8] These studies become critical when tumours present in unusual age groups or locations, and when unusual morphological variants or aberrant immunoreactivity are encountered. As a result of recent advances in technology, fluorescence *in situ* hybridisation (FISH)[9–12] and reverse transcriptase polymerase chain reaction (RT-PCR)[12–16] assays can now be performed reliably on paraffin-embedded tissue. Tumour cells can be also be retrieved from fixed tissue by laser capture microdissection and subsequently analysed by RT-PCR for the signature translocations.[17] This is particularly important when frozen tissue is not available, as in the case of small biopsies or outside referral cases.

Soft tissue sarcomas constitute 5–8% of childhood tumours. They often pose significant diagnostic challenges because of their infrequent occurrence and histological diversity. The pitfalls in diagnosis of soft tissue sarcomas can be divided into five main categories (Table 1). Each will be considered in turn, with reference to the relevant specific soft tissue tumours.

CLASSIFICATION OF SARCOMAS

The diagnosis of the precise type of sarcoma has major therapeutic significance. Paediatric soft tissue sarcomas are classified as rhabdomyosarcomas (RMS), non-rhabdomyosarcomatous (NRSTS) and undifferentiated soft tissue sarcoma (USTS). The NRSTS group includes a large number of clinically and histologically diverse tumours. The relative frequencies of the histotypes vary with age. For example, infantile fibrosarcoma is common in children less than 2 years of age, while synovial sarcoma and malignant peripheral nerve sheath tumour most commonly affect adolescents. USTS indicates a high-grade mesenchymal tumour which fails to demonstrate a specific line of differentiation by the pathological and molecular investigations.[18]

RHABDOMYOSARCOMA

Rhabdomyosarcoma (RMS) is the most common sarcoma, accounting for 50–60% of the soft tissue sarcomas in childhood. It is a primitive mesenchymal

Table 1 Difficulties in the diagnosis of soft tissue tumours

Potential pitfalls	Specific tumours
Misclassification of specific sarcomas	RMS versus non-RMS Alveolar versus embryonal RMS Synovial sarcoma versus other adult-type of RMS
Benign lesions misdiagnosed as sarcoma	Rhabdomyoma Plexiform (multinodular) cellular schwannoma Pseudosarcomatous myofibroblastic tumours Infantile myofibroma/ myofibromatosis
Sarcomas misdiagnosed as benign lesions	Embryonal RMS Low-grade fibromyxoid sarcoma Myofibrosarcoma
Misgrading of sarcoma	IMT as embryonal RMS Infantile fibrosarcoma as malignant spindle-cell tumour Angiomatoid fibrous histiocytoma as RMS, EFT or MFH
Non-soft tissue tumours misdiagnosed as soft tissue sarcomas	Deep juvenile xanthogranuloma Non-Hodgkin lymphoma Granulocytic sarcoma

RMS, rhabdomyosarcoma; EFT, Ewing family of tumours; MFH, malignant fibrous histiocytoma; IMT, inflammatory myofibroblastic tumour.

tumour that recapitulates the phenotypic and biological features of skeletal muscle differentiation. Around two-thirds of the paediatric cases are diagnosed before the age of 10 years.

Features associated with outcome include age at diagnosis, site, stage, clinical group and histology. Typing into embryonal and alveolar RMS is of extreme importance as alveolar RMS displays adverse outcome.[3]

The WHO recognises embryonal, alveolar and pleomorphic types of RMS.[6] Although pleomorphic RMS occurs in children,[19] it is rare. The international classification of RMS used currently places RMS into three prognostic groups.[20] The superior prognostic group includes the botyroid and spindle-cell variants of embryonal RMS. Embryonal RMS, not otherwise specified, has an intermediate prognosis. Alveolar RMS, in contrast, has a poor prognosis. Typing is not recommended on a poor-quality or small sample; in such cases, the term RMS, not otherwise specified, should be used.

The two main types, embryonal RMS and alveolar RMS, differ in their clinical, pathological and genetic aspects (Table 2). Mixed-RMS, composed of both the types, is classified as alveolar RMS. Embryonal RMS is a spindle-cell tumour, while alveolar RMS is the archetypal small round cell tumour. They can both be accurately diagnosed by immunohistochemistry using a panel of antibodies (Tables 3 and 4). Karyotypic and molecular cytogenetics are valuable adjuncts, and vital in specific situations such as unusual clinical settings and difficult cases (Table 5).

More than 95% of RMSs show expression of myogenic transcription factors (Myogenin/myf4 and myoD1/myf3).[21,22] The extent and intensity of staining of Myogenin and myoD1 can be used as an aid in distinguishing between the

Table 2 Clinical, pathological and genetic differences between the two main types of rhabdomyosarcoma (RMS)

	Embryonal RMS	Alveolar RMS
Five-year survival	~80%	~38%
Incidence	80%	20%
Age	up to 50% < 5 yr; 85% < 10 yr	Mean 9.0 yr
Location	Head and neck 47% Genito-urinary tract 28%	Extremities 45% Head and neck 22%
Histology	Stellate or spindle-cell usually Myxoid stroma	Round-cell Fibrous septa
Cytogenetic analysis	Loss of heterozygosity Chromosome 11 p15.5	t(2; 13) or t(1; 13)

Table 3 The basic panel of antibodies used for identification of small round-cell tumours by immunohistochemistry[38]

	CD45	NB84	CD99[a]	Myogenin[b]	WT1[b]	CKand/or EMA	INI1[b39]
Rhabdomyosarcoma	−	−	−	+	−	+, <10%	+
EFT	−	+[#]	+	−	−	+, < 7%	+
DRCT	−	+[##]	−	−	+	+	+
MRT	−	NK	+	−	NK	+	−
NHL[c]/ALL	+	−	+	−	+[d]	+**	NK
Neuroblastoma	−	+	−	−	−	−	NK
Blastemal component of WT	−	−	−	−[e]	+	+	+

[a]Membranous pattern of staining.
[b]Nuclear expression.
[c]NHL (anaplastic large cell lymphoma) positive for EMA.
[d]Positive in acute myeloid leukaemia.
[e]Positive in areas of skeletal muscle differentiation.
[#]20%; [##]50%.
IHC, immunohistochemistry; EFT, Ewing sarcoma family of tumours; DRCT, desmoplastic round cell tumour; MRT, malignant rhabdoid tumour; NHL, non-Hodgkin lymphoma; ALL, acute lymphoblastic leukaemia; WT, Wilms tumour; EMA, epithelial membrane antigen; CK, cytokeratin; WT1, Wilms tumour gene product; NK, not known.

Table 4 Immunohistochemical reactivity of spindle-cell sarcomas – percentage positivity

	Myogenin	CK 7	EMA	S100	Nestin[30]
RMS	95	< 10	< 1	< 10	NK
SS	10	60	90	48	0
MPNST	0	0	13, weak	55	78
FS	20	0	0	< 5	NK

RMS, rhabdomyosarcoma; SS, synovial sarcoma; MPNST, malignant peripheral nerve sheath tumour; FS, fibrosarcoma; CK, cytokeratin; EMA, epithelial membrane antigen.

Table 5 Genetic abnormalities in soft tissue sarcomas and their detection

Soft tissue tumour	Chromosomal re-arrangement	FISH	Chimeric fusion transcripts	RT-PCR
ARMS	t(2; 13)(q35; q14)	P[11]	PAX3–FKHR	RT-PCR[14,17]
	t(1; 13)(p36; q14)		PAX7–FKHR	Q-PCR[13]
EFT	t(11; 22)(q24; q12)	P[12]	EWS–FLI	RT-PCR[14]
	t(21; 22)(q22; q12)			
DRCT	t(11; 22)(p13; q12)	F	EWS–WT1	RT-PCR[14]
	t(21; 22)(p22; q12)			
SS	t(X; 18)(p11.23; q11)	P[10]	SYT–SSX1	RT-PCR[14]
	t(X; 18)(p11.21; q11)		SYT–SSX2	Q-PCR[14,15]
IFS	t(12; 15)(p13; q25)	F, P	ETV6–NTRK3	RT-PCR[14]
IMT	t(1; 2)(q25; p23)	P[9]	TPM3–ALK	RT-PCR
	t(2; 19)(p23; q13)		ALK–TPM2	
LGFMS	t(7; 16)(q34; p11)		FUS/CREB3L2	RT-PCR[35]
Extrarenal MRT	del(22q)(11.2)		hSNF/INI1 del	

ARMS, alveolar rhabdomyosarcoma; EFT, Ewing sarcoma family of tumours; DRCT, desmoplastic round cell tumour; SS, synovial sarcoma; IFS, fibrosarcoma; IMT, inflammatory myofibroblastic tumour; LGFMS, low-grade fibromyxoid sarcoma; MRT, malignant rhabdoid tumour.
F, frozen; P, paraffin.

two main types of RMS. Most alveolar RMSs display extensive (> 50%) nuclear staining for Myogenin, whereas embryonal RMSs typically show a focal pattern of staining.[22] Myogenin expression is reliable in separating RMS from malignant peripheral nerve sheath tumour (MPNST),[22] although it can be expressed in MPNST which show rhabdomyosarcomatous differentiation (malignant Triton tumour).[7] Its expression is also useful in excluding nodular fasciitis, inflammatory myofibroblastic tumour as well as benign and malignant smooth muscle and neural tumours.[22]

However, Myogenin expression should be interpreted with caution because its immunoreactivity, albeit focal, is also seen in blastemal component of Wilms tumour, synovial sarcoma and infantile fibrosarcoma.[22] Myogenin immunopositivity may be seen in isolated benign nuclei in lymph nodes.[21] Moreover, the non-neoplastic, entrapped or regenerating skeletal muscle fibres show expression of Myogenin and myoD1.[21,22] This is a potential pitfall, and should be kept in mind when assessing immunoreactivity at the infiltrative edges of a round- or spindle-cell tumour.

Several other immunocytochemical markers have been identified in RMSs and can lead to diagnostic errors if interpreted out of the context of the clinical and histological findings. These include desmin, CD99, anaplastic lymphoma kinase, CD56, smooth muscle actin, cytokeratin, S100 and neurofilament protein.

Embryonal rhabdomyosarcoma

Embryonal RMSs show cytological characteristics that range from primitive stellate or fusiform mesenchymal cells to well-differentiated forms with extensive rhabdomyoblastic differentiation. Hypercellular areas, typically concentrated around the blood vessels, alternate with mucoid matrix-rich, hypocellular areas. Adequate sampling is crucial, as a wide variety of benign and malignant myxoid tumours[7] can mimic hypocellular embryonal RMS.

Spindle cell variant of embryonal rhabdomyosarcoma

The spindle cell variant of embryonal RMS arises in the paratesticular and head and neck regions. It is composed of cells that resemble smooth muscle cells arranged in intersecting fascicles, although they may display a benign fibrous histiocytoma- or neurofibroma-like pattern. This subtype may also be mistaken for leiomyosarcoma, from which it can be distinguished by positive Myogenin and negative h-caldesmon immunoprofile.

Botyroid variant of embryonal rhabdomyosarcoma

The botyroid variant of embryonal RMS arises in the hollow cavities of the genito-urinary, biliary, auditory and upper aerodigestive tract. Making a definite diagnosis requires the demonstration of the subepithelial cellular 'cambium layer' of neoplastic rhabdomyoblasts (Fig. 1). Its endoscopic, grape-like or polypoid appearance may be mimicked by fetal rhabdomyoma and inflammatory myofibroblastic tumour (IMT).

Fetal rhabdomyoma, a benign skeletal muscle tumour, also overlaps with embryonal RMS in age at diagnosis, location and histology.[6,7] The head and neck are a common site for both. It can be distinguished from embryonal RMS by an absence of cellular pleomorphism. In submucosal tumours, the absence of cambium layer, which is the defining feature of the botyroid subtype of embryonal RMS, should resolve the diagnostic dilemma.

In addition to the similarity in gross appearance, other features of IMT may contribute to an overdiagnosis of embryonal RMS. For example, its infiltrative growth pattern can cause concern for malignancy. The constituent myofibroblastic/fibroblastic cells may show a high mitotic count, moderate

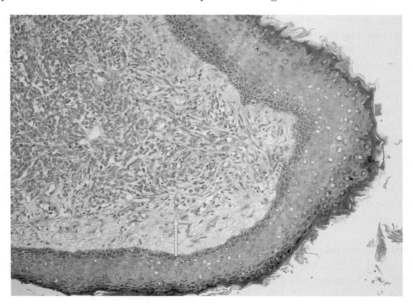

Fig. 1 Embryonal RMS with cambium layer (arrow) presenting as a nasal polyp.

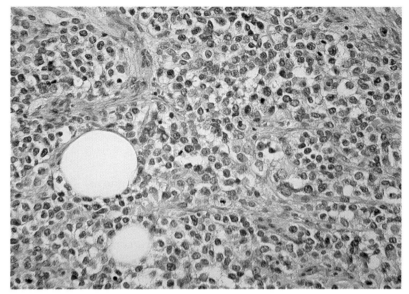

Fig. 2 Solid alveolar RMS composed of undifferentiated small round cells.

atypia and vascular bulging. IMT may show desmin[6] and embryonal RMS may show ALK[9] immunoreactivity, causing further confusion in diagnosis. IMT can be distinguished from embryonal RMS by a mixture of three growth patterns, an absence of atypical mitotic figures and Myogenin expression.[22]

Alveolar rhabdomyosarcoma

Alveolar RMS is defined by the cytological appearance of round cells with frequent mitoses, hyperchromatic nuclei, coarse chromatin pattern, and

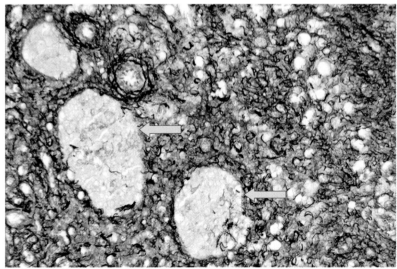

Fig. 3 Reticulin stain outlining the solid alveolar component (arrow) of a mixed embryonal and alveolar RMS.

distinct smooth nuclear membrane. The classic variant of ARMS consists of anastomosing fibrous septa, which delineate aggregates of discohesive cells, while the solid type shows a paucity of fibrous septa (Fig. 2). The reticulin stain is particularly helpful as it encircles the variably-sized, solid aggregates of tumour cells (Fig. 3). It is important to emphasise that a single focus of alveolar morphology is sufficient to type it as alveolar RMS. However, the alveolar component may not be represented or may be difficult to appreciate in a small biopsy, necessitating molecular genetic studies in certain clinical situations.[13]

Anaplastic variant of rhabdomyosarcoma
The anaplastic variant of RMS has a poor prognosis. It shows large hyperchromatic nuclei and multipolar mitotic figures. Although it can be seen in both the types of RMS, it is more common in embryonal RMS.

Sclerosing, matrix-rich subtype of rhabdomyosarcoma
Recently, the sclerosing, matrix-rich subtype of RMS has also been reported in children, although its precise clinical relevance remains uncertain.[23] It is rare, and usually located in the head and neck. It causes difficulties in diagnosis because the abundant stroma obscures the smaller component of small, blue, tumour cells, often resulting in a micro-alveolar architecture resembling angiosarcoma or carcinoma. Most cases show mixed embryonal and alveolar histology. The normal pattern of immunostaining of myogenic transcription factors is reversed as the alveolar component shows relatively strong diffuse MyoD1 staining while the embryonal component shows stronger Myogenin staining.

PAEDIATRIC NON-RHABDOMYOSARCOMATOUS SOFT TISSUE SARCOMAS

In children and adolescents, the non-RMS round cell soft tissue sarcomas include the Ewing sarcoma family of tumours and desmoplastic round cell tumour. The epithelioid group of tumours is represented by malignant rhabdoid tumour.

Ewing sarcoma family of tumours
The Ewing sarcoma family of tumours (EFT) encompasses extra-osseous Ewing, its variants and peripheral primitive neuro-ectodermal tumours (pPNET). It constitutes the second most common soft tissue sarcoma in childhood, accounting for up to 20% of paediatric sarcomas. It usually occurs in the chest wall, followed by paraspinal tissues and the abdominal wall.

These round cell tumours show a range of appearances depending on the degree of neural differentiation. Ewing sarcoma represents the undifferentiated end of the spectrum, while pPNET shows varying degrees of neural differentiation. A large number of histological variants of Ewing sarcoma, such as adamantinoma-like, sclerosing-type and spindle-cell type have been reported,[24] presenting a potential diagnostic trap for the unwary.

Immunoreactivity for CD99 and FLI-1 is seen in over 90% of these tumours.[24] As neither CD99 nor FLI-1 is specific for EFT, they should be used as part of a panel of antibodies to exclude haematolymphoid, neuroblastic and myogenic tumours.

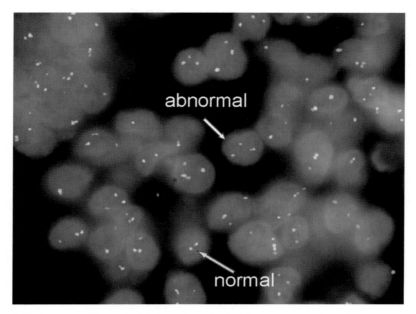

Fig. 4 FISH on paraffin-embedded section of primitive neuroectodermal tumour showing normal and split signal of t(11; 22).

Lymphoblastic lymphoma is notorious for its mimicry of EFT as it displays the uniform, strong membranous reactivity of CD99 and nuclear reactivity of FLI-1. Moreover, lymphoblastic lymphomas can be negative for CD45 (leukocyte common antigen). A combination of immunohistochemical reactivity for various haematolymphoid markers, such as TdT, CD43, CD34, CD10 and CD79a, can distinguish lymphoblastic lymphoma from EFT. Neuroblastomas are negative for CD99. This is a useful discriminator because NB84, a neuroblastoma marker, shows immunoreactivity with 20% of EFT.[25] It is also useful to remember that EFT can be positive for cytokeratin, CD117, CD31 and, rarely, for desmin.

As there are no specific histological, immunohistochemical or electron microscopic features, cytogenetic or molecular genetic confirmation of the characteristic translocations (Fig. 4) and gene fusion transcripts are valuable.[12,14] It is critical when EFT presents in visceral locations or when rare morphological variants of EFT are encountered.

Desmoplastic round cell tumour

Desmoplastic round cell tumour (DRCT) is a highly aggressive, well-defined clinicopathological entity primarily of young adults, but has also been reported in children. DRCT displays striking diversity in location, which is reflected in the clinical presentation.

The histological spectrum is also wide, with several morphological variants and polyphenotypic immunoreactivity.[6,7] Immunostaining for the carboxy-terminus of WT1 is the most sensitive, followed by others such as desmin, EMA, cytokeratin and NB84. In difficult cases, confirmation of the specific chromosomal re-arrangement and chimeric transcript should be sought by various techniques (Table 5).

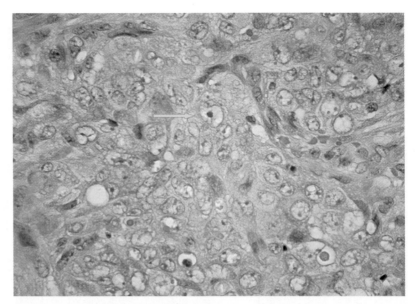

Fig. 5 Extrarenal malignant rhabdoid tumour displaying undifferentiated cells, some with large eosinophilic nucleoli (arrow).

Malignant rhabdoid tumour

Malignant rhabdoid tumour (MRT) is a very aggressive neoplasm of infancy and childhood with a propensity for wide-spread metastases.[6,26] In addition to the renal and central nervous system MRTs, which are well-established entities, the clinicopathological spectrum includes involvement of other organs, extrarenal soft tissue and a congenital disseminated form.[27] Rare examples have been described in adults. Irrespective of location, MRT characteristically demonstrates abnormalities of 22q11, and mutations and homozygous deletions of the *INI1(hSNF5)* gene are detected in about 80% of cases.[26]

The hallmark 'rhabdoid cell' has large, round or oval nuclei, with conspicuous central eosinophilic nucleoli and abundant cytoplasm (Fig. 5). Inclusions in the form of paranuclear cytoplasmic globules are seen in some cells. The cells are typically arranged in patternless sheets or cords. However, MRTs may display a variety of cytological and architectural features such as small, round cells and a myxoid or collagenous stroma.

MRT shows a complex immunophenotype, with co-expression of vimentin and at least one epithelial marker such as cytokeratin or epithelial membrane antigen. A wide variety of other neuro-ectodermal and mesenchymal markers, including smooth muscle actin, may also be present.

The morphological variability and immunohistochemical profile of MRT presents challenges in differential diagnosis, particularly with rhabdomyo-sarcoma, desmoplastic round cell tumour, Ewing sarcoma family of tumours, epithelioid sarcoma, synovial sarcoma and other primitive malignant neoplasms. Recent availability of the antibody against the gene product INI1/BAF1 has greatly facilitated the diagnosis of MRT. Normal cells show nuclear reaction to INI1/BAF1 (Fig. 6). Neoplasms which display the 'rhabdoid' phenotype of MRT

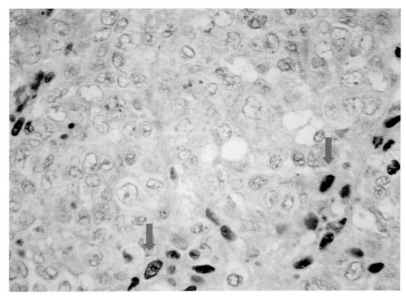

Fig. 6 Loss of INI1/BAF1 immunostaining in extrarenal malignant rhabdoid tumour, but preservation of normal nuclear staining in the stromal cells (arrows).

but lack deletions and mutations of *INI1(hSNF5)* show normal immuno-reactivity,[28] while MRT shows an absence of nuclear reaction (Fig. 6).

ADULT-TYPE NON-RHABDOMYOSARCOMATOUS SOFT TISSUE SARCOMAS

'Adult-type' NRSTS are a heterogeneous group of tumours, and include entities which are usually seen in adults.[27] Synovial sarcoma, malignant peripheral nerve sheath tumour, liposarcoma, epithelioid sarcoma, leiomyosarcoma and adult-type fibrosarcoma constitute around 70% of 'adult-type' NRSTS in children.[27] Gastrointestinal stromal tumours (GISTs) comprise about 2% of soft tissue sarcomas.[28]

Synovial sarcoma

After RMS and EFT, synovial sarcoma is the most common sarcoma, accounting for one-third of adult-type soft tissue sarcomas in children.[27] It occurs most commonly in the second decade. However, it has been reported in younger children and even in newborns. Like its counterpart in adults, it usually occurs in the extremities, although in the recent years it has been reported in a number of visceral sites as well as the mediastinum.

The histological features seen in children and adults are similar, with biphasic and monophasic types which show immunoreactivity for cytokeratin and epithelial membrane antigen (EMA). The monophasic spindle-cell type comprises about 70%, and the remainder are the biphasic type.[29] Monophasic epithelial type is extremely uncommon.

Its classic biphasic pattern, comprising the spindle and epithelial cells forming glands, is easy to recognise. Malignant peripheral nerve sheath tumour (MPNST) is the most important tumour in the differential diagnosis of biphasic synovial sarcoma because it may also show glandular differentiation. A characteristic feature of MPNST is the presence of intestinal-type epithelial differentiation with goblet-cells and microvilli in the glands, which is not seen in synovial sarcoma.

The monophasic spindle-cell type of synovial sarcoma has to be distinguished from MPNST and other spindle-cell sarcomas, particularly fibrosarcoma. This can be very difficult. A thorough search should be made for the epithelial component and foci of calcification, which are more common in synovial sarcoma than in fibrosarcoma. Cytokeratin and/or EMA positivity in both the spindle and epithelial cells is the most reliable indicator of synovial sarcoma in this context.

Histological variants in which poorly-differentiated, myxoid, or haemagiopericytomatous comprise the predominant population, may be difficult to recognise as synovial sarcoma in biopsies. The poorly-differentiated variant, which comprises about a quarter of the synovial sarcoma in one series,[29] shows a strong resemblance to small, round cell tumours of childhood or MPNST. The myxoid variant has to be distinguished from embryonal RMS. Of particular relevance is the haemangiopericytomatous synovial sarcoma. It must be distinguished from infantile haemangiopericytoma, which falls within the morphological spectrum of infantile myofibroma and is a benign lesion. Routine histology and IHC may not distinguish between the two on a small sample, underscoring the importance of genetic studies for demonstration of the specific translocation t(X;18) in synovial sarcoma.

Malignant peripheral nerve sheath tumour

Malignant peripheral nerve sheath tumour (MPNST) represents about 15% of adult-type sarcomas in children and, like synovial sarcoma, usually presents in the second decade of life. Essential criteria for its diagnosis include association with neurofibromatosis type 1 (NF1), peripheral nerve or pre-existing neurofibroma.

MPNSTs are histologically heterogeneous tumours and, as mentioned earlier, have to be distinguished from synovial sarcoma and other spindle cell sarcomas. In a recent study comparing the immunoreactivity of monophasic synovial sarcoma and MPNST, nestin emerged as the most sensitive and specific neural marker.[30]

MPNSTs in childhood differs from those in adults by the presence of prominent neuro-epithelial foci and primitive cells.[5,7] Due to the high likelihood of sampling error, caution should be exercised before making the diagnosis of MPNST on a Tru-Cut biopsy.

An important tumour to consider in the differential diagnosis of paediatric MPNST is plexiform (multinodular) cellular schwannoma. It is a rare type of benign peripheral nerve sheath tumour which may be mistaken for malignancy because of its rapid growth and locally aggressive behaviour.[31] Surgical difficulty in obtaining clear margins and its tendency for local recurrence may lead also to a misleading impression of a malignant tumour. Histological features that cause concern for MPNST are the lack of a capsule, uniformly high cellularity and increased mitotic activity.

In contrast to MPNSTs, plexiform schwannomas occur most commonly in the first decade, and half present as congenital tumours. They do not show an association with NF1 or evidence of a co-existing neurofibroma or schwannoma. These tumours are superficial, and typically located in the subcutis of extremities. Moreover, tumour cells are uniformly positive for S100 and do not express p53 protein. Electron microscopy shows a uniform population of well-differentiated Schwann cells.[31]

BENIGN TUMOURS MISDIAGNOSED AS SARCOMA

In addition to fetal rhabdomyoma and plexiform schwannoma, other benign tumours which may cause difficulties are pseudosarcomatous fibroblastic/myofibroblastic lesions and infantile myofibroma/myofibromatosis.

PSEUDOSARCOMATOUS FIBROBLASTIC/MYOFIBROBLASTIC LESIONS

Pseudosarcomatous fibroblastic/myofibroblastic lesions represent about 12% of soft tissue tumours in childhood. This group of benign tumours includes nodular fasciitis and its variants, and proliferative fasciitis/myositis. An alarming clinical finding is that these lesions often grow rapidly over a few days to several weeks to form sizeable tumours. Pathologically, they also comprise a significant group as florid examples often show a disturbing degree of cellularity, nuclear pleomorphism and mitotic activity. The overlap with the myogenic immunophenotype can also cause confusion. Indeed, in the setting of second-opinion consultation practice, 45% of the tumours in this category were submitted as sarcoma in a recent study.[32]

Nodular fasciitis
Nodular fasciitis is a typical example of this group of tumours with clinical and histological features that mimic malignancy. About 20% of nodular fasciitis occurs in childhood, although it is rare in infancy. The head and neck region is a common site in children, followed by extremities and the trunk. Cranial fasciitis occurs in the temporoparietal soft tissues in the first 2 years of life.

Nodular fasciitis displays a zonal pattern composed of a central hypocellular myxoid area juxtaposed to extravasated red blood cells and loosely-arranged myofibroblasts, which in turn are surrounded by plump- and spindled-fibroblasts. Features that are likely to contribute to an overdiagnosis of malignancy include its occurrence in unusual extracranial locations, erosion of the underlying bone, invasion of the adjacent skeletal muscle, nerves and lymph nodes, nuclear pleomorphism and abundant mitoses in densely cellular areas. In children, it may mimic a spindle cell sarcoma, such as embryonal rhabdomyosarcoma, synovial sarcoma, dermatofibrosarcoma protuberans or fibrosarcoma.

Helpful features for recognition of nodular fasciitis are the small size (usually less than 4 cm), an awareness of various histological subtypes and variants and an absence of atypical mitotic figures. Demonstration of the myofibroblastic immunotype (vimentin, muscle-specific actin, smooth muscle actin-positive, desmin-positive) combined with negative Myogenin,[22] cytokeratins and/or EMA and CD34, can help in excluding other spindle-cell sarcomas. Nodular fasciitis may regress spontaneously, and recurrence should prompt reconsideration of the diagnosis. Cranial and extracranial fasciitis are less cellular, more myxoid and more uniform than typical nodular fasciitis. The immunophenotype is similar.

Proliferative fasciitis and myositis

These entities, although closely related to nodular fasciitis, are rare in childhood. Like their counterparts in adults, they are located within the subcutaneous tissue and superficial fascia of skeletal muscle, and characterised by the presence of large basophilic ganglion-like cells or histiocytoid myofibroblasts. However, there are differences between the childhood and adult lesions, which may lead to a misdiagnosis of embryonal rhabdomyosarcoma or ganglioneuroblastoma.[7] Those presenting in childhood display increased cellularity, necrosis and numerous mitotic figures but contain less collagen and myxoid matrix. They also lack the delicate fibroblastic component, which is a feature of the adult-type lesion.

INFANTILE MYOFIBROMA/MYOFIBROMATOSIS

Infantile myofibroma/myofibromatosis (IM) constitutes around 20% of the fibroblastic–myofibroblastic lesions in children and adolescents. The majority of these tumours occur before the age of 2 years, and 60% are present at birth. IM occurs in solitary, multicentric and generalised forms, all of which show similar histology but different clinical and prognostic features. The generalised form is associated with visceral involvement such as heart, lungs and gastrointestinal tract, and is the one most likely to cause progressive disease and death.

The macroscopic appearance is distinctive, with a red or yellow soft centre surrounded by white and firm areas. Histologically, these features are also reflected in a zonal pattern. The central part resembles a haemangiopericytoma while the peripheral part is composed of spindle-shaped myofibroblasts arranged in interlacing fascicles.

Four features may be responsible for its misdiagnosis as infantile fibrosarcoma. These are increased cellularity and mitotic activity, infiltration of the myofibroblasts into the adjacent uninvolved tissue and intravascular growth simulating vascular invasion. Multicentric involvement may be interpreted as a sign of metastases. Distinguishing between the two may be particularly difficult if the lesion has been biopsied, precluding an appreciation of the characteristic zonal pattern. IHC is usually unhelpful in distinguishing between the two lesions. Both are focally positive for Myogenin.[22] In this scenario, genetic studies may be necessary to exclude infantile fibrosarcoma (Table 5).

SARCOMAS MISDIAGNOSED AS BENIGN LESIONS

Myxoid tumours comprise one of the most treacherous group which account for misdiagnosis in paediatric soft tissue tumours. The clinical spectrum ranges from reactive, benign lesions to high-grade sarcomas such as embryonal RMS and myofibrosarcoma.

MYOFIBROSARCOMA

The malignant myofibroblastic tumour myofibrosarcoma is rare in children. It can arise in the bone or soft tissue, and has predilection for the head and neck.[33] It can metastasise even after a relatively long period.

It shows an infiltrative pattern of spindle cells arranged in a herring-bone fashion against a collagenous background. The tumour cells show cytological features ranging from low-grade to high-grade. As in the case of embryonal RMS, foci of low cellularity may be misleading as to the grade of the lesion, particularly in small samples.

LOW-GRADE FIBROMYXOID SARCOMA/HYALINISING SPINDLE CELL TUMOUR WITH GIANT ROSETTES

These intermediate-grade tumours represent a morphological spectrum of the same entity as they share a common translocation t(7;16)(q34;p11), which has been characterised only recently. The majority of cases occur in young to middle-aged adults, although no age group is exempt. About 20% occur under 18 years of age.[6] The usual presentation in adults is that of a slowly growing deep soft tissue mass most commonly arising in the shoulder or extremity. The metastatic rate is around 5%, and late metastases are a recognised feature of this neoplasm. By contrast to the adult tumours, the superficial form is more common in children,[34] and is not associated with metastases.

These tumours are composed of a mixture of fibrous and myxoid tissues (Fig. 7), which may show an abrupt transition or blend imperceptibly with each other.[34] Collagen rosettes are an inconsistent component. Uniform spindle cells with small, hyperchromatic nuclei and a pale eosinophilic cytoplasm are present in both the components. These cells are set in a variable collagenous

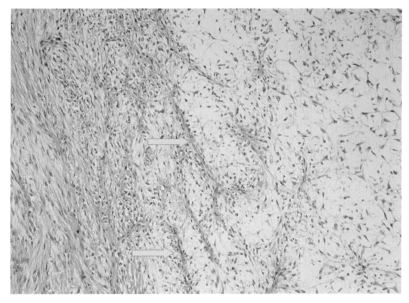

Fig. 7 Low-grade fibromyxoid sarcoma showing compact fibrous and myxoid components, the latter showing the arcading blood vessels (arrows).

stroma, and may be arranged in a swirling pattern. Arcades of curvilinear blood-vessels are a characteristic feature (Fig. 7).

Low-grade fibromyxoid sarcoma shows a bland appearance because of low cellularity, infrequent mitoses and an absence of nuclear pleomorphism. These features together with its well-circumscribed borders add to its deceitful resemblance to benign tumours such as nodular fasciitis or benign nerve sheath tumour.[34] A lack of awareness of LGFMS and its rarity also contribute to its misdiagnosis.

The superficial form is usually less than 5 cm in size. Deep location and large size (9–10 cm) are important pointers toward a high-grade sarcoma. A diligent search for the two distinct components and collagen rosettes will aid recognition and prevent diagnostic errors. Virtually all LGFMSs are characterised by chimeric FUS/CREB3L2 gene, and its transcripts can be detected by RT-PCR.[35]

MISGRADING OF SARCOMAS

Fibroblastic/myofibroblastic neoplasms of intermediate (borderline) biological potential may recur locally, but rarely metastasise. Inflammatory myofibroblastic tumour and infantile fibrosarcoma are two examples of such tumours, which may overdiagnosed as malignant sarcomas.

INFLAMMATORY MYOFIBROBLASTIC TUMOUR

Inflammatory myofibroblastic tumour (IMT) can occur at any age and in virtually any anatomical location. Most IMTs occur in the first two decades of life, and 90% arise in the abdomen, genito-urinary and upper respiratory tract. One-third of patients have associated systemic symptoms and polyclonal hyperglobulinaemia.

IMT is composed of a lymphoplasmacytic-rich population mixed with spindle-shaped myofibroblasts and collagen. Variable amounts of these components result in three histological patterns: nodular fasciitis-, fibrous histiocytoma- and scar-like patterns. Large ganglion cell-like myofibroblasts are seen in the first two patterns.[6] The myofibroblasts generally lack atypical mitoses and significant atypia.

The cellular fibrous histiocytoma-like pattern is the most likely to be misdiagnosed as a high-grade spindle-cell sarcoma, from which it can be distinguished by IHC (Table 4). The distinction between IMT and embryonal RMS has also been discussed earlier. Other tumours in the differential diagnosis include leiomyosarcoma and gastrointestinal stromal tumour, both of which are extremely rare in childhood,[28] and can be excluded by absence of h-caldesmon and diffuse membranous CD117 staining, respectively.

Chromosomal re-arrangement of 2p23 and *ALK* (anaplastic lymphoma kinase gene) occurs in about 50% of IMTs. ALK protein can be demonstrated within the myofibroblasts by IHC and the cytogenetic abnormality by FISH on paraffin-embedded tissue. ALK is not specific.[9]

Approximately 25% of IMTs recur. Recurrent IMT may undergo a round cell or sarcomatoid histological transformation. There are no definite clinical or histological criteria for distinguishing between the two. The presence of necroses, large highly atypical cells resembling ganglion cells or Reed–Sternberg cells and p53 expression, are probably indicative of malignancy.

INFANTILE FIBROSARCOMA

Infantile fibrosarcoma (IFS) presents in children mainly under one year of age, and at least half of the cases are congenital. It occurs in the deep soft tissues of the distal extremities and, occasionally, in the head and neck, or axial sites. Although they are microscopically identical to the adult-type fibrosarcoma, the natural history is more favourable. The 5-year survival rate is > 90%, the recurrence rate is 30% and < 10% metastasise. Spontaneous regression has been observed. Local excision is the treatment of choice and chemotherapy is also effective. Adult-type fibrosarcoma occurs uncommonly in children, and is usually encountered after the age of 10 years. Rapid growth to a large size, erosion of the bone and growth around neurovascular structures are reasons for clinical concern.

IFS shows a broad histological spectrum, ranging from small immature fibroblasts without fascicular arrangement to that resembling fibromatosis and adult type fibrosarcoma. The latter pattern comprises a solid growth of mitotically active spindle cells, which are arranged in a herring-bone fashion. It must be distinguished from other spindle cell sarcomas of childhood by IHC (Table 3).

Because of the histological and immunophenotypic similarities, the differentiation of IFS from infantile fibromatosis is more problematic and may be virtually impossible in some cases. In the younger age group, differentiating between these two entities may not be necessary since the treatment of choice for both is wide local excision.

IFSs which show a predominantly myxoid pattern must be distinguished from myxoid mesenchymal tumour of infancy.[36] This is a recently described fibroblastic–myofibroblastic tumour of intermediate or low-grade malignant biological potential. Unlike IFS, it is a multinodular tumour and the primitive tumour cells are embedded in a uniformly myxoid stroma with branching blood vessels. The interlacing cellular fascicles are present only focally, and at the periphery of nodules. It is locally aggressive and displays poor chemosensitivity.

In contrast to the adult-type fibrosarcoma, fibromatosis and myxoid mesenchymal tumour of infancy, almost all IFSs show a characteristic translocation t(12;15)(p13;q25) which results in *ETV6–NTRK3* fusion and chimeric transcripts. Genetic confirmation, either on fresh or archival tissue, may be critical in difficult cases,[16] particularly as IFS does not show a specific immunophenotypic profile.

NON-SOFT TISSUE TUMOURS MISDIAGNOSED AS SOFT TISSUE SARCOMAS

An awareness of the atypical presentations of histocytic and haemato-lymphoid disorders should prevent misinterpretation as childhood sarcomas.

DEEP JUVENILE XANTHOGRANULOMA

Juvenile xanthogranuloma (JXG) is the most common non-Langerhans histocytic disorder. Typically it occurs in neonates and young children, either

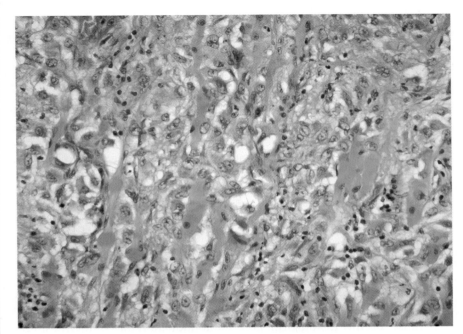

Fig. 8 Mononuclear cells of juvenile xanthogranuloma infiltrating skeletal muscle.

as solitary or multiple skin lesions in the head and neck. It can also occur in subcutaneous tissue or parenchymal organs. Deep JXG is a benign self-limited lesion which is treated with a conservative surgical procedure.

The diagnosis is easy when JXG shows the classic picture comprising varying proportions of lipidised and non-lipidised, multinucleated Touton cells and inflammatory cells. The main difficulty is recognising it when located in the deep soft tissues and skeletal muscle.[37] Solitary skeletal muscle involvement may be seen in up to 5% of cases. The deep lesions are poorly-circumscribed and grow rapidly, raising concerns about a sarcoma.[37] They are composed of a homogeneous population of non-lipidised, mononuclear histiocyte-like cells (Fig. 8). The characteristic Touton giant cells may be absent, or present in decreased numbers, and the histiocytes may show atypia and mitotic activity. JXG should be kept in mind as a possible diagnosis in infants and young children who present with a histiocytic disorder in the soft tissue with or without skin or visceral involvement. An extensive panel of antibodies is generally unnecessary for its diagnosis, which can be established by demonstration of CD68 and FXIIa, and non-reactivity or weak and patchy staining with S100 and CD1a.

HAEMATOLYMPHOID MALIGNANCIES

In contrast to adults, children show a higher proportion of extranodal non-Hodgkin lymphomas. Extramedullary myeloid tumours are also common in children, and should be considered in the differential diagnosis of round cell tumours.

ACKNOWLEDGEMENTS

The contribution of Figure 4 by Eileen Roberts and her cytogenetics team at Southmead Hospital is gratefully acknowledged. The author would also like to thank Professor C. Fisher and Dr Salim Anjarwalla for their helpful comments on the text.

Points for best practice

- Soft tissue sarcomas are rare and diverse biologically, clinically and pathologically.

- Benign myofibroblastic/fibroblastic tumours are the largest group involving misdiagnosis.

- Rhabdomyosarcoma is the most common soft tissue sarcoma in childhood. There are strict criteria for the diagnosis of the types and variants, each of which has therapeutic significance.

- Extrarenal soft tissue malignant rhabdoid tumour shows morphological and immunophenotypic variability. It can be diagnosed easily by immunohistochemistry because of the recent availability of commercial antibody to the *INI1/BAF* gene product.

- Extensive immunohistochemistry may be necessary for accurate identification of round-cell and spindle-cell tumours, but none of the antibodies are specific. A panel of antibodies is recommended, and the pathological findings should be interpreted in the context of clinical and radiological findings.

- Genetic studies provide valuable support to pathological diagnosis, particularly for tumours which have no specific histological features. They are critical when soft tissue tumours present in unusual clinical settings or when rare morphological variants or aberrant immunoreactivity is encountered. With recent advances in technology and the commercial availability of break-apart re-arrangement probes, RT-PCR and FISH assays can now be performed reliably on paraffin-embedded tissue.

References

1. Steliarova-Foucher E, Stiller C, Lacour B, Kaatsch P. International Classification of Childhood Cancer, third edition. *Cancer* 2005; **103**: 1457–1467.
2. Steliarova-Foucher E, Stiller C, Kaatsch P, Berrino F, Coebergh JW. Trends in childhood cancer incidence in Europe, 1970–99. *Lancet* 2005; **365**: 2088.
3. Stevens MC. Treatment for childhood rhabdomyosarcoma: the cost of cure. *Lancet Oncol* 2005; **6**: 77–84.
4. Robison LL, Green DM, Hudson M *et al.* Long-term outcomes of adult survivors of childhood cancer. *Cancer* 2005; **104 (Suppl)**: 2557–2564.
5. Coffin CM. *Pediatric soft tissue tumours: a clinical, pathological, and therapeutic approach*, 1st edn. Baltimore. MD: Williams & Wilkins, 1997.
6. Fletcher CD, Unni K, Mertens F. (eds) *WHO Classification of Tumours: pathology and genetics. Tumours of soft tissue and bone*, 4th edn. Lyon: IARC, 2002.

7. Weiss SW, Goldblum JR. (eds) *Enzinger's and Weiss' soft tissue tumours*, 4th edn. St Louis, MO: Mosby, 2001.

8. Lazar A, Abruzzo LV, Pollock RE, Lee S, Czerniak B. Molecular diagnosis of sarcomas: chromosomal translocations in sarcomas. *Arch Pathol Lab Med* 2006; **130**: 1199–1207.

9. Cessna MH, Zhou H, Sanger WG *et al*. Expression of ALK1 and p80 in inflammatory myofibroblastic tumor and its mesenchymal mimics: a study of 135 cases. *Mod Pathol* 2002; **15**: 931–938.

10. Terry J, Barry TS, Horsman DE *et al*. Fluorescence *in situ* hybridization for the detection of t(X; 18)(p11.2; q11.2) in a synovial sarcoma tissue microarray using a breakapart-style probe. *Diagn Mol Pathol* 2005; **14**: 77–82.

11. Nishio J, Althof PA, Bailey JM *et al*. Use of a novel FISH assay on paraffin-embedded tissues as an adjunct to diagnosis of alveolar rhabdomyosarcoma. *Lab Invest* 2006; **86**: 547–556.

12. Bridge RS, Rajaram V, Dehner LP, Pfeifer JD, Perry A. Molecular diagnosis of Ewing sarcoma/primitive neuroectodermal tumor in routinely processed tissue: a comparison of two FISH strategies and RT-PCR in malignant round cell tumors. *Mod Pathol* 2006; **19**: 1–8.

13. Hostein I, Andraud-Fregeville M, Guillou L *et al*. Rhabdomyosarcoma: value of Myogenin expression analysis and molecular testing in diagnosing the alveolar subtype: an analysis of 109 paraffin-embedded specimens. *Cancer* 2004; **101**: 2817–2824.

14. Hill DA, O'Sullivan MJ, Zhu X *et al*. Practical application of molecular genetic testing as an aid to the surgical pathologic diagnosis of sarcomas: a prospective study. *Am J Surg Pathol* 2002; **26**: 965–977.

15. Coindre JM, Pelmus M, Hostein I, Lussan C, Bui BN, Guillou L. Should molecular testing be required for diagnosing synovial sarcoma? A prospective study of 204 cases. *Cancer* 2003; **98**: 2700–2707.

16. Argani P, Fritsch M, Kadkol SS, Schuster A, Beckwith JB, Perlman EJ. Detection of the ETV6–NTRK3 chimeric RNA of infantile fibrosarcoma/cellular congenital mesoblastic nephroma in paraffin-embedded tissue: application to challenging pediatric renal stromal tumors. *Mod Pathol* 2000; **13**: 29–36.

17. Jin L, Majerus J, Oliveira A *et al*. Detection of fusion gene transcripts in fresh-frozen and formalin-fixed paraffin-embedded tissue sections of soft-tissue sarcomas after laser capture microdissection and RT-PCR. *Diagn Mol Pathol* 2003; **12**: 224–230.

18. Somers GR, Gupta AA, Doria AS *et al*. Pediatric undifferentiated sarcoma of the soft tissues: a clinicopathologic study. *Pediatr Dev Pathol* 2006; **9**: 132–142.

19. Furlong MA, Fanburg-Smith JC. Pleomorphic rhabdomyosarcoma in children: four cases in the pediatric age group. *Ann Diagn Pathol* 2001; **5**: 199–206.

20. Newton Jr WA, Gehan EA, Webber BL *et al*. Classification of rhabdomyosarcomas and related sarcomas. Pathologic aspects and proposal for a new classification – an Intergroup Rhabdomyosarcoma Study. *Cancer* 1995; **76**: 1073–1085.

21. Morotti RA, Nicol KK, Parham DM *et al*. An immunohistochemical algorithm to facilitate diagnosis and subtyping of rhabdomyosarcoma: the Children's Oncology Group experience. *Am J Surg Pathol* 2006; **30**: 962–968.

22. Cessna MH, Zhou H, Perkins SLTSR, Layfield L, Daines C, Coffin CM. Are Myogenin and MyoD1 expression specific for rhabdomyosarcoma? A study of 150 cases, with emphasis on spindle cell mimics. *Am J Surg Pathol* 2001; **25**: 1150–1157.

23. Chiles MC, Parham DM, Qualman SJ *et al*. Sclerosing rhabdomyosarcomas in children and adolescents: a clinicopathologic review of 13 cases from the Intergroup Rhabdomyosarcoma Study Group and Children's Oncology Group. *Pediatr Dev Pathol* 2004; **7**: 583–594.

24. Folpe AL, Goldblum JR, Rubin BP *et al*. Morphologic and immunophenotypic diversity in Ewing family tumors: a study of 66 genetically confirmed cases. *Am J Surg Pathol* 2005; **29**: 1025—1033.

25. Miettinen M, Chatten J, Paetau A, Stevenson A. Monoclonal antibody NB84 in the differential diagnosis of neuroblastoma and other small round cell tumors. *Am J Surg Pathol* 1998; **22**: 327–332.

26. Oda Y, Tsuneyoshi M. Extrarenal rhabdoid tumors of soft tissue: Clinicopathological and molecular genetic review and distinction from other soft-tissue sarcomas with rhabdoid

features. *Pathol Int* 2006; **56**: 287–295.
27. Ferrari A, Casanova M, Collini P *et al*. Adult-type soft tissue sarcomas in pediatric-age patients: experience at the Istituto Nazionale Tumori in Milan. *J Clin Oncol* 2005; **23**: 4021–4030.
28. Cypriano MS, Jenkins JJ, Pappo AS, Rao BN, Daw NC. Pediatric gastrointestinal stromal tumors and leiomyosarcoma. *Cancer* 2004; **101**: 39–50.
29. Hill DA, Riedley SE, Patel AR *et al*. Real-time polymerase chain reaction as an aid for the detection of SYT–SSX1 and SYT–SSX2 transcripts in fresh and archival pediatric synovial sarcoma specimens: report of 25 cases from St Jude Children's Research Hospital. *Pediatr Dev Pathol* 2003; **6**: 24–34.
30. Olsen SH, Thomas DG, Lucas DR. Cluster analysis of immunohistochemical profiles in synovial sarcoma, malignant peripheral nerve sheath tumor, and Ewing sarcoma. *Mod Pathol* 2006; **19**: 659–668.
31. Woodruff JM, Scheithauer BW, Kurtkaya-Yapicier O *et al*. Congenital and childhood plexiform (multinodular) cellular schwannoma: a troublesome mimic of malignant peripheral nerve sheath tumor. *Am J Surg Pathol* 2003; **27**: 1321–1329.
32. Arbiser ZK, Folpe AL, Weiss SW. Consultative (expert) second opinions in soft tissue pathology. Analysis of problem-prone diagnostic situations. *Am J Clin Pathol* 2001; **116**: 473–476.
33. Fisher C. Myofibroblastic malignancies. *Adv Anat Pathol* 2004; **11**: 190–201.
34. Billings SD, Giblen G, Fanburg-Smith JC. Superficial low-grade fibromyxoid sarcoma (Evans tumor): a clinicopathologic analysis of 19 cases with a unique observation in the pediatric population. *Am J Surg Pathol* 2005; **29**: 204–210.
35. Mertens F, Fletcher CD, Antonescu CR *et al*. Clinicopathologic and molecular genetic characterization of low-grade fibromyxoid sarcoma, and cloning of a novel FUS/CREB3L1 fusion gene. *Lab Invest* 2005; **85**: 408–415.
36. Alaggio R, Ninfo V, Rosolen A, Coffin CM. Primitive myxoid mesenchymal tumor of infancy: a clinicopathologic report of 6 cases. *Am J Surg Pathol* 2006; **30**: 388–394.
37. Janssen D, Harms D. Juvenile xanthogranuloma in childhood and adolescence: a clinicopathologic study of 129 patients from the Kiel pediatric tumor registry. *Am J Surg Pathol* 2005; **29**: 21–28.
38. Ramani P, Gordon A, Shipley J. Solid tumour pathology and molecular diagnostics. In: Pinkerton R, Plowman PN, Pieters R. (eds) *Paediatric Oncology*, 3rd edn. London: Arnold, 2004; 52–82.
39. Hoot AC, Russo P, Judkins AR, Perlman EJ, Biegel JA. Immunohistochemical analysis of hSNF5/INI1 distinguishes renal and extra-renal malignant rhabdoid tumors from other pediatric soft tissue tumors. *Am J Surg Pathol* 2004; **28**: 1485–1491.

Phillip Cox Helen L. Whitwell

10

Sudden unexpected
death in infancy

Despite changes to the advice given to new parents about sleeping position and environment in recent years (*e.g.* 'Back to Sleep Campaign', UK 1994), some 600 infants per year still die suddenly and unexpectedly in the UK of causes other than congenital malformation, antepartum or peripartum injury, or prematurity.[1] In the majority of cases of sudden unexpected death in infancy (SUDI), a definitive cause of death is not reached and such cases may be designated 'sudden infant death syndrome' (SIDS) or 'unascertained' depending on the findings, circumstances and preference of the pathologist, coroner or other professionals.[2] The rate of sudden infant death syndrome/unascertained deaths is about 0.5 per 1000 live births.[3] Rates of SUDI are broadly similar across the industrialised world.

The range of possible causes of the approximately 30% of these cases that are unexpected but explained is wide and, beside a vast range of recognised natural causes of death, a small proportion of cases are the result of accidental or malicious harm.[4] In order to maximise the chances of identifying the cause of death, it is essential that cases of SUDI are investigated by a multidisciplinary team following a standard protocol.[5,6] This team should include the police, social services, a specialist paediatrician and a pathologist with expertise in paediatric deaths, either alone or with the aid of a forensic pathologist.

TERMINOLOGY

The field of sudden death in the infant period is littered with acronyms and terms that can lead to a degree of confusion between professionals and the public.

Phillip Cox MBBS PhD FRCPath (for correspondence)
Consultant Perinatal Pathologist, Birmingham Women's Healthcare NHS Trust, Metchley Park Road, Birmingham B15 2TG, UK
E-mail: phillip.cox@bwhct.nhs.uk

Helen L. Whitwell MBChB FRCPath DMJPath FACBS FFFLM
Professor and Consultant Home Office Accredited Forensic Pathologist, West Midlands Forensic Centre, Sandwell District General Hospital, West Bromwich, West Midlands B71 4HJ, UK

INFANCY

Infancy is the period from birth to the end of the first year of life. The majority of unexpected deaths of young children occur between 1 week and 6 months of age.

SUDDEN UNEXPECTED DEATH IN INFANCY (SUDI)

SUDI is a descriptive term without a precise definition, denoting the way in which death occurred. It indicates that the child, of less than 1 year of age, was either healthy or at least was not thought to have a life-threatening disease prior to death. It also suggests that death occurred rapidly: this may have been as an observed collapse, or during a period of sleep, with the child being found lifeless. SUDI is not a recognised cause of death, although it has been suggested that it might replace 'unascertained' or 'not ascertained' (see below).[6] This would seem likely to create confusion with SIDS, which is currently acceptable for purposes of death certification.

SUDDEN INFANT DEATH SYNDROME (SIDS)

To qualify as 'sudden infant death syndrome', a death must fit the definition laid down by Beckwith and subsequently subjected to some minor revision:[7] 'SIDS is the sudden death of an infant under one year of age which remains unexplained after a thorough case investigation, including performance of a complete autopsy, examination of the death scene, and review of the clinical history'.

Even with this definition, there is variation in the interpretation between pathologists and other professionals with regard to what can and cannot be included as SIDS. For example, some prefer to exclude all co-sleeping deaths,[4] whilst for others the mere fact of that an infant is co-sleeping with a parent is not an exclusion criterion.[8] This may, at least in part, explain the variation in the rates of SIDS as the cause of death between different areas and year on year.

NOT ASCERTAINED/UNASCERTAINED

This is used as the cause of death when the death is not explained after full investigation, but the case cannot be classed as SIDS because:

1. The child is older or younger than acceptable for SIDS.
2. There are atypical features in the history.
3. There are atypical, but unexplained, pathological features, *e.g.* abundant pulmonary siderophages.

Some authors, and indeed the authors of the Kennedy report,[6] suggest that these cases should be classified as SUDI.

EXPLAINED NATURAL INFANT DEATH

CLASSIFICATION OF INFANT DEATHS

Sudden deaths in infancy can be classified in a number of ways, *e.g.* natural or unnatural, by cause, *etc.* When considering what the cause of infant deaths

Expected

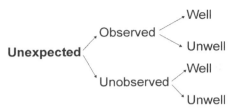

Fig. 1 Classification of SUDI by presentation. Unexpected observed deaths are likely to be explained whether the child was apparently well or unwell prior to collapse. Unexpected unobserved deaths are more likely to be explained if the child was symptomatic prior to death, than if apparently well.

may be, it can be helpful to consider cases by the mode of death (Fig. 1). Cases can first be divided according to whether death was expected or unexpected. Unexpected deaths may be either observed or unobserved, and the infant may have been previously completely well or have had some preceding symptoms.

The majority of unexpected, observed deaths will be explained, whilst amongst the unobserved deaths (cot deaths) more of the previously unwell babies will be found to have a specific cause than those babies who showed no prior symptoms. A cause will also be more likely to be found in babies dying in the first few weeks of life than those over 1 month of age.

CLASSIFICATION BY CAUSE

Infection and cardiac disease are the commonest explanations of sudden death in infancy. However, any system can harbour the cause of death and the list of possible causes is long.[4]

Infection

Bacterial infection is a common cause of death in infancy accounting for about one-quarter of post-neonatal infant deaths.[1] Overwhelming pneumonia, septicaemia and meningitis should be considered in cases of SUDI. Group B streptococcus (GBS), pneumococcus and meningococcus are all frequently isolated and can lead to very rapidly progressive infection in previously healthy babies. Group A streptococci, *Staphylococcus aureus* and *Escherichia coli* are also found on occasion. Bacterial pneumonia may be preceded by minor respiratory symptoms and is one of the causes of unobserved death (cot death) in apparently previously well babies. Inflammation may not be histologically prominent in the early stages and there may just be an eosinophilic exudate containing bacteria accompanied by scanty neutrophils.

Epiglottitis due to *Haemophilus influenzae* was once a fairly common illness, but since the advent of the Hib immunisation programme it is now rare in the UK.

Primary septicaemia may result from infection with GBS, pneumococcus, meningococcus, group A streptococcus and occasionally other organisms. In these cases, the source of infection may not be found. Infants with asplenia are particularly prone to pneumococcal septicaemia.

Babies with meningitis generally show some symptoms; however, these may be vague and non-specific. Causative organisms include, meningococcus, pneumococcus, GBS, *E. coli* and *H. influenzae*. As noted above, *H. influenzae* is now rare due to immunisation in the UK. Acute encephalitis may lead to sudden collapse through involvement of vital structures in the brain stem.

Peritonitis may also occasionally present as sudden death in a child with vague symptoms. Underlying pathology includes volvulus, Hirschsprung's disease, meconium ileus, intussusception, congenital bands, *etc*. Primary peritonitis, typically due to pneumococcus, may also occur in patients with asplenia.

Problems in interpretation may arise when bacterial cultures taken after death, either in the casualty department or at post-mortem examination, are positive, but no macroscopic or histological evidence of infection is found. On the whole, mixed cultures are likely to be due to post-mortem bacterial overgrowth or contamination. In some cases, a pure growth of a single pathogen is isolated. These cases require careful evaluation with clinical colleagues, to try to determine whether death should be attributed to overwhelming infection or should be regarded as SIDS/unascertained.

Viral infection is less frequently identified as a cause of sudden death in infants. However, myocarditis, pneumonitis and encephalitis may all be fatal. Myocarditis may be acquired congenitally or after birth. Congenital myocarditis is most frequently due to enteroviruses, in particular type B coxsackieviruses (Fig. 2), and the organism may be detected by PCR.[9] Maternal symptoms may be minimal and the baby may appear non-specifically unwell, prior to its collapse in the first few weeks of life. Enteroviruses may also lead to myocarditis in later infancy, along with a host of other viruses, bacteria and other organisms.

Viral pneumonitis, *e.g.* respiratory syncytial virus (RSV), is generally symptomatic, although carers and health professionals may not appreciate the child's grave condition until it is too late. RSV may lead to apnoea in very young infants, in particular those born prematurely and with predisposing conditions such as cardiac disease.[10,11] Occasional overwhelming, rapidly

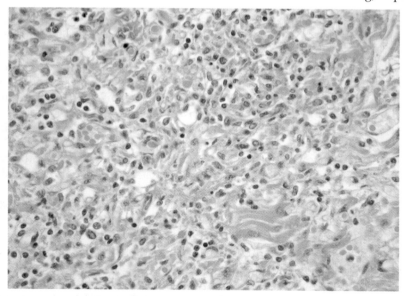

Fig. 2 Myocarditis due to coxsackie virus type B in an infant aged 15 days who collapsed unexpectedly whilst feeding. Haematoxylin and eosin stain.

progressive, viral infections do occur, particularly with enteroviruses and adenoviruses.

Viral encephalitis is usually symptomatic, but the baby may die before reaching hospital, having been non-specifically unwell. Herpes simplex, is commonest after 6 months of age, whilst enteroviruses predominate in the first 3 months of life. Other herpes viruses, adenoviruses, measles, mumps and rubella may all also be implicated.[12]

Gastroenteritis may cause death as a result of dehydration, which may not be recognised by the family, or rarely due to septicaemia. There are always preceding symptoms of vomiting, diarrhoea or both. Hyponatraemia can result if lost fluid is replaced with water rather than with electrolyte solution.

In cases of overwhelming infection, the possibility of an underlying congenital or acquired immune deficit should always be considered. This is particularly true for pneumococcal infection and overwhelming viral infections. Investigation after death, beyond histology, is problematic; however, in view of the genetic implications, recognition of a possible immune defect is important.

Cardiac disease

Myocarditis has already been discussed above.

Despite advances in antenatal screening, undiagnosed congenital heart malformations remain a common cause of death in the first week of life. Affected babies are often poor feeders and parents may observe that they are 'not quite right'. Death is frequently an observed collapse, rather than a 'cot death'. Common lesions include: aortic stenosis/atresia; other causes of hypoplastic left ventricle; and transposition of the great arteries – although a variety of complex lesions may occur. Anomalous origin of one or more coronary arteries is a recognised cause of sudden collapse. This may occur in association with congenital heart disease, but may be an isolated finding.

Infantile cardiomyopathy is a further cause of SUDI, again usually as an observed collapse. At post-mortem examination, the heart is usually severely hypertrophic rather than dilated. The possibility of an underlying metabolic (*e.g.* glycogen storage disease, long-chain 3 hydroxyacyl CoA dehydrogenase deficiency) or mitochondrial disease should be considered and appropriate samples taken.[13] Oncocytic (histiocytoid) cardiomyopathy may be focal and, therefore, several samples of myocardium should be taken. This is thought to be an abnormality of the conducting tissue, although some cases show mutations in mitochondrial DNA.[14] Endocardial fibro-elastosis typically presents as fetal hydrops, but occasional cases may lead to SUDI. The cause of this disorder is uncertain, but metabolic disease should be considered,[15] and there is an association with maternal autoimmune disease, in particular anti-Ro and anti-La antibodies.[16]

Cardiac tumours may lead to arrhythmias and severe cardiac enlargement. Multiple rhabdomyomas are the commonest cardiac tumour and alert to the possibility of tuberous sclerosis.

Disorders of the cardiac conducting system may lead to SUDI, but are unlikely to be recognised unless there is a history pointing in that direction. If there is a family history of sudden death in infants or in children and young adults, the possibility of an ion channelopathy, leading to long QT syndrome and arrhythmias, should be considered. Some groups believe this to be a major cause of SUDI/SIDS deaths (see below). Diagnosis is problematic after death, but other family members should be offered ECG screening; storage of DNA for genetic analysis is important.

Respiratory tract

Infections of the respiratory tract have been discussed above. Structural malformations of the upper airways may be associated with respiratory obstruction. Disorders include choanal atresia, laryngomalacia and tracheomalacia. Noisy breathing or stridor may be apparent and the condition may be exacerbated by concurrent respiratory infection. A careful examination of the respiratory tract is essential.[17]

Respiratory failure may result from neuromuscular disease, including congenital myopathies, polymyositis, viral myositis and anterior horn cell disease. These may be first diagnosed at post-mortem examination and disease may be confined to the diaphragm.[18]

Metabolic disease

Metabolic disease generally presents as an unwell child who collapses suddenly, rather than as 'cot death'. Onset is usually in the early neonatal period, or else follows an infectious illness, most often gastroenteritis. In the latter situation, the baby typically starts with gastroenteritis, but then deteriorates, becomes drowsy and collapses. This is typically seen with medium-chain acyl coenzyme A dehydrogenase (MCAD) deficiency, but may also occur with other fatty acid oxidation defects and mitochondrial disease. Fat stains of liver, kidney, muscle and heart should, therefore, be routine in the investigation of SUDI (Fig. 3), ideally combined with biochemical screening of blood, bile or both by tandem mass spectrometry.[19] Children with known metabolic disease are at increased risk of sudden cardiac collapse and seizures.

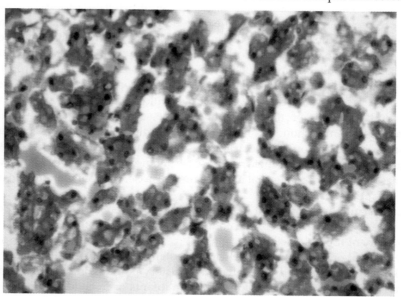

Fig. 3 Severe fatty liver in an infant aged 4 weeks presenting as SUDI (sudden observed collapse). Oil Red O stain.

Tumours

Various tumours may be associated with SUDI. In addition to cardiac rhabdomyomas (see above), various other cardiac tumours are also reported in cases of sudden death. Brain tumours may occasionally present as sudden death due to massive intracranial haemorrhage. The authors have also personally encountered congenital leukaemia, and a prostatic ectomesenchymoma presenting as SUDI; many other fatal tumours are described.

Miscellaneous

Epileptic seizures in infants with known epilepsy may result in sudden, unobserved death. Typical features may not be apparent at post-mortem examination. Death is more likely in infants with underlying neurological disease than with idiopathic epilepsy.[20] Samples should be taken for anticonvulsant levels.

Pulmonary vascular disease is difficult to diagnose in early infancy because vascular remodelling is still taking place. It is typically associated with congenital heart disease but may occur in isolation, or in association with other syndromes, *e.g.* Smith Lemli Opitz syndrome. Williams syndrome is associated with supravalvular aortic stenosis and abnormal peripheral pulmonary vessels and sudden death may result.

CURRENT THEORIES ON THE CAUSATION OF SIDS

Most unexpected, unobserved infant deaths remain unexplained, despite a full post-mortem examination and consideration of all the circumstances.[8] These cases are classified as 'SIDS' or 'not ascertained'. However, there must be a cause for each of these deaths; it is just that current techniques do not allow the precise cause to be identified. All cases currently classed as SIDS are unlikely to have the same aetiology. The lack of a clear cause of death in these cases has led to a profusion of theories, for which there are varying degrees of supporting evidence. The currently favoured theories are: (i) respiratory arousal/brainstem development; (ii) inflammatory mediators/bacterial toxins; and (iii) cardiac arrhythmia.

Epidemiological studies have identified parental smoking and co-sleeping, particularly on a sofa, as the major risk factors for SUDI.[8] In most cases of co-sleeping, however, there is no firm evidence to indicate that death was a result of accidental smothering or overlaying. In addition, cot death is not more common in societies where co-sleeping is the norm. Similarly, many smoking families claim not to smoke in the house or around the child. Research studies have tried to link these risk factors to the theories of causation of cot death.

RESPIRATORY AROUSAL/BRAINSTEM DEVELOPMENT

Some investigators have produced evidence that cot death is the result of failure of normal respiratory arousal in response to an adverse sleeping environment. Studies of respiratory physiology show immaturity in the arousal response to hypoxia in the first 6 months of life and there is evidence to suggest a reduced arousal response in SIDS.[21] Two groups, in particular have focused on subtle abnormalities of development in the brainstem affecting cardiorespiratory control centres, such as the medullary arcuate nucleus, which they suggest are present in at least 50% of SIDS cases. Abnormal prenatal development or prenatal damage to these areas is postulated to lead to failure of respiratory arousal in adverse sleeping environments.[21] Others have cast doubts on the validity of this theory,[22] and personal experience suggests that if structural abnormalities exist, they are not readily identified in routine material.

INFLAMMATORY MEDIATORS

It has been suggested that SIDS victims show evidence of immune activation, such as increased inflammatory cells in the lungs, thymic enlargement and raised levels of cytokines. Studies of genetic polymorphisms of cytokine genes have shown an excess of certain high-activator alleles of interleukin-10 (IL-10), which have been suggested to lead to an abnormal cytokine response in response to minor infection.[23] Polymorphisms in vascular endothelial growth factor (VEGF) and IL-6 have also been found to be associated with SIDS;[24] it may be that several unfavourable cytokine genotypes or combinations of different genotypes may lead to abnormal responses to minor infection.

There is also some evidence for a role of bacterial and viral infection as a trigger for SIDS, possibly through toxin production. This may be linked to inappropriate cytokine response as a result of genetic polymorphism and other risk factors.

CARDIAC ARRHYTHMIAS

Sudden death in young adults and older children may be the result of mutations in a number of genes coding for membrane ion channels. These mutations lead to the long QT syndrome (LQTS), which predisposes to fatal cardiac arrhythmias. This has led to the suggestion that some (if not many) SIDS cases are a consequence of LQTS.[25] A number of studies have looked for mutations in the various LQTS genes and it appears that possibly 5% of cases, otherwise classified as SIDS, carry mutations.[26] The most likely candidate gene, *SCN5A*, can lead to sudden death in sleep. Polymorphisms in other LQTS genes may be also present with increased frequency in SIDS but it is unclear whether these polymorphic alleles have pathogenic effects. With the current state of knowledge, it is probably not necessary to test all cases of SIDS for LQTS channel gene mutations. However, if there is a family history of sudden unexplained death or features in the history, which point in the direction of a cardiac death, it may be appropriate to offer genetic testing of the affected child or ECG screening of the close family.

FORENSIC ASPECTS

SUFFOCATION

This is one of the most difficult problems in young infants. Recent, high-profile cases have illustrated the problems in this area,[27,28] as well as highlighting the importance of expert witnesses confining their evidence to their area of expertise. This is particularly so where there are multiple deaths. There is still considerable confusion in the literature over the precise classification of natural and unnatural deaths where there is more than one death in a family. The study by Carpenter *et al.*[29] identified 87% in their series as natural; however, this has been challenged by others on the basis that a number of indeterminate deaths or unnatural deaths were reclassified as natural suggesting that the true incidence of proven natural deaths may be lower.[30]

The pathological appearances of suffocation in the young infant are commonly identical to those in a true SIDS – essentially a negative autopsy. Suffocation may be accidental, such as in cases of overlaying, or inflicted; this includes suffocation with a pillow, cushion or other mechanism such as a hand placed over the mouth. Rarities include obstruction of the airway by a foreign object. As with all infant deaths, a careful history with a detailed external examination of the infant are essential. If there are concerns about the possibility of abuse or neglect, the forensic pathologist should take the lead role assisted by the paediatric pathologist.[6]

External findings of concern include facial and conjunctival petechiae; however, it should be realised these are not specific for upper airway obstruction. Features such as facial bruising, pressure marks and abrasions need an explanation; a history of resuscitation needs to be excluded as injuries such as bruising and finger-type abrasions are recorded during medical procedures.[31] Similarly, frenulum injury, which is well recognised to occur in the spectrum of non-accidental injury, may need careful interpretation if intubation has been performed.

Frank bleeding from the upper airways is unusual in the context of SIDS; resuscitation injury should be borne in mind. Likewise, natural causes such as an infection or vascular lesion should be excluded.[32] The possibility of suffocation should be considered whether this is in the context of a co-sleeping death or inflicted injury.[33]

INTERNAL FINDINGS

These are frequently indistinguishable from true SIDS deaths. The presence or absence of petechiae – whether thymic, cardiac or pleural – has no diagnostic significance (Fig. 4).

There has been considerable debate over the issue of pulmonary haemorrhages – both acute and older where haemosiderin macrophages are identifiable. Alveolar haemorrhage was investigated by Yukawa *et al.*[34] and it was suggested that significant intra-alveolar haemorrhage may be an indicator of airway obstruction such as in overlaying or suffocation. However, intra-alveolar haemorrhage may occur in the younger age group (under 4 weeks in age) as well as in a background of resuscitation.[35] It is recognised to be a feature of co-sleeping deaths, but the mechanism of death (overlaying or other) remains unclear. There are considerable difficulties in estimating the degree of haemorrhage present.

The presence of haemosiderin-laden macrophages (Fig. 5) has been suggested as a marker of previous upper airway obstruction.[36,37] However, careful analysis of the available literature does not provide enough evidence to substantiate this.[38] This, as with intra-alveolar haemorrhage, is a factor that should be evaluated carefully in each case along with other information.

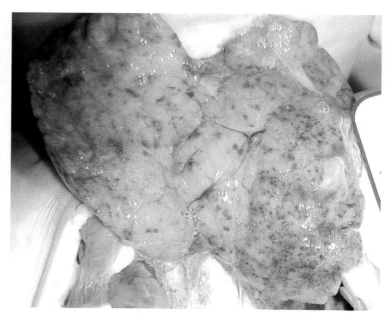

Fig. 4 Thymic petechial haemorrhages in an infant presenting as SUDI (unexpected, unobserved death). Early bilateral pneumonia on histology.

Natural causes need to be excluded, including pulmonary haemosiderosis, bleeding disorders and cardiac disease.

A common artefact that may be seen in these infant deaths is epidural haemorrhage around the spinal cord. This should not be mistaken for either genuine trauma or as an indication of suffocation. It appears to be caused by congestion of the epidural fat network and may well be post-mortem artefact.[39]

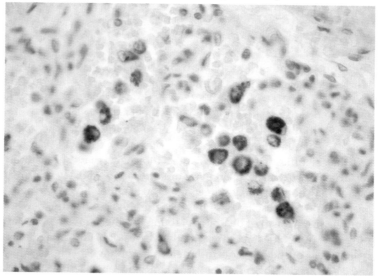

Fig. 5 Haemosiderin in alveolar macrophages. The infant, aged 7 weeks, presented as SUDI (unexpected, unobserved death). No suspicious features were identified at post-mortem examination or by other agencies involved (Perls').

CO-SLEEPING DEATHS

This group has shown an increased incidence with parental co-sleeping and smoking. Legal issues may arise if the carer was under the influence of alcohol or drugs. It appears some infants are particularly vulnerable to transient airways obstruction.

MUNCHAUSEN SYNDROME BY PROXY

This topic has generated considerable debate over the last few years. It was originally described by Meadow with further subsequent reports.[40] The carer – commonly the mother – causes harm to the infant or child to bring it to the attention of the medical authorities. Rare cases are described in male carers. The identification of such cases is extremely difficult. Infants may present with apparent life-threatening events (ALTEs) but poisoning and other conditions may occur. In infants, there may be a history of apnoeic episodes before a sudden death. The pathology may be identical to SIDS as the commonest proposed mechanism is external airway occlusion, although attention should be paid any injuries identified. Toxicological analysis is essential – it should be carried out as a routine in all cases of sudden unexpected death in infancy.

Points for best practice

- Investigation of SUDI requires a multidisciplinary team, including paediatrician, police, specialist paediatric pathologist and social services. In cases with potentially suspicious factors, a forensic pathologist should also be involved.
- Case review by the team can be helpful in refining the diagnosis.
- The range of causes of explained SUDI is very wide and a full post-mortem examination should be undertaken to an agreed protocol, including a range of ancillary tests. Tissue should be stored in case DNA is required for genetic tests.
- Long QT syndrome is not a common cause of SUDI, but the diagnosis should be considered if there is a family history of sudden death.
- The cause of SIDS remains unknown. However, current theories highlight the possible role of poor respiratory arousal, inflammatory response/infection and LQTS.
- Suffocation, either accidental or deliberate, is difficult to diagnose in this young age group.
- The significance of fresh alveolar haemorrhage and haemosiderin macrophages needs to be judged in the light of all of the findings and circumstances of the death.
- Fresh spinal epidural haemorrhage may be a post-mortem artefact.
- Toxicological testing should be a routine part of the post-mortem examination in SUDI.

References

1. <http://www.statistics.gov.uk/STATBASE/ssdataset.asp?vlnk=9519>.
2. Limerick SR, Bacon CJ. Terminology used by pathologists when reporting on SIDS. *J Clin Pathol* 2004; **57**: 309–311.
3. Corbin T. Investigation into sudden infant deaths and unascertained deaths in England and Wales, 1995–2003. *Health Statistics Quarterly* 2005; **27**: 16–23.
4. Howatson AG. The autopsy for sudden unexpected death in infancy. *Curr Diagn Pathol* 2006; **12**: 173–183.
5. American Academy of Pediatrics: Committee on Child Abuse and Neglect. Distinguishing sudden infant death syndrome from child abuse fatalities. *Pediatrics* 2001; **107**: 437–441.
6. Multiprofessional Working Party on the Investigation of Sudden Death in Infancy. *A multi-agency protocol for care and investigation after the sudden unexpected death of an infant or child*. London: Royal College of Pathologists and Royal College of Paediatrics and Child Health, 2004.
7. Willinger M, James LS, Catz C. Defining the sudden infant death syndrome (SIDS): deliberations of an expert panel convened by the National Institute of Child Health and Human Development. *Pediatr Pathol* 1991; **11**: 677–684.
8. Fleming P, Bacon C, Blair P, Berry PJ. (eds) *Sudden unexpected deaths in infancy. The CESDI SUDI series 1993–1996*. London: The Stationery Office, 2000.
9. Inwald D, Franklin O, Cubitt D, Peters M, Goldman A, Burch M. Enterovirus myocarditis as a cause of neonatal collapse. *Arch Dis Child* 2004; **89**: F461–F462.
10. Pickens DL, Schefft GL, Storch GA, Thach BT. Characterization of prolonged apneic episodes associated with respiratory syncytial virus infection. *Pediatr Pulmonol* 1989; **6**: 195–201.
11. Church NR, Anas NG, Hall CB, Brooks JG. Respiratory syncytial virus-related apnea in infants. Demographics and outcome. *Am J Dis Child* 1984; **138**: 247–250.
12. Modlin JF. Perinatal echovirus and group B coxsackievirus infections. *Clin Perinatol* 1988; **15**: 233–246.
13. Gilbert-Barness E. Metabolic cardiomyopathy and conduction system defects in children. *Ann Clin Lab Sci* 2004; **34**: 15–34.
14. Andreu AL, Checcarelli N, Iwata S, Shanske S, DiMauro S. A missense mutation in the mitochondrial cytochrome b gene in a revisited case with histiocytoid cardiomyopathy. *Pediatr Res* 2000; **48**: 311–314.
15. Bennett MJ, Hale DE, Pollitt RJ, Stanley CA, Variend S. Endocardial fibroelastosis and primary carnitine deficiency due to a defect in the plasma membrane carnitine transporter. *Clin Cardiol* 1996; **19**: 243–246.
16. Nield LE, Silverman ED, Taylor GP *et al*. Maternal anti-Ro and anti-La antibody-associated endocardial fibroelastosis. *Circulation* 2002; **105**; 843–848.
17. Sivan Y, Ben-Ari J, Schonfeld TM. Laryngomalacia: a cause for early near miss for SIDS. *Int J Pediatr Otorhinolaryngol* 1991; **21**: 59–64.
18. Sundararajan S, Ostojic NS, Rushton DI, Cox PM, Acland P. Diaphragmatic pathology: a cause of clinically unexplained death in the perinatal/paediatric age group. *Med Sci Law* 2005; **45**: 110–114.
19. Loughrey CM, Preece MA, Green A. Sudden unexpected death in infancy (SUDI). *J Clin Pathol* 2005; **58**; 20–21.
20. Callenbach PM, Westendorp RG, Geerts AT *et al*. Mortality risk in children with epilepsy: the Dutch study of epilepsy in childhood. *Pediatrics* 2001; **107**: 1259–1263.
21. Kinney HC. Abnormalities of the brainstem serotonergic system in the sudden infant death syndrome: a review. *Pediatr Dev Pathol* 2005; **8**: 507–524.
22. Guntheroth WG, Spiers PS. The triple risk hypotheses in sudden infant death syndrome. *Pediatrics* 2002; **110**: e64.
23. Opdal SH, Rognum TH. The sudden infant death syndrome gene: does it exist? *Pediatrics* 2004; **114**; 506–512.
24. Dashash M, Pravica V, Hutchinson IV, Barson AJ, Drucker D. Association of sudden infant death syndrome with VEGF and IL-6 gene polymorphisms. *Hum Immunol* 2006; **67**: 627–633.

25. Schwartz PJ. QT prolongation and SIDS – from theory to evidence. In: Byard RW, Krous HF. (eds) *Sudden Infant Death Syndrome. Problems, progress and possibilities*. London: Arnold, 2001; 83–95.
26. Skinner JR. Is there a relation between SIDS and long QT syndrome? *Arch Dis Child* 2005; **90**: 445–449.
27. R-v- Sally Clark [2000] EWCA Crim 54 at 115-6.
28. R-v- Angela Cannings [2004] EWCA Crim 1.
29. Carpenter RG, Waite A, Coombs RC *et al*. Repeat sudden unexpected and unexplained infant deaths: natural or unnatural? *Lancet* 2005; **365**: 29–35.
30. Gornall J. Was message of sudden infant death study misleading? *BMJ* 2006; **333**: 1165–1168.
31. Leadbetter S. Resuscitation injury. In: Rutty GN. (ed) *Essentials of Autopsy Practice*, Vol 1. London: Springer, 2001: 42–63.
32. Krous HF, Nadeau JM, Byard RW, Blackbourne BD. Oronasal blood in sudden infant death. *Am J Forensic Med Pathol* 2001; **22**: 346–351.
33. Beercroft DM, Thompson JM, Mitchell M. Nasal and intrapulmonary haemorrhage in sudden infant death syndrome. *Arch Dis Child* 2001; **85**: 116–120.
34. Yukawa N, Carter N, Rutty G *et al*. Intra-alveolar haemorrhage in sudden infant death syndrome: a cause for concern? *J Clin Pathol* 1999; **52**: 581–587.
35. Berry PJ. Intra-alveolar haemorrhage in sudden infant death syndrome: a cause for concern? (comment) *J Clin Pathol* 1999; **52**: 553–554.
36. Beecroft DM, Lockett BK. Intrapulmonary siderophages in sudden infant death: a marker for previous imposed suffocation. *Pathology* 1997; **29**: 60–63.
37. Milroy CM. Munchausen syndrome by proxy and intra-alveolar haemosiderin. *Int J Legal Med* 1999; **112**: 309–312.
38. Forbes A, Acland P. What is the significance of haemosiderin in the lungs of deceased infants? *Med Sci Law* 2004; **44**: 348–352.
39. Rutty GN, Squier WM, Padfield CJ. Epidural haemorrhage of the cervical spinal cord: a post mortem artefact? *Neuropathol Appl Neurobiol* 2005; **31**: 247–257.
40. Meadow R. Munchausen syndrome by proxy. The hinterland of child abuse. *Lancet* 1977; **2**: 343–345.

Ian S.D. Roberts, Marta C. Cohen,
Emyr W. Benbow

11

The non-invasive or minimally invasive autopsy

There is much international variation in the autopsy rate, reflecting differences in medicolegal systems, available resources, and religious and cultural attitudes towards post-mortem dissection. In England and Wales, about 20% of deaths are followed by autopsy and the great majority of these are performed for medicolegal reasons on the instructions of a coroner. Autopsy rates have declined over several decades; in recent years, public resistance to conventional autopsy has been fuelled by the organ retention scandals at Alder Hey and Bristol. In addition, there are religious objections to post-mortem dissection, from the Jewish and Muslim communities in particular. This has led to consideration of non-invasive or minimally invasive alternatives to the traditional autopsy that may fulfil the legal requirements to identify the cause of a sudden death and investigate unnatural causes.

We shall discuss the various non-invasive techniques available, the evidence regarding their diagnostic accuracy and their potential roles in an autopsy service. The adult and the fetal, perinatal and paediatric autopsies are considered separately because they present very different diagnostic challenges.

FETAL, PERINATAL AND PAEDIATRIC AUTOPSY

The purposes of the fetal, perinatal and paediatric autopsy include determination of the cause and manner of death of a baby, infant or child, the

Ian S.D. Roberts BSc MBChB FRCPath (for correspondence)
Consultant Pathologist, Department of Cellular Pathology, John Radcliffe Hospital, Headley Way, Headington, Oxford OX3 9DU, UK
E-mail: ian.roberts@orh.nhs.uk

Marta C. Cohen MD CCPM
Consultant Pathologist, Sheffield Children's Hospital NHS Trust, Western Bank, Sheffield S10 2TH, UK

Emyr W. Benbow BSc MB ChB FRCPath
Senior Lecturer in Pathology, University of Manchester and Honorary Consultant Histopathologist, Department of Histopathology, Manchester Royal Infirmary, Oxford Road, Manchester M13 9WL, UK

identification of unsuspected additional lesions, the description of new pathogenic mechanisms and diseases, evaluation of the accuracy of clinical diagnoses, and provision of information to support parental counselling. The autopsy also provides a gold standard against which to audit antenatal ultrasound and the management of pregnancy. In the setting of a fetal, perinatal or neonatal death, autopsy findings may help with counselling about the probabilities of recurrence in future pregnancies.

Different investigators have reported that new information is obtained at autopsy in 34–48% of cases.[1,2] In many instances, the autopsy is the only investigation that provides information about the cause of death, often crucial information for genetic counselling. In 1988, a joint working party of the Royal College of Obstetricians and Gynaecologists and the Royal College of Pathologists recommended that a perinatal autopsy rate below 75% was unacceptable, and that the ideal was 100%. Nearly two decades later, and following the 'organ retention scandal', the autopsy rate in the UK is still far below this standard.[3] There remains a reluctance to obtain, and unwillingness to grant, consent for autopsy and for the retention of tissue for histological examination in non-coronial cases; fewer histological examinations inevitably threaten autopsy quality. There has been a clear decline in the rate of requests for autopsies by clinicians, and a change in the public perception of autopsy, after the 'organ retention scandal'.

In 1990, Ros et al.[4] were the first to describe the use of post-mortem magnetic resonance imaging (MRI) as a possible means of compensation for declining autopsy rates in the US. Since then, the role of MRI has progressed from being an ancillary, novel, pre-autopsy technique to one that has become an acceptable adjunct to the autopsy itself; some authors advocate the replacement of the traditional autopsy with post-mortem MRI.[5] They argue that MRI can be an excellent substitute for the traditional autopsy, especially where autopsy is not permitted by religions such as Islam or Judaism, unless demanded by law.

In this section, we review the literature and describe experience gained in the use of imaging in fetal, perinatal and paediatric post-mortem examinations in Sheffield, UK.

IMAGING

The use of imaging studies in fetal, perinatal and paediatric autopsies was, until a decade ago, limited to the conventional radiograph. In Sheffield, the standard operational procedure for autopsies includes full-body radiographs of all cases, with additional views in specific circumstances. Radiographs allow the pathologist to identify bone age, detect skeletal abnormalities that suggest specific syndromes, and discover or confirm skeletal fractures in birth trauma or child abuse. Radiographs are taken in the mortuary using a Faxitron apparatus with a low kilovolt technique by a standardised procedure for fetuses, stillborns and neonates, or using a movable X-ray machine for older children; they are always reported by a paediatric radiologist. A population-based study of post-mortem perinatal radiography revealed abnormalities in 30% of cases imaged, though in only 3.1% of the cases did the abnormal radiographs provide new information that was essential in establishing the

Table 1 Fetal and paediatric MRI sequences

Fast spin echo T2-weighted images	
TR*	11.460 ms
TE	92 ms
Flip angle	90
Echo train length	32
Band width	20.8
Slice thickness	2 mm
Gap	0
Field of view	10 cm
Matrix (phase/read)	256/256
Signal averages	4
Gradient echo T1-weighted 'volume' images	
TR	15 ms
TE	4.47 ms
Flip angle	25
Band width	31.25
Slice thickness	0.8 mm
Gap	0
Field of view*	205 mm
Matrix (phase/read)	256/256
Signal averages	1

*May need to be altered depending on the size of the fetus being imaged.

cause of death.[6] Radiography may also indicate the skeletal growth stage, specifically bone length, presence of ossification centres, and the relationship between length and ossification stage, as indirect indicators of fetal growth.[7]

MRI, on the other hand, depends on the presence of protons (hydrogen nuclei) within the water content of the body, and radiofrequency pulse sequences and gradient magnetic fields are applied within the main static magnetic field. MRI is motion sensitive, and thus the best resolution is obtained in immobile subjects, making it ideal for post-mortem work, where it offers non-invasive, high-resolution imaging of soft tissues. MRI also provides a permanent, comprehensive digital record of each case for future reference.

MRI scanners are usually optimised for adults and older children, and the approach generally needs to be adapted when imaging the fetus or the newborn, with adjustments to the coils and sequences to ensure maximum quality. The current fetal and paediatric MRI imaging sequences used by Sheffield's radiologists are provided in Table 1; the team uses a 1.5 T magnet (Eclipse; Phillips Medical Systems, Best, The Netherlands) and the wrist, knee or head coil depending on the size of the fetus; the technique has been reported elsewhere.[8] The smallest coil the fetus can fit into is best, in some cases a wrist coil; if the fetus is too small, saline bags can be placed within the coil to provide enough signal to image the fetus.

CENTRAL NERVOUS SYSTEM POST-MORTEM MRI

The diagnostic sensitivity of post-mortem MRI is higher for central nervous system (CNS) abnormalities, which account for 20% of fatal congenital

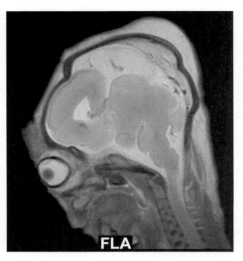

Fig. 1 Post-mortem MRI sagittal image of a 21/40 weeks' gestation fetus, featuring a single ventricle in alobar holoprocencephaly.

abnormalities, than for other body regions. This contrasts with cardiac abnormalities, which present particular difficulties on imaging, but account only for 4% of severe congenital malformations.

The fetal brain softens quickly after intra-uterine death, and thus may be very difficult to handle and easily destroyed during dissection. The dissection process disturbs tissue compartments and modifies spatial relationships; MRI can be an excellent way of overcoming these technical difficulties.

Traditionally, the brain is subjected to 3–4 weeks' fixation in 20% buffered formalin to produce sufficient hardening for further handling. Parents who consent to autopsy often now insist on a rapid restoration of all the organs to the body for burial or cremation. Although we have responded by introducing a method that facilitates rapid fixation, the brain is still sometimes incompletely fixed when examined. The introduction of post-mortem MRI was expected to complement the autopsy and overcome difficulties with dissection of incompletely fixed brains, and was deemed better than computed tomographic (CT) scan because MRI provides better demarcation of grey matter from white matter,[9] even in fetuses with little myelination.

An initial comparison between standard autopsy, and MRI of the brain and spine,[9] in 40 stillborn infants provided good quality MRI in 32 (80%) cases, with agreement between the procedures in 31/32 (97%) cases (Fig. 1); in the remaining eight, structural information from autopsy was limited because the unfixed tissue was difficult to examine. In only four cases was there disagreement between the MR images and autopsy. A joint review of these cases resulted in a consensus diagnosis: in three cases, the MRI provided information not available at the autopsy, and in one case the MRI was incorrect. Autopsy may fail to detect pathology due to the nature of the abnormality, for instance a small encephalocele, alobar holoprocencephaly or hydrocephalus with maceration of the brain.

The radiologists in Sheffield have gained confidence with experience,

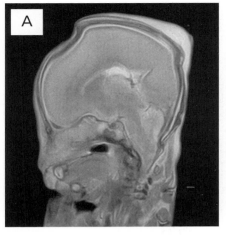
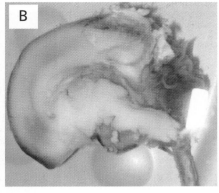

Fig. 2 (A) Post-mortem MRI featuring the presence of a small cerebellum in the posterior fossa and (B) post-mortem examination of the brain and spine with disruption and apparent 'vanishing' of the cerebellum.

rapidly learning to identify migrating neurons, the development of the sulci and gyri, and normal variations. There have been a few cases in which there was disagreement between the MRI and the autopsy interpretation, but such occasions have underlined the advantage of a combined approach. One recent example of such discrepancy was the unexpected finding of a complete absence of cerebellum due to autolysis at autopsy in a fetus with a Dandy–Walker variant malformation. Although small, a cerebellum was clearly demonstrated at the antenatal ultrasound scan and MRI, as well as post-mortem MRI (Fig. 2).

In Sheffield, post-mortem MRI is currently used in fetuses beyond 12 weeks' gestation, in stillborns and in neonatal deaths. To date, the unit has investigated over 250 fetuses and children by MRI prior to autopsy. This has not been performed as a cohort study but rather there has been selection of cases that would potentially most benefit. Experience with early paediatric deaths (before 5 years) is more limited. The MRI provides good-quality information on the morphology of the CNS and also allows us to plan the best approach for the autopsy. When dealing with lesions of the posterior fossa, we have found it useful to remove the occipital plate in order to visualise the cervical cord and cerebellar structures *in situ*. It is often useful to remove the brain under water to minimise disruption of the anatomical relationships.

MRI has proved itself to be a valuable tool for the evaluation of CNS malformations,[10] not only as an adjunct to the autopsy but also to *in utero* ultrasonography after 19 weeks' gestation, particularly with abnormalities of the posterior fossa.[11]

FULL-BODY MRI

Full-body post-mortem MRI was first reported in 1990, in three stillborn infants, one infant and two adults.[4] MRI alone proved to be less useful than the

A

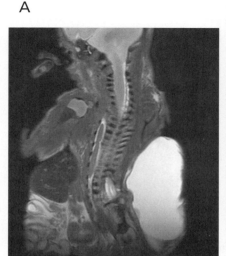

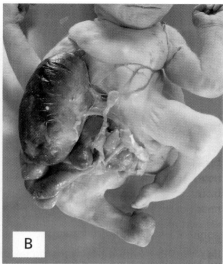

B

Fig. 3 (A) Post-mortem MRI, depicting CSF and neural tissue from a lumbar myelo-meningocele and an omphalocele containing liver and bowel in a case of OEIS complex. (B) Post-mortem examination of the same case, showing the large omphalocele with imperforate anus and ambiguous genitalia.

autopsy in detecting minor pathology or abnormalities not usually seen by cross-sectional imaging, such as an ileal atresia with bowel malrotation. Microscopic findings such as small infarcts, micro-abscesses, petechiae or areas of small haemorrhage are usually missed on MRI.[4]

Fetal anatomy can be demonstrated in great detail as early as 14 gestational weeks: organs easily visualised from this stage include heart, lungs, liver, gall bladder, stomach, small bowel, adrenals, and kidneys. Woodward and colleagues[12] imaged 26 fetuses (whole body) and the findings of three radiologists were compared to formal autopsy, performed without knowledge of the MRI results. The 26 subjects had 47 major and 11 minor malformations. All three radiologists correctly identified 37 (79%) of the major malformations on the MRI and one detected 43 (91%) of them. Only one of the 11 minor malformations was identified by any reviewer. There were six false-positive diagnoses, but in two cases with major CNS malformation, MRI was superior to autopsy.

One area where post-mortem MRI is especially useful is in studies of conjoined twins,[13] defining the anatomy of shared organs and facilitating the planning of dissection.[8] Recently, the Sheffield unit was the first to report the use of MRI in the diagnosis of OEIS complex,[14] a distinct clinical entity comprising of a combination of anomalies, including omphalocele, exstrophy of the cloaca, imperforated anus and spinal defects. In our case, consent for autopsy was refused and only external examination, karyotype investigations and MRI were allowed. MRI showed a large omphalocele that contained liver, a kidney, bowel and a fluid-filled structure thought to represent an exstrophic bladder/cloaca; the other kidney was pelvic. There was a large myelomeningocele at the upper lumbar level that contained cerebrospinal fluid (Fig. 3). In case 2 of the study, a full autopsy was consented and the diagnosis of OEIS complex

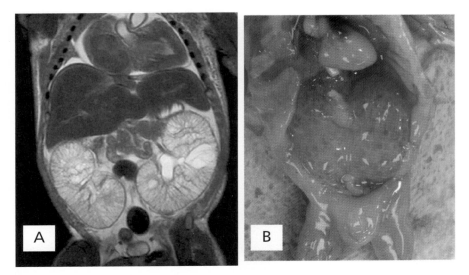

Fig. 4 Polycystic kidneys in a case of Meckel–Gruber syndrome as seen on post-mortem MRI (A) and at the post mortem examination (B).

was made more easily. These cases indicate that, in the absence of autopsy, fetal MRI scan should be offered to parents to facilitate accurate counselling for subsequent pregnancies.

A significant disadvantage of MRI as the sole instrument in post-mortem studies is that histological examination cannot be performed. Important information regarding timing of intra-uterine death, determination of gestational age or causation of malformations might never be disclosed without a formal autopsy. A recent investigation conducted in Sheffield to evaluate the impact of ancillary investigations, including MRI, in 100 fetal autopsies revealed that MRI and autopsy had a 54% agreement and that MRI provided relevant information in 24% of cases. However, if MRI had been the only investigation, essential information would have been lost in 17 of 24 (71%) cases where a full autopsy, including placental examination, was crucial to provide the cause of death or the aetiology of the malformation.

KIDNEY MRI

In a full-body MRI investigation,[12] renal anomalies were the most common major malformation found and they were easily identified in all cases. On T2-weighted images, the kidney has a low-signal intensity cortex and a high-signal intensity medulla. They are easily distinguished from the adjacent adrenal gland, which has lower signal intensity. Although post-mortem MRI is highly sensitive in detecting renal malformations, the kidneys degenerate relatively slowly after death, and there is generally little need of MRI in their characterisation. We have recently used post-mortem MRI in a case of Meckel–Gruber syndrome, a condition characterised by the presence of occipital encephalocele, low-set ears, polydactyly of the right hand and cystic kidneys (Fig. 4).

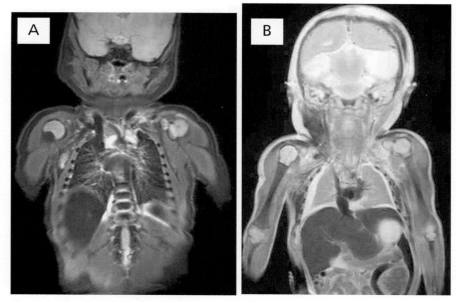

Fig. 5 Post-mortem MRI, demonstrating aerated lungs in a live-born baby (A) and lack of aeration in a stillborn baby (B).

CARDIAC MRI

As indicated above, post-mortem MRI is less sensitive for cardiac abnormalities, compared with CNS malformations, though it might improve with the acquisition of three-dimensional datasets and further experience. This possibility was raised by Deng *et al.*,[15] who were able to perform 3-D reconstruction of the post-mortem fetal heart using MRI. Their images are of high quality, and most of the details of the cardiac structures are depicted.

The use of post-mortem MRI proved useful in a recent case affected by Pentalogy of Cantrell. This is a specific combination of congenital ventral midline defects and includes at least two of the following: midline supra-umbilical abdominal defect, defect of the lower sternum, deficiency of the diaphragmatic pericardium, deficiency of the anterior diaphragm and congenital cardiac anomalies.

LUNG MRI

Post-mortem MRI has proved valuable in detecting pulmonary hypoplasia,[10] and the presence of pneumothorax, meconium aspiration and non-expanded lungs in a case of intra-uterine fetal demise.[4] The expansion of the lungs is crucial when determining stillborn versus 'born alive', a distinction with major legal implications in certain circumstances (Fig. 5).

Congenital cystic malformation of the lung comprises a heterogeneous group of developmental lesions that usually manifest within the first year of life, and should be differentiated from diaphragmatic hernia. Accurate diagnosis of cystic lung disease, either congenital or acquired, poses a challenge to obstetricians, paediatricians, radiologists and pathologists. Post-mortem MRI of the lungs is potentially a useful tool for diagnosis, but conventional autopsy remains the gold standard.

ADULT AUTOPSIES

The non-invasive or minimally invasive techniques available for the investigation of adult deaths include:

- external examination
- thorough clinical history combined with a study of the medical records
- imaging techniques, including plain X-ray, ultrasound, MRI, CT, angiography and other radiocontrast studies
- aspiration of blood, urine or other fluids for analysis (toxicology, biochemistry, microbiology, serology, immunology)
- fine-needle aspiration cytology or needle biopsy and histology
- laparoscopy and thoracoscopy.

An incomplete autopsy using the above tools alone, or in combination, usually provides incomplete information, when compared to a full, conventional autopsy. However, there is a gathering body of evidence that non-invasive techniques may, in some circumstances, be a valid alternative to a full autopsy and can, on occasion, provide information that is superior to dissection. If these techniques are to be used appropriately, an understanding of their strengths and limitations is required. The evidence is incomplete at present but, on the basis of data available, we shall define as far as possible the potential of non-invasive autopsies.

The uses of non-invasive techniques are best considered according to the circumstances of the death, and the questions being asked of the post-mortem examination. We shall discuss separately sudden deaths of unknown cause, traumatic/violent deaths, and deaths where the medical history and circumstances of death raise specific clinical questions.

SUDDEN DEATHS OF UNKNOWN CAUSE

In England, Wales and Northern Ireland, sudden deaths of unknown cause are referred to a coroner and, in the majority of instances, the coroner will request an autopsy; this is, therefore, the commonest indication for autopsy. However, in many other countries, including Scotland, the standard approach to these deaths is a detailed review of the circumstances of the death and medical records, together with an external examination of the body by a forensic pathologist. This will frequently reveal a likely cause of death and full autopsy is avoided. This 'view and grant' system is probably efficient at excluding unnatural deaths but risks systematic errors in death certification. Common causes of death, such as ischaemic heart disease, are likely to be over-diagnosed, as the system is based on probability (*i.e.* an educated guess), whereas unexpected or less common conditions will often be missed. It will be the experience of all pathologists that major pathologies, completely unpredictable on the basis of the clinical history, are frequently found at autopsy. An approach based on a 'verbal autopsy', combined with external examination, is likely to have a high inaccuracy rate, similar to that of clinical death certificates, in the absence of autopsy.[16] It could, however, be argued that identifying the precise cause of a natural death is of secondary importance and that a system that simply identifies unnatural deaths, and unlawful killing in particular, is sufficient.

Imaging techniques, especially MRI and CT, have been used to diagnose causes of sudden adult death. As in paediatric work, image quality is excellent, often superior to that obtained ante-mortem, because movement artefacts are excluded. There are, however, a number of peri- and post-mortem changes that may cause difficulties and over-diagnosis of ante-mortem pathology. For example, the heart is relatively dilated after death, irrespective of cardiac disease,[17] gas accumulates in the cardiovascular system, particularly following cardiopulmonary resuscitation,[18] and gas also accumulates in the peritoneal cavity. The latter may result in a false positive diagnosis of perforated viscus.[19]

Post-mortem MRI

Post-mortem MRI has been used in England as an alternative to conventional coroner's autopsy, in cases where there are religious objections to post-mortem dissection. A series of 53 such cases were reported by Bisset et al.[20] Only six of these, in which MRI findings were inconclusive, were followed by conventional autopsy, the findings of which were largely predicted by the radiology and clinical history. Studies directly comparing post-mortem MRI with full, conventional autopsy are currently limited. Of six cases reported by Patriquin et al.,[19] there were major discrepancies in three, with MRI missing two coronary artery occlusions and a myocardial infarct. Roberts et al.[21] reported 10 MRI autopsies that were reported independently by four radiologists. An abnormality relating to the cause of death was identified by at least one radiologist in eight cases but only in one case were all radiologists able to provide a confident correct cause of death. This study identified important weaknesses of post-mortem MRI: coronary artery lesions were not visualised, post-mortem clot in the pulmonary artery was mistaken for ante-mortem thrombo-embolism, and bronchopneumonia with pulmonary consolidation could not be reliably differentiated from pulmonary oedema secondary to cardiac failure. Together, these pathologies account for a large proportion of sudden adult deaths, and these diagnostic weaknesses, that partly relate to lack of spatial resolution, need to be overcome before MRI is considered a reliable alternative to conventional autopsy. The authors are

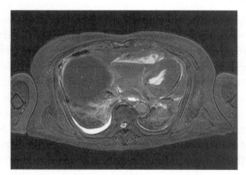

Fig. 6 Post-mortem MRI of the thorax, demonstrating non-dependent 'consolidation' (the radiological description of fluid in alveolar spaces). Features favouring pulmonary oedema rather than pneumonia are the wide-spread bilateral changes with hilar accentuation and bilateral pleural effusions.

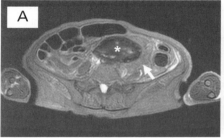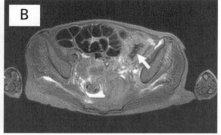

Fig. 7 Post-mortem MRI of the abdomen, demonstrating (A) rupture of a large aortic aneurysm (asterisk) with retroperitoneal haemorrhage (arrow) and (B) an incidental finding of a large adenocarcinoma of the sigmoid colon (arrow) in the same patient.

currently undertaking a prospective study of over 300 adult deaths, in which post-mortem MRI and CT are followed by full autopsy. It is hoped that this will better define the appropriate use of post-mortem imaging and overcome some of the drawbacks encountered in earlier series. An example of this is seen in Figure 6, where a confident radiological diagnosis of pulmonary oedema was made in a patient who died one week following myocardial infarction.

Recent studies suggest that, with greater experience, some of the diagnostic weaknesses described above can be overcome. Jackowski *et al.*[22] described cardiac findings in a series of 80 cases in which post-mortem CT and MRI was compared to conventional autopsy. This group used their experience to improve imaging sequences and interpretation, resolving some of the diagnostic difficulties described above. For example, hypo-intensity within the myocardium secondary to post-mortem lividity can be distinguished from pathological causes, such as myocardial infarction, by comparing with hypostasis in other organs. Post-mortem clot was seen to produce a layering appearance on T2-weighted MRI and, in contrast to ante-mortem thrombi, did not show haemosiderin-induced loss of signal.

Post-mortem MRI in adults does have certain strengths: it is exceedingly sensitive to CNS pathology, often providing superior information to that obtained by dissection, and is excellent at defining mass lesions caused by haemorrhage or tumour (Fig. 7).

Post-mortem CT

There has been greater experience comparing conventional autopsy with post-mortem CT than with MRI. Poulson *et al.*[23] have recently described 525 medicolegal autopsies in which CT was followed by conventional autopsy. This procedure is routine in their centre, as in several other forensic pathology units, and these cases represent a single year's experience. Unlike the MRI investigations described above, the CT examinations were performed by a single forensic pathologist who had no specific training in radiology. Many were traumatic deaths (see below); of the non-traumatic pathologies, CT reliably identified haemorrhages such as haemo-pericardium, aneurysms and pulmonary tumours if over 10 mm in diameter. However, a number of weaknesses were highlighted. Post-mortem hypostasis and putrefaction within the lungs were commonly mistaken for pneumonia, which was overdiagnosed by 48%, although this did improve with observer experience. Pleural effusions could not be differentiated from haemothorax or pyothorax. Atherosclerosis could not be visualised unless the affected vessels were heavily calcified. Within the abdomen, fluid was only detected by CT if the volume was great, and hepatic fibrosis was missed in 40% of cases.

Shiotani et al.[24] described pulmonary findings in 150 non-traumatic deaths in which CT was performed within 2 h of confirmation of the fact of death. The cause of death was usually based on clinical and CT findings; conventional autopsy was performed in only 16 cases. CT-autopsy correlation in these cases demonstrated that dependent density on CT was a common but non-specific finding, whereas a ground-glass appearance of the lungs on CT corresponded to pulmonary oedema. Post-mortem CT could not reliably differentiate between pneumonia and pulmonary oedema. Yamazaki et al.[25] reported a series of 10 cases of sudden death with abdominal injury or disease in which post-mortem CT was followed by autopsy. Ascites on CT scan was found to be a more reliable indicator of a perforated small bowel than the presence of free gas in the peritoneal cavity. Hepatic-portal venous gas was a common and, therefore, non-specific post-mortem finding, although it was most evident following trauma.

Needle biopsy

Needle biopsy and histology may be used to improve the quality of information obtained by post-mortem imaging, and is generally acceptable to groups who express religious or cultural objections to full autopsy. Whereas blind needle biopsy of the major organs frequently fails to identify cause of death, or even obtain the correct tissue,[26] imaging-guided biopsies appear to be a relatively reliable tool in post-mortem diagnosis. In a series of 100 cases reported by Farina et al.,[27] ultrasound-guided biopsy provided a concordant diagnosis to full autopsy in 83 cases. This technique appeared sensitive for the detection of diffuse pulmonary lesions, such as pneumonia, and for myocardial infarcts, but some cardiac pathologies, pulmonary embolism and small malignant tumours were, however, missed. Farina and colleagues now use ultrasonographic autopsy alone when consent for full autopsy is refused, and these account for 22% of all post-mortem examinations in their centre.[28] More recently, CT fluoroscopy has been successfully used to guide needle biopsy,[29] but the first report of this technique includes only three cases, and greater experience is required to determine its value.

TRAUMATIC DEATHS AND THE FORENSIC AUTOPSY

Imaging techniques have long been used to provide supplemental information to the conventional autopsy in the identification of bony injuries. Plain X-rays may be superior to dissection in the identification of some fractures, particularly if combined with 3-D imaging techniques.[30] Radiographs also aid identification and are particularly valuable for the incinerated or decomposed body, and for the investigation of major incidents with multiple fatalities and separated body parts. Additionally, the routine use of X-ray fluoroscopy prior to physical examination of a body in military fatalities enables the identification of live munitions.

CT provides more detailed information than plain X-ray and is excellent for the localisation of foreign bodies such as bullets. Three-dimensional computerised reconstruction of injuries facilitates their interpretation. CT has the added advantage that evidence is not destroyed by imaging: fractures are demonstrated *in situ* with little or no post-mortem artefact, whereas following dissection, bone fragments may fall apart and create difficulties in interpretation. Furthermore, the scans are available for review without disadvantage to the defence in criminal cases.

Poulsen *et al.*[23] found CT excellent for the identification of pelvic and limb fractures, although non-displaced basal skull fractures were sometimes missed on imaging. In a series of 40 forensic cases examined by multislice CT (MSCT), Thali *et al.*[31] reported that 26 of 47 partly combined causes of death were found only on imaging data. CT was superior to dissection in identifying some cases of cranial, skeletal and soft tissue injuries. The same group studied five cases of upper cervical spine injury with MSCT and MRI, finding that imaging was superior to neck dissection for forensic reconstruction.[32] In a further three cases of fatal blunt head injury, MSCT and MRI enabled the diagnosis of cerebellar tonsillar herniation prior to autopsy.[33]

Laparoscopy[34] and thoracoscopy[35] have been used in a single centre in Tel Aviv, primarily to satisfy the preference for minimal interference with the body and rapid burial. These provided useful information in a small study, mainly of patients who had died from trauma. Unfortunately, these methods are unlikely to be useful in jurisdictions where the delay before autopsy is routinely much more than 24 h because the increasing tissue rigidity associated with refrigeration would hamper the gas insufflation that precedes the procedure.

SPECIFIC CLINICAL QUESTIONS

As discussed above, in many cases of sudden adult death of unknown cause, there are few clues in the medical history of circumstances of death to indicate a probable cause of death. If non-invasive investigations are to be used as an alternative to conventional autopsy in such cases, they must be able to detect a wide range of pathologies in any organ system. Whilst MRI and CT, in particular, may be able to achieve this in the future, current experience indicates that they cannot. However, in cases where the clinical history and ante-mortem investigations have limited the likely cause of death to a single organ or pathology, non-invasive techniques may be used to answer specific questions. Often this is a request for confirmation or refinement of the clinical cause of death and the use of non-invasive techniques may avoid the need for full autopsy. Some of these situations will be discussed here.

Drug-related deaths

When the circumstances of the death point strongly to drug toxicity, such as death following intravenous injection of diamorphine, external examination together with aspiration of femoral blood and urine for drug analysis may confirm the diagnosis without full autopsy. Some coroners in England sanction this approach if there is a known infective hazard, such as HIV infection or hepatitis C. Additional use of post-mortem imaging may exclude injury in such cases and, at least in theory, might identify complications of drug misuse such as endocarditis.

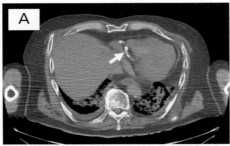 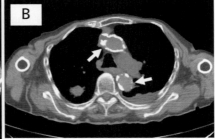

Fig. 8 Post-mortem CT, demonstrating calcification (arrowed) within atheromatous coronary arteries (A) and aorta (B).

Cerebrovascular disease

Post-mortem MRI is excellent for the detection of many intracranial pathologies, including haemorrhage and other mass lesions. Acute cerebrovascular pathology, including vasospasm-induced segmental narrowings, may be demonstrated by post-mortem cerebral angiography, which is also able to localise the source of haemorrhage following ruptured intracranial aneurysms.[36] Karhumen and Servo[37] reported a series of 63 patients who died following neurosurgery for intracranial aneurysms. Post-mortem angiography demonstrated operative haemorrhage in 25% and clip-induced obstruction of cerebral arteries in 11% of patients. In one patient, angiography demonstrated occlusion caused by arterial kinking associated with a properly placed aneurysm clip. The latter may be difficult to demonstrate with conventional autopsy, as dissection during brain removal may result in unkinking of the affected vessel. Saimanen *et al.*[38] compared post-mortem cerebral cast angiography with autopsy in the investigation of cerebrovascular pathology in 144 deaths following cardiac surgery. Full autopsy demonstrated new cerebral infarcts in 15.3% of patients. Angiography detected recent infarcts associated with main cerebral artery thrombosis with a sensitivity of 92%, but was less effective in detecting small recent infarcts, with 60% sensitivity, and did not detect any of six old infarcts.

Coronary heart disease

Initial experience with post-mortem MRI has demonstrated a low sensitivity in detecting fatal coronary heart disease. Ante-mortem CT may be used to demonstrate coronary artery calcification and has been found to be of prognostic value in identifying patients at risk of myocardial infarction and sudden death.[39] Similarly, post-mortem CT may be used to confirm extensive coronary artery disease in cases of suspected sudden cardiac death, but this does still not equate to identification of individual stenosing lesions (Fig. 8). Estimation of coronary artery stenosis at conventional autopsy is often highly subjective and, in the presence of calcified vessels, it may be impossible to accurately quantify stenosis. Post-mortem angiography has been used to give an accurate and permanent record of coronary artery disease.[40] Post-mortem blood clots are unusual in the coronary arteries and do not prevent filling of the vessels by contrast medium. However, this has largely been performed as an open procedure; non-invasive post mortem coronary angiography presents greater technical challenges.

Malignant disease

Minimally invasive techniques may be used when ante-mortem investigations have suggested malignancy but a histological or cytological diagnosis has not been obtained, or when a metastatic tumour is detected but the site of the primary is unknown. As discussed above, MRI in particular is excellent for the detection of clinically significant tumours, although it may still miss smaller tumours. A histological diagnosis may be obtained by combining imaging with needle biopsy or fine needle aspiration cytology.

SUMMARY AND FUTURE DIRECTIONS

Imaging studies already provide relevant and valuable information in the investigation of fetal and peri-natal deaths, but remain an adjunct to, rather than a replacement for, the traditional autopsy. Some investigators see MRI as an ideal substitute of the traditional autopsy, particularly when the parents, for religious or personal reasons, do not consent to the autopsy, and clinicians may find it easier to request consent for the less invasive investigation. However, such an approach would have the disadvantage of a reduction rather than an improvement in the overall quality of the autopsy. It is clear that, even if a biopsy is taken under MRI guidance, there may be sampling error. Besides, needle biopsy or fine-needle aspiration can never provide better quality than samples taken under direct vision. Histopathologists and radiologists should work closely together to allow new techniques to develop and to complement each other.

The situation is less well developed for MRI and CT scans in adult autopsies. A small number of forensic units are using them on a routine basis, but invariably as an adjunct to conventional autopsy, and much of the evidence about their value is anecdotal, based on case reports and small series. There are small studies of the role of MRI in more routine coroner's autopsies, and CT scanning in the investigation of traumatic deaths, but current evidence suggests that, in this situation too, imaging is likely to prove to be a valuable adjunct to, rather than a substitute for, conventional autopsy.

In 2004, the UK Department of Health published the document *Less invasive autopsy: the place of magnetic resonance imaging*.[41] Recommendations included setting up comparative trials of post-mortem MRI against conventional autopsy for adults and fetuses or infants separately. It is expected that the role of MRI and CT as an adjunct or substitute for the traditional autopsy will be influenced by the outcome of such investigations. These are due to be completed in 2009. Any future expansion of the non-invasive autopsy has major cost implications and raises a number of clinical governance issues. For example, who (radiologists or pathologists) will perform and interpret post-mortem imaging, how will they be trained and their competency tested and maintained, and who will select the type of examination to be performed for each case? As the use of non-invasive techniques becomes more wide-spread, it is important that these questions are addressed and that each new application of a non-invasive procedure be fully validated.

ACKNOWLEDGEMENTS

The authors would like to thank radiologists Steve Lee, Rob Bisset, Alan Jackson, Zoe Traill and Nigel Cowan for their collaboration with the adult autopsies, and Elspeth Whitby and Paul Griffiths for their collaboration with the fetal and perinatal post-mortem examinations, and for their assistance with the preparation of this manuscript. We are also grateful to Sue Blakey and Trudy Donn in Sheffield, and Anthony McIntyre, Lindsay Dainton and Sheena Thomas in Oxford, for their technical support.

Points for best practice

- Religious objections to post-mortem dissection and recent organ scandals in the UK have led to a search for non-invasive alternatives to the traditional autopsy.

- Post-mortem imaging is becoming an important adjunct to the autopsy by dissection, but diagnostic weaknesses have so far restricted its use to a limited number of situations.

- In the fetal and perinatal autopsy, MRI is a valuable tool in the identification of congenital abnormalities when consent for full autopsy is withheld, and is particularly accurate in identifying CNS pathology.

- In adults, post-mortem MRI has been used to diagnose the cause of sudden death when there have been religious objections to full medicolegal autopsy. Initial validation studies have, however, highlighted important weaknesses, particularly its inability to visualise coronary arteries, and to differentiate thrombus from post-mortem clot and pulmonary oedema from pneumonia.

- Post-mortem CT is a powerful tool in the forensic autopsy, identifying bone fractures, bullets and other foreign bodies before dissection has disturbed the site of injury. These images are open to review and 3-dimensional techniques allow virtual reconstruction of wounds.

- Diagnostic accuracy has been increased by combining imaging techniques (ultrasound, CT and MRI) with fine-needle aspiration cytology or needle-core biopsy and histology. The information obtained is, however, frequently incomplete when compared to full conventional autopsy.

References

1. Laing IA. Clinical aspects of neonatal death and autopsy. *Semin Neonatol* 2004; **9**: 247–254.
2. Weston MJ, Porter HJ, Andrews HS *et al*. Correlation of antenatal ultrasonography and pathological examination in 153 malformed fetuses. *J Clin Ultrasound* 1993; **21**: 387–392.
3. Burton JL, Underwood JCE. Necropsy practice after the 'organ retention scandal': requests, performance, and tissue retention. *J Clin Pathol* 2003; **56**: 537–541.
4. Ros PR, Li KC, Vo P *et al*. Preautopsy magnetic resonance imaging: Initial experience. *Magn Reson Imaging* 1990; **8**: 303–308.
5. Whitby EH, Paley MN, Cohen M, Griffiths PD. Post mortem MR imaging of the fetus: An adjunct or a replacement for conventional autopsy? *Semin Fetal Neonatal Med* 2005; **Oct**: 475–483.
6. Olsen ØE, Espeland A, Maartmann-Moe H *et al*. Diagnostic value of radiography in cases of perinatal death: a population based study. *Arch Dis Child* 2003; **88**: F521–F524.

7. Olsen ØE, Lie RT, Maartmann-Moe H *et al*. Skeletal measurements among infants who die during the perinatal period: new population-based reference. *Pediatr Radiol* 2002; **32**: 667–673.
8. Whitby EH, Paley MNJ, Cohen M, Griffiths PD. Post-mortem fetal MRI: what do we learn from it? *Eur J Radiol* 2006; **57**: 250–255.
9. Griffiths PD, Variend D, Evans M *et al*. Postmortem MR imaging of the fetal and stillborn central nervous system. *Am J Neuroradiol* 2003; **24**: 22–27.
10. Brookes JAS, Hall-Craggs MA, Sams V, Lees WR. Non-invasive perinatal necropsy by magnetic resonance imaging. *Lancet* 1996; **348**: 1139–1141.
11. Whitby E, Paley MN, Davies N *et al*. Ultrafast magnetic resonance imaging of central nervous system abnormalities *in utero* in the second and third trimester of pregnancy: comparison with ultrasound. *Br J Obstet Gynaecol* 2001; **108**: 519–526.
12. Woodward PJ, Sohaey R, Harris EP *et al*. Postmortem fetal MR imaging: comparison with findings at autopsy. *Am J Radiol* 1997; **168**: 41–46.
13. Manzano AC, Morillo AJ, Vallejo JM, Bayona MP. Necropsy by magnetic resonance in a case of conjoined thoracopagus twins. *J Magn Reson Imaging* 2001; **13**: 976–981.
14. Vasudevan PC, Cohen MC, Whitby EH *et al*. The OEIS complex two case reports that illustrate the spectrum of abnormalities and the utility of the MRI in the diagnosis. *Prenat Diagn* 2006; **26**: 267–272.
15. Deng J, Brookes JAS, Gardener JE *et al*. Three-dimensional magnetic resonance imaging of the post-mortem fetal heart. *Fetal Diagn Ther* 1996; **11**: 417–421.
16. Hill RB, Anderson RE. *The Autopsy – Medical Practice and Public Policy*. London: Butterworths, 1988.
17. Shiotani S, Kohno M, Ohashi N *et al*. Dilatation of the heart on post-mortem computed tomography (PMCT): comparison with live CT. *Radiat Med* 2003; **21**: 29–35.
18. Shiotani S, Kohno M, Ohashi N, Atake S, Yamazaki K, Nakayama H. Cardiovascular gas on non-traumatic post-mortem computed tomography (PMCT): the influence of cardiopulmonary resuscitation. *Radiat Med* 2005; **23**: 225–229.
19. Patriquin L, Kassarjian A, O'Brien M *et al*. Postmortem whole-body magnetic resonance imaging as an adjunct to autopsy: preliminary clinical experience. *J Magn Reson Imaging* 2001; **13**: 277–287.
20. Bisset RAL, Thomas NB, Turnbull IW, Lee S. Postmortem examinations using magnetic resonance imaging: four year review of a working service. *BMJ* 2002; **324**: 1423–1424.
21. Roberts ISD, Benbow EW, Bisset RAL *et al*. Accuracy of magnetic resonance imaging in determining cause of death in adults: comparison with conventional autopsy. *Histopathology* 2003; **42**: 424–430.
22. Jackowski C, Schweitzer W, Thali M *et al*. Virtopsy: post-mortem imaging of the human heart *in situ* using MSCT and MRI. *Forensic Sci Int* 2005; **149**: 11–23.
23. Poulsen K, Simonsen J. Computed tomography as routine in connection with medico-legal autopsies. *Forensic Sci Int* 2006; Epub ahead of print.
24. Shiotani S, Kohno M, Ohashi N *et al*. Non-traumatic post-mortem computed tomographic (PMCT) findings of the lung. *Forensic Sci Int* 2004; **139**: 39–48.
25. Yamazaki K, Shiotani S, Ohashi N *et al*. Comparison between computed tomography (CT) and autopsy findings in cases of abdominal injury and disease. *Forensic Sci Int* 2006; **162**: 163–166.
26. Foroudi F, Cheung K, Duflou J. A comparison of the needle biopsy post mortem with the conventional autopsy. *Pathology* 1995; **27**: 79–82.
27. Farinnna J, Millana C, Fernandez-Acennnero MJ *et al*. Ultrasonographic autopsy (echopsy): a new autopsy technique. *Virchows Arch* 2002; **440**: 635–639.
28. Farinnna J, Millana C, Fernandez-Acennnero. Ultrasonographic autopsy. *Histopathology* 2004; **45**: 298.
29. Aghayev E, Thali MJ, Sonnenschein M, Jackowski C, Dirnhofer R, Vock P. Post-mortem tissue sampling using computed tomography guidance. *Forensic Sci Int* 2006; Epub ahead of print.
30. Myers JC, Okoye MI, Kiple D *et al*. Three-dimensional (3-D) imaging in post mortem examinations: elucidation and identification of cranial and facial fractures in victims of homicide utilising 3-D computerised imaging reconstruction techniques. *Int J Legal Med* 1999; **113**: 33–37.

31. Thali MJ, Yen K, Schweitzer B *et al*. Virtopsy, a new imaging horizon in forensic pathology: virtual autopsy by postmortem multislice computed tomography (MSCT) and magnetic resonance imaging (MRI) – a feasibility study. *J Forensic Sci* 2003; **48**: 386–403.

32. Yen K, Sonnenschein M, Thali MJ *et al*. Postmortem multislice computed tomography and magnetic resonance imaging of odontoid fractures, atlantoaxial distractions and ascending medullary edema. *Int J Legal Med* 2005; **119**: 129–136.

33. Aghayev E, Yen K, Sonnenschein M *et al*. Virtopsy post-mortem multi-slice computed tomography (MSCT) and magnetic resonance imaging (MRI) demonstrating descending tonsillar herniation: comparison to clinical studies. *Neuroradiology* 2004; **46**: 559–564.

34. Avrahami R, Watemberg S, Hiss Y *et al*. Laparoscopic vs conventional autopsy: a promising perspective. *Arch Surg* 1995; **130**: 407–409.

35. Avrahami R, Watemberg S, Hiss Y *et al*. Thoracoscopy vs conventional autopsy of the thorax: a promising perspective. *Arch Surg* 1995; **130**: 956–958.

36. Karhunen PJ, Servo A. Sudden fatal or non-operable bleeding from ruptured intracranial aneurysm. Evaluation by post-mortem angiography with vulcanising contrast medium. *Int J Legal Med* 1993; **106**: 55–59.

37. Karhunen PJ. Neurosurgical vascular complications associated with aneurysm clips evaluated by post-mortem angiography. *Forensic Sci Int* 1991; **51**: 13–22.

38. Saimanen E, Jarvinen A, Pentitila A. Cerebral cast angiography as an aid to medico-legal autopsies in cases of death after adult cardiac surgery. *Int J Legal Med* 2001; **114**: 163–168.

39. Thompson GR, Partridge J. Coronary calcification score: the coronary-risk impact factor. *Lancet* 2004; **363**: 557–559.

40. Thomas AC, Davies MJ. Post-mortem investigation and quantification of coronary artery disease. *Histopathology* 1985; **9**: 959–976.

41. Parker A. *Less invasive autopsy: the place of magnetic resonance imaging*. London: Department of Health, 2004. <http://publications.doh.gov.uk/cmo/program/organretention/mri_report.pdf>.

Sebastian Lucas

Bioterrorism

Although bioterrorist attacks have taken place over the last two decades (see Box 1), many doctors, including pathologists, in the UK and elsewhere are unaware of their medical aspects. However, pathologists and anatomical pathology technologists (APTs) in the mortuary are likely to be involved more closely than many other medical and paramedical staff. This chapter outlines the history of bioterrorism, the responses of government, and the likely agents and their clinical pathologies, medicolegal aspects, and what mortuary workers should be prepared for. A more detailed account is published elsewhere.[1]

The episode in 2001 of anthrax-contaminated letters in the US mail focused minds.[2-4] The civil and criminal investigation responses to that event are well documented,[5] but the role of pathology in that investigation needs emphasising.[6-8]

Bioterrorism is defined as:[9] 'the use or threatened use of biologic agents against a person, group, or larger population to create fear or illnesses for purposes of intimidation, gaining an advantage, interruption of normal activities, or ideologic activities. The resultant reaction is dependent upon the actual event and the population involved and can vary from a minimal effect to disruption of ongoing activities and emotional reaction, illness, or death.'

THE MOTIVES FOR BIOTERRORISM

Broadly, the purposes of bioterrorism are to: (i) cause morbidity and mortality; (ii) disrupt health services; (iii) induce fear in the population; (iv) disrupt society; and (v) force change of government and/or government policies.

Sebastian Lucas BM BCh FRCP FRCPath
Professor, Department of Histopathology, KCL School of Medicine, St Thomas's Hospital, London SE1 7EH, UK
E-mail: sebastian.lucas@kcl.ac.uk

Box 1 Bioterrorism events

USA, 1984 Contamination of salad bars with *Salmonella typhimurium*, apparently for local political purposes.[5,10] A total of 751 persons affected; no deaths

Iraq, 1990s Following the first Gulf War in 1991, it became evident that the country had prepared and stockpiled vast quantities of botulinum toxin, aflatoxin, and anthrax spores.[4,27,28] These were never found (presumed to have been destroyed on site) by the subsequent US and European science teams that went in search of weapons of mass destruction

Japan, 1995 When the attack on the Tokyo metro with the neurotoxic sarin gas by the Aum Shinrikyo cult was investigated, it emerged that members had visited Zaire in order to obtain samples of Ebola virus for bioterrorism purposes.[10] They were not successful. They had also attempted to disseminate *Clostridium botulinum* toxin, unsuccessfully.[27]

USA, 1996 Contamination of food in a laboratory staff rest-room with *Shigella dysenteriae*; motive unknown.[5] Twelve people became ill; no deaths

USA, 2001 About 10 g of anthrax spores was sent in multiple envelopes by post, by person(s) unknown, which resulted in 22 cases. The presumed intended targets were news media and government personnel.[29] The index case had anthrax meningitis.[6] Twenty of the victims handled mail, and one person was probably accidentally infected by indirect letter-to-letter contamination. Eleven cases were cutaneous anthrax (all survived); 11 cases were inhalational or meningeal anthrax of whom 5 died.[5,7,22] Thirty-two thousand people received antibiotic prophylaxis.

BIOTERRORISM POTENTIAL: THE ANTHRAX SCENARIO

In a densely populated country such as the UK, deliberate release could leave 5 million people exposed, particularly if there were multiple, simultaneous attacks in urban areas.

Perhaps 10% (~500,000 people in the UK) would be at significant risk of infection (quantified as > 0.1% risk), and 2% (~100,000 people in the UK) would be at high risk of infection (> 1%). Thus, without prophylactic antibiotic therapy, about 7500 of those exposed could become infected. The risk of infection could extend to 50 km downwind of the point of release.

Many people would present to hospitals during the following week or so. How they would be managed will depend on:

- whether the attack was overt or covert
- how many present and to how many health centres
- how rapidly the diagnosis is made in those living
- how rapidly the diagnosis is made from those dying, if not made before death
- the facilities available at the healthcare centres
- the polices drawn up in preparation for such events.

Once it became public that an anthrax bioterrorism event had occurred, a larger number of people within the target and downwind zone would present to healthcare centres, or contact health phone lines for advice:

- well but worried

- chronically ill with another disease, but perceive themselves at high risk from anthrax
- symptomatic although the cause is more likely to be something else
- symptomatic, due to anthrax.

There will also be a greater number of people who could not have been exposed but are concerned for their health, and those who have been in contact with people within the target zone. They would swamp the health centres and divert resources from the routine disease management processes.

There would be demands for antibiotic prophylaxis and vaccination (although there are no available vaccines for the public). Without stockpiles, there would not be enough antibiotics. Public anger at perceived ill preparation on the part of the government and the health systems could result in public disorder.

Because anthrax spores would be distributed over the ground, through air-conditioning systems, and get into immediate water supplies, infrastructures, such as public transport and schools, would be closed for decontamination. This would disrupt the social economy as well as the business and financial economies, and reduce the active workforce (child-minding, workplaces closed). The objectives of the terrorists will have been achieved.

THE MEANS AND COSTS OF TERRORISM

The four physical means of terrorism (conventional weaponry, biological, chemical, nuclear) have different consequences for societies and their preparations. Assuming a bioterrorism attack is covert, it would be days to weeks before anything was noticed and, by then, the effects would be wide-spread. Bioterrorism is the cheapest means of terrorism, costing approximately US$1 to kill 50% of the population in a given area per square kilometre.[10]

THE POTENTIAL AGENTS FOR BIOTERRORISM

There is no ideal bioweapon. A list of criteria characterising the ideal agent includes:

1. Easily available from other laboratories or easily prepared from local materials.
2. Safe to generate and weaponise.
3. Easily and safely disseminated as an aerosol of 1–5 μm-size particles.
4. Long-lasting and stable in the environment to prolong infectivity.
5. Readily transmitted from person to person (contagious secondary spread).
6. High infectivity, virulence and mortality rate.
7. No effective treatment of those with clinical disease.
9. No effective prophylaxis for infected, asymptomatic people (chemotherapy and/or vaccine).
10. Requires special action for public health agencies.

In the late 1990s, the US Centers for Disease Control and Prevention (CDC), drew up a consensus list of the most likely and dangerous agents that bioterrorists might use — the Category A list (Table 1)[3,9] comprising: smallpox

Table 1 Properties of biological agents in Category A

Agent/disease	ACDP hazard group	Survival in nature	Infectious dose	Transmission	Incubation period	Person-to-person transmission	Case fatality	Specific therapy
Smallpox	4	2 days	10–100	Contact; inhalation	10–16 days	Yes	15–95%	?
Viral haemorrhagic fevers	4	2 days	Unknown	Inhalation; inoculation; ingestion	1–21 days	Yes	20–90%	for Lassa only
Anthrax	3	40 years	$LD_{50} \sim 10,000$, but may be 10–100	Inhalation; inoculation; ingestion	1–10 days, but may be up to 6 weeks	Not in life, but possible during autopsy	20–90%	Yes
Plague	3	4 h	100–500	Inhalation; inoculation by infected flea	1–4 days via inhalation	Yes, from pneumonic plague	33–95%	Yes
Tularaemia	3	Long	10–50	Inhalation; inoculation; ingestion	2–5 days	Not in life but possible at autopsy	30–50%	Yes
Botulinum toxin	3	2 days	~1 ng/kg	Inhalation; ingestion	3–4 days	No, although it is just possible from an externally contaminated cadaver	?	No

Data from multiple US and UK public health sources.
ACDP, Advisory Committee on Dangerous Pathogens (UK).

(variola), anthrax (*Bacillus anthracis*), plague (*Yersinia pestis*), tularaemia (*Francisella tularensis*),botulism toxin (*Clostridium botulinum*), and viral haemorrhagic fevers (Ebola, Lassa, Marburg viruses).

Two further categories of infective agents were considered, that might be used in bioterrorism attack, but carry a lower mortality than the Category A list agents. The Category B list comprises: Q fever (*Coxiella burnettii*),[11] brucellosis (*Brucella spp.*), glanders (*Burkolderia mallei*), arthropod-borne encephalitis (Venezuelan, Eastern and Western), and water- and food-borne gut pathogens (*Salmonella* and *Shigella spp., Escherichia coli, Vibrio cholerae, Cryptosporidium parvum*).

The Category C list includes emerging or re-emerging pathogens that might be engineered for mass dissemination, are easily available, and have potentially high mortality. They include: Nipah virus, hantaviruses, tick-born haemorrhagic fevers, tick-borne encephalitis, Yellow fever virus, and multidrug resistant tuberculosis (*Mycobacterium tuberculosis*).

AVAILABILITY, WEAPONISATION AND DISSEMINATION OF THE PROPOSED AGENTS

With the exception of smallpox, all the agents in Categories A, B and C cause disease naturally and are present in nature, globally or locally. In addition, there are freeze-dried preparations in many laboratories. Apart from smallpox, the most difficult to obtain by terrorists would be Ebola virus, as it is not clear in which animal reservoir the virus resides in the wild in Central Africa.[12] However, there are isolates in several laboratories.

To establish a laboratory capable of manufacturing bioterrorism agents on a large scale is not difficult, and the estimated cost of setting up the facility is about $100,000.[2,10]

The various means of dissemination of bioterrorism agents include: aerosol dispersion, contamination of food, contamination of water supplies, contamination of milk tankers, and direct inoculation into people. The consensus is that aerosol dissemination is most likely to be used for mass bioterrorism attacks.

AEROSOL DISPERSION

All Category A agents can be disseminated in a fine particle aerosol of 1–5 µm size. This is invisible, and small enough to be inhaled into the alveoli without filtering and capture. The means of spreading the agents are various, and include: paint-sprayers, fogging machines used to disseminate insecticides, hand-held perfume atomisers, hand-held drug delivery devices (like asthma inhalers), and aeroplanes, as for crop-dusting

BIOTERRORISM TERMINOLOGY AND RESPONSES FROM PUBLIC HEALTH ORGANISATIONS

The UK Health Protection Agency (HPA) has issued guidelines for action in the event of deliberate release of a range of chemical, nuclear and biological agents (see <www.hpa.org.uk/infections/topics_az/deliberate_release/menu.htm>).

For the biological agents, the HPA guidelines include comprehensive sections on biology of the agent, epidemiology, transmission, communicability, clinical features, mortality, antimicrobial sensitivity, clinical procedures, treatment, infection control, immunisation, decontamination, protection of healthcare workers, post-exposure prophylaxis, laboratory diagnosis, public health procedures, and contact names and addresses. Autopsy is considered briefly, stressing that it should not be performed if the infection is suspected.

There is more detail in *Initial investigation and management of outbreaks and incidents of unusual illnesses – a guide for histopathologists*.[13] As well as specific advice on what samples to take and where to refer them for confirmation, the role of the coroner is acknowledged in the autopsy process. An update on microbiological sampling has been issued.[14] 'Unusual illnesses' are described as being in or of:

- patients presenting with signs and symptoms which do not fit any recognisable clinical picture, or
- known aetiology but not usually expected to occur in the UK or a setting where it has been observed, or
- known aetiology that does not behave as expected, *e.g.* failure to respond to standard therapy, or
- unknown aetiology.

Thus pathologists have a crucial role to play in identification of covert releases. Previously unrecognised syndromes may also be due to new or emerging or re-emerging conditions. New infections would be those previously unknown, or known in animals but not known to affect man (most significant human infections arose this way, from animal-to-man transmission[15]).

MORTUARY PLANS AND PROVISIONS

Bioterrorism cases can arrive at any mortuary, with or without prior known diagnosis or of unknown cause of death before autopsy. What happens after it is established that a bioterrorism outbreak is definite or likely will depend on scale. If there are only a few identified or suspected cases, then they will probably be handled at the place of arrival or in a specialist referral unit for autopsy.

However if the outbreak is larger and is designated as a 'disaster', then many local authorities will institute established plans and concentrate all cases in one designated public mortuary in an area, or go further and create a temporary multi-agency 'resilience mortuary'.

THE DISEASES THAT MAY PRESENT AS BIOTERRORISM

Smallpox and anthrax are described in some detail. Colour images of the clinical, gross and histopathological features of all the infections are on the US CDC and the UK HPA websites.

SMALLPOX

Smallpox is a Category A infection considered likely to be used in a bioterrorism attack. The following account of the disease exemplifies the aspects of which an involved pathologist needs to be aware.[16–18]

Transmission is usually by inhalation of droplet aerosols from infected persons. Direct skin-lesion-to-skin contact can transmit, as can contact with infected body fluids. The most infectious period in a patient is after the incubation period, during the first week of the rash, when virus is released from the respiratory tract.

Clinical features

During the asymptomatic first week, there is viraemia and dissemination to the lymphoreticular system. A second viraemia commences about 8 days after infection and is associated with the characteristic illness:

- sudden high fever
- macular rash 1–3 days later in the oropharynx, then face, forearms and trunk
- the rash becomes papular 2 days later, then vesicular after another 1–2 days. Typically, it is more severe on the face and extremities – centrifugal pattern
- the vesicles become pustular after another 2–3 days, forming scabs 5–8 days after the onset of the rash
- the scabs separate leaving characteristic pitted scarring, most prominent on the face.

Smallpox can have less common atypical patterns that have caused late diagnosis through confusion. The two forms are:

1. Haemorrhagic smallpox – with haemorrhage into the mucosal and skin lesions.
2. Malignant smallpox – the lesions do not develop to the pustular stage but remain soft and flat

Differential diagnosis of smallpox

The classic differential diagnosis has been chickenpox (varicella-zoster virus). Other skin rashes that could be confused with smallpox, and almost inevitably will be so in the event of an outbreak, include:[16]

- monkeypox
- generalised vaccinia
- herpes simplex virus
- molluscum contagiosum
- measles
- parvovirus (B19)
- rubella
- enteroviral infections
- hand-foot-and-mouth disease
- syphilis
- impetigo
- drug eruptions and Stevens–Johnson syndrome

- atypical forms of skin lesions in immunosuppressed persons (*e.g.* anergic cutaneous cryptococcosis in advanced HIV disease can resemble herpetic and smallpox rashes in the pustular stage).

For atypical smallpox, the differential diagnosis is meningococcal sepsis and haemorrhagic chickenpox.

The World Health Organization has produced training materials to help healthcare workers recognise smallpox and its differential diagnosis (see <www.who.int/emc/diseases/smallpox/slideset/index/htm>).

Treatment

There are no proven antiviral drugs effective against smallpox. Cidofovir is active against other orthopox viruses and would be tried if cases arose. It has to be administered intravenously and is potentially nephrotoxic.

Vaccination

Stocks of smallpox vaccine have been depleted since 1980, but are now being regenerated because of the threat of bioterrorism. It is most effective before exposure, but vaccination does reduce the clinical attack rate if given after exposure. Vaccine 'effectiveness' means reducing the attack rate to < 10% and mortality to < 1%.

In the UK, stocks of vaccine are limited; only a few laboratory staff and emergency service personnel (but not pathologists or mortuary workers to date) have been vaccinated. Supply is controlled by the Department of Health (England). There are vaccination complications including:[19] generalised vaccinia, progressive vaccinia, post-vaccination encephalitis, fetal vaccinia, and myopericarditis.

These complications are uncommon, but sufficient to advise a cost–benefit approach as to who needs vaccination. A new issue is the susceptibility of HIV-infected persons to complications. Whether potential vaccinees should have an HIV test or be screened by questioning for HIV risk factors and knowledge of their HIV status awaits clarification.[20]

Diagnostic procedures and the autopsy

In life, there are protocols on clinically suspecting smallpox and how to confirm or exclude it. In the laboratory, the diagnosis will be made by real-time polymerase chain reaction (PCR) and electron microscopy.[16]

For those who die, the HPA guidance is fairly specific:[18]

1. If the diagnosis is already known, there is no requirement for autopsy.

2. If smallpox is suspected, the examination procedure can be kept to a minimum of invasiveness to reduce the likelihood of infection to pathologists and APTs. There is no need to open the cadaver to prove smallpox.

3. All staff involved in an autopsy must be vaccinated.

4. Full respiratory protection must be used, in addition to the standard universal precautions in dress.

5. Skin samples can show the virus through standard virological techniques.

6. Post-mortem blood through cardiac puncture is a useful source of virus.

7. The samples must be transported to the reference centre laboratory in leak-proof secondary containers, complying with the UN602 standard packaging, and labelled 'BIOHAZARD'.

The pathology of smallpox[8]

Skin. Histopathologically, there is intra-epidermal oedema, ballooned epidermal cells and necrosis. The characteristic Guaneri bodies are intracytoplasmic granular, basophilic viral inclusion bodies in epidermal cells. There is marked dermal inflammation.

Heart. In fatal cases of smallpox, there is a myocarditis.

Lung. In fatal cases, there is often a direct smallpox pneumonitis and secondary bacterial infections.

The impact in the mortuary

What would happen in the mortuary should a case be autopsied, without anyone realising at the outset that it was smallpox, is unpredictable? If the pathologist or APT suspects the diagnosis, then the diagnostic and logistic procedures follow. But the staff are unlikely to have been vaccinated, and there will probably be some panic. Occupational health units will be involved and vaccines would have to be obtained from the Department of Health (England) rapidly. In a public mortuary environment, there are usually no such on-site health advice facilities, and tissue sampling is also more problematic.

If the diagnosis was not suspected by the end of the gross autopsy examination, either: (i) the diagnosis is not made at all, no tissue having been retained and another cause of death provided; or (ii) the diagnosis becomes evident later on histopathological and/or microbiological analyses.

If only histopathology is used, it is likely to be days to weeks before the diagnosis is suspected and confirmed. The opportunity to protect the staff by vaccination will either be lost or made too late, unless the diagnosis becomes evident sooner for other reasons (*e.g.* review of clinical history).

ANTHRAX

This is an aerobic Gram-positive bacillus, readily grown on artificial media. Once the growth is saturated, it forms spores; this also happens when bacilli in man are exposed to air. Infection is by the spores which are 2 µm diameter. In nature, many animals are normally infected from spores in the soil where they remain viable for decades.[21]

There are three routes of infection for *B. anthracis* – inhalational, cutaneous, and gastrointestinal. The clinical presentation includes meningitis; half the autopsied victims of the 1979 Sverdlovsk anthrax outbreak also developed meningitis.[2,4] An index case of anthrax meningitis suggests deliberate release.

Clinical presentation

For inhalational anthrax, the incubation period is usually 2–10 days. The initial symptoms are non-specific fever, non-productive cough and malaise. Then, sudden shortness of breath, hypotensive shock, stridor and cyanosis develop, and within a day or so death occurs, despite intensive care. Radiologically, the critical finding is widening of the mediastinum and pleural effusions.

Inhalation anthrax is suspected clinically in a previously healthy person if there is:

1. Rapid onset of severe unexplained febrile illness of febrile death.

2. Rapid onset of severe sepsis not due to a predisposing illness, or respiratory failure with a widened mediastinum.

3. Severe sepsis with Gram-positive bacilli or *B. anthracis* identified in the blood, chest effusions or cerebrospinal fluid and judged not to be a contaminant.

Pathologically, this is not a pneumonia, but a haemorrhagic effusion involving the mediastinal lymph nodes and pleura. There is necrosis of the lymph nodes with immunoblast proliferation, abundant Gram-positive bacilli, but little acute inflammation. The lung parenchyma shows oedema and haemorrhage and acute lung injury. If the patient has been treated with chemotherapy for 72 h or more, the Gram-positive bacilli may not be visible, but are evident immunohistochemically.[22]

The meningitis is also haemorrhagic. Cerebrospinal fluid examination reveals features of acute bacterial meningitides with abundant Gram-positive bacilli.

Cutaneous lesions developed in half of the 2001 US anthrax patients. These are ulcers that become eschars. The clinical differential diagnosis includes skin haematoma and non-specific erosions.[22] Histologically, there is epidermal and dermal oedema and necrosis, acute inflammation, and characteristic Gram-positive bacilli; treatment reduces their number, but immunocytochemistry identifies the antigens.

Autopsy in cases of known or suspected anthrax in the UK is discouraged.[21] However, if autopsy is essential, then full protective clothing and equipment must be used.

SURVEILLANCE FOR BIOTERRORISM

What is the optimum means of identifying bioterrorism attacks, either before they have affected anyone, or early after people become ill? The consensus is that local reporting systems are the most likely to be useful and efficient. The pathologist has a role both as surgical biopsy and autopsy diagnostician, and the important aspects are: (i) awareness of the differential diagnoses that include bioterrorism agents; and (ii) ability to confirm or exclude them.

Table 2 presents the commoner clinicopathological scenarios that may present to the mortuary that include the possibility of a bioterrorism-related disease, alongside commoner infectious and non-infectious causes.

STANDARDS OF AUTOPSY PRACTICE

In the circumstance of a pandemic bird influenza epidemic,[23] it is agreed that once the initial cases have been identified from clinical pre-mortem investigation and autopsy investigation, subsequent cases will be identified syndromically and not require positive identification of the infecting agent. Syndromic diagnosis will suffice for medicolegal purposes and death certification.

However, deaths from proven bioterrorist attacks are homicide,[8,9] so consideration is given to the extent and thoroughness of autopsy examination; compromise may affect the stringency of evidence in cases required to bring a successful prosecution against alleged perpetrators at a criminal trial.

Table 2 The syndromic approach to surveillance for bioterrorism agents

Clinico-pathological syndrome	Common causes, including infections of public health interest	Potential bioterrorism illness
Vesicular skin rash	Varicella, immunological blistering disorders	Smallpox
Diffuse haemorrhagic skin rash	Measles, rickettsioses, meningococcaemia, dengue, toxic shock syndrome, enterovirus, other thrombocytopenias, leukaemia	Viral haemorrhagic fever, smallpox
Community-acquired pneumonia	*Strep. pneumonia*, *Legionella*, influenza, hantavirus pulmonary syndrome, tuberculosis, other bacterial and viral pneumonias	Plague, tularaemia, Q fever
Haemorrhagic mediastinitis and pleural effusion	Carcinoma and mesothelioma, pulmonary leptospirosis	Anthrax. *If Gram-positive bacilli present, highly likely*
Sepsis syndromes, including disseminated intravascular coagulation[26]	Streptococcal and staphylococcal infections, meningococcaemia, malaria, leptospirosis, yellow fever, rickettsioses, tuberculosis, haemophagocytic syndrome, lymphoma, HIV	Plague, tularaemia, viral haemorrhagic fever, anthrax
Haemorrhagic meningitis	Herpes simplex encephalitis	Anthrax. *If Gram-positive bacilli present, highly likely*
Encephalitis, meningitis	Viral, bacterial, fungal and parasitic meningitis and encephalitis	Venezuelan equine encephalitis, Nipah virus
Swallowing, muscle movement, eye movement, and breathing difficulties	Myasthenia gravis, Eaton–Lambert syndrome, Guillain–Barré syndrome, rabies	Botulinum toxin
Hepatitis, fulminant hepatic necrosis	HBV, HCV, septic shock	Brucellosis, viral haemorrhagic fevers
Haemorrhagic colitis	Bacillary dysentery, infarction	*E. coli*, *Shigella*, gastrointestinal anthrax
Pharyngitis, epiglottitis	Common viral and streptococcal sore throat	Viral haemorrhagic fever (Lassa)

Expanded from Guarner and Zaki[6] and Nolte *et al.*[9]

FORENSIC EPIDEMIOLOGY

The recent concept of 'forensic epidemiology' has emerged when public heath investigations overlap with criminal investigations. Because the training and experience of epidemiologists is quite different from that of criminal investigators, there are different priorities and perhaps conflicts when the two groups interact. Forensic epidemiology is defined as:[5] 'the use of epidemiological methods as part of an ongoing investigation of a health problem for which there is suspicion or evidence regarding possible intentional acts of criminal behaviour contributing to the health problem'.

In the US, a standard training programme is being introduced (see CDC website <www.bt.cdc.gov/>). In brief, the important issues when investigating an outbreak of infectious disease focus on:

1. Understanding how public health investigations proceed by: (i) defining exposed populations; and (ii) providing prophylaxis to exposed persons.

2. Identifying the source, *i.e.* perpetrators or reservoir.

3. Recognising that certain unusual or unnatural findings in a disease investigation may suggest intentional action.

4. Identifying procedures and mechanisms to communicate suspicion of intentionality to law enforcement officials.

5. Understanding how a public health investigation differs from a criminal investigation.

6. Assessment and credibility of a threat.

7. The laws surrounding entry into and obtaining samples within homes and workplaces.

8. Establishing chain of custody of evidence.

PERSONAL PROTECTION DURING AUTOPSY IN BIOTERRORISM CASES

Historically, pathologists have acquired a range of infections from autopsy: streptococcal sepsis, tuberculosis, tularaemia, diphtheria, glanders, scrub typhus, systemic mycoses, toxoplasmosis, HIV-1, hepatitis B and C, rabies, smallpox, and viral haemorrhagic fever.[24] Deaths have occurred among prosectors from these infections, which include agents in the bioterrorism Category A–C lists.

The threat of bioterrorism is likely to reinforce the historical trend amongst mortuary workers to use greater levels of personal protection against accidental infection. Both in the US and UK, the standard recommended dress for all exposed staff for all autopsies is:[24,25]

- surgical scrub suit
- hat
- water-impermeable gown covering arms, trunk and upper legs
- plastic apron over the gown

- respiratory protection
- eye protection
- reinforced rubber boots
- multiple glove layers, ideally latex gloves either side of a cut-resistant neoprene glove.

Respiratory protection prevents inhalation of aerosols and contamination of the mucosa by droplets. Standard surgical masks provide protection against droplet splashes, but finer aerosols readily get round the sides. When there is a risk from inhaling a pathogenic aerosol, respirators that prevent nearly all particles ≥ 1 μm getting into the lungs are necessary.[24] There are two basic types:

1. Modified disposable mask (N-95 respirator in US; EN149 FFP3 respirator in UK).

2. Powered air-purifying respirator (PAPR) with high-efficiency particulate air (HEPA) cartridge filters. These are ventilated hoods that cover the head; they may be part of a whole body suit, or applied on top of a separate suit. In the UK, the standard PAPR is the EN12941 with PP3 filters.

It is intuitive that PAPR would be preferred when dealing with suspected bioterrorism agents such as smallpox and viral haemorrhagic fevers;[24] however, there is no evidence for such a statement, and there is no official public health service guidance on the issue, in either the US or the UK. At present, it is a matter of preference and equipment resource.

GENERIC PROTOCOL FOR THE AUTOPSY AND SPECIMEN COLLECTION IN SUSPECTED BIOTERRORISM CASES

The protocol includes (see also Table 3):[14]

1. Autopsies should be performed within 24 h of the patient's death, to increase the validity of culture and PCR results.

2. Aseptic techniques must be applied as rigorously as possible to minimise contamination, from within and without the body.

3. All samples should be collected in duplicate for histopathology (fixed in formalin) and microbiology (unfixed in sterile containers, fresh and frozen).

4. Normally site-sterile samples, whenever possible.

5. Tissues to be sampled include: local inflammatory lesions or abscesses, liver, spleen, lung, heart, kidney, lymph nodes, bone marrow, and other organs with gross pathological abnormality.

6. The tissue fragments for microbiology should be ~10 mm cubes.

7. Samples for microbiology should be both fresh and frozen at −70°C.

8. Heart blood samples, whole in one tube and spun for post-mortem serum in a separate tube.

Table 3 Checklist if an autopsy is performed on a Category A infection case

	Anthrax	Smallpox	Plague	Viral haemorrhagic fever	Tularaemia	Botulinum toxin
FFP3 respiratory protection	Yes	Yes	Yes	Yes	Yes	No
Samples for microbiology	Lung, pleural fluid, spleen, lymph node	Skin, blood	Lung, spleen, lymph node	Blood, liver, spleen	Lung, spleen, lymph node	Blood, faeces
Samples for histopathology	Standard set including skin	Standard set	Standard set	Standard set	Standard set	Standard set
Vaccinate staff	No	Yes	No	No	No	No
Antibiotic prophylaxis for staff, assuming universal precautions used during autopsy	Yes	No	Yes	No. Only if direct skin contact with infected material	Yes	No
Anti-toxin for staff	n/a	n/a	n/a	n/a	n/a	No
Decontaminate body and surfaces with hypochlorite	Yes	Yes	Yes	Yes	Yes	No
Embalm body	No	No	No	No	No	No
Cremate body	Yes	Yes	Yes	Yes	Yes	Yes
Autoclave instruments	Yes	Yes	Yes	Yes	Yes	No

9. Cerebrospinal fluid (fresh and frozen).

10. Urine (frozen).

11. Gut contents, for microbe and toxin detection.

12. Cytological preparations from tissue smears done at the time of autopsy.

13. Samples labelled with patient's name, date of autopsy and site of sample.

14. Chain of custody of sample evidence ensured.

This sample list is necessarily exhaustive and is hardly likely, or required, to be followed in every instance. The nature of the case and the material actually available will determine what is taken. The mortuaries undertaking autopsies of this nature must be equipped with necessary facilities and material. These include:

- good ventilation, lighting and water provision
- sterile specimen containers and labels
- formalin fixative
- sterile instruments
- centrifuge
- freezer
- storage facilities for specimens
- skilled anatomical pathology technologists
- personal protective equipment
- protocols for safe practice in the mortuary.

PATHOLOGICAL IDENTIFICATION OF BIOTERRORISM AGENTS

The clinicopathological syndrome is the starting point for consideration.[6] Table 2 sets out the syndromes that could present as bioterrorism-related illness, with the other common causes of such disease. If a bioterrorism infection is suspected, confirmation or exclusion depends on the scenario and what material is available. Fresh tissue for microbiological analysis is obviously optimal. But formalin-fixed, paraffin-embedded material can be precisely categorised in many cases, using haematoxylin and eosin (H&E), empirical special stains, immunocytochemistry, and (potentially) molecular diagnostics.

H&E stains identify viral inclusion bodies, but do not necessarily enable a more specific diagnosis. The histological special stains most useful in evaluation of bioterrorism infections and their differential diagnosis are: Gram, Grocott silver, Ziehl–Neelsen, and Warthin–Starry.[8] Immunocytochemical antibodies are not generally available for specific typing of the relevant infectious agents, at least in the UK. The US CDC, however, does maintain a large panel of antibodies that can reliably identify most of the bioterrorism agents.[6] Molecular technology is increasingly the gold standard for microbiological identification in fresh material.[7]

Points for best practice

- Bioterrorism attacks are probably going to happen in the UK and elsewhere.

- The likely infections include anthrax, smallpox and plague.

- Awareness of the possibility and the types of presentation in cadavers is critical.

- Sensible precautions and personal protection will minimise risk to mortuary healthcare staff.

- Much practical guidance is available on public health websites.

References

1. Lucas SB. Bioterrorism. In: Rutty GN. (ed) *Essentials of Autopsy Pathology*. London: Springer, 2007; in press.
2. Henderson DA, Borio LL. Bioterrorism: an overview. In: Mandell GL, Bennet JE, Dolin R. (eds) *Mandell, Douglas and Bennett's Principles and Practice of Infectious Diseases*. Pennsylvania: Elsevier Churchill Livingstone, 2005; 3591–3601.
3. Centers for Disease Control and Prevention. Biological and chemical terrorism: strategic plan for preparedness and response. *MMWR* 2000; **49**: 1–14.
4. Lucey DR. Anthrax. In: Mandell GL, Bennet JE, Dolin R. (eds) *Mandell, Douglas and Bennett's Principles and Practice of Infectious Diseases*. Pennsylvania: Elsevier Churchill Livingstone, 2005; 3618–3624.
5. Goodman RA, Munson JW, Dammers K, Lazzarini Z, Barkley JP. Forensic epidemiology: law at the intersection of public health and criminal investigations. *J Law Med Ethics* 2003; **31**: 684–700.
6. Guarner J, Zaki SR. Histopathology and immunocytochemistry in the diagnosis of bioterrorism agents. *J Histochem Cytochem* 2006; **54**: 3–11.
7. Shieh W-J, Guarner J, Paddock C *et al*. The critical role of pathology in the investigation of bioterrorism-related cutaneous anthrax. *Am J Pathol* 2003; **163**: 1901–1910.
8. Marty AM. Anatomic laboratory and forensic aspects of biological threat agents. *Clin Lab Med* 2006; **26**: 515–540.
9. Nolte KB, Hanzlick RL, Payne DC *et al*. Medical Examiners, Coroners, and Biologic Terrorism. A guidebook for surveillance and case management. *MMWR* 2004; **53** (RR08): 1–27.
10. Aggrawal A. Terrorism: nuclear and biological. In: Payne-James J, Byard RW, Corey TS, Henderson C. (eds) *Encyclopaedia of Forensic and Legal Medicine*. Oxford: Elsevier, 2005; 277–290.
11. Parker NR, Barralet JH, Bell AM. Q fever. *Lancet* 2006; **367**: 679–688.
12. Lahm SA, Kombila M, Swaenpoel R, Barnes FW. Morbidity and mortality of wild animals in relation to outbreaks of Ebola haemorrhagic fever in Gabon, 1994–2003. *Trans R Soc Trop Med Hyg* 2007; **101**: 64–78.
13. Health Protection Agency Centre for Infections. *Initial investigation and management of outbreaks and incidents of unusual illnesses*. Version 3. Colindale: HPA, 2004; 1–42.
14. Health Protection Agency Centre for Infections. *Protocol for the investigation of microbiologically unexplained serious illness and death*. Version 1. Colindale: HPA, 2006; 1–17.
15. Palmer S, Brown D, Morgan D. Early qualitative risk assessment of the emerging zoonotic potential of animal diseases. *BMJ* 2005; **331**: 1256–1260.
16. Moore ZS, Seward JF, Lane M. Smallpox. *Lancet* 2006; **367**: 425–435.
17. Rotz LD, Cono J, Damon I. Smallpox and bioterrorism. In: Mandell GL, Bennet JE, Dolin R. (eds) *Mandell, Douglas and Bennett's Principles and Practice of Infectious Diseases*. Pennsylvania: Elsevier Churchill Livingstone, 2005; 3612–3617.

18. Health Protection Agency Centre for Infections. Smallpox. Interim guidelines for action in the event of a deliberate release. Version 5.2. Colindale: HPA, 2005; 1–24.
19. Auckland C, Cowlishaw A, Morgan D, Miller E. Reactions to small pox vaccine in naive and previously-vaccinated individuals. *Vaccine* 2005; **23**: 4185–4187.
20. Bartlett JG. Smallpox vaccination and patient with HIV infection or AIDS. *Clin Infect Dis* 2003; **36**: 468–471.
21. Health Protection Agency Centre for Infections. *Anthrax. Guidelines for action in the event of a deliberate release.* Version 5.8. Colindale: HPA, 2007; 1–22.
22. Guarner J, Jernigan JA, Shieh W-J *et al*. Pathology and pathogenesis of bioterrorism-related inhalational anthrax. *Am J Pathol* 2003; **163**: 701–709.
23. Department of Health and Health Protection Agency. *Guidance for pandemic influenza: infection control in hospitals and primary care settings.* London: Department of Health, 2005; 1, 68.
24. Nolte KB, Taylor DG, Richmond JY. Biosafety considerations for autopsy. *Am J Foren Med Pathol* 2002; **23**: 107–122.
25. Royal College of Pathologists. *Guidelines for Autopsy Practice.* London: RCPath, 2002.
26. Lucas SB. The autopsy pathology of sepsis-related death. *Curr Diag Pathol* 2007; in press.
27. Bleck TP. Botulinum toxin as a biological weapon. In: Mandell GL, Bennet JE, Dolin R. (eds) *Mandell, Douglas and Bennett's Principles and Practice of Infectious Diseases.* Pennsylvania: Elsevier Churchill Livingstone, 2005; 3624–3625.
28. Zilinskas RA. Iraq's biological weapons: the past as future? *JAMA* 1997; **278**: 418–424.
29. Atlas RM. Bioterrorism: from threat to reality. *Annu Rev Microbiol* 2002; **56**: 167–185.

Index

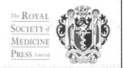
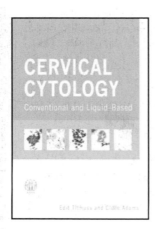

Immigration and the Nation-State

The United States, Germany, and Great Britain

CHRISTIAN JOPPKE

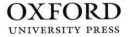

OXFORD
UNIVERSITY PRESS

OXFORD

UNIVERSITY PRESS

Great Clarendon Street, Oxford OX2 6DP

Oxford University Press is a department of the University of Oxford
It furthers the University's objective of excellence in research, scholarship,
and education by publishing worldwide in

Oxford New York

Athens Auckland Bangkok Bogotá Buenos Aires Calcutta
Cape Town Chennai Dar es Salaam Delhi Florence Hong Kong Istanbul
Karachi Kuala Lumpur Madrid Melbourne Mexico City Mumbai
Nairobi Paris São Paulo Singapore Taipei Tokyo Toronto Warsaw

with associated companies in Berlin Ibadan

Oxford is a registered trade mark of Oxford University Press
in the UK and in certain other countries

Published in the United States
by Oxford University Press Inc., New York

British Library Cataloguing in Publication Data

Data available

Library of Congress Cataloging in Publication Data
Joppke, Christian.
Immigration and the nation-state: The United States, Germany, and
Great Britain / Christian Joppke.
1. United States—Emigration and immigration—Government policy.
2. Citizenship—United States. 3. Germany—Emigration and
immigration—Government policy. 4. Citizenship—Germany.
5. Great Britain—Emigration and immigration—Government policy.
6. Citizenship—Great Britain. I. Title.
JV6483.J66 1999 325.73—dc21 98–46622
ISBN 0–19–829428–X
ISBN 0–19–829540–5 (Pbk)

1 3 5 7 9 10 8 6 4 2

Typeset by Hope Services (Abingdon) Ltd.
Printed in Great Britain
on acid-free paper by
Bookcraft (Bath) Ltd
Midsomer Norton, Somerset

Une fois encore, pour Catherine

Preface

This book contributes to the growing macro-sociological and political science literature on immigration, citizenship, and the nation-state. It compares the postwar politics of immigration control and immigrant integration in the United States, Germany, and Britain, three liberal states characterized by sharply distinct nationhood traditions and immigration experiences. Besides mapping out these variations, the book focuses on the impact of immigration on two generic principles of the nation-state, sovereignty and citizenship. Regarding sovereignty, which is at stake in immigration control, I argue that liberal states are self-limited by interest-group pluralism, autonomous legal systems, and moral obligations toward particular immigrant groups, the relative weight of these factors differing across states. Regarding citizenship, which is at stake in immigrant integration, I show the continued relevance of national citizenship for incorporating immigrants, though modified by nationally distinct schemes of multiculturalism. This book thus sets a counterpoint to current diagnoses of nation-states diminished by the external forces of globalization and international human rights regimes and discourses. At least in the face of immigration, nation-states have proved remarkably resilient.

This is a synthetic work, whose point is not the discovery of new data but the broad comparison of macro-configurations that may have escaped more specialized authors writing about a particular policy, country, or period. Its spirit is 'quaterny', as Abram de Swaan characterized his *In Care of the State* (1988), a synthesis, across a wider comparative canvas, of smaller-scale, country-specific synthetic analyses and interpretations. The huge literature already piled up about immigration in Western states is therefore a plus, not a minus. It helped me to produce a type of argument that presupposes the empirical groundwork laid by other authors. However, whenever possible I tried to incorporate primary and secondary sources, such as records of parliamentary debates and public hearings in the forefield of important legislation, the texts of landmark court rules, the grey literature produced by non-governmental organizations, and newspaper accounts of significant immigration-related events. Most importantly, I conducted sixty-seven interviews with policy-makers and -advisers, immigration lawyers, and leaders of ethnic immigrant organizations. These interviews were equally skewed to the capitals, in which national immigration policy is made: Washington, Bonn, and London, and to locales of heavy immigrant concentration plagued by integration problems: Los Angeles, Frankfurt and Berlin, and London. While they rarely show in the text, the interviews gave me a feel for the country-specific immigration problematiques, and the confidence to write about them.

Research was supported by generous funding from the Research Council of the European University Institute. Imco Brouwer, Jessica Ter Wal, Hans-Jörg Trenz, and Kerstin Ullrich provided valuable research assistance. Rogers Brubaker read parts of an earlier draft and gave excellent advice.

Christian Joppke

San Domenico di Fiesole
March 1998

Contents

1

Immigration and the Nation-State

International migration is commonly experienced in the developed societies of the West as 'immigration', which depicts states as passive receivers of voluntary migrants from afar. This optic obscures the constitutive role of the modern state in international migration. Only in a world made up of sovereign states, each exercising final control over a bounded territory and populace, is there international migration, which by definition includes a 'transfer of jurisdiction' (Zolberg, 1981: 5). But the modern state is not only definitionally involved in the making of international migration. The modern state's principle of territorial rule frees individuals from the ascriptive ties and personal bondage that once locked them into a concrete place and community, providing incentives for physical and social mobility (Preuss, 1996: 22). Moreover, modern states are not monads, but exist as part of an interactive, comprehensive system of states, which requires regularized, constant communication and boundary exchanges. International migration is enabled by and feeds upon the communicative, expansive grid of the modern state system. Finally, states have actively created transborder movements, as nationalizing states that expel unwanted religious, ethnic, or political groups, as colonizing states that set up dependencies overseas, or, in reverse, as labour-recruiting states that either force or invite foreigners to fill jobs for which domestic workers cannot be found.

While states have been part in creating international migration, they are also dependent on restricting it. This is because international migration violates the principle of sedentariness underlying the modern state system, which differentiates world society into a multiplicity of territorially bounded, self-reproducing units. As Rogers Brubaker (1992: ch. 3) has shown in his discussion of the origins of state membership in Prussia, sedentariness codified as nationality (*Staatsangehörigkeit*) is administratively convenient, dividing up international state responsibility for certain categories of people (such as the migrant poor). But the expectation of sedentariness, and ensuing restrictiveness of entry, also springs from the cultural fundament of modern states, their nationness. As nations, modern states are political communities invested with the right of self-determination. An expression of this right is the admission, or rejection, of new members. As Michael Walzer (1983: 52) outlined, 'the members of a political community have a collective right to shape the resident population'. Otherwise political communities (or nations) could not be 'communities of character' (ibid. 62). While constrained by moral obligations to those who can claim a right of place and to refugees, decisions over new membership are discretionary and not subject to considerations of justice. Inclusionary and democratic to the inside, nation-states are necessarily exclusionary and undemocratic to the outside, rocks of facticity that defy universal justice and human rights.[1]

The relationship between international migration and modern states is thus ambivalent: it is one of mutual conditioning and exclusion at the same time. This ambivalence has grown and intensified over time (see Zolberg, 1978). Under mercantilism, labour scarcity had motivated absolutist states to prohibit exit, limiting migration to the forced incorporation of slaves or indented labour. With exit prohibited, entry (and thus, immigration) could not even be an issue. Mercantilism gave way to a brief period of liberalism, in which the removal of barriers to exit coincided with non-existing restrictions on entry. Liberalism was the classic hour of immigration, with unprecedented population movements within and outside Europe, the outside movement giving rise to the transoceanic new settler nations of Canada, Australia, and the United States. But the 'liberal moment' (Zolberg, 1992: 322) in international migration was short. By the 1880s, nation-building concerns moved all Western states, including the settler nations, to impose restrictions on entry. This established today's fundamental contradiction of how states deal with international migration: a generalized commitment to the freedom of exit is combined with severe restrictions on entry.

After the fall of communism (the last regional regime to prohibit exit) and with the rise of globalization, in which most barriers to the movement of capital, goods, information, and (certain categories of) people have melted away, the contradiction of free exit and restricted entry has become more conspicuous than ever. Cosmopolitan intellectuals denounce the evils of factual boundaries that stand in the way of universal justice and human rights. On the other hand, aggrieved majorities resort to parochial nationalisms to find halt in a disorderly world. The control of entry becomes one of the few domains in which states can still be strong—'renationalizing' immigration policies as antidote to the 'denationalizing' logic of globalization (Sassen, 1996: ch. 3). But in a discursively postnational West, the justification of exclusiveness is growing thin, being reduced to a factual defence of First-World riches against mobilized Third-World poverty. Globalization fuels the free exit versus restricted entry dualism, and brings into the open the 'fundamental tension between the interests of individuals and the interests of society' (Zolberg, 1981: 7) that has always characterized international migration in the modern state system.

Recent macro-studies have drawn radically opposite scenarios of how immigration is tied up with the development and transformation of modern nation-states. Rogers Brubaker's (1992) comparison of citizenship and nationhood in France and Germany sees even the most recent immigration and citizenship policies conditioned by entrenched 'cultural idioms' of nationhood that, once in place, have proved resistant to change.[2] His is a vestigial view in which the nation-state is the only feasible form of political organization in the modern world; the nation-state is not wholeheartedly embraced but accepted for 'lack of a coherent and persuasive alternative' (Brubaker, 1989: 4 f.). Characteristically, Brubaker registers postwar migrations as a 'fundamental challenge' to the nation-states of the West, which have 'compelled these countries . . . to reinvent themselves . . . *as* nation-states' (ibid. 1; emphasis supplied). New forms of state membership for migrants are taken as 'conspicuous deviation' (ibid. 5) from the model of national citizenship, which will have to be corrected in the long run.

Yasemin Soysal's (1994) study of migrant rights in postwar Europe has come to the opposite conclusion. Shifting the nation-state from independent to dependent variable, she argues that recent migrations have helped put into place a permanent, alternative 'postnational' model of membership anchored in a world-level discourse of human rights. What Brubaker took for a deviation subject to correction, Soysal endows with the dignity of a new institutional form that 'transgresses the national order of things' (p. 159). In her view, nation-states have undergone fundamental transformation: states are increasingly instruments for implementing international human-rights conventions and norms, thus dissociating them from the nations they still claim to represent.[3] Obviously the exercise of postnational migrant rights remains 'tied to specific states and their institutions' (p. 157), but as a matter of organizational exigency only, not of legitimacy. Realizing that states will continue to exist, Soysal sees the global system characterized by the 'institutional duality' of national sovereignty and universal human rights. This is a merely pragmatic concession to the factually entrenched state system. Her suggestion is clear: in a globalized world, states have run out of ideas to justify their boundaries.

This study takes an empirically grounded middle position between nation-state defenders and nation-state bashers. Neither is the nation-state simply reaffirmed by recent migratory challenges, nor is it undergoing fundamental transformation. We can observe both, a stubborn insistence of states to maintain control over their borders *and* increasing human-rights constraints on traditional sovereignty; a proliferation of membership categories *and* pressures to remould them as unitary citizenship; a persistence of distinct national models of handling (and containing) ethnic diversity *and* multicultural pressures on the monocultural texture of nations.

Against Brubaker, I argue that immigration is as much conditioned by as it is involved in redefining nationhood. His 'cultural idiom' approach to nationhood leaves too little room for contingency and contestation. For instance, Germany, which Brubaker sees forever locked into an ethnocultural mode of citizenship and nationhood, is moving toward civic-territorial citizenship in order to better integrate her second- and third-generation immigrants. Against Soysal, I argue that human rights norms and obligations do not meet nation-states from the outside. Rather than hovering in abstract 'global' space, the protection of human rights is a constitutive principle of nation-states qua liberal states. Postwar migrations have driven a wedge between the principle of human-rights protection and a second constitutive principle of nation-states, popular sovereignty.[4] Accordingly, the adequate root image is not nation-states meeting external human-rights obligations, but nation-states undergoing internal conflict between their human rights and popular sovereignty dimensions.

Sovereignty and Citizenship

Assessing the persistence or transformation of nation-states requires a clearer understanding which aspects of the nation-state are entangled with immigration. Both Brubaker's and Soysal's are studies of citizenship, thus omitting a second key dimension of the nation-state challenged by immigration: sovereignty.

Sovereignty refers to the stateness of modern nation-states: final control over a bounded territory and populace. Sovereignty is the legacy of absolutism, in which the feudal fragmentation of authority and the religious strife of the reformation period was put to rest by the establishment of one secular authority within a given territory.[5] Sovereignty makes territory, rather than persons, the basic reference point of rule.[6] This implies control over access to and stay within territory, which is the domain of immigration policy. Every state divides the world into 'nationals' who have a right of entry and stay, and 'aliens' to whom entry and stay may be denied. Accordingly, sovereignty was never absolute, but limited to the exclusion of aliens.[7] A recent development is that even the capability of states to exclude aliens has come under attack. An expression of this is the phenomenon of unwanted immigration: illegal immigration, asylum-seeking, and (in Europe) family reunification of labour migrants. In these cases, limitations on a state's right to exclude aliens do not spring from the interdependence of states, but from elementary human rights that aliens are invested with. This raises the question where these rights, and subsequent limitations on sovereignty, are situated: at the domestic level of nation-states, or in a global human-rights regime. I will argue in Part I that restricted state sovereignty over the entry and stay of aliens has predominantly domestic roots. Otherwise the new immigrant-receiving states in the Middle East or South-East Asia would do what Western states (normally) do: respect the rights of migrants.[8]

While the institution of sovereignty has pre-democratic roots, it has been reinterpreted since the French Revolution as popular sovereignty. Accordingly, the insistence on sovereign entry and residence controls is on behalf of the national collectivity from which the state derives its legitimacy. This entails a confounding of the established political Left vs. Right continuum: in immigration control, the rightist call for tight border controls is on popular demand, while the leftist defence of migrant rights tends to decouple the state from its people. In short, democracy is a threat to migrants. The major dilemma of immigration control is to reconcile the popular constraints of states with their parallel, inherently unpopular, mandate to protect the human rights of migrants.

Citizenship refers to the modern state not as a territorial organization, but as a membership association. Since the French Revolution, citizenship has been the unitary membership category of democratic states, replacing the multiple, stratified subject categories (estates) of the *ancien régime*. If sovereignty is linked to the (pre-democratic) stateness of modern nation-states, citizenship is linked to their (demo-cratic) nationness. As long as there is no democratic world state, the nation demarcates the boundaries of a community of citizens. Citizenship is thus 'internally inclusive' and 'externally exclusive' (Brubaker, 1992: ch. 1): a set of rights and obligations bestowed equally on all members of the community, but also a mechanism of closure, separating members from non-members. In a world of limited resources, the internal and external dimensions of citizenship are interdependent: because rights are costly, they cannot be for every-body. In the tradition of T. H. Marshall (1992), citizenship has been addressed in its internally inclusive aspect, as normative claim of workers, women, and other disadvantaged groups to achieve full inclusion in the national community.

Immigration has opened up a post-Marshallian view of citizenship, which stresses its externally exclusive dimension, the drawing of boundaries between members and non-members. Empirically, immi-gration has multiplied the membership categories in Western societies, defying the citizen–alien dualism of either full or no membership at all. Many immigrants today settle for something less than full citizenship. As 'permanent resident aliens' (in US parlance) they enjoy equal civil rights and welfare entitlements. Only their political rights are severely restricted. There is disagreement among post-Marshallian citizenship analysts about the implications of this. Is non-citizen membership, or 'denizenship' (Hammar, 1990: 22), a temporary deviation from mem-bership as citizenship, or is it a new model of membership in its own right that entails the decline of traditional citizenship? An answer to this question refers back to the initial question where the rights of migrants are ultimately situated: at the national or supranational levels. If denizenship, both in its implementation and legitimation, is situated at the level of nation-states, as I shall suggest, it would be precipitate to celebrate it as a new model of postnational membership. In absence of a supranational polity with implementation force, the exclusion of denizens from the national polity is not to be slighted, because then denizenship is an inherently vulnerable status. Current citizenship debates in Germany and the United States provide much evidence that denizenship is a vulnerable 'second-class' membership status in need of correction. Michael Walzer (1983: 62) is right: 'No community can be half-metic, half-citizen and claim that its admissions policies are acts of self-determination or that its politics is democratic.'

Citizenship is not only a legal status but also an identity (see Kymlicka and Norman, 1994: 369). As an identity, citizenship depends on and reinforces shared values and understandings, that is, a common culture. While we are used to denounce the nationalizing practices of modern states as retrogressive and repressive, we often overlook the evolutionary achievement of a single culture shared by all members of a society. As Ernest Gellner (1983) famously elaborated, the penetration of society by one high culture and ensuing universal literacy have been a fundamental prerequisite of modern industrial society, enabling mobility and communication across large spaces. In this view, the modern world appears as composite of large, separate breathing chambers, with culture as their medium, and states as control devices to check their temperature and oxygen: 'Not the guillotine but the doctorat d'état is the main tool of state power' (ibid. 34). Beyond Gellner, monoculture may be looked at as not only a cognitive but also a moral achievement. For John Stuart Mill, democracy was not possible without a commonly shared culture. And for Durkheim and Parsons, commonly shared norms and values were the glue that kept even functionally differentiated societies together.

However fictitious the scenario of a world differentiated into separate monocultures may be, it is evident that immigration must be a profound challenge to it. In fuelling ethnic diversification, international migrations challenge the principle of modern nationhood, according to which political and cultural boundaries shall be congruent. The centrifugal thrust of international migrations is further aggravated by current claims of multiculturalism, which reject traditional assimilation and demand that the cultural difference of migrant groups is to be maintained in the receiving society—in the extreme, as a matter of public policy, not just of private initiative. There are a number of reasons why multicultural programmes are popular today. On the pull side, Western states are liberal states that hesitate to impose particular cultural ways on their members; all that liberal states expect is commitment to the same civic rules. Such procedural liberalism is historically situated: after Nazism and World War II all forms of racism and nationalism have been outlawed and delegitimized, at least in Western Europe and North America. This created a cultural vacuum that was easily filled by multicultural claims. On the push side, today's migrants are less prepared to assimilate. This is because today's migrations occur in an established nation-state system, characterized by entrenched national loyalties that are not easily abandoned. Moreover, due to advanced transport and communication technologies, migrations are no longer 'one-way trips', which T. Todorov (1993: 346) considered the basis of the classic immigrant's willingness to become assimilated.[9] Modern technology makes the diaspora the dominant and permanent life-form for immigrants. I will show in Part II that, contrary to its self-presentation as oppositional movement, multiculturalism has become thoroughly institutionalized in liberal states, though in distinct national colours.

Case Selection

Sovereignty and citizenship are two generic principles of the modern nation-state that are challenged by immigration. But the nation-state exists only in distinct historical incarnations, each characterized by distinct immigration experiences. This study compares the responses of three Western nation-states: the United States, Germany, and Great Britain, to large-scale immigration after World War II. Taking on three cases seeks to fill a lacuna in immigration research, which is either single-case oriented and thus too narrow in scope or swallowing country-specific detail by considering too many cases.[10] Choosing *these* three cases is meaningful in several regards. First, all three represent distinct types of nationhood. The United States is the world's classic settler nation, where the experience of immigration has been a nation-founding myth. On the opposite side, Germany is the classic type of ethnic nation, defined by common blood rather than a common creed, which erects extraordinarily high barriers for the admission of new members. Britain shares elements of both: a civic creed overlaying and encompassing multiple ethnicities, but a history of emigration rather than immigration. Britain is distinguished from both Germany and the United States by its paradoxical dual existence as nation-state and empire. Restricting immigration from its colonies was in fact one major (and tortuous) avenue by which Britain devolved from empire to nation-state proper.

Partially reflecting these distinct legacies of nationhood, all three countries established distinct immigration regimes. They exhaust the variety of immigration experiences in the West: a settler regime recurrently recruiting new permanent members (United States); a guest-worker regime recruiting temporary labour migrants, which quickly faces the problem of adjusting to the permanent settlement of migrant workers (Germany); and a postcolonial regime attuned to restricting, while thoroughly integrating, the inflow of migrants from former colonial possessions (Britain).

Most similar in their liberal stateness, the United States, Germany, and Britain are thus most diverse in their nationhood traditions and immigration experiences. In opening itself to immigration from the Third World, the United States has returned to its roots as a non-ethnic, universal 'new nation' that recurrently remakes itself through immigration. As we will see, this has not been done without conflict and new paradoxes, such as the delegitimation of boundaries, and thus of nationhood, altogether. The immigration experience in Germany and Britain has been radically different: underneath the different logics of postcolonial and guestworker immigration, immigration is considered a non-recurrent, historically unique event whose conse-quences are not yet fully mastered, and which is unlikely to be repeated in the future. 'Immigration' is therefore a misnomer in Europe, still officially denied in Germany, and associated with routine passenger controls at the ports of entry in Britain. Rogers Brubaker (1989: 7) has got it right: 'The massive immigration of the last quarter-century has not transformed European countries into countries of immigration in the classical North American sense.' Accordingly, the distinction between 'endogenous nations' and 'nations of immigrants' is not moot, as Zolberg and Long (1997: 8) erroneously assume, but has life in it yet.

The three cases exhibit shifting sets of communalities and differ-ences that allow meaningful comparisons. The United States and Germany are the world's two largest immigrant-receiving countries, yet they differ fundamentally in their responses—one acknowledging (even celebrating), the other denying the reality of immigration. Britain is distinguished from the United States and Germany in its obsessive thrust toward zero-immigration, which has brought down new entries to a trickle. Both Germany and Britain are, and will con-tinue to be, European non-immigrant nations for whom postwar immigration has been a disturbing novelty, exacting great adjustment costs. If the United States handled its postwar immigration in the spirit of generosity, the joint European response has certainly been a pettier restrictiveness. While pedantically restrictive like perhaps no other European state, Britain has built a remarkably liberal regime of man-aging race relations that took its clues from the American race experi-ence, and she abandoned the idea that immigrants had to assimilate long before the notion of multiculturalism was invented.

The three cases also exhibit distinct problematiques on the two nation-state dimensions challenged by immigration. With regard to sovereignty over entry and exit, there is a clear dividing line between Britain, commonly referred to as 'exceptionally' effective in control-ling immigration (Layton-Henry, 1994), and the United States and Germany, both of which have succumbed to large-scale unwanted immigration. Several factors are responsible for this outcome, not the least of which is the 'splendid' geographic isolation of Britain, which allows for effective controls at a few ports of entry. But a key difference is the absence of constitutional and judicial constraints on the executive, which allows the Home Office to devise and execute immigration policy as it sees fit. By contrast, aliens enjoy extensive constitutional rights in the United States and Germany, enforced by independent courts that constrain the executive in immigration policy. The most obvious failure of effective immigration control in the United States is the vexing problem of illegal immigration. As I will demonstrate, cross-cutting domestic interests, a general aversion to internal state controls, and a culture of non-discrimination have stood in the way of controlling illegal immigration. In Germany, a similar failure of immigration control has occurred in the area of mass asylum-seeking. In this case, a traumatic national past, which tabooed the questioning of the redemptive constitutional right of asylum, has obstructed effective immigration control.

The challenge to citizenship as a legal status has been most dramatic in Germany. As long as citizenship was vicariously held open for the German diaspora in the communist East and tied to the constitutional mandate to achieve national unification, it was deliberately withheld from immigrants. The unresolved national question allowed (West) Germany to perpetuate the long-standing tradition of citizenship by descent (*jus sanguinis*). But it also led to the prolongation of non-citizen status into the second and third immigrant generations. If postnational membership advocates were right, the non-citizen status of later generation immigrants should not matter much. This is indeed the case for descendants of European Union citizens, privileged members of the only existing supranational polity with implementation force. It is not the case for Turks, the largest foreigner group in Germany. Their campaign for eased access to citizenship attests to the unbroken relevance of national citizenship. In Germany, immigration is not about to diminish the importance, but the meaning of national citizenship: the introduction of as-of-right naturalization in 1993 has decoupled the acquisition of citizenship from a cultural assimilation test, and there is now a contested but unstoppable trend from citizenship by descent toward territorial citizenship (*jus soli*).

In Britain and the United States, the challenge to legal citizenship has been less severe. In Britain, postwar immigrants from the New Commonwealth arrived with quasi-citizenship (as subjects of the Crown), so that citizenship acquisition or non-citizen membership never emerged as a problem. Britain underwent a reverse dynamic of narrowing down membership by instituting national citizenship, in order to shield herself from potentially massive postimperial immigration. The manipulation of membership was thus intricately tied up with immigration control. In the United States, an expansive constitution and the anti-discriminatory culture of the civil-rights era have almost equalized the status of permanent resident alien to that of citizen. As the Supreme Court has famously decreed, alienage (at the state level) is, like race or gender, a 'suspect classification' that must not entail disadvantages in education, employment, and public benefits. After *Plyler* v. *Doe*, even illegal immigrants are equal to citizens in crucial respects, such as the right of public education. In light of increasingly equalized alienship, some immigration scholars have diagnosed the 'devaluation' of American citizenship (Schuck, 1989). But this does not matter much, because second-generation immigrants are automatic citizens via *jus soli*, and because only Hispanics have naturalized in numbers far below those of traditional immigrant groups. More importantly, the very devaluation of citizenship has helped set into motion a reverse trend of 're-evaluated' citizenship (Schuck, 1998). Since Republican legislators have discovered the vulnerability of alienage at the federal level, restricting federal welfare benefits and family unification rights for permanent resident aliens, the naturalization rates of entitled aliens (including Hispanics) have reached historic heights. However instrumentally acquired, national citizenship in the United States shows no sign of decline.

Finally, the challenge to citizenship as an identity has been expressed in distinct national versions of multiculturalism and ethnic politics. In the United States, ethnicity and race have long been central cleavage lines of politics, similar to the centrality of class cleavages in Europe. New is the strategy of immigrant groups, especially Hispanics and Asians, to depict themselves as racial minorities entitled to compensatory 'affirmative action' privileges. This goes along with a roots-oriented politics of identity that contradicts the future-oriented, transethnic texture of American nationhood. There is a tension in American multiculturalism between redefining American nationhood, that is, further radicalizing its universalistic bent, and denouncing nationhood altogether as falsely homogenizing and repressive.

In Europe, multiculturalism has been free of restitutive 'affirmative action' connotations, reflecting the absence of race-based domestic slavery. Instead, multiculturalism is meant to pluralize ethnic nationhood, something more modest yet more difficult to achieve. This is especially the case in Germany, where the notion of multicultural society is addressed to the majority population, and consists of the moderate request to respect the very fact of ethnic diversity brought about by immigration. But the matter is complicated by the peculiarly post-national thrust of German multiculturalism, which feeds on the general delegitimation of nationhood after the Nazi regime. German multiculturalism is an intra-German affair in which ethnic immigrant groups are only marginally involved. British multiculturalism originates from liberal élites, perhaps plagued by guilt over colonialism but unwittingly prolonging some aspects of colonial indirect rule on the British mainland. As younger immigrant activists took over the race-relations institutions, shallow official multiculturalism was quickly abandoned in favour of more militant anti-racism. However, the small number of coloured immigrants, and their effective insulation from national politics, has prevented a larger debate over British nationhood. British nationhood, always vague and fragile, has never been more precarious than today. But immigration has little to do with it.

Overview

Part I, 'Embattled Entry', is about immigration policy proper, that is, the determination of rules of entry and stay. Control over borders is one of the key prerogatives of sovereign states. Yet throughout the West, there is a dramatic sense of control crisis, of an increasing incapacity of states to stop especially unwanted immigration. Human rights obligations are one reason why liberal states accept unwanted immigrants, in particular family members of settled labour migrants and refugees. I shall argue that such constraints are more domestic than international. Chapter 2, 'A Nation of Immigrants, Again: The United States', describes America's reopening to large-scale immigration, both legal and illegal, stressing the pivotal importance of the civil-rights culture of non-discrimination and expansive interest group politics. Chapter 3, 'Not a Country of Immigration: Germany', refers the continued acceptance of immigration despite zero-immigration policies after 1973 to the influence of independent courts and an emergent moral élite consensus to deal humanely with the recruited guest-workers. Chapter 4, 'The Zero-Immigration Country: Great Britain', explains why Britain has been more effective than Germany in implementing her zero-immigration policies, focusing on the absence of legal and moral constraints on a restriction-minded executive.

Part II, 'Multicultural Integration', shifts from the front- to the back-end of the politics of immigration. The aspect of the nation-state under challenge in this respect is citizenship as a legal status and as an identity, with different emphases in different states. I compare the state responses to the multiplication of membership statuses, and the different national versions of multiculturàlism and ethnic politics. Underneath a multiplicity of citizenship problematiques, we will observe one communality: the rejection of assimilation, and respect for the cultural identities of immigrants. Chapter 5, ' "Race" Attacks the Melting-Pot: The United States', argues that a colour-conscious civil-rights law and discourse has provided incentives for ethnic leaders to conceive of their immigrant constituencies in terms of racial minorities. Chapter 6, 'From Postnational Membership to Citizenship: Germany', depicts an integration debate that has moved from giving foreigners all the rights that Germans have to making them citizens. Chapter 7, 'Between Citizenship and Race: Great Britain', looks at foreigners arriving with (*de facto*) citizenship, and an integration approach torn between Marshallian citizenship universalism and racial group particularism.

Chapter 8, 'Conclusion: Resilient Nation-States', reassesses the two immigration challenges to the nation-state: the challenges to sovereignty and citizenship. On both dimensions, current diagnoses of the decline of the nation-state are premature. At least in regard to immigration, nation-states have proved remarkably resilient.

PART I

Embattled Entry

Introduction to Part I

Immigration policy, which deals with the admission and exclusion of non-members of a state, is a prime expression of the sovereignty of states. Michael Walzer (1983: 61 f.) further pointed out that the distribution of membership is related to elementary national self-determination, and as such cannot be subject to considerations of justice: 'The distribution of membership is not pervasively subject to the constraints of justice . . . Admission and exclusion are at the core of communal independence. They suggest the deepest meaning of self-determination. Without them, there could not be *communities of character*, historically stable, ongoing associations of men and women with some special commitment to one another and some special sense of their common life.' While discretionary admission may be questioned on a normative plane,[1] it is the acknowledged principle and practice in the international state system. It follows that immigration policy is notionally tied to the national interest, and not just to the special interests of well-organized subsections of the population.[2]

However, Gary Freeman (1995*a*: 881) has noted that, contrary to their restrictionist function of stabilizing and sustaining the boundaries of nation-states, the immigration policies of Western states are in reality 'broadly expansionist and inclusive'. Freeman explains this disjunction between principle and reality with the help of J. Q. Wilson's concept of client politics. The costs of immigration, such as unemployment or overpopulation, are widely diffused, while its benefits, such as cheap labour or family reunification, are highly concentrated. This poses a classic collective-action dilemma, in which the organized beneficiaries of concentrated benefits will prevail over the unorganized bearers of diffused costs. Accordingly, the expansive interests of organized employers and ethnic groups will outcancel the restrictionist leanings of the non-mobilized and underinformed public. The logic of client politics is backed up by a 'strong antipopulist norm' (ibid. 885), which prohibits political élites from addressing the

ethnic and racial composition of migrant streams, and urges them to
consensually take immigration off the political agenda. Freeman concludes: 'The typical mode of immigration politics . . . is client politics, a form of bilateral influence in which small and well-organized
groups intensely interested in a policy develop close working relationships with officials responsible for it. Their interactions take
place largely out of public view and with little outside interference.
Client politics is strongly oriented toward expansive immigration
policies' (ibid. 886).

Not only a rare attempt to inject political science into usually
descriptive accounts of immigration policy, Freeman's model of immigration policy as client politics also delivers a convincing counter-
picture to allegedly 'restrictionist' immigration policies in Western
states. But the following comparison of immigration policies in the
United States, Germany, and Britain suggests some modifications to
Freeman's model. These modifications build upon Freeman's own
insight that the model of client politics works best in the case of the
United States, a classic settler nation, in which immigration has coincided with nation-building and is accordingly well-entrenched and
institutionalized. Client politics is more temporary, if not absent at all,
in European guestworker and postcolonial regimes, in which immigration has postdated nation-building, is accordingly less well-
entrenched, and even follows an altogether different logic.

First, Freeman fails to identify the legal process as a separate source
of expansiveness and inclusiveness toward immigrants. The political
process in electoral democracies is endemically vulnerable to the populist pressure of majority opinion. By contrast, judges are shielded
from such pressures, and only obliged to the non-discriminatory and
universalistic principles of modern law. As Virginie Guiraudon (1998)
has sharply observed, most rights for immigrants were not achieved in
the open arena of democracy, but behind the closed doors of bureaucracy and the courtroom. The legal system is the true province of the
'antipopulist norm' rightly identified (but not properly located) by
Freeman as backing up client politics. Distinguishing more clearly
between the political and legal processes will allow us to explain why
Germany, in which the impact of client politics was much weaker than
in the United States, but where even stronger constitutional protections for non-citizens existed, ended up similarly expansive and inclusive toward immigrants. Reversely, the absence of both client politics
and legal-constitutional politics will help explain the exceptional
restrictiveness of British immigration policy.

Secondly, as already pointed out by Rogers Brubaker (1995) and Ted Perlmutter (1996*a*), Freeman has exaggerated the strength of the 'antipopulist norm', especially in the non-immigrant countries of Europe. The degree of politicization and range of nasty solutions to immigration dilemmas, even within mainstream political forces, was greater than Freeman would have it. In an interesting debate, Freeman (1995*b*) has derived antipopulist constraints from the logic of liberal democracy, whereas Brubaker (1995: 906) sees them as only 'conjunctural features of particular discursive fields'. Perlmutter (1996*a*) has added that only in unitary states with strong party leaderships will immigration be off the political agenda, whereas in federalist polities with mixed coalition parties and governments there will be endemic incentives to politicize immigration. There are elements of truth in all three propositions. The following comparison suggests a fourth proposition. The relative reluctance to address the ethnic and racial composition of migrant streams is dependent upon the underlying model of nationhood. There is a clear dividing line between the United States, in which the principles of non-discrimination and source-country universalism have fully flourished, and Germany and Britain, in which these principles remained weaker or could not take hold at all. This is because a politically constituted nation of immigrants cannot prioritize one ethnic immigrant group over another, whereas the ethnic nations of Europe can, and have in fact done so in blatantly discriminatory ways. A prime example is ethnic priority immigration. Abandoned in all settler nations since the 1960s, ethnic priority immigration has not only continued to exist in Europe (in the form of Britain's patrials or Germany's *Aussiedler*), but even received a new mainstay within the internal free movement regime of the European Union. Moreover, the non-immigrant nations of Europe developed a sense of special obligation toward its historical immigrants, which allowed them to be (more or less) generous toward particular immigrant groups, while closing themselves to the rest.

This suggests, thirdly, to draw even sharper lines than Freeman does between classic settler nations, in which immigration is a willed, recurrent event, and the non-immigrant nations of Europe, in which immigration has been acquired largely by default, and is considered a non-recurrent, historical episode. Once the latter decided to close down postcolonial or guestworker immigration, they found themselves confronted with settlers who had never been wanted, and whose communal and family ties were spinning forth new and ongoing immigration. From that point on, which in Britain preceded and in

Germany coincided with the first oil crisis of 1973, all new immigration to Europe has been unwanted immigration. This unwanted immigration cannot be understood within the logic of client politics. European states now reconnected notional non- or zero-immigration policies to their perceived national interest, while being obliged to respect the residence and family rights of already admitted immigrants. These obligations are both legal and moral, stemming from the statutory and constitutional rights of immigrants variously developed in the national legal systems, but also from a more informal political élite obligation toward the actively recruited or at least passively tolerated migrants. Tackling these legal and moral obligations, European states developed a language of primary versus secondary immigration that is altogether unknown in the United States, with the non-immigration maxim commanding a narrowing of obligations toward the outer immigration layers. This is especially visible in the handling of family reunification, which has been more generous toward primary than secondary immigrants. Family reunification has generally followed a different logic in Europe and the United States. In Europe, family reunification is framed within a discourse of rights, which pits the immigrant against an executive that would rather not admit more immigrants. In the United States, family reunification proceeds within a discourse of negotiated quotas, which, among other factors, are dependent on the strength of organized ethnic groups. Exempted from quota limitations, nuclear family reunification follows a nominal as-of-right logic, but it rarely clashed with a recalcitrant executive.[3] In a settler nation, family reunification is not a front to stop unwanted immigration, but the routine mechanism of recruiting new wanted immigrants.

Fourthly, the following comparison suggests a clearer intra-European differentiation between a guestworker and a postcolonial immigration policy, which are misleadingly lumped together by Freeman. The German guestworker policy started as an extreme case of client politics, but switched toward national-interest politics after the oil crisis. British immigration policy never was client politics, but was from the start a negative policy to close down New Commonwealth immigration. To put it bluntly, New Commonwealth immigrants had at no point been wanted; they had to be tolerated for the sake of a secondary goal, the maintenance of the British Empire. This minimized the élite sense of moral obligation toward its primary and secondary immigrants alike, and helped Britain build its extraordinarily effective zero-immigration regime.

Returning to the central theme of sovereignty challenged by immigration, I suggest in the following three chapters that most limitations on state discretion to admit or exclude non-members are self-induced. Self-limited sovereignty, not externally diminished sovereignty, characterizes the state in an age of international migration. Externally diminished sovereignty is the diagnosis by globalists (Sassen, 1996) and human rights internationalists (Soysal, 1994; Jacobson, 1996), who argue that the twin forces of global capitalism and a world-level discourse of human rights have incapacitated states to admit or reject migrants as they see fit. The notorious problem of this line of reasoning is a hyperbolical baseline of strong sovereignty that never was (except perhaps in the late nineteenth-century moment of high imperialism). There have always been *some* limitations on state discretion over entry and exit, such as the obligation to accept nationals or the principle of non-discrimination (as elaborated by Goodwin-Gill, 1978: ch. 5), and there has been no significant expansion of such limitations in the era of globalization. Moreover, an inquiry why states have to accept certain categories of unwanted immigrants: guestworkers as settlers, family immigrants, illegal immigrants, and asylum-seekers,[4] will almost always identify domestic, rather than external, causes. In Europe, the chief dynamic is fully discretionary primary admissions limiting the state's discretion over secondary admissions (in the sense of continued residence or new family immigration), which have to follow for moral and legal reasons.[5] In the United States, the control of illegal immigration has crashed over the logic of client politics and a culture of strict non-discrimination, which is anchored in its paradoxical self-description as a universal nation of immigrants. Regarding mass asylum-seeking, a major source of unwanted immigration in all Western states, the original constraint is external, in terms of the non-refoulement obligation of the Geneva refugee convention. But, as the German and American cases will show, the substantive resource for asylum-seekers is domestic constitutions protecting human rights. Perhaps because the original constraint regarding asylum-seekers is external, this has been the field of unrelenting experimentation by states to circumvent their obligation.

The case of Britain does not fully fit the theorem of self-limited sovereignty. It is no small irony that the country that once championed the breakup of princely absolutism now sticks to an archaic notion of parliamentary absolutism, which has prevented the judiciary from taking a more active role in the control of the executive. European courts have stepped into the vacuum left by the absence of a written constitution and of judicial review. All effective censoring of Britain's harsh family immigration rules and asylum practice has originated from the European plane. The question of British exceptionalism is tied up with the question of European exceptionalism. Here a unique polity is in the making where sovereignty is divided and no clear distinction can be drawn between the domestic and non-domestic, 'international' spheres. Globalists argue that Europe's multiple-level polity is a blueprint to be emulated elsewhere (see Soysal, 1994; also Schmitter, 1991). But the evidence for this is thin, and it is more reasonable to assume that a unique historical constellation has given rise to a unique reconfiguration of political space, in which nation-states have abandoned authority on some dimensions only to gain new strength on others (see Milward, 1992). European Union constraints are not truly external, because they are grounded in the voluntary agreements of member states. In this sense, also Britain's sovereignty constraints are lastly self-induced. Europe may well be the trick to provide Britain with what other Western states have long had: effectively divided powers, a bill of rights, and judicial review.

2

A Nation of Immigrants Again:
The United States

In 1958, the young Senator John F. Kennedy published an inconspicuous little book, *A Nation of Immigrants*. It attacked the National Origins Act of 1924 that had restricted immigration to a few Northern European source countries: 'Such an idea is at complete variance with the American traditions and principles that the qualifications of an immigrant do not depend on his country of birth, and violates the spirit expressed in the Declaration of Independence that "all men are created equal" ' (Kennedy, 1964: 75). More than a book, *A Nation of Immigrants* was a programme for the reopening of America to large-scale immigration. Linking immigration to the American founding myth of an 'asylum of all nations' (G. Washington) or 'nation of nations' (W. Whitman) has been the enduring motif of this reopening, which was shared across party lines. Two decades after Kennedy's opening salvo, when the public mood was already turning sour over illegal immigration and mass asylum-seeking, the Republican presidential candidate Ronald Reagan invoked the same liberal founding myth to defend the acceptance of anti-communist 'freedom-fighters': 'Can we doubt that only a Divine Providence placed this land, this island of freedom, here as a refuge for all those people in the world who yearn to breathe free?' (in Cose, 1992: 145).

However, the 'nation of immigrants' formula, which framed America's reopening to mass immigration, is less self-evident and interest-transcendent than it may appear. First, as Rogers Smith (1993) correctly pointed out, there are multiple traditions in America. Next to the liberal tradition of a nation defined by an abstract political creed and immigration, there has been an illiberal tradition of 'ascriptive Americanism', which hypostasizes an ethnic core of protestant Anglo-Saxonism that is to be protected from external dilution. A restrictive concept of national community, anti-catholic, anti-radical, and racially nativist, had in fact undergirded the national-origin-based immigration regime in place until 1965 (see Higham, 1955). The recovery of the 'nation of immigrants' formula therefore has to be placed into a historical context that had delegitimized racial nativism: a war that was won against a country that had carried racism to the murderous extreme, Nazi Germany; a new awareness for the interdependence of nations and the international obligations of a superpower, which obviated inward-looking isolationism; and, perhaps most importantly, the domestic civil-rights revolution that outlawed discriminatory racial and national origins distinctions.

Secondly, Kennedy's selective reappraisal of 'American traditions' served a concrete interest: to cover the stigma of Catholicism in this first presidential bid of a non-Protestant, and to build a Catholic-Jewish coalition against the Protestant establishment regarding immigration reform. As John Higham (1984: 6) pointed out, 'immigrants' proper are bearers of a foreign culture, who are to be distinguished from the original 'settlers' who created a new society and laid down the terms of admission for the others. Kennedy's 'nations of immigrants' was a South-Eastern European fighting term, attacking an imbalance within the existing immigration system, which favoured the British and Irish, but locked out the Italians, the Polish, and the Greeks.

However situated in a concrete historical and interest context, the 'nation of immigrants' formula built upon and radicalized the liberal-universalist streak of American nationhood. By the same token, the 'nation of immigrants' formula provides no criteria for the drawing of legitimate boundaries, without which no nation could exist, and whose reinforcement is the very task of immigration policy. Pre-1965 immigration policy could rely on such boundaries, but ones that were no longer legitimate: the boundaries of race, infamously enshrined in the Chinese Exclusion Act of 1882, which barred Chinese labourers from entering the United States and proscribed the naturalization of those Chinese who already legally resided there (see Salyer, 1995: ch. 1). The dilemma of post-1965 immigration policy has been the lack of a legitimate concept of national boundaries, from which clear criteria for entry and stay, membership and non-membership could be derived. As Peter Schuck (1985) realized, liberalism and nationalism are incompatible: the universal thrust of liberalism contradicts the concept of bounded national community. Bereft of legitimate national boundaries, the trend in US immigration law and policy in the liberal civil-rights era has been toward the empowerment of non-members: increase the number of legal immigrants (with no consideration of their national origins), include rather than exclude illegal immigrants, and provide even first-time entrants, such as asylum-seekers, with constitutional due process protection.

The 1965 Immigration Reform and its Unintended Consequences

The Hart–Celler (Immigration Reform) Act of 1965, which abolished the national-origins system of 1924, changed America like few other legislations in this century. By establishing source-country universalism in the admission of immigrants, it opened the door for the large-scale immigration from Asia and Latin America, which is dramatically transforming the texture of American society. As conservative immigration foes correctly point out, this has been a transformation by design, originating in an identifiable political decision (Auster, 1990: 10–26; Brimelow, 1995: ch. 4). But it must be stressed that the opening of America to Third-World immigration was the unintended consequence of moderate, even restrictive legislation, whose purpose was to redress an intra-European imbalance of immigrant stock, and to realign law and actual policies. Regarding the latter, by the early 1960s two-thirds of legal immigration occurred outside the national-origins quota, mostly through special legislation for persons 'displaced' by World War II and Cold War refugees 'paroled in' by the Attorney General (Reimers, 1983: 14). Moreover, American overseas commitments and wartime alliances had put cracks in the racial exclusion of Asians—Chinese exclusion was repealed in 1943, and the War Brides Act of 1945 for the first time made Asian women eligible for admission. Already before the civil-rights revolution would outlaw racial discriminations, the 1952 McCarran–Walter Act's perpetuation of national origins quotas and tacit prolongation of Asian exclusion in the 'Asia-Pacific Triangle' provision had incensed the liberal conscience,[1] and the act was passed by Congress only over President Truman's veto.

When President Kennedy first introduced a bill to abolish the national-origins system in July 1963, intra-European discrimination was key. The old quota system's explicit purpose had been to reproduce the ethnoracial features of the American populace, allotting immigrant visas to nationals proportional to their nationality's representation in the US populace in the 1920 census. This led to gross inequities of national quotas, favouring countries with sizeable immigrant stock in 1920, and discrepancies between countries with huge backlogs and countries that did not even use up their quotas. In 1963, among the most disfavoured countries were Greece, with a quota of only 308 and a backlog of 97,577, Italy (quota: 5,666, backlog: 122,706), Portugal (quota: 438, backlog: 46,659), and Poland (quota: 6,488, backlog: 55,429). On the other hand, Britain used only 25,000 of its 65,361 allotted visas, Ireland 5,500 of 17,756.[2] As a result of this imbalance, almost half of the annual total number of 156,700 immigrant slots had remained unfilled in 1962. Much like the Hispanic MALDEF or National Council of La Raza today, Jewish and Italian ethnic organizations sought to reshape immigration policy in their interest.[3] The final act of 1965 thus must be seen as a triumph of the older South-European immigrants, who were well-entrenched as the urban constituents of the Democratic Party and pursued immigration reform as a 'politics of recognition' to achieve equal standing in the American nation.[4]

As incontestable as the concept of source-country universalism may appear today, it aroused strong opposition at the time. The American Coalition of Patriotic Societies defended the quota system as a true reflection of the American people: 'The national-origins system is like a mirror held up before the American people and reflecting the proportions of their various foreign national origins.'[5] It took two years for the Presidential bill to be signed into law, and the final version included important modifications that were to moderate the new legislation's impact. Most importantly, the first Presidential bill had advocated a skill-based preference system; this was in line with moving from ascription to achievement in the selection of immigrants. The final bill, however, gave first priority to family members of US citizens and residents. Only a bill that lessened the chance of ethnic change was sellable to Congress, whose legislators could then depict themselves less as revolutionaries than as 'extended family'.[6] Democrat Edmund Celler, the sponsor of the House bill, was blunt about the purpose of shifting from skills to family reunification: 'There will not be . . . many Asians or Africans entering this country . . . Since the people of Africa and Asia have very few relatives here, comparatively few could immigrate from those countries because they have no family ties in the U.S.' (in Reimers, 1983: 16).

A second, restrictionist modification of the original bill was the introduction of a cap for Western hemisphere immigrants. Before 1965, immigration from Latin America and Canada was unrestricted; after 1965, it was limited to 120,000 per year. This was also a concession to labour, which had already pushed hard for the abolition of the Bracero guestworker programme in 1964, which was seen as undercutting domestic wages. Like all major immigration legislation in the last thirty years, the 1965 reform was a 'package deal', in which anti-immigrant conservatives had to be appeased—in this case, by excluding Hispanics, especially Mexicans. This most intensely debated aspect of the bill had far-reaching implications: it literally created the phenomenon of illegal immigration over the open Mexican–US land border, which would inflame the heated debate over 'uncontrolled' immigration two decades later.

Given these modifications, President Johnson's understated words during the ceremonial enactment of the bill near the Statue of Liberty seem utterly justified: 'This . . . is not a revolutionary bill. It does not affect the lives of millions. It will not reshape the structure of our daily lives, or really add importantly to either our wealth or our power . . . (Yet) it does repair a very deep and painful flaw in the fabric of American justice . . . The days of unlimited immigration are past. But those who come will come because of what they are—not because of the land from which they sprung' (in Reimers, 1983: 17). The new act established an Eastern hemisphere ceiling of 170,000 new immigrant visas per year (complemented by 120,000 visas for the Western hemisphere), distributed according to a seven-category preference system prioritizing family reunification, and stipulating that from no country the total number of new immigrants was to exceed 20,000.[7] By abolishing the Asia-Pacific Triangle provision, the legacy of racial exclusion had been swept away, and each country in the world was put on an equal footing. Testifying before House Immigration subcommittee members, Attorney General Robert Kennedy famously malpredicted the numerical impact of this measure: 'I would say for the Asia-Pacific Triangle it [immigration] would be approximately 5,000, Mr. Chairman, after which immigration from that source would virtually disappear; 5,000 immigrants would come in the first year, but we do not expect that there would be any great influx after that' (in Reimers, 1985: 77).

Initially, immigration patterns from Europe changed as intended. For a decade after 1965, Italy became the leading European sending nation with about 20,000 new immigrants per year (Reimers, 1983: 19). Yet by the mid-1970s the Southern European visa backlogs were depleted, and the economic reconstruction of Europe eased the pressure for new-seed immigration. By 1980, only 5 per cent of legal immigration came from Europe. Of the 570,000 legally admitted newcomers that year, Asians (primarily Filipinos, Koreans, Vietnamese and Indians) accounted for nearly half, while migration from Latin America (mainly Mexico) made up about 40 per cent.[8]

What had happened? Latin Americans, the truly disadvantaged by the 1965 reform, simply shifted from open to restricted immigration, crowding the relatively small country quotas that were in no correlation with historically high Western hemisphere immigration (especially from Mexico). Asians had arrived either as resettled refugees, as did 500,000 Indo-Chinese after the American withdrawal from Vietnam and Cambodia in 1975, or as 'third preference' new-seed immigrants in the skills category, who then multiplied their number through resorting to the generous family reunification provisions. This phenomenon became known as 'chain migration'. It accounts for the self-perpetuation of Third-World immigration once it had been kicked off, and for the relative absence of European immigration once the family backlog had been cleared. The 1965 act reserved 74 per cent of annual new immigrant visas for the reunification of families, limiting skill-based visas to 20 per cent (the remaining 6 per cent were reserved for refugees from communist countries). With 24 per cent of all immigrant visas, the largest (and oddest) preference category is the fifth preference, which allows naturalized immigrants to sponsor their (married) brothers and sisters. Congressman Peter Rodino had pushed for the fifth preference on behalf of the family-oriented Italians—accordingly, the 1965 act has been nicknamed the 'Brothers and Sisters Act'. But by the late 1980s, the largest demand for fifth-preference admissions originated from Mexicans and Filipinos. There is evidence that Asian countries especially 'press the legal immigration system for all it is worth' (Goering, 1989: 804), for instance, circumventing the crowded fifth preference by sponsoring their (non-quota) parents, who as naturalized immigrants can then petition for other offspring. Of course, the effect of the 'immigration multiplier' built into the family preference system is limited by country and preference category limits. As John Goering (ibid. 809) concludes, 'there is no solid evidence that the multiplier in the first or second decade after an admission ever approaches the theoretical maximums or indeed even a small fraction of that limit.' But this should not obscure the larger irony: a family-based immigration system that was designed to minimize the possibility of ethnoracial transformation has actually maximized such transformation, stabilizing and perpetuating America's Third-World immigration of today.

The Problem of Illegal Immigration: The Immigration Reform and Control Act of 1986

Several observers have pointed out that, in contrast to European restrictionism after the first oil crisis, US immigration policies have remained 'remarkably liberal and expansive' (Schuck, 1992: 39; see also Tichonor, 1994). There is no better proof of this than the legislation that bore the word 'control' in its name and was to resolve the vexing problem of illegal immigration. The Immigration Reform and Control Act (IRCA) of 1986, passed after five years of intense, if not Byzantine, Congressional bickering and deal-making, legalized the status of about three million undocumented immigrants in the country, while failing to stop the inflow of new illegal immigrants. Why have the United States been incapable of controlling illegal immigration? First, like all immigration policies in the USA, policies dealing with illegal immigration are 'client politics' (Freeman, 1995a), in which the organized potential recipients of 'concentrated benefits' prevail over the non-organized carriers of 'diffuse costs'. The one restrictionist group, the Federation of Americans for Immigration Reform (FAIR), which was close to the pulse of a public disgruntled about uncontrolled large-scale immigration, had virtually no impact on legislation. On the contrary, Hispanics concerned about the discriminatory impact of employer sanctions and Western growers interested in cheap immigrant labour managed to transform initially restrictive into eventually expansive legislation. Secondly, the range of restrictive immigration policy was severely limited by the civil-rights imperative of non-discrimination. As Alan Simpson, for twenty years the Republican leader of immigration reform in Congress, put it, 'any reference to immigration reform or control turns out, unfortunately, to be a code word for ethnic discrimination.'[9] Because Hispanics (especially Mexicans) have formed the majority of illegal immigrants in the USA, any policy directed against illegal immigration had to appear as 'anti-Hispanic'.[10] To avoid even the slighest connotation of ethnic discrimination, IRCA was softened by an elaborate set of 'anti-discrimination' provisions that effectively neutralized it as an instrument of immigration control.

When new immigration reached record levels in the 1980s,[11] the parallel surge of illegal immigration came to symbolize a general 'loss of control' over the nation's borders. Even the liberal Select Commission on Immigration and Refugee Policy, which laid the groundwork for the immigration reforms of the 1980s, presumed that immigration policy was 'out of control', targeting the containment of illegal immigration as a first step toward 'regain[ing] control over U.S. immigration policy' (Select Commission, 1981). This perspective, stipulating a sequence of loss and recovery, is misleading. There never had been a Golden Age of control. The problem of illegal immigration is a byproduct of the attempt to build a uniform national system of immigration control, which no longer exempted Western hemisphere immigration. When the Eastern hemisphere preference system and country limits were first extended to Western hemisphere countries in 1976, Mexico suddenly faced a severe backlog, with 60,000 applications for 20,000 available visas. Since an elaborate immigration network, with established pathways, settlement, and seasonal employment patterns, already existed, the nationalization and standardization of US immigration policy simply transformed a legal (or at least tolerated) into an illegal immigrant stream.

Immigration control at America's southern land border has historically been lax, with intermittent shows of toughness, such as Operation Wetback in 1954, in which over a million Mexicans without residence or work permits were rounded up and deported back to Mexico. Mexican sojourners were an indispensable part of agriculture in the American South-West. The notorious expression of this was the so-called Texas Proviso in the 1952 Immigration and Nationality Act. Wanted by Texan growers, it stated that employing illegals did not constitute the criminal act of 'harboring'—accordingly, it was legal to employ illegal immigrants, while the latter were still subject to deportation. Only, such deportations were rarely implemented, and the INS Border Patrol would 'dry out' illegal 'wetbacks' by escorting them back to the Mexican border, having them step to the Mexican side, and bringing them back as legal guestworkers, or even 'parole' illegal immigrants directly to prospective employers (Calavita, 1994: 59). 'The whole process had the appearance more of a sad joke than of serious deterrence policy', complains Vernon Briggs (1992: 153). Labour unions were the first to find fault with cheap foreign labour. In 1964, they moved Congress to abandon the Bracero guestworker programme with Mexico, which had been originally established in the early 1940s to deal with war-conditioned labour shortages. In conjunction with the 1965 Act, the end of Bracero illegalized established immigration flows and networks between Mexico and the American South-West. After 1964, apprehension figures—widely used as indicators for the stock and flow of illegal immigrants—rose steeply, until they passed the one million mark in 1977. This is when the problem of illegal immigration was first framed as a national crisis, and President Carter established the Select Commission on Immigration and Refugee Policy to seek out political remedies. But it is important to see that the problem of illegal immigration is not due to a 'loss' of control, but is the product of the opposite attempt to establish first-time control over the southern land border. On this premiss, this border may still be inherently difficult to control for a liberal state. As Nathan Glazer (1988: 17) described the uniqueness of the US–Mexican border, 'nowhere else in the world is there a land border between the developed world and the developing world'.

However, domestic politics, not geography, ultimately prevented the United States from controlling illegal immigration. Driven into action by rising numbers of apprehended illegal immigrants and, above all, the pressure of organized labour, Democrat Peter Rodino, chair of the House Judiciary's subcommittee on immigration, introduced two employer sanctions bills in the early 1970s. While both bills passed the House easily, they died in the Senate—Judiciary Committee boss James Eastland, likewise a Democrat but a cotton planter beholden to Southern agricultural interests, refused to hold hearings on the issue. The lesson was to attach an amnesty provision to the employer sanctions bill, in order to garner support from both liberal immigrant rights advocates and business advocates interested in cheap immigrant labour. President Carter asked Congress in August 1977 to pass a combined sanctions/amnesty bill, but committee leaders Peter Rodino and Edward Kennedy were unenthusiastic to move on legislation that did not bear their signatures. Most importantly, immigration reform proved divisive for the Democratic Party, which became caught in the crossfire between Hispanics and organized labour (Fuchs, 1990). So it was best to remove immigration reform from partisan politics. The vehicle for this was the Select Commission on Immigration and Refugee Policy, established by President Carter in October 1978, which was to study the issue thoroughly and create consensus as a prerequisite of bipartisan reform.

The Select Commission, which included members of Cabinet and Congress and representatives of societal groups active on immigration (the Catholic Church, Labor, Hispanics, and Asian-Americans), epitomizes the liberal and expansive cloth out of which immigration reform in the 1980s was made. This is especially clear if one compares the 1978 Select Commission with the 1907 Dillingham Commission, which had laid the groundwork for the restrictive National Origins

Act of 1924 (Fuchs, 1983). Whereas all the members of the Dillingham Commission were descendants of English and Scottish settlers, half of the membership of the Select Commission had ancestors whom the Dillingham Commission had tried to keep out—Italians, Poles, East European Jews. Most importantly, the Dillingham Commission's obsession with the ethnic and racial features of immigrants was absent in 1978. Father Theodore Hesburgh, a noted civil-rights advocate and chair of the Select Commission, insisted from the start on a 'policy as free of racial or ethnic bias as we can make it' (ibid. 63). On the contrary, ethnic diversity, repudiated in 1907, was celebrated in 1978 within the 'nations of immigrants' formula: 'It is a truism to say that the United States is a nation of immigrants . . . New immigrants benefit the United States and reaffirm its deepest values' (Select Commission, 1981). At the same time, the Select Commission's final report conceded that the United States could not 'become a land of unlimited immigration', and that immigration policy must be guided by 'the basic national interests of the people of the United States' (ibid.). Targeting the problem of illegal immigration, the Select Commission gave out the marching order of immigration reform in the 1980s: 'We recommend closing the back door to undocumented/ illegal immigration, [and] opening the front door a little more to accommodate legal migration in the interests of this country' (ibid.). With regard to controlling illegal immigration, this proposal included employer sanctions (backed by an effective system to determine employment eligibility), legalization of the undocumented immigrant population, and rejection of any guestworker scheme, with the negative European experience firmly on the Commissioners' minds.

The Select Commission's uncertainty of denominating 'undocumented/illegal' immigration reveals a larger ambivalence about immigration control. Illegal aliens were no longer treated as either lawbreakers or growers' fodder, as in the 1950s, but as discriminated-against and vulnerable people living in the 'shadows of American life', deserving equal membership status (Tichonor, 1994: 341). The Select Commission's exterior 'control' rhetoric was thus offset by its redemptive anti-discrimination agenda—the legalization provision, for instance, was partial 'acknowledgment that . . . our society has participated in the creation of the problem [of illegal immigration]' (Select Commission, 1981). The same ambivalence is inherent in the notion of national interest, which appears in the title of the Select Commission's final report, *U.S. Immigration Policy and the National Interest*. 'National interest' conveys that immigration policy should be an expression of sovereignty, and flow from the shared interests of the members of the American nation. However, the national interest so defined has had only a marginal impact on the actual immigration policies that were crafted on the basis of the Select Commission's recommendations. This is because the national interest, which is inherently status-quo oriented and exclusive, contradicted the reigning view of the United States as a nation of immigrants, which is forever unfinished and inclusive. Tellingly, the one organization that purported to represent the national interest in immigration policy, FAIR, has been restrictionist, and its agenda of 'maintaining the integrity of our sovereignty'[12] failed to have an imprint on any legislation in this period. On the opposite side, the component members and profiteers of the nation of immigrants, denounced by FAIR as 'special interests', shaped legislation, undermining the control intention that had brought the Select Commission into existence.

The Select Commission's dual recommendation of imposing employer sanctions and granting an amnesty for illegal immigrants became the key element of a concerted congressional bill named after its sponsors, Senator Alan Simpson (R-Wyoming) and Congressman Roman Mazzoli (D-Kentucky). Simpson and Mazzoli were veterans of the Select Commission, and as delegates from low-immigration states sufficiently aloof from pressure groups to produce legislation in the national interest. Crafted in the spirit of bipartisan consensus, the Simpson–Mazzoli bill was on paper an 'ingenious trade-off between liberals and conservatives' (Zolberg, 1990: 323), sanctions appealing to organized labour and restrictionists, the amnesty appealing to Hispanics and civil-rights advocates. However, what seemed like a classic package-deal initially left out the agricultural employers, the major users of illegal immigrant workers; and it posed the risk that a group opposing a particular aspect of the bill might try to block the bill altogether. Accordingly, the rocky career of the Simpson–Mazzoli bill, from its first incarnation in 1982 to its passing as IRCA in 1986, may be reconstructed as two separate battles: a first battle over employer sanctions, which were opposed by an odd coalition of Hispanics and civil-rights groups, on the one hand, and the Chamber of Commerce and agricultural growers, on the other; and a second battle over the insertion of a guestworker programme to accommodate the interests of agricultural employers. To secure the passage of the bill, employer sanctions had to be softened to the point of being merely 'symbolic' (Calavita, 1994), while the guestworker programme had to be transformed into a second amnesty for temporary workers. What had started as an attempt to control immigration in the national interest turned out as an effort to further expand immigration, in order to accommodate the group interests that were instrumental for passing any legislation.

In retrospect, the most significant aspect of the battle over employer sanctions is the rise of Hispanics as a political force capable of blocking federal legislation detrimental to their perceived interest. Twice, in 1982 and 1983, the Hispanic lobby succeeded in stalling the House version of the Simpson–Mazzoli bill, after the latter had won comfortable majorities in the Senate. As the Democratic House majority leader Tip O'Neill defended his refusal to hold a vote on the second Simpson–Mazzoli bill in October 1983, 'it has to be acceptable to the Hispanic Caucus'.[13] Why wasn't the bill acceptable to Hispanics? Briefly, Hispanics feared that sanctions on the employers of illegal immigrants would lead to discriminatory hiring practices, in which Hispanic-looking job applicants would be rejected upfront or be subjected to humiliating special identity checks. Interestingly, Hispanic leaders carefully framed their opposition to employer sanctions as being in the interest of 'Hispanic citizens' or legal residents, in order to avoid the appearance of disloyalty and pan-national fraternizing.[14]

The Hispanics were joined by civil-rights advocates, who feared that the introduction of an employment verification system (dubbed a 'national ID card') would be detrimental to civil liberties in general, and lead to a 'culture of suspicion'.[15] A leading conservative columnist branded the introduction of an 'ID card' as 'this generation's largest step toward totalitarianism', concluding that 'it is better to tolerate the illegal movement of aliens and even criminals than to tolerate the constant surveillance of the free'.[16] In his refusal to have a vote on the second Simpson–Mazzoli bill, Democrat Tip O'Neill struck a similar chord: 'Hitler did this to the Jews, you know. He made them wear a dog tag' (in Cose, 1992: 167). Against such wide opposition, which fed upon the traditional American distrust of the state, the plan of a standardized employment verification scheme had to be dropped, inflicting a first severe crack on the control dimension of IRCA.

Eventually, the Hispanic opposition to Simpson–Mazzoli came to be viewed as obstructionist, and its influence waned. A member of the congressional Hispanic Caucus admitted that 'we . . . failed to come up with a realistic alternative that could pass'.[17] At the same time, agricultural employers switched their strategy from obstruction to compromise-seeking, thus opening the battle over the adding of a guestworker programme to Simpson–Mazzoli. In a remarkably well-orchestrated campaign, western growers secured the support of liberal

Democratic Congressman Leon Panetta to add an amendment to the House version of Simpson–Mazzoli, which would have authorized the attorney general to admit about 250,000 foreign crop-pickers per year on three-day's notice, outside the established H–2 temporary visa programme. In June 1984, the House finally passed this version of the bill, with the slenderest of margins (216 to 211). But this was a hollow victory, because intense Hispanic lobbying had moved all three Democratic contenders for the 1984 Presidential elections to come out strongly against Simpson–Mazzoli. Without backing by the Democratic leadership, the final negotiations in the House-Senate conference collapsed, and Simpson–Mazzoli was dead once again.

The mutual charges as to who was responsible for this disappointing outcome, blowing to pieces three years of intense negotiation, show the complexity of an immigration reform that had to reconcile incompatible interests.[18] Because the Panetta amendment was dropped in conference in favour of an expanded H–2 programme, the American Farm Bureau Federation switched from support to opposition; also AFL-CIO opposed the conference compromise, but for the opposite reason that the concessions to agricultural employers were going too far. Conservative Republicans were unhappy about strong civil-rights protections for legal aliens, pushed through by House Democrat Barney Frank, and accepted by Simpson only with 'the gravest reservations'. The final blow came from the Reagan Administration, which disliked the federal reimbursement of states for amnesty-related costs. Epitomizing the divided views about Simpson–Mazzoli, a distinguished immigration historian bemoaned the loss of 'a more liberal measure than any we've had in 90 years', while a no less distinguished fellow historian found the bill 'identical with the restrictive legislation of the 1920s, when we were trying to keep certain groups out of the country'.[19]

In April 1985, the indefatigable Simpson tried again, perhaps aware that his imprint on history would depend on successful immigration reform. But the third version of his immigration bill was different. Thriving on a growing public groundswell in favour of clamping down on illegal immigration, which was now increasingly related to crime and drug trafficking, Simpson for the first time laid hands on the amnesty programme, suggesting making it contingent upon the prior improvement of immigration controls. Decoupling the amnesty from employer sanctions was an unconcealed warning to the liberal opponents of Simpson–Mazzoli that continued obstruction might lead to the abandonment of the entire amnesty provision, for which there was no public support anyway.[20] This moved uncompromising Hispanic groups like MALDEF to opt out altogether, its leader Antonia Hernandez preferring to 'go down in flames' than make agreements she presumed disastrous for her constituents (in Cose, 1992: 179). But other immigrant advocacy groups like the National Immigration Forum, the National Council of La Raza, or the League of United Latin American Citizens (LULAC) opted for improving the bill that was now deemed unavoidable. Similarly, Peter Rodino, the grey 'Mr Immigration' eminence in the House, abandoned his previous reserve and jumped into the fray, aware that any further delay could only lead to more restrictionist legislation.

In this final round of the Simpson–Mazzoli saga, the attempt of agricultural growers to install a guestworker programme was again key. In addition to an already granted transitional programme that allowed growers to hire illegal immigrants for three more years, Senator Pete Wilson (R-California) pushed for a guestworker amendment to the Senate bill, which closely resembled the Panetta amendment a year earlier. This would allow for 350,000 workers to harvest perishable fruits and vegetables for up to nine months a year, their movement restricted to a particular region, and 20 per cent of their wages held back until their departure from the United States. In line with the Select Commission's recommendations, Simpson rejected such a guestworker scheme. 'The greed of the growers . . . is insatiable,' Simpson lashed out in obvious irritation about the growers' unrelenting campaign, 'there is no way they can be satisfied. Their entire function in life is that when the figs are ready, the figs should be harvested and they need four thousand human beings to do that' (in Fuchs, 1990: 123). Naturally, organized labour and Rodino disliked the Wilson amendment, dubbed a 'de facto slave labor programme' (in Calavita, 1994: 67). But since the time for a liberal immigration bill was seemingly running out, a compromise had to be found.

The compromise arrived in the form of the Schumer proposal, worked out in eight months of intense negotiation between liberal Congressman Charles Schumer, a Democrat from New York, and representatives of organized labour and the growers. A 'remarkable feat of congressional horse-trading' (Zolberg, 1990: 330), the Schumer proposal essentially transformed the guestworker programme into a second amnesty: it provided permanent resident status, and eventually citizenship, for illegal aliens who worked in American agriculture for at least 90 days in the year preceding May 1986; the same possibility was granted to 'replenishment' workers in the future. Lawrence Fuchs

(1990: 124) called the Schumer proposal revolutionary: 'For the first time in American history . . . outsiders brought in to do difficult, temporary jobs would be given the full Constitutional protections and many of the privileges of insiders.' The proposal broke the last deadlock over Simpson–Mazzoli. Aware that a more liberal law could not be had at the time, even five of the eleven members of the Hispanic Caucus voted in favour of this last version of Simpson–Mazzoli (which by now had become 'Simpson–Rodino'). Only the restrictionists around FAIR, in whose hope of gaining control over the nation's borders, legislation on illegal immigration had originally been launched, were dismayed: 'We wanted a Cadillac, we were promised a Chevy, and we got a wreck' (in Fuchs, 1990: 124).

Signed into law in early November 1986, the Immigration Reform and Control Act was certainly a 'left-centre bill',[21] in which the 'control' aspect was barely visible. Putting to an end the Texas proviso, IRCA imposed a sanction scheme on employers who knowingly hired illegal immigrants. But in a concession to Hispanics and employers, sanctions would be abolished if the General Accounting Office were to find discrimination or undue burdens on employers in the future. Most importantly, IRCA included a far-reaching anti-discrimination provision that added the concept of 'alienage' to Title VII of the Civil Rights Act, prohibiting employment discrimination on the basis of citizenship. This amounted to the 'only expansion of civil rights protection in the whole Reagan era'.[22] On the amnesty side, a sequence from temporary resident status to citizenship was provided for illegal immigrants who had resided in the United States continuously since before 1 January 1982. Reflecting the Schumer proposal, the same possibility of citizenship was granted to the participants of a seven-year special agricultural workers (SAW) programme. Finally, IRCA authorized $1 billion annually for four years beginning in 1988 to reimburse state governments for costs of public assistance, health, and educational services for newly legalized immigrants (Bean and Fix, 1992: 44), which amounted to federal support for local immigrant advocacy networks in regions of high immigration density.

No wonder that a representative of La Raza called IRCA 'probably the best immigration legislation possible under current political conditions' (in Fuchs, 1990: 126)— perhaps under *any* conditions, if one considers that the purpose of this legislation had been control, not expansion. Of its dual legalization-sanctions agenda, only the legalization component of IRCA worked as intended. Nearly 1.8 million illegal immigrants applied for legal status under the general legalization programme, and 1.3 million under the Special Agricultural Worker (SAW) programme. But IRCA failed to reduce the stock and flow of illegal immigrants. After a temporary drop of apprehension figures in 1987 and 1988, attributable less to the effectiveness of sanctions than to a 'wait and see' response among potential immigrants, by 1989 the illegal flow was back to pre-IRCA levels.[23] In 1993, the size of the illegal population in the United States was estimated to be as high as ten years before—between three and four million persons (Papademetriou, 1993: 325).[24]

IRCA's failure to control illegal immigration is attributable to multiple factors. To begin with, IRCA does not even touch the problem of visa overstayers, which accounts for over 60 per cent of the undocumented population (Martin, 1995: 3). But most importantly, the 'odd coalition' pressure of Hispanics and employers has yielded a toothless sanctions scheme. From early on, a 'good faith' clause had been inserted into the Simpson–Mazzoli bill, which released employers from any obligation to check the authenticity of shown employees' documents: a document check conducted in 'good faith' constituted an 'affirmative defense' that the respective employer had not committed the 'knowing hire' misdemeanour (see Calavita, 1994: 71). In effect, employers were immune from punishment if they filled out and filed away routine I–9 forms that attested the document check. Because the introduction of a national ID card had been blocked, some twenty-nine documents, including easily faked US birth certificates (so-called 'breeders'), served to satisfy the control requirement. The positive 'affirmative defense' incentive was complemented by a negative 'anti-discrimination' incentive: demanding a *specific* ID constituted an 'unfair immigration-related employment practice', so that employers were better off accepting the document passively offered by the prospective employee. As David Martin (1995: 6 f.) put it, IRCA's sanctions scheme 'tells employers that it is more important to avoid even an appearance of discrimination than it is to wind up employing unauthorized workers'. Evidently the civil rights imperative of non-discrimination has stood in the way of effective immigration control.

'Avoiding Choices by Expanding the Pie': The Legal Immigration Act of 1990

After the (however incomplete) closing of the illegal back door, legislative attention turned to the opening of the legal front door, as suggested by the Select Commission in 1981. The original impulse behind the reform of legal immigration was twofold: first, to strengthen the component of skills within an immigration system that prioritized family-based immigration, which was increasingly linked to a deterioration of the educational and occupational quality of new immigrants; and, secondly, to redress an imbalance in the national origins of post-1965 immigration, which was skewed toward a few Third-World countries, with European immigration having virtually ceased. Both impulses taken together amounted to a subterranean, never openly articulated attack on the dominance of Hispanics and Asians in US immigration. Epitomizing the ironically inverted positions in this conflict, advocates of European immigration would rally behind the Third-World notion of 'diversity', whereas Hispanic and Asian leaders would brand as 'racist' attacks on the existing system of family reunification, which had once been installed to minimize the possibility of ethnoracial change. Invoking civil-rights language, Senator Edward Kennedy deplored the 'discrimination . . . against Irish and other European immigrants' who constituted 'the "old seed" source of our heritage' (in Cose, 1992: 198). On the other side, a House member speaking on behalf of Japanese-Americans suspected that the impulse against family reunification 'really is a bias against the Pacific Rim and Latin America'.[25]

Eventually, the system of family reunification proved too deeply entrenched to allow restrictions in favour of skill-based immigration, and the initial attempt of reducing one component at the cost of the other gave way to a 'strategy of conflict-suppressing expansion' (Schuck, 1992: 88). As a close observer-participant of the 1990 reform characterized the outcome, 'we avoided choices by expanding the pie'.[26] Hurriedly passed during the last hours of the 101st Congress, and almost unnoticed by the public, the Legal Immigration Act of 1990 would increase legal immigration to the United States by almost 40 per cent, and basically reaffirm the priority of family-based immigration as established in 1965.

Even more than IRCA, in which the perceived need to control illegal immigration was at least notionally tied to a group-transcending national interest, the Legal Immigration Act must be seen as the outcome of pure client politics, with very little public involvement. The national-interest dimension was reduced to attempts by Senator Alan Simpson to introduce, for the first time since 1924, an absolute cap on legal immigration, and to his overall objective to tie the admission of immigrants closer to labour-market needs, at the cost of family reunification—both of which were eventually defeated. From a national-interest perspective, the system of family reunification appeared as 'nepotism', the selection of immigrants according to random family ties, 'rather than 'on the basis of the talents and skills needed in this country'.[27] However, even if backed by academic evidence that post-1970 immigrants were characterized by decreased skill levels (Borjas, 1990), a national-interest line on legal immigration was difficult to take. It abstracted from the way immigration had historically occurred and found sediment in the collective experience of Americans. 'Isn't that the way people have always come here, that they have left people behind; that they have come and tried to put down roots and become economically viable and then bring their families?' retorted Bruce Morrison, the House immigration subcommittee leader, to FAIR's 'nepotism' charge. 'Certainly, members of my family did that'.[28] The nepotism charge also did not resonate well with the celebration of 'family values' during the Republican Bush administration. In their defence of family reunification, ethnic groups shrewdly exploited their discursive advantage: 'By making the family the focus of our system, the Nation lives up to its highest ideals while providing a strong network that helps immigrants adjust to their new lives in the United States'.[29]

A joint Senate bill, introduced by Alan Simpson and Edward Kennedy in early 1988, set the baseline for the final Legal Immigration Act, both positively and negatively. On the positive side, the Simpson–Kennedy bill was built upon a compromise between Simpson's agenda of increasing skill-based immigration in the 'national interest', and Kennedy's agenda of promoting source-country 'diversity', especially in the interest of his Irish constituency. But on the negative side, this compromise was achieved at the cost of reducing family-based immigration, which had to arouse the opposition of Hispanics and Asians. The Simpson–Kennedy bill contained three main provisions: first, it limited the Fifth Preference to unmarried siblings of US citizens, which would cut the annual immigrant intake in this category from almost 65,000 to just 22,000; second, it would increase from 55,000 to 120,000 the number of skill-based immigrants per year, and introduce a new category of 'independent worker', selected on a points system that honoured age, education, occupation, and English language competency; and third, it introduced an absolute ceiling of 590,000 legal immigrants per year, which included the previously exempted immediate family members of naturalized US citizens.[30] Each of these provisions had to be an affront to ethnic groups with a stake in family reunification. Slashing the Fifth Preference disadvantaged the Asians, who by 1987 received 56 per cent of all visas in this category (Cose, 1992: 200). Honouring English language competency in the 'independent worker' category was a code word for preferring Western European (especially Irish) immigrants, thus indirectly reintroducing the maligned national-origins discrimination. And an absolute cap on legal immigration meant that the immediate family categories would squeeze out the distant family categories, which were heavily used by Hispanics and Asians alike. A leader of the American Jewish Congress criticized the Simpson–Kennedy bill: 'The bill allows for the admission of skilled newcomers, many of whom are Europeans, at the expense of fifth preference, many of whom are Asian-Hispanic. Applying a preference of skilled immigrants over family reunification could produce unnecessary ethnic strife'.[31] Predictably, the House, more beholden to ethnic constituency pressure than the Senate, refused to consider the bill.[32]

After ethnic group campaigning was on, even the Senate moved into rough water. The second Simpson–Kennedy bill, introduced in July 1989, passed with only three important modifications: first, an amendment proposed by Senators Orrin Hatch (R-Utah) and Dennis DeConcini (D-Arizona) established a floor of 216,000 visas allocated for non-immediate family, which was the level under current law; if the demand for immediate family visas exceeded the total number of 480,000 family visas, the cap would become 'piercable'—and be no cap at all. Second, at the insistence of Senator Paul Simon (who was known to be friendly with Asian constituencies) the Fifth Preference restrictions were withdrawn. And thirdly, after emotional debate in the Judicial Committee, the 'English fluency' criterion in the independent worker category had to be dropped.[33] These were three important victories for the non-European ethnic groups with a stake in the maintenance of the existing family reunification system, and who also took a symbolic interest in an immigration policy based on strict non-discrimination.

But there were omissions in the Senate bill that would have to be addressed head-on in the House, such as the business demand for more temporary visas for skilled workers and professionals (which was opposed by labour unions), or a clearer separation between skill-based and 'diversity' immigration. In the House, Bruce Morrison, a young and ambitious Democrat from Connecticut who had taken Mazzoli's post of immigration subcommittee chair in 1989, opted for an expansive logrolling strategy of satisfying both business and the diverse 'old' and 'new' ethnic groups by increasing the numbers in all admission categories.

The extensive House hearings held in 1989 over legal immigration reform show the bewildering variety of interests that had to be reconciled in such a logroll. The older European ethnic groups, such as the Italians or Irish, had little to gain from the existing family reunification provisions. But they were also unhappy with the 'independent worker' approach of the 1988/9 Senate bills, because they feared to be 'outskilled' by other (English-speaking) workers from India, Pakistan, or Hong Kong. Instead, European ethnic groups advocated 'regional ceilings' that brought the latent tension between European and Third-World immigrant groups to the open. A leader of the American Committee on Italian Migration argued against 'discrimination in reverse': 'We want the Asiatics to continue to participate in the benefits of the (immigration) law, but we claim the same fairness of treatment for our potential immigrants from Europe'.[34] Defending a regionally targeted 'diversity visa' programme, the leader of the Irish Immigration Reform Movement complained no less explicitly that 'it is fundamentally wrong to exclude . . . the nations of those countries which have contributed so greatly to our culture and society in the past as part of our Nation's historical immigration stream'.[35] On the opposite side, a leader of the Hispanic National Council of La Raza demanded improvements in the family reunification provisions, most notably abolishing the Second Preference (spouses and minor children of permanent residents), easing the family reunification of the Hispanics legalized under IRCA, and increasing the visa contingent for 'contiguous countries', which meant that Mexico and Canada would receive higher numerical ceilings than other countries. At the same time, she warned that a point system for 'selected immigrants' was to be on a trial-basis only, and that it 'should not even give the appearance of favoring some parts of the world over others'.[36] Campaigning for more skill-based immigration, a representative of the US Chamber of Commerce attacked an inflexible, restrictive system of admitting professional non-immigrant workers, which hampered 'the ability of American companies to compete in foreign markets'.[37] Some interest groups, such as the American Immigration Lawyers Association, with its feet firmly in both the ethnic group and business camps, anticipated the eventual logroll by embracing both the business need to 'compete in an increasingly competitive global economy' and the ethnic group demands for maintaining the Fifth and abolishing the Second Preference, which would remove the admission of the spouses and children of permanent residents from numerical restrictions.[38] Similarly, a leader of the American Jewish Congress stipulated that new-seed immigration had to be 'in addition to, rather than in competition with, family-based immigration',[39] which in fact describes the essence of the final deal.

Tellingly entitled 'Family United and Employment Opportunity Immigration Act', the House bill, sponsored by Bruce Morrison, had little in common with the original Simpson–Kennedy bill, including vastly increased numbers and generous family reunification provisions.[40] In order to get both labour and business aboard, the bill held to a restrictive line on temporary employment visas, but further increased the number of permanent employment visas. Placating the European ethnic groups, a regionally concentrated 'diversity' category was now clearly separated from the universal 'skills' category. To clear backlogs on family reunification, the Second Preference category was doubled in size (from 70,000 to 140,000 annual visas), three-quarters of which were to be distributed on a first-come first-serve basis, thus waiving the 20,000 country ceiling—this was especially good for Mexican-Americans. Human-rights groups, whose voice was liberal Congressman Barney Frank, achieved a provision that would prohibit the executive from excluding would-be entrants because of their ideological or sexual orientations, which was the dismal legacy of the McCarthy-period McCarran–Walter Act of 1952. A sarcastic observer characterized the ensuing hotchpotch as a 'Christmas Tree, a tree that everybody puts their own ornaments on'.[41]

Signed into law by President Bush in November 1990, the Immigration Act of 1990 amounted to the most extensive reform of US immigration law since 1924 (Lawson and Grin, 1992: 255). By increasing the intake of legal immigrants to 700,000 during the next three years, and 675,000 thereafter, which was about 40 per cent above the present level, the 1990 Act was indeed, as a *New York Times* editorial hailed it, 'a monument . . . to a nation of immigrants'.[42] These large numbers reflected the nature of a positive-sum logroll between business and ethnic groups. In retrospect, it is astonishing to see that the philosophically restrictive Immigration Reform and Control Act (IRCA) was passed during a period of economic expansion and job growth, while the philosophically expansive Immigration Act of 1990 came right at the onset of a serious recession. Obviously, US immigration policy, which is contingent upon a bewildering variety of conflicting client interests, follows its own, inert momentum that is different from the exigencies of the business cycle. 'Nobody liked the

1990 Act', says a perplexed US immigration expert in retrospect.[43] While the 1990 Act may be understood as the culmination of a nation rebuilding itself as a 'nation of immigrants' after 1965, the obscurity and clientelistic mode of its making cast doubt on its longevity. As one of the 1990 Act's best chroniclers put it, 'The public was not exactly clamoring for such a bill. Nor, outside the community of experts, was America even much aware that such legislation was taking shape' (Cose, 1992: 208). Peter Schuck (1992: 91) is therefore right to conclude that the 1990 Act may simply reflect 'a particular logroll at a particular point in time', and be no indication for a 'broad consensus in favor of an expansionist future'.

Transformation of Immigration Law

Not just the political, but also the legal process has been remarkably expansive towards aliens. Legal expansiveness rests upon a fundamental 'transformation of immigration law' (Schuck, 1984) since the 1960s.[44] Classical immigration law, which was formulated in the restrictionist 1880s, fused the principles of consent-based obligation, strong sovereignty, and restrictive national community. Consent-based obligation modelled the relationship between government and alien along the private-law relationship between a landowner and a trespasser, in which the former owed no obligation to the latter except those explicitly consented to. The principle of strong sovereignty was formulated by the Supreme Court in 1892: 'It is an accepted maxim of international law, that every sovereign nation has the power, as inherent in sovereignty, and essential to self-preservation, to forbid the entrance of foreigners within its dominions, or to admit them only in such cases and upon such conditions as it may see fit to prescribe' (quoted in Schuck, 1984: 6). Applied to the institutions of government, strong sovereignty meant the unfettered, 'plenary power' of the political branches of government over the admission, expulsion, and naturalization of aliens. Finally, strong sovereignty was exerted on behalf of a restrictive national community, in which the main dividing-line was race. The benchmark of classical immigration law is the Chinese Exclusion Case of 1889, in which the Supreme Court refused to overturn legislation that had barred Chinese labourers from entry to the United States. As the Court infamously reasoned, '[if Congress] considers the presence of foreigners of a different race in this country, who will not assimilate with us, to be dangerous to its peace and security, . . . its determination is conclusive upon the judiciary' (ibid. 14).

Since the 1960s, following a larger 'communitarian' (Schuck, 1984) or 'participation'[45] turn of public law, immigration law has moved away from the classical model. Postclassical immigration law abandons the individualistic principle of consent-based obligation, and 'grants the alien rights according to an ascending scale as her identification with society deepens'.[46] In the new communitarian model, individuals are seen as invested with inalienable human rights and social ties that must be respected and protected by government. No longer allowed to get tough with aliens as illicit trespassers, government 'owes legal duties to all individuals who manage to reach America's shores, even to strangers whom it has never undertaken, and has no wish, to protect' (ibid. 4). This has entailed a cautious but steadily increasing assertiveness of courts, which refused to defer to the plenary power of Congress and executive branch in immigration affairs, and invoked constitutional and statutory norms to protect the rights of aliens. Motivated by the anti-discriminatory impetus of the civil-rights era, courts have extended constitutional protections beyond the national community, to include legal resident aliens, undocumented immigrants, and even first-time entrants, such as asylum-seekers. However, this extension did not go without strains. As Peter Schuck (1984: 90) has pointed out, the legal empowerment of aliens has undermined the very possibility of national self-definition, which necessarily implies the exclusion of non-members: 'If the American community's power to define its common purposes and obligations is no greater than the power of strangers to cross our borders undetected and to acquire interests here, our capacity to pursue liberal values—to decide as individuals and as a society what we wish to be—may be critically impaired.'

The major resource for the legal empowerment of aliens has been a constitution that grants broad equal protection and due process rights to 'persons', not just to 'citizens' (see Bickel, 1975: ch. 2). Here one must distinguish between three classes of aliens who have successively been brought under constitutional protection: legal permanent residents, illegal immigrants, and first-time entrants. Legal permanent residents (LPRs) now enjoy rights and benefits that are essentially equal to those of US citizens.[47] This has not always been so, as under classical immigration law the states could invoke the legal 'special public interest' doctrine to prohibit aliens from owning or acquiring land, working on public laws projects, or receiving welfare benefits. In

Graham v. *Richardson* (1971), the Supreme Court put an end to this, ruling that states cannot discriminate against resident aliens in providing welfare benefits unless there is a 'compelling state interest'. Applying the language of civil-rights law, the Court argued that LPRs were a 'discrete and insular minority', victims of 'irrational discrimination' and politically powerless, so that classification based on alienage—much like classification based on race—was 'inherently suspect' and 'subject to close judicial scrutiny'.[48] In a typical example of communitarian reasoning, the Court emphasized that aliens were active members of society who, like citizens, paid taxes and contributed with their work and capital to the public welfare.[49]

The second class of aliens to enter the orbit of constitutional protection are illegal immigrants. In *Plyler* v. *Doe* (1982), the Supreme Court invalidated a Texas statute that withheld free public education from the children of illegal immigrants. This most famous of all US court rules on aliens' rights argued that the 14th Amendment's Equal Protection clause referred to all 'persons' within a state's jurisdiction,[50] so that aliens, whatever their legal status, had to be included: 'Whatever his status under the immigration laws, an alien is surely a "person" in any ordinary sense of that term.'[51] Procedural due process protections, for instance, in deportation proceedings, had been granted to illegal aliens already before *Plyler*; the novelty was to extend substantive entitlements normally reserved to lawful residents to illegal aliens. In an expansive reading, *Plyler* marked a decisive break with the principles of classical immigration law, because it enlarged the national community to uncertain dimensions and patently disregarded the parallel congressional policy to contain illegal immigration. In this reading, as Peter Schuck (1984: 58) put it, '*Plyler* [is] the most powerful rejection to date of classical immigration law's notion of plenary national sovereignty over our borders.'[52]

With first-time entrants, such as asylum-seekers, we reach the 'outermost ring of membership' (Martin, 1983: 216) in which the degree of constitutional protection is at its nadir. As the anonymous author of 'Developments in the Law' (p. 1309) emphasizes, the postclassical participation model of immigration law only marginally applies in this case, because 'the entering alien . . . has no preexisting stake in the community upon which a grant of rights might be based'. Indeed, the exclusion of entering aliens is inherently linked with elementary national self-definition, and accordingly has remained, however besieged, a bastion of sovereignty in which the plenary power doctrine is firmly in place (see Legomsky, 1985; 1995). 'Over no conceivable subject is the legislative power of Congress more complete,' the Supreme Court argued in 1909. Plenary power over the admission of aliens was reaffirmed as late as 1977 in *Fiallo* v. *Bell*, where the Supreme Court held that 'policies pertaining to the entry of aliens . . . are peculiarly concerned with the political conduct of government'.[53] However, since the onset of mass asylum-seeking in the early 1980s lower courts have openly challenged the plenary-power doctrine and tried to bring first-time entrants also under the umbrella of the constitution. Discussing the lower court challenge to plenary power, Peter Schuck (1984: 70) appropriately characterizes the 'emergent law of asylum' as an exemplar of communitarian immigration law, '[enabling] any alien to acquire rights against the government to which the latter has not expressly consented'.

The new phenomenon of mass asylum-seeking from Cuba and Haiti caused a serious 'due process crisis' (Martin, 1983: 168) regarding excludable aliens. Facing the arrival of 125,000 Marielito Cubans and of 15,000 Haitian boat people in 1980 alone, the Reagan government ended the previous generous policy of 'paroling' asylum-seekers into the country,[54] and went over to an extremely restrictive mass detention and expulsion policy. This policy was perhaps commanded by the imperative of containing illegal immigration, but it entailed extraordinary hardship for those subjected to it, such as prolonged incarceration under harsh and oppressive conditions, the summary denial of asylum claims, and erratic and discriminatory treatment by the INS. As Peter Schuck (1984: 68) remarked, the denial of elementary due process rights to the innocent victims of economic deprivation, civil war, and political persecution has 'seared the judicial conscience as few events since the civil rights struggles of the 1950s and 1960s have done'. In a sometimes explicit, more often implicit challenge to the plenary power doctrine, lower courts have acknowledged due process claims raised by human-rights and public-interest lawyers on behalf of detained or rejected asylum-seekers, holding prolonged detention invalid, prescribing elaborate legal procedures for asylum hearings, and rebuking the INS for discriminating on the basis of national origin and race.

David Martin (1983: 171) has castigated as 'procedural exuberance' the inclination of lower courts to apply constitutional due process and equal protection rules 'to anyone in the world who presents himself at our borders'. The dilemma is clear: continuing to treat excludables as non-persons, as stipulated by the old Knauff–Mezei doctrine,[55] violates the liberal and communitarian values of postclassical immigration law; but granting the constitutional status of 'person' to excludables would extend constitutional protection to literally everyone in the world, and stand in the way of effective immigration control.

Scrutinizing the lower-court challenge to plenary power, one can detect at least three patterns. First, there were variable, often contradictory, lines of court reasoning. These variations partially depended on the national origins of the plaintiffs: regarding Haitians, who were automatically detained and categorized as 'economic' refugees ineligible for asylum (while most Cubans were generously paroled into the country), some courts would point at national origin and racial discrimination; regarding detained Marielito Cubans, an alternative line of reasoning was to consider detention not as an immigration measure, but as 'punishment' that was subject to constitutional due process control. Secondly, contrary to the impression given by David Jacobson (1996: ch. 5), courts were disinclined to resort to international law as a protection for asylum-seekers; the major thrust has been to bring the latter under the roof of the constitution. Thirdly, the application of constitutional norms to excludable asylum-seekers has remained a lower court phenomenon; the Supreme Court has refused to deliver an equivalent to *Plyler* v. *Doe* for excludable aliens.[56]

Regarding the second pattern, which is relevant for my argument of the primacy of domestic over international human-rights norms, consider the following detention case. In *Fernandez* v. *Wilkinson* (1980), a Cuban, who had arrived as part of the Mariel Boat lift in spring 1980 and was deemed non-admittable because of a criminal history, claimed that his prolonged detention was tantamount to cruel and unusual punishment prohibited by the 8th Amendment, and a violation of the due process clause of the 5th Amendment. The district court of Kansas concluded that the plaintiff's status of excludable alien prohibited recourse to the constitution, thus reaffirming Knauff–Mezei: 'We have declared that indeterminate detention of petitioner in a maximum security prison pending unforeseeable deportation constitutes arbitrary detention. Due to the unique legal status of excluded aliens in this country, it is an evil from which our Constitution and statutory laws afford no protection' (quoted in Hassan, 1983: 71). However, the court decided that arbitrary detention was a violation of customary international law, ordering the government to release the Cuban on these grounds within ninety days. Celebrated by international human-rights advocates (Martineau, 1983; Hassan, 1983), this was the only time that a US court based a detention or asylum decision on international law. But, as a legal commentator pointed out (Hahn, 1982: 964

f.), this was also a questionable decision. As the Supreme Court ruled in *Paquete Habana* (1900), international law is the law of the land only interstitially, 'in the absence of any treaty or other public act of . . . government in relation to the matter'. Accordingly, the validity of the respective detention depended on whether or not it was undertaken without presidential approval—which was never considered by the court.

Without commenting on the district court's reasoning, the Tenth Circuit Court of Appeals, in *Rodriguez-Fernandez* v. *Wilkinson* (1981), upheld the claimant's release from detention, but on starkly different grounds. The appeals court argued that indeterminate detention in a federal prison, which resulted from Cuba's refusal to take the plaintiff back, was no longer part of the process of exclusion under immigration law; rather, it amounted to punishment, for which constitutional protection under the 5th and 8th Amendments applies. Interestingly, the court based its ruling on the sub-constitutional ground that the INS lacked statutory authority for indefinite detention. But, in Motomura's terms (1990), the court used 'phantom constitutional norms' favourable to aliens in its statute interpretation—'serious constitutional questions [would be] involved if the statute were construed differently', argued the court (quoted in Hassan, 1983: 75). Overall, the thrust of *Rodriguez-Fernandez* was to redefine detention as punishment, and thus to bring the respective would-be entrant under the roof of the constitution; the role of international law was diminished from that of a 'controlling' to a 'definitional' device (Martineau, 1983: 104), as one (among several) guidelines for the definition of what process was due.

Toward Source-Country Universalism in Asylum Policy

Until the late 1980s, US asylum and refugee policy had remained a bastion of state sovereignty within an immigration regime where strong sovereignty had long been in retreat. In summarily granting refugee status to individuals fleeing communist regimes while denying asylum claims of individuals fleeing dictatorial yet 'friendly' regimes, asylum and refugee policy represented a curious anomaly within an immigration regime that had abandoned national discriminations in favour of source-country universalism. The trajectory of asylum and refugee policy was thus to a large degree a catching-up with the non-discriminatory principles of immigration law and policy. Rescuing asylum and refugee policy from foreign policy tutelage, which was not completed before the end of the Cold War and the fall of communism, appeared itself as the curiously anomalous liberalization of a policy area that in Western Europe was then falling to the sway of illiberal restrictionism.

US asylum policy proper is the result of a double differentiation: first, of refugee from immigration policy; and secondly, of asylum from refugee policy. In the 1965 Immigration Act, refugee policy was still an integral part of immigration policy. The Seventh Preference category of the Act reserved 6 per cent of Eastern hemisphere immigrant visas to refugees from 'communist-dominated countries' or the Middle East—thus inaugurating the ideological, discriminatory bias of US refugee policy after World War II (see Loescher and Scanlan, 1986: 73). In addition, the Attorney General, acting on behalf of the President, had discretionary 'parole' power to admit refugees outside the normal immigration process—a power first used by Eisenhower to 'parole in' 40,000 Hungarian refugees after the Soviet crackdown in 1956. Only the Refugee Act of 1980 clearly separated refugee from immigration policy. It first established the regular legal status of refugee and—consonant with the principles of an immigrant nation— the subsequent expectation of refugees to acquire citizenship, along with generous resettlement benefits to ease the transition. In incorporating the 1951 UN refugee definition and non-refoulement obligation, the Act's purpose was to overcome the ideological bias of US refugee policy, and to achieve more Congressional control over the executive's erratic parole authority. Finally, in a more subterranean yet momentous change for asylum-seekers, the Refugee Act levelled Knauff–Mezei's sharp distinction between 'excludable' aliens at the borders, with no statutory and constitutional rights, and 'deportable' aliens on US territory, endowed with constitutional due process protection (Dinh, 1994). Compliant with the non-refoulement obligation, the exclusion process was henceforth framed by extensive statutory and due process rights for aliens, including access to federal courts.

While the 1980 Refugee Act formally introduced the right to apply for political asylum on US territory or at the borders, this remained essentially 'an afterthought' (Meissner, 1988: 60). For the United States, refugees have traditionally been an overseas phenomenon, relevant only if it touched upon foreign policy interests or obligations. As in the Indo-Chinese refugee crisis that followed the American withdrawal from Cambodia and Vietnam in the mid-1970s, refugee policy meant the screening and selection of refugees in camps overseas, with at best loose application of UN convention refugee criteria, and their resettlement in the United States. Such refugee policy was not antithetical to, but a direct outgrowth of state sovereignty, because it reflected unforced, proactive state action toward non-nationals to which the United States, as one of the world's two superpowers after World War II, felt special obligations and responsibilities.

Mass asylum-seeking, and with it the differentiation of asylum from refugee policy, first became an issue with the Mariel Boat Lift, a few weeks after the passing of the Refugee Act in March 1980. As Doris Meissner (1988: 61) put it, 'asylum, the sleeper of the new legislation, emerged as the dragon lady, center stage'. In an obvious attempt to embarrass the US government, Castro allowed some 125,000 Cubans to sail freely, on rigged-up rafts and boats, to the shores of Florida, among them a good portion of criminals and mentally disturbed. While met with considerable ambivalence, most Marielitos were allowed to enter without individual screening for refugee status, privileged by the Cuban Adjustment Act of 1966 that allowed Cubans to apply for permanent resident status after a short period on US territory. No such privileged reception was granted to a parallel flotilla of 15,000 Haitian refugees who arrived in Florida at about the same time, but whose departure from the notoriously ruthless yet 'friendly' Duvalier regime led the government to label them 'illegal immigrants' without legitimate asylum claims. This opened up the debate about a discriminatory 'double standard' in US asylum policy, which operated on the simple principle of 'Cuba, yes. Haiti, no.'[57]

The double standard was further aggravated by the general denial of refugee status to new land-based arrivals from civil-war torn Central America (especially El Salvador), whom the government likewise labelled 'illegal immigrants' subject to deportation (see Romig, 1985; Barnett, 1985). In fact, the linkage between asylum-seeking and illegal immigration cannot be dismissed wholesale. The vast majority of asylum applications are not made at the borders and ports of entry, but while already on US territory. This is because applying for asylum is a no-cost game for illegal entrants to avoid deportation. Federal courts have furthered this rational strategy by insisting that the INS must inform detained illegal aliens about their right to apply for asylum. In turn, generous asylum-granting had to have bad precedence effect for historically high illegal immigration from the Western hemisphere. Finally, the Reagan government held 'friendly' relationships with right-wing military regimes in Central America, and subsequently denied regime-compromising and destabilizing asylum claims from the region's migrants, because it feared to be overwhelmed by refugees in case of Marxist guerilla takeovers. As Reagan outlined, 'the result [of Marxist dictatorships coming to power in Central America] could be a tidal wave of refugees—and this time they'll be feet people, not boat people—swarming into our country seeking a safe haven from Communist repression to our south' (quoted in Romig, 1985: 316).

Strictly speaking, the anomaly of US asylum policy was not the generally restrictionist response to mass asylum-seeking at the country's land and sea borders, which was in line with the practice of other Western states, and intricately linked to the parallel fight against illegal immigration. Instead, it was the preferential treatment for Cubans and other refugees from communist regimes that was anomalous.[58] In rejecting pleas to grant 'extended voluntary departure' (temporary safe haven) status to illegal Salvadorians in the US, a government official could credibly point at the bad precedence effect of such a measure for 'all other migrants from poor, violent societies to our south'.[59] But why had this status been granted to 5,000 Poles during martial law?[60] This imbalance created a double dynamic of asylum advocates trying to lift up the general asylum practice to the generosity displayed to refugees from communism, and of a government cautiously but steadily abandoning its preferential treatment for some categories of asylum-seekers. Already the Marielitos were not unequivocally welcome, and one of the uglier asylum battles of the early 1980s was to detain and deport thousands of them whose criminal or medical records did not make them eligible for entry in the first place, or whose 'parole' status had been forfeited by crimes committed while in the United States.[61] Curiously, a Cuban advocate wondered aloud whether it was 'just' if Cuban hijackers were no longer welcomed as heroes but sent back to Havana, complaining that 'today's Cubans must file their requests for asylum with the rest of the world'.[62] In fact, the Marielitos' privileged transition from temporary parole ('Cuban-Haitian entrant') status to permanent residence, by means of the Cuban Adjustment Act, which so blatantly left out the Haitians, was forced by a federal court rule upon a government that would have preferred to settle jointly the legal status of both groups within the Simpson–Mazzoli bill.[63]

Throughout the 1980s, hard-nosed government measures of mass detention, deportation, and high-sea interception were undercut by increasingly activist courts which no longer deferred to the traditional 'plenary power' of Congress and the President over immigration, and brought to bear the communitarian impetus of immigration law on the new field of asylum. In this respect, the decade is marked by a string of legal victories for asylum-seekers. Next to limiting the detention and deportation power of the executive, courts have eased the burden of proof for asylum applicants, for instance, in no longer using false documentation or witness as automatic grounds for dismissal of a case (see Anker and Blum, 1989). More importantly still, in *INS* v. *Cardoza-Fonseca* (1987), the Supreme Court ruled that the Reagan Administration's demanding 'clear probability' of persecution standards for deciding asylum claims had to be replaced by the looser 'reasonable possibility' of persecution standards, pointing out that a one-in-ten chance of persecution would qualify as a legitimate asylum claim (Porter, 1992: 234 f.). Finally, there has been a tendency toward broadening the grounds on which individuals can raise asylum-claims. For instance, in *Bolanos-Hernandez* v. *INS* (1984), a court stipulated that 'political neutrality' also constituted a 'political opinion' subject to persecution.[64] A 'gender-conscious' judiciary has even been willing to grant asylum to homosexuals who claim to be persecuted for their sexual orientation.[65]

The court-driven liberalization of asylum culminated in new asylum rules given out by the Justice Department in 1990. They replaced the uneven, politically driven 'interim rules' that had guided the administrative asylum process since 1980.[66] In addition, a corps of professional asylum officers trained in international relations and human-rights law was established, with the mandate to make politically neutral asylum decisions, unimpaired by State Department prerogatives. According to the new rules, work permits and the help of lawyers were to be granted routinely to asylum-seekers. Most importantly, the new rules gave asylum-seekers the benefit of the doubt. Claimants no longer needed to prove that they were individually singled out for persecution; it was enough to show 'a pattern or practice of persecuting the groups of persons similarly situated'[67]—a refugee definition considerably looser than the UN convention refugee definition. Moreover, aliens now qualified for asylum on the basis of their own statements, without objective corroboration, if the testimony was 'credible in light of general conditions' in the home country (to be ascertained by means of a newly established documentation centre). In David Martin's (1988) terms, this new policy moved from 'deterrence' to 'fair adjudication', and as such it stood out in the Western world.

The double standard was officially put to rest in a subsequent court settlement, in which the government agreed to stop detaining and deporting illegal aliens from El Salvador and Guatemala, granting new asylum hearings for all 150,000 applicants denied since 1980 and for 350,000 illegal aliens who had never applied previously.[68] The settlement averted a trial of the government's 'discriminatory' denial of asylum to Salvadorans and Guatemalans,[69] who claimed violation of their constitutional rights to free speech, equal protection, and due process. The government now explicitly obliged itself to rule out foreign policy, border control, and the applicant's country of origin as criteria of asylum determination. This was a major victory for the 'sanctuary movement' of church leaders, social workers, and human-rights lawyers, who had filed the suit in May 1985. This movement, which included not just 200 churches and synagogues but entire cities like Los Angeles and Sacramento declaring themselves 'sanctuaries' for Central American refugees, epitomizes the normative cloth out of which US asylum liberalization was made: not abstract human-rights principles hovering above nation-states, but—as a church leader put it—'the deepest values of our United States traditions of being a place of refuge, a place to where persecuted people can come.'[70]

Closing the Golden Door? Proposition 187 and After

Since 1965, US immigration policy has followed a path of 'relentless liberalization' (Freeman, 1996: 1). The 1980 Refugee Act applied the principle of source-country universalism to refugee and asylum policy; the notionally restrictionist Immigration Reform and Control Act of 1986 turned 3 million illegal into legal immigrants; and the 1990 Immigration Act increased legal-quota immigration by one-third. An expansive political process under the sway of client politics was undergirded by the communitarian turn of immigration law, which inflicted cracks on traditional state sovereignty ('plenary power') and amounted to the legal empowerment of aliens. In a counterpoint to this liberalization, which spurred the biggest wave of mass immigration since the turn of the century,[71] American public opinion turned increasingly restrictionist. According to annually held Gallup polls, the proportion of Americans who opted for 'decreasing' the current immigration levels has grown steadily, from 33 per cent in 1965 to 42 per cent in 1977, 49 per cent in 1986, and 65 per cent in 1993.[72] A *Newsweek* poll of August 1993 found a majority of 59 per cent of the belief that immigration had been a good thing in the past, but only a minority of 29 per cent who thought it was still a good thing today.[73] No wonder, when provided with the vote, the public came out strongly against the expansive immigration policies of the élites.

In November 1994, Californian voters overwhelmingly passed Proposition 187, dubbed as the 'Save Our State' (SOS) initiative, which would bar illegal aliens from most state-provided services, including non-emergency health care and school education. This was nothing less than a political earthquake. Transmitted by the most conservative Congress in half a century, with both houses falling to Republican control in the same November 1994 elections, the aftershock was immediately felt in Washington. A sweeping overhaul not only of illegal, but also of legal immigration seemed to be in the making. Two years later, the earthquake has been reduced to a ripple, unable to overturn the 'incremental expansionism' (Freeman, 1996: 5) that had characterized US immigration policy since the mid-1960s. The planned restriction of legal immigration was shelved, perhaps indefinitely. Until it was signed into law as the Immigration Control and Financial Responsibility Act of 1996, an initially drastic proposal to combat illegal immigration was watered down significantly. Once again, client politics came in the way of 'put[ting] the interests of America first'.[74]

This outcome is doubly astonishing, given that the popular challenge was accompanied by a formidable academic challenge to the expansionist orthodoxy. Certainly outside the realm of 'respectable' academic discourse but with tremendous public impact, the Republican-leaning financial journalist Peter Brimelow (1995: p. xvii) dared question the changing 'racial and ethnic balance' due to Third-World immigration, which would turn the white majority into a near-minority by the year 2050.[75] Michael Lind (1995) sought to reclaim a restrictionist stance toward immigration from a liberal perspective, advocating 'zero-net immigration' (p. 321 f.) as in the interest of American workers and the black underclass. Nathan Glazer (1995) summarized the joint liberal-conservative anti-immigration chorus, giving five reasons why the United States in the 1990s differed from the United States in the 1920s (the end of the previous wave of mass immigration): first, in a more densely populated country there was no demographic need for a further population increase; secondly, regionally concentrated immigration raised environmental concerns; thirdly, immigration became decoupled from the business cycle, whose lulls had dampened immigration in the past; fourthly, the United States was now a mature welfare state, whose benefits were contingent upon limiting their claimants; and fifthly, multicultural identity politics overcharged the assimilatory force of American nationhood. 'These changes', Glazer cautiously concludes, 'do nothing to support an argument for more immigration' (p. 55). The new scepticism of intellectuals was bolstered by economist George Borjas's disturbing finding that immigrant households were more likely to be in the welfare system than native households, and that the case for immigration had to be made on political rather than economic grounds.[76] Even the popular argument that immigrants displace native workers is no longer routinely rejected (as in Muller, 1993: ch. 5). Sociologist Roger Waldinger, no immigrant foe he, argued in prominent place that low-skilled blacks do suffer from immigration, because immigrant groups create their own job niches and networks that exclude blacks, and because employers prefer immigrants over blacks as more docile and productive workers.[77]

It is no accident that the popular anti-immigrant earthquake had its epicentre in California. Not only does this state, initially rural and settled by white farmers' flight from the 'dust-bowl' misery of the 1930s Mid-West, lack the 'nation of immigrants' insignia of the East Coast cities, with the Statue of Liberty and the like. More importantly, the problem of illegal immigration, the root cause of America's immigration debate, is more ardently felt in California than elsewhere: almost half of the estimated national total of four million illegal immigrants resides here. The Urban Institute calculated that they cost the state almost $2 billion per year in education, emergency medical services, and incarceration. Against this, the $732 million in state revenues from sales, property, and income taxes on illegal aliens appear paltry (Schuck, 1995: 88). California epitomizes three problems of contemporary immigration to the United States. First, this immigration is extremely regionally concentrated, with three-quarters of immigrants ending up in just six states (40 per cent of them in California). Secondly, disproportionate costs are incurred by some state governments and municipalities, while the main benefits in terms of federal taxes and social security payments are reaped by the federal government. 'The smaller the jurisdiction, the larger the burden', concluded the California Senate Office of Research (1993: 6). Sixty per cent of immigrants' taxes land in federal coffers, while counties receive just 3 per cent. Accordingly, a 1992 Los Angeles County study showed that despite a total tax income of $4.3 billion from (legal and illegal) immigrants, the county still suffered a net loss of $808 million in public services (ibid.). Eric Rothman and Thomas Espenshade (1992: 410) characterized the federal–local imbalance as a result of 'bumping rights', in which higher levels of government deflect costs to the next lower one: 'Because local governments have nowhere else to turn, they end up paying most of the costs of immigration.' Moreover, because the costs of federal immigration are not fully internalized, 'the immigration door is open wider than it would otherwise be' (ibid.). In response, since 1994 a bipartisan movement of state governors has sued the federal government for carrying the costs of its expansionist policies.[78] Thirdly, and related to this, in the wake of Proposition 187 the economic focus of the US immigration debate has shifted from the labour market to the negative fiscal implications. As Governor Pete Wilson maliciously calculated, the $1.8 billion that California spent each year on educating the 355,000 children of its illegal immigrants could be used for hiring 51,000 new teachers, building 2,340 new classrooms, or installing 1 million new computers in the state's battered and under-equipped schools.[79] While the draconian core of Proposition 187 was rejected even by many Republicans, a bipartisan consensus emerged that immigrants, illegal or legal, should be excluded from most welfare state services, such as Aid for Families with Dependent Children (AFDC) or Medicaid. The one novelty of post-1994 restrictionism is to use the field of immigrant integration, so far one of 'benign neglect' in the United States, for purposes of 'exclusion' (Fix and Zimmermann, 1995: 36).

It was clear upfront that Proposition 187, which openly defied the Supreme Court rule in *Plyler* v. *Doe*, would be blocked by the courts. Within hours after the polls had closed, a flurry of court-suits were filed, and instant restraining orders blocked the controversial education provision.[80] In November 1995, the US District Court of Los Angeles found the measure in breach of the Constitution, and in violation of the federal prerogative to control immigration.[81] However, supported even by one-third of Latino and the majority of Asian and black voters, Proposition 187 was essentially a 'symbolic message' (Schuck 1995: 92) to the political élites who had so recklessly evaded realities and responsibilities for years.[82] And if Congress picked up the ball at the national level—this was the more-than-symbolic reasoning of the initiative leaders—the Supreme Court might be led to a reconsideration of *Plyler* v. *Doe* and eventually uphold the restrictionist state law.

Congress picked up the ball indeed, without delay. The federal Commission on Immigration Reform, originally established to review the impact of the 1990 Immigration Act, immediately proposed drastic changes of existing immigration law and policy. The full weight of the restrictionist challenge is indicated in the fact that the Commission was headed by Barbara Jordan, the former black Congresswoman from Texas with impeccable liberal credentials, and spiked with some of the very same liberal pro-immigrant politicians and academics who had been responsible for the expansionist immigration policies of the 1980s.[83] In its March 1995 report, the Commission recommended cutting legal immigration by one-third. This included the scrapping of most extended family categories, including the old Fifth Preference prioritizing the married brothers and sisters of naturalized citizens, which had already been under serious attack in 1990. In addition, and supported by the labour-friendly forces in the Clinton administration,[84] it should become more difficult and costly for employers to hire foreign professionals. In contrast to Brimelow (1995) and Lind (1995),[85] the Commission did not touch the 'nation of immigrants' myth: 'The U.S. has been and should continue to be a nation of immigrants.'[86] But this proposal went even further than Proposition 187 and California's Governor Pete Wilson, who had targeted only illegal immigration. Regarding illegal immigration, the Commission had advocated already in late 1994 a national employment verification system, which would compile the names and social security numbers of all citizens and legal aliens authorized to work in the United States, and make it mandatory for employers to call it up before hiring new workers. This stopped short of introducing a national ID card, which continues to be anathema in the United States. But it became opposed, predictably, by a plethora of ethnic, civil-rights, and business organizations as being just that: a national ID card in disguise.

The Commission's recommendations became incorporated in similar House and Senate bills, introduced by Lamar Smith, a Republican Congressman from Texas, and Senator Alan Simpson, the Republican immigration veteran from Wyoming. Both bills centred around three measures: cutting legal immigration by slashing the non-nuclear family categories and reducing skilled immigration; combating illegal immigration by screening the workplace more tightly and fortifying the borders; and, in a windfall from the parallel Congressional effort to reform the welfare system, making even legal aliens ineligible for most public services. Hardly was the ink dry, when the machine of client politics was set in motion. An unusually broad 'Left–Right Coalition on Immigration' included not just the usually odd immigration bedfellows of employers and ethnic and civil-rights groups, but also the Home School Network, a Christian fundamentalist group rallying against the 'anti-family' measures to curtail legal immigration;

Americans for Tax Reform, who disliked—along with Microsoft, Intel, and the National Association of Manufacturers—having employers pay a heavy tax on each foreign worker they sponsored; and the National Rifle Association, upset by the employment verification system—'If you're going to register people, why not guns?'[87] Richard Day, the chief counsel to the Senate Judiciary Subcommittee, characterized this unusual line-up as 'Washington groups' against 'the American people', who had asked for 'some breathing space' from immigration.[88] Such is the logic of immigration policy as client politics.

The first success of the client machine was to split the omnibus bill into two. The client machine was helped in this by divisions within the Republican Party. A large section of free-market and family-value Republicans (such as Jack Kemp, William Bennett, and Dick Armey) favoured legal immigration. In addition, Republicans from California, where the problem of illegal immigration was most pressing, feared that rifts over legal immigration would improperly delay the eagerly awaited crackdown on illegal immigration. In March 1996, the Senate Judiciary Committee, with the parallel House committee following suit, decided to postpone legislation on legal immigration, and to concentrate on illegal immigration first. The Big One had suddenly shrunk to a rather smallish immigration earthquake. Only a few months earlier, Republican Lamar Smith had boasted that 'the question is no longer whether legal immigration should be reformed, but how it should be reformed'.[89] Now he lay flattened by the client machine. 'Congress has listened to lobbyists more than public opinion,' wrote an angry immigration foe.[90]

After cracking the omnibus bill, the effort of the pro-immigration lobby concentrated on smoothing out some drastic features of the remaining bill on illegal immigration. One target was the employment verification system, denounced by a libertarian critic as 'dialing "1–800 Big Brother" '.[91] An amendment by Senator Edward Kennedy softened the proposed verification system from being nationwide and mandatorily in place within eight years to a variety of voluntary pilot programmes in high-immigration states, to be reviewed by Congress after three years.[92] This meant, without new legislation, no nationwide employment verification system. This was an important step back from the recommendation of the Commission on Immigration Reform, which had called a mandatory national verification system 'the linchpin' of combating illegal immigration.[93] In addition, an amendment by Senator Orrin Hatch, the pro-immigration Republican from Utah, eliminated a hefty increase of fines against employers who knowingly hired illegal aliens—this was a victory for small business owners.[94]

When signed into law by President Clinton in early October 1996, the 'Maginot line against illegal immigration' (D. Papademetriou)[95] looked more like a Swiss cheese, with big holes eaten into it by America's clients of immigration policy. The drastic Gallegly amendment in the House (named after its sponsor, California Republican Elton Gallegly), which would allow states to bar the children of illegal immigrants from public schools and thus turn into national law California's Proposition 187, was dropped from the final bill, also because of a safe Presidential veto. A watered-down employment verification system is unlikely to fix the biggest deficit of illegal immigration control, ineffective workplace screening and employer sanctions. The control impetus in the new law thus boils down to stricter border enforcement, doubling the number of border patrol agents to 10,000 by the year 2000, requiring the INS to build a 14-mile-long, 10-foot high, triple steel fence south of San Diego, and imposing stiff penalties on the flourishing business of smuggling aliens into the United States. This only reinforces existing policy. As in its various border operations 'Gatekeeper' or 'Hold the Line', the Democratic Clinton administration had cleverly pre-empted Republicans from occupying the immigration control discourse during the 1996 Presidential election campaign.

The one novelty of the 1996 Immigration Control and Financial Responsibility Act is to adjust unabated mass immigration to a welfare state under siege. Already a new welfare law, passed three months earlier, had made most legal immigrants ineligible for federally funded, means-tested welfare benefits, such as Supplemental Security Income (SSI) and food stamps.[96] The new immigration law added to this the concept of 'deeming', which requires the sponsors of family immigrants to have an income 125 per cent above the poverty line, and holding the sponsor legally responsible for supporting the immigrant in the case of neediness. This could significantly diminish the size of legal immigration in the future. However, a much more drastic proposal to deport legal immigrants who had become 'public charges' was dropped from the final bill. The Golden Door has certainly narrowed a bit, but the attempt to have it slammed shut has been averted.

This chapter described America's reopening to large-scale immigration after World War II, in the spirit of the civil rights revolution. The focus was on why the United States, in contrast to Europe's excluding new immigration after the first oil crisis, continued expansive open-door policies, which manifested themselves in the double legislative reforms on illegal and legal immigration in 1986 and 1990. I adduced two factors to explain this outcome: first, the civil-rights imperative of non-discrimination seized the immigration field, which prohibited effective controls of illegal immigration and (necessarily) Third-World targeted cuts of legal immigration. Secondly, immigration policy maintained low visibility throughout the 1980s, which helped a strange coalition of ethnic groups, agricultural producers, and free marketeers to shape legislation—a classic case of small but well-organized interests prevailing over the large but diffuse interests of the public. Even in asylum policy, the thrust has been liberalizing rather than restrictive, driven by the principle of source-country universalism and aggressive courts invoking constitutional norms to challenge harsh detention and expulsion measures of the federal government. The slim successes of the current movement for restricting legal and illegal immigration suggest that America will not stop being a nation of immigrants any time soon.

3

Not a Country of Immigration: Germany

Compared to the United States, whose reopening for mass immigration after World War II was framed by its emphatic self-definition as a nation of immigrants, Germany appears as the exact opposite. In the same period, (West) Germany became one of the largest immigrant-receiving countries in the world: between 1950 and 1993, the net migration balance has been an astounding 12.6 million, accounting for 80 per cent of the country's population growth (Müme and Ulrich, 1995: 3). But as of today, successive governments have stubbornly stuck to the maxim that Germany is 'not a country of immigration' (*kein Einwanderungsland*). The discrepancy between *de facto* immigration and its political denial is the single most enduring puzzle in the German immigration debate. However, the numerous critics of the 'not a country of immigration' formula have overlooked its normative character, and its grounding in national self-definition.[1] As such, the no-immigration formula is overdetermined by history and culture. As in all European nations, large-scale immigration postdated the nation-building experience in Germany. Accordingly, immigration has not become part of national self-definition. Like France, Germany had large-scale immigration before World War II. But this past has been (conveniently) forgotten, helped by the multiple and dramatic regime changes and accompanying breaks of memory.[2] No country in Europe conceives of itself as a 'nation of immigrants', US-style. From this angle, the puzzle is not why Germany doesn't do so, but why it should.

While Germany is not alone in Europe in not defining itself as a nation of immigrants, it is the only country that has not become tired of repeating it, elevating the no-immigration maxim to a first principle of public policy and national self-definition. Britain, for instance, pursued the same zero-immigration policies, but did not feel compelled to make much noise about it. This requires additional explanation. When it was first officially adopted by the federal government in 1977,[3] the no-immigration maxim already flew in the face of four million foreigners in Germany, who showed no sign of leaving. In fact, the no-immigration imperative is conditional upon the context of *de facto* immigration, because otherwise there would be no point of raising it. Extolling the no-immigration maxim was part of the Federal Republic's response to its guestworker immigration: as a historical episode that was not to be repeated.

But why this eagerness to close and historicize the guestworker episode? Recurrent immigration was at odds with the ethnocultural mode of German nationhood. While in principle delegitimized by its racist aberrations under the Nazi regime, ethnocultural nationhood was indirectly reinforced and prolonged by the outcome of World War II, with the division of Germany and the scattering of huge German diasporas in communist Eastern Europe and the Soviet Union. Against this backdrop, the Federal Republic defined itself as a vicarious, incomplete nation-state, home for all Germans in the communist diaspora. This mandate is expressed in the preamble to the Basic Law: 'The entire German people remains asked to complete the unity and freedom of Germany in free self-determination.' Much like Israel was the homeland of all Jews (West) Germany was the homeland of all Germans, and it prioritized the immigration of co-ethnics. This is enshrined in Article 116 of the Basic Law, which assigns automatic citizenship to ethnic German refugees from communism. Opening the national community to foreigners would have posed the risk of a redefinition of national identity, and of diluting the Federal Republic's historical obligation to its dispersed and repressed co-ethnics in the East. Kay Hailbronner (1983: 2113) put it this way: 'Conceiving of the Federal Republic as a country of immigration with multiple national minorities would contradict the Basic Law's conception of a provisional state geared toward the recovery of national unity.'

This implies that only the recovery of national unity and the end of communism have allowed a more relaxed attitude toward the no-immigration maxim. Tellingly, the resettlement of ethnic Germans has since been restricted by quota, approximating it to 'normal' immigration, while the calls for a self-conscious immigration policy have gained ground (see Bade, 1994*b*). To be sure, the space for such manœuvres is limited, especially in a European zero-immigration context. But after 1990 the grounding of the compulsively reiterated no-immigration maxim in incomplete nationhood is no more.

Given their opposite national self-descriptions and policy intentions, it is astounding that Germany and the United States have been
similarly expansive toward immigrants. In fact, shortly after the no-
immigration maxim was officially adopted, an influential legal study
drily concluded that 'the previous policy of "no immigration country" is no longer possible for constitutional reasons' (Schwerdtfeger,
1980: A131). The no-immigration rhetoric in the political arena has
always been counteracted by extensive rights and protections for foreigners granted by the legal system. The Basic Law tames sovereign
state power with a catalogue of universal human rights, such as liberty and family rights. They have helped transform the precarious
guestworker status into a secure permanent-resident status, which
equals that of citizens. Constitutional court rules on the staying of
deportation orders, the routine renewal of residence permits, and
family reunification rights have prevented the political executive
from following through on its no-immigration maxim (see Neuman,
1990).

This is not to say that after the recruitment stop of 1973 a radical
roll-back of the guestworker population has ever been seriously tried.
Next to legal constraints, moral constraints kept the political élite
from doing this. When the post-oil-shock recession was fuelling mass
unemployment, the federal government still declared that 'no legally
employed foreign worker . . . shall be forced to return home', while
rejecting the introduction of a rotation system.[4] The various schemes,
introduced in the early 1980s, to induce especially unemployed guestworkers and their families to return home have been strictly voluntary.
The political élite developed a sense of special obligation toward the
guestworker population, which it had brought into the country and
now could not be disposed of at will. Rebuffing a right-wing proposal
for a 'reasonable and humane rotation system' in the early 1980s, the
liberal Minister of the Interior made this moral obligation explicit:
'(The foreign workers) have not come here spontaneously. Instead, we
have brought them into this country since 1955 . . . Even if they are
without jobs, we have obligations toward them.'[5] To be sure, the
boundaries of such special obligations were contested, and drawn differently according to the issue at stake. Regarding family reunification, an unconditional right for settled foreigners to bring in their
spouses was granted only to the first generation, while restrictions
were imposed on the second generation, also to close a major loophole
for recurrent immigration.[6] Regarding integration measures, such as
easing the acquisition of citizenship, second- and third-generation for-

eigners were prioritized, because they were deemed to have cut all ties with their country of ancestry.

To sum up, legal and moral constraints on political élite discretion eventually converged not just to stabilize, but to increase the number of settled foreigners in Germany, recruitment stop and no-immigration maxim notwithstanding.

Foreigner Law and Policy

In assessing German foreigner law and policy, one has to be aware of their feeble origins. A legal-political framework for dealing with the more-than-temporary presence of foreigners originally did not exist. It had to be invented, by means of incremental steps. In the beginning, foreigner policy was labour-market policy. To counteract the inflationary pressure of a full employment economy, the federal government had signed recruitment agreements (*Anwerbeabkommen*) with a number of Mediterranean countries, beginning with Italy in 1955, followed by agreements with Spain and Greece in 1960, Turkey in 1961, Portugal in 1964, Tunisia and Morocco in 1965, and finishing with Yugoslavia in 1968. A pure form of client politics followed, devoid of parliamentary involvement or public debate, which involved only employers, the labour-recruiting government bureaucracy, and trade unions (whose initial reservations were quietened by securing the primacy of the domestic workforce in the filling of job openings, and by guaranteeing equal wages and social benefits to the recruited foreign workers). Upon the recruitment agreements, the Federal Employment Office opened field offices in Athens, Verona, Madrid, Istanbul, Belgrade, Lisbon, Casablanca, and Tunis to select suitable applicants, provide them with work and residence permits, and organize their collective transportation in specially chartered trains directly to their future employers—in a process whose bureaucratic precision one commentator found 'chillingly reminiscent of the 1930s and 1940s' (Katzenstein, 1987: 221).

The assumption that these 'guestworkers' would eventually return was initially shared on all sides. The guestworkers' provisional status was symbolized by their accommodation in army-style employer-provided mass quarters (see Herbert, 1986: 202–4). In fact, the assumption of return migration is the very rationale of a guestworker regime, which sees foreign labour as a conjuncturally disposable commodity without social reproduction and education costs. This assumption was reaffirmed as late as 1966–7, when the first postwar recession motivated between 300,000 and 500,000 foreign workers to leave the Federal Republic voluntarily (Katzenstein, 1987: 216).

During the first ten years of the guestworker era, the Nazi *Ausländerpolizeiverordnung* of 1938 provided the meagre legal framework for handling the presence of foreign workers in Germany. The introduction of a new Foreigner Law in 1965 was praised at the time as part of a 'liberal and cosmopolitan foreigner policy facilitating the conditions of entry and stay' (quoted in Hailbronner, 1984: 4). But it inherited the disposition of its predecessor to conceive of foreigners as a threat to the home population.[7] As Werner Kanein (1973: 729) put it, the Foreigner Law was a 'national special law (*nationales Sondergesetz*) limited to (the regulation of) the beginning, duration, and end of the presence of foreign nationals'. Whereas its Nazi predecessor had made the entry and stay of foreigners contingent upon their subjective 'worthiness', the new Foreigner Law shifted to the objective criterion of state interest. Paragraph 2(1) of the Foreigner Law stipulates: 'A residence permit may be issued if the presence of the foreigner does not harm the interests of the Federal Republic of Germany.' This increased the sovereignty of the state in issuing residence permits, because the individual could no longer effect a continuation of her stay by 'worthy' behaviour (see Dohse, 1981: 233–8). As Fritz Franz (1980: 162) outlines the rationale, 'with the "worthiness" clause of the old law immigration could not be prevented, while it could be prevented with the "interest" clause of the new law.'

Enshrining the supremacy of state interests, the Foreigner Law makes the issuance of residence permits virtually 'acts of grace' (Kanein, 1973) by the state. Extreme discretion on part of the executive and the complete absence of rights on part of the foreigner has been a (heavily criticized and eventually reformed) aspect of German foreigner law. To be sure, such executive discretion could go either way: liberal or restrictionist, and in conjunction with German-type 'co-operative federalism' (Katzenstein, 1987) it accounts for huge regional variations in foreigner policy.

A second deficit of German foreigner law is the initial lack of differentiated residence permits, and the absence of provision for more-than-temporary stays on German territory. Only in 1978, the introduction of the so-called 'permanence regulation' (*Verfestigungs-regelung*) stipulated conditions under which unrestricted residence permits could be issued: after five years of continuous residence, an unrestricted residence permit (*unbefristete Aufenthaltserlaubnis*) could be granted; after eight years stay, a furthergoing residence entitlement (*Aufenthaltsberechtigung*) could be awarded on demand, contingent upon proven language competence and a high degree of socioeconomic integration. The permanence regulation first introduced a residence status akin to US legal permanent resident status. To be sure, the new rules did not amount to individual rights that could be held against the state, and they left administrative discretion fully intact. But their introduction, by means of a largely unnoticed routine 'administrative order' (*Verwaltungsvorschrift*), was still a momentous event. Before 1978, long-term residence could be taken by a permit-granting local foreigner office as a reason not to renew a residence permit, because it contradicted the official 'no-immigration' policy after the recruitment stop. After 1978, long-term residence strengthened, rather than threatened, the legal status of the foreigner. A legal commentator concludes that with the introduction of permanence regulation '[the Federal Republic] has acknowledged that immigration has irrevocably taken place' (Heinrich, 1987: 983).[8]

A third deficit of the Foreigner Law was the complete absence of rules for family reunification. This was within the logic of a guest-worker regime, which conceived of the foreigner as a return-oriented, isolated carrier of labour power, devoid of family ties. Only in 1972, the foreign spouses of German nationals were granted unconditional residence rights that outcancelled the priority of 'state interests' in the Foreigner Law.[9] Detailed rules for reunifying foreign families were not devised before 1981. Introduced in order to close a major source of unwanted immigration after the recruitment stop, family reunification rules would remain a major stake in political conflict throughout the 1980s.

These residence-permit and family-reunification provisions, meant to fill the most glaring loopholes of the Foreigner Law, had only the status of administrative rule changes or federal government recommendations, respectively. They did not have the status of law. The absence of legislative reform, from 1965 to the passing of a new Foreigner Law in 1990, has been among the most striking peculiarities of German foreigner policy. As a legal scholar had complained already in 1980, 'the gravest deficiency [in German foreigner law] is the absolute passivity of the law-maker (*Gesetzgeber*), who has stolen himself out of his responsibility for years' (Tomuschat, 1980: 1079). Reviewing the deficiencies of the old Foreigner Law, Kay Hailbronner (1980: 231) similarly concluded that 'legal security has to replace the largely undetermined discretion of the administration'. Before a

modicum of such legal security was introduced in the new Foreigner
Law of 1990, foreigner policy was guided by *ad hoc* decisions of the
Conference of Interior Ministers, Cabinet recommendations, or
Bund-Länder agreements, all put into practice by means of federal and
state administrative rules (Meier-Braun, 1988: 59). Legislative absti-
nence may be explained by a variety of factors, such as sheer inattention, but perhaps also the attempt not to politicize unnecessarily a
delicate issue from which no direct constituency gains were to be
drawn.

Whatever the reasons for legislative passivity, a foreigner policy
based on administrative decree had to entail huge regional variations.
This is because German-style 'co-operative federalism' grants extreme
powers to the states. There are no federal agencies like the US
Immigration and Naturalization Service (INS), with its own field
offices throughout the states. In Germany, the local foreigner offices
that fulfill similar functions of issuing residence permits or ordering
deportations are liable to the *Land*, not the federal government. And
different *Land* governments, depending on the party in power and the
exposure to foreign migration, have pursued radically different foreigner policies. In general, the CDU/CSU-governed southern states of
Bavaria and Baden-Württemberg have pursued a restrictionist line, for
instance, imposing tougher family reunification rules than recommended by the federal government, while SPD-ruled Hesse and
Bremen have followed a liberal line, allowing more foreign family
members to join their relatives in Germany than recommended by the
federal government (see Meier-Braun, 1988: ch. 4). All federal policies
of inducing return migration or limiting ongoing immigration flows in
the 1980s have been first concocted by restrictionist state governments, most notably Baden-Württemberg. As a result of the regional
dispersal of authority in foreigner policy, foreigners living in
Hamburg, Munich, or Berlin faced radically discrepant chances of
having a residence permit renewed, a deportation stayed, or a spouse
and children joining them from the country of origin.

Federal fragmentation aggravated a final key characteristic of
German foreigner policy: the lack of an overarching conception. Still
in 1996, a leading politician demanded that 'Germany needs an overall
conception for immigration and integration.'[10] While the explicit reference to 'immigration' indicates a changed mindset *vis-à-vis* the 'not
a country of immigration' maxim, this is still an astonishing statement
to make after five decades of continuous foreign migration to
Germany. In his comparison of 'national models' of handling immi-

gration in some major Western states, James Hollifield (1994: 24) had to conclude that Germany did not have such a model, only a variety of *ad hoc* rules and policies that did not add up to a coherent whole.

Basic Law to the Rescue

Judged by the principles of German foreigner law and policy alone, the status of settled foreigners in Germany would be exceedingly precarious. Fortunately, this is not the case. Filling the vacuum created by the passiveness of the political branches of government, activist courts have expansively interpreted and defended the rights of foreigners. They could do this on the basis of a constitution that drew two fundamental lessons from recent German history, especially the history of the Third Reich: first, the subordination of state power to the rights of individuals; and secondly, granting the most fundamental of these rights without respect to nationality. Regarding the latter, the first seven articles of the Basic Law protect universal human rights, independent of national citizenship. As Josef Isensee (1974: 74) writes, 'the broken nation of the Basic Law seeks to find its spiritual unity and self-consciousness on the basis of human-rights universalism.' This is most emphatically expressed in Article 1 of the Basic Law, which stipulates that 'the dignity of the individual is untouchable'. Article 1 also introduces the principle of limited sovereignty, in obliging the state to 'respect' and 'protect' the dignity of the individual. In a conscious departure from the German state tradition, the German Basic Law puts the individual first, the state second; it is conceived in the spirit of limiting state sovereignty by individual rights.[11]

Applied to the immigration context, the limited sovereignty of the German state is expressed in the absence of a US-style plenary power doctrine. The admission and expulsion of aliens and the overall regulation of foreign migration is not deemed a prerogative of the political branches of government, in principle out of reach of judicial review. As Gerald Neuman (1990: 74–85) outlined, the greater reach of constitutional limitations on German (*de facto*) immigration policy is due to a number of factors: most importantly, the specific delegitimation of unfettered state sovereignty by Nazism; but also the general advantage of a young constitution written in the era of universal human rights, and untainted by older international law doctrines of absolute state sovereignty; and, finally, the absence of foreign policy considerations in German immigration policy.

While German foreigner law and policy is thus in principle subject to judicial review, this does not imply that state interests are thereby cancelled out. The supremacy of state interests in the Foreigner Law and of individual rights in the Basic Law are the two antipodes that courts had to reconcile in concrete decisions. This could be achieved, for instance, by means of the legal principle of proportionality (*Verhältnismässigkeit*), which stipulates that restrictions of individual rights had to be in proportion with the public good to be achieved.

The legal empowerment of foreigners in Germany had two pillars: legal scholarship, which carved out the doctrinary principles of constitutional protection for foreigners; and actual court rules putting these principles into practice. Regarding the former, the two most important legal statements are by Isensee (1974), who deduced the rights of foreigners from the principle of self-limited state sovereignty, and by Schwerdtfeger (1980), who postulated that over time the constitutional rights of foreigners approximated those of Germans.

Josef Isensee's report *The Constitutional Status of Foreigners in the Federal Republic of Germany*, presented at the 1973 Convention of the Society of Constitutional Lawyers in Mannheim, is based on an important distinction: regarding the first admission of foreigners, state sovereignty reigns supreme; but once a foreigner has been admitted to German territory, the equal protection of the law applies also to her, and state discretion is subsequently limited. According to Isensee (1974: 74 f.), the human-rights universalism of the Basic Law precludes two classical topoi of foreigner law: unfettered sovereignty and the treatment of foreigners according to a special 'guest law' (*Gastrecht*). Blowing to pieces the 'guestworker' construction of German foreigner law and policy, Isensee states: 'In the age of human rights the foreigner does not enjoy guest but home rights' (p. 75).

Accordingly, foreigners are entitled to extensive civil and social rights. Even the constitutional rights limited to Germans only, such as the rights of association, free movement and residence, or occupation, are not in principle foreclosed to foreigners. In this respect, Article 2(1) of the Basic Law, which protects the 'free development of personality', functions as a general 'residuary right' (*Auffanggrundrecht*) that endows the foreigner with legitimate claims even in those spheres that transcend the basic human rights.[12] For instance, once the state has admitted foreigners to the labour market, the principles of equal protection of the law and self-limited state power prohibit certain discriminations, such as higher taxes, bans on joining unions, or the priority hiring of Germans. In sum, the Basic Law 'empowers the foreigner with increasing status rights, to which on the side of the state corresponds a system of progressing self-limitation' (p. 85).

Gunther Schwerdtfeger's *Recommendations to Improve the Legal Status of Foreigners in Germany*, presented at the 1980 German Lawyers Convention in Berlin, radicalizes and systematizes an idea first introduced by Isensee: with the increasing length of stay on German territory, foreigners come to share with German nationals the 'legal fate of dependency' (*Rechtsschicksal der Unentrinnbarkeit*), so that their constitutional rights must approximate those of Germans. In non-legal terms: because they have nowhere else to go, settled foreigners must be treated like Germans. Accordingly, the degree of constitutional protection increases with the length of residence. Surveying the legal status of foreigners in crucial areas such as residence rights, welfare-state benefits, and labour-market participation, Schwerdtfeger concludes: 'With increasing length of residence the foreigners of the first generation, as well as their children who have grown up in Germany, reach a constitutional status that is equal or close to that of Germans' (p. A26). Like Isensee, Schwerdtfeger interprets the constitutional Article 2(1) expansively as a general *Auffanggrundrecht*, which allows foreigners to enjoy the rights normally reserved to Germans (such as residence and occupational rights).[13] But its material protection is dependent on the length of residence: 'The longer the stay in the Federal Republic, and the more the foreigner is dependent on developing his personality only in the Federal Republic [*Rechtsschicksal des Unentrinnbaren*], the more grows the material protection for the foreigner according to Article 2(1) of the Basic Law' (p. A32).

This does not rule out the possibility of restricting individual rights in light of state interests, according to the principle of proportionality. But from a certain point on, the constitutional claims of settled foreigners have become so strong that only parliamentary legislation could legitimate such restrictions (see ibid. A132). This was a clear hint that a restrictive foreigner policy as administrative decree policy was unconstitutional. The state was free to deny the first entry and settlement of new-seed immigrants. But once they had been let in, and the moment of practising strict rotation had slipped away, there was no going back: 'After the state has allowed the "guestworker wave" to happen, the automatism of constitutional law steps in. Already for constitutional reasons a return to the status quo ante is no longer possible' (p. A45).

Isensee and Schwerdtfeger's programmatic statements about the legal status of foreigners both reflected and further incited actual court rules. The three most important of these rules, issued between 1973 and 1987, concerned the residence status of foreigners and their right to be joined by family members. Taken together, these court rules ratified that the temporary guestworker programme had turned into permanent, even self-reinforcing immigration, undermining the restrictionist foreigner policy after the recruitment stop.

Enjoying the broad civil and social rights guaranteed by the constitution and the territoriality principle of the welfare state[14] is contingent upon a secure residence status, originally the Achilles' heel in the life of *de facto* immigrants in Germany.[15] Two landmark rules of the Constitutional Court (*Bundesverfassungsgericht*) severely limited the discretion of the state to deport foreigners or deny them a renewed residence permit. The so-called Arab case, decided in July 1973, concerned the issue of deportation.[16] Previously, the primacy of state interests in the Foreigner Law had allowed easy routine deportations, in which settled foreigners who had committed a small delinquency like drunk driving or petty theft were ordered to leave the Federal Republic immediately (see Dohse, 1981: 240–4). In the Arab Case, the Constitutional Court declared such deportations unconstitutional. The case concerned two Palestinian students, who had been living in the Federal Republic since the early 1960s. After the Palestinian terrorist attack on Israeli athletes during the Munich Olympic Games in 1972, administrative courts ordered the students' immediate expulsion as 'security risks', because both had been members of a Palestinian student organization suspected of harbouring contacts with terrorists. The Constitutional Court ruled that the immediate expulsion orders violated the plaintiffs' constitutional liberty rights according to Article 2(1) and the principle of legal stateness, guaranteed by Article 19(4) of the Basic Law.[17] Since the two students were not accused of any personal wrongdoing, and the risk of their committing a terrorist act during the court consideration of the appeal was negligible, their personal liberty interests outweighed the public interest in their immediate removal. This was a momentous court rule. For the first time, the Constitutional Court affirmed that foreigners had rights protected by the constitution, which—according to the principle of proportionality—could outweigh the interests of the state (see Pietzcker, 1975). As the Court argued, the 'public interest [has to be] balanced against the private interests of the respective foreigner, that is, the impact of the deportation on his economic, professional, and private life, . . . as well as on his other social ties' (Arab Case, 1974: 401).

A second landmark rule, the so-called Indian Case, decided in September 1978, concerned the renewal of residence permits.[18] According to the Foreigner Law, there is no legal difference between a first and a renewed residence permit. Paragraph 21(3) of the Foreigner Law stipulates: 'An appeal [against a denied residence permit] has no staying effect [*aufschiebende Wirkung*]. The same holds for a foreigner's application for a renewed residence permit.' First and renewed residence permits are essentially acts of grace, in which the principle of proportionality does not apply, and in which the previous length of stay makes no difference (see Dohse, 1981: 240). In the Indian Case, the Constitutional Court found this equalization of first and renewed residence permits unconstitutional. The case involved an Indian national, who had first entered the Federal Republic in 1961 as an apprentice in the metal industry, and since 1967 was continuously employed by a construction firm, all on the basis of routinely renewed residence permits. In September 1973, the local foreigner office declined to renew his residence permit, arguing that his further presence would harm the interests of the Federal Republic because he was seeking permanent settlement in Germany, beyond his original purpose of seeking occupational training. A state administrative court upheld this decision in reference to the federal government's no-immigration policy. In overturning the lower court rule, the Constitutional Court argued that the non-renewal of the residence permit was in violation of Article 2(1) of the Basic Law, in conjunction with the principle of legal stateness. More concretely, the Court held that the previous routine renewals had created a constitutionally protected 'reliance interest' (according to the principle of *Vertrauensschutz*) in continued residence. The Court famously added that this reliance interest outweighed the no-immigration maxim of public policy: 'For a rejection of the residence permit renewal it is not sufficient to point to the general maxim that the Federal Republic is not a country of immigration' (Indian Case, 1979: 186). The Indian decision entailed a significant limitation on the government's options in foreigner policy: a policy of expulsion and forced repatriation was ruled out for constitutional reasons.[19]

The Arab and Indian decisions of the Constitutional Court secured the residence rights of *de facto* immigrants, effectively prohibiting the government to return to the status quo ante by means of deportation and termination of residence permits.[20] In a third landmark decision, the Turkish and Yugoslav Case of 1987, the Court turned to the issue of family reunification.[21] This was a much trickier terrain, because it did not involve the rights of established residents but the initial grant of new residence permits. Since the recruitment stop of 1973, the chain migration of families of guestworkers was (next to asylum) one of two major avenues of ongoing migration flows to Germany, in patent contradiction of the official no-immigration policy. Since December 1981, the federal government recommended that the responsible states severely restrict the entry of foreign spouses of second-generation guestworkers, and make such family reunification contingent upon an eight-year residence minimum of the resident spouse and a post-marital waiting period of one year. Characteristically, the states implemented this recommendation highly unevenly. Liberal Hesse lowered the residence requirement to five years; restrictionist Bavaria increased the waiting period for spouses to three years; and hyper-restrictionist Baden-Württemberg even broke the existing élite consensus of not limiting first-generation family reunification by extending the three-year rule from second- to first-generation guestworkers.

One Yugoslav and two Turkish parties challenged these restrictive rules on family reunification, arguing that they violated Article 6 of the Basic Law, which protects the integrity of marriage and the family. In a complicated decision that betrays a hesitation to restrict the state's capacity to control a major source of recurrent immigration, the Court held that Article 6 did not imply a constitutional right of entry for non-resident spouses. But non-resident family members still possessed family rights under Article 6 that foreigner law and policy had to respect, according to the principle of proportionality. In this light, the Court upheld the challenged eight-year residence requirement and the one-year waiting rule, arguing that these measures were necessary to guarantee the social and economic integration of the resident spouse and to prevent sham marriages, respectively. But Bavaria and Baden-Württemberg's three-year waiting rule was found disproportionate, because of its destructive effect on young marriages. Interestingly, the Court criticized especially Baden-Württemberg's extension of the three-year waiting rule to the first generation: 'The Federal Republic of Germany has shouldered a special degree of responsibility toward the [directly] recruited [guestworkers], which is violated by the three-year waiting rule' (Turkish and Yugoslav Case, 1988: 70).

The Court's Turkish and Yugoslav decision may be read as 'retrenchment from earlier, more protective attitudes' (Neuman, 1990: 63).[22] Apart from invalidating Baden-Württemberg and Bavaria's three-year rules, the Court rule granted a 'wide space of action' to the political branches of government (Weides and Zimmermann, 1988: 1415). Denying a right of entry for non-resident spouses, the Court reaffirmed the basic sovereignty of the state to control the entry of aliens: '. . . legislature and executive are free to decide in which number and under which conditions aliens may enter the Federal Republic' (Turkish and Yugoslav Case, 1988: 47). The Court furthermore approved some family-related pressure in order to provide incentives for return migration, and even approved the wide variations in the *Länder* regulations of family reunification. But a less restrictive Court rule, such as construing a right of entry according to Article 6, would have amounted to mandating a generation-spanning, recurrent immigration process, in direct opposition to the government's attempt to prevent just that. While less assertive than in its rules on the rights of settled foreigners, the Court's decision on family reunification still went far beyond the most liberal decisions of the US Supreme Court in this area, first in constraining the government's power to regulate family-based immigration at all, and secondly in rejecting a quota system as unconstitutional and applying constitutional protection also to aliens not residing on German territory (see Motomura, 1995: 13–19). Most importantly, in deducing a modicum of family reunification rights from Article 6, the Court decreed that *de facto* immigration could not remain limited to the directly recruited guestworker population, but had become a recurrent, self-reproducing process for constitutional reasons alone.

Emergent Moral Élite Consensus: The Failed Campaign Against Family Reunification

Turning from the legal to the political process, the German case exhibits some striking differences from the US case. First, the relative weight of the legal and political processes is exactly the reverse in each case. In Germany, the legal process is key to explaining the expansiveness and inclusiveness toward foreigners; as the analysis of the long-winded making of the new Foreigner Law of 1990 will show, the political process only caught up with positions that had long been established and determined by the legal process. By contrast, in the United States the political process had been key to explaining expansive immigration policies, whereas the reach of judicial review was limited by the plenary power doctrine. Much follows from this crucial difference. For constitutional reasons, the space for implementing the political 'no immigration' maxim was limited, to say the least, and much noisy manœuvring about repatriation, rotation, or prohibiting family reunification belongs to the realm of shadow boxing, or 'symbolic politics' as political scientists prefer to say.

The distinction between legal and political processes, and a comparison of their different constellations across polities, adds an important nuance to Gary Freeman's (1995*a*) correct finding of the inherently expansive and inclusive thrust of liberal democracies toward immigrants. Freeman's focus on convergent outcomes partially obscures the radically different processes that lead to them. In particular, a look at the German case forces one to modify the anti-populist, anti-discriminatory norm that Freeman found equally strong across liberal polities.[23] The range of drastic solutions in a European non-settler nation, however futile in the end, was more extreme and more mainstream-based than Freeman would predict. Getting tough on 'foreigners' was clearly not as tabooed in Germany as getting tough on 'immigrants' in the United States, where even legitimately tough stances on illegal immigrants were tempered by the racism verdict. Even at the legal plane, German foreigner law violates non-discriminatory norms and the principle of source-country universalism in drawing categorical distinctions between non-privileged foreigners and privileged foreigners (such as EU nationals and special-treaty nationals), which would never pass constitutional muster in the United States (see Neuman, 1990: 73). At the political plane, Turks were singled out as an undesired, 'difficult' foreigner group, which went far beyond concerns about 'unassimilable' Hispanics in the United States. These different stances are grounded in different national self-understandings. 'Foreigners' could never be part of 'us' in an ethnic nation, opening up the possibility of drastic solutions, and limiting even a liberal solution to a 'fair compromise' [*fairer Ausgleich*] between two separate collectivities.[24] By contrast, 'immigrants' in a self-described 'nation of immigrants' were already part of 'us', radically limiting the range of drastic solutions and reinforcing the imperative of non-discrimination.

The story of the German political process regarding foreigners after the recruitment stop is one of the successive cancelling out of drastic solutions, culminating in the liberalized Foreigner Law of 1990. Why and how were drastic solutions cancelled out? First, political élites have not been unaware of the legal impossibility of forced repatriation or rotation schemes, limiting such calls to fringe voices within the major parties and political institutions. Secondly, the drastic solutions that were tried out did not work. For instance, denying work permits to young foreigners who had belatedly joined their parents in Germany threatened to create a demoralized, crime-prone subproletariat in the inner cities; accordingly, this restrictive measure had to be quickly abandoned. Thirdly, and most importantly, within the political élite a consensus developed of a special obligation toward the recruited guestworker population. This allowed a historical closing of the guestworker episode. Getting tough on sources of recurrent immigration, such as asylum-seekers and the outer family layers of resident foreigners, could be legitimized by being generous to those foreigners toward whom a direct moral obligation existed. Such generosity was the best way of realizing the no-immigration intention. Fourthly, moral obligations toward foreigners in Germany, not just the historical guestworkers, were powerfully reinforced by a liberal public and an increasingly organized foreigner lobby of churches, charity organizations, and unions, which first demonstrated its clout in the debate leading to the new Foreigner Law of 1990.

In a further difference from US immigration policy, after the recruitment stop German foreigner policy abandoned its character of client politics. Employer interests now diverged from the principles and direction of foreigner policy, which was forged by relatively autonomous state élites. Despite massive campaigning by the Federation of German Employers (*Bund deutscher Arbeitgeber*, BDA) for seasonal guestworker schemes or even a *Karenzzwang*-type rotation system, the recruitment stop remained firmly in place.[25] This meant putting up with severe employment impasses in economic sectors that were highly dependent on foreign workers, such as agriculture, the hotel and restaurant sector, and the mining and steel industries.[26] For the federal government, the recruitment stop was commanded by domestic security considerations alone—the problem of urban ghettoization and lacking social integration, which had been completely neglected during the first two decades of guestworker recruitment, and the problem of growing domestic unemployment at the end of the postwar boom, which fed the resentment of Germans against the foreigners.

Between 1973 and 1978 the migration balance had been mostly negative. But from 1979 onwards the number of foreigners began to rise sharply. This suddenly shifted attention to the problem of unregulated family reunification. The gravity of this problem is demonstrated by statistics that show the changing demographic composition of the foreigner population after the recruitment stop. Between 1973 and 1980, the number of foreign workers fell from 2,595,000 to 2,070,000; but at the same time, the absolute number of foreigners increased from 3,966,200 in 1973 to 4,450,000 in 1980, accounting for 7.5 per cent of the total population (Herbert, 1986: 188). Subtracting asylum-seekers, whose number remained negligible until the late 1970s, only family reunification could account for this increase, in obvious defiance of recruitment stop and the no-immigration policy of the government.

And more were yet to come. A government-commissioned study of 1981 estimated the as yet unrealized potential of family reunification at 1.35 million, including 500,000 children under 18 living in non-EU states, 250,000 spouses living in non-EU states, and 600,000 potential spouses of second- and third-generation foreigners approaching adulthood by 2000.[27] In late 1981, the federal government estimated that 450,000 foreigners had entered on the family-reunification ticket during the last three years. If these trends were to continue, the number of foreigners in Germany could exceed the 7 million mark by the year 2000.[28] This prospect pushed the federal government to finally tackle one of the major sources of recurrent immigration, family reunification.

When family reunification became the focus of foreigner policy in the early 1980s, the conditions for a generous solution did not exist. At this time, the Federal Republic was undergoing its first society-wide backlash against foreigners. A survey showed that the share of Germans who favoured the return migration of foreigners increased from 39 per cent in November 1978 to 66 per cent in December 1981.[29] The reasons for this backlash are manifold. When the second oil crisis pushed the unemployment rate toward the 2 million mark, the perfect symmetry of 2 million unemployed Germans and 2 million employed guestworkers was tailor-made for populist agitation. Secondly, in 1980 the number of asylum-seekers reached the unprecedented number of over 100,000, opening up a second front of foreigner-related concerns, and creating the spectre of cataclysmic, uncontrolled mass immigration. Thirdly, the ethnic composition of the foreigner population was for the first time subjected to public scrutiny. This is because Turks had meanwhile become the largest foreigner group, with 1.4 million in 1981, having increased by over 30 per cent during the previous three years. In fact, of all foreigner groups in Germany the Turkish was the only one which was still growing, rather than shrinking. Not just in dubious circles, a perception took hold that 'the foreigner problem . . . is a Turkish problem'.[30] A conservative opinion leader warned against the 'Orientalization of Europe',[31] but also the social-liberal

coalition government expressed its concern that the foreigner population was increasingly dominated by nationalities that 'stand at greater
distance from our culture'. If this development continued unchecked,
as the government justified its planned restrictions on family reunification, 'the point could be reached from which the resentment of large
parts of the German population turns into open hostility. The result
would be social and political tensions that threaten the societal peace
in the Federal Republic'.[32] As always since the recruitment stop,
domestic-security concerns, rather than the logic of client politics,
drove the government's foreigner policy.

But the concrete dynamics of resorting to restrictive measures were
more hideous still. In a clear example of the politicizing effect of federalism in German foreigner policy, the social-liberal federal government was pushed into action by the conservative *Länder* governments
of Baden-Württemberg, Berlin, and Schleswig-Holstein, which had
issued restrictive rules on family reunification in the second half of
1981 (see Meier-Braun, 1988: 166–9). Most drastic was the so-called
Lummer Decree of Berlin (named after its author, the hardline Interior
Senator Heinrich Lummer, CDU), which included measures such as
deporting unemployed second-generation foreigners. Under such
pressure the federal government issued the drastic statement that 'the
family reunification of non-EU nationals has to be stopped by all legal
means compatible with the Basic Law' (ibid. 19).

However, the government's Decree on the Socially Responsible
Regulation of Family Reunification, issued in early December 1981,
was a good deal mellower than might have been expected. Regarding
children, the cut-off age of family reunification was lowered from
eighteen to sixteen years; furthermore, children were no longer permitted to join a single parent, or parents who were students. However,
spouses were considered the more serious source of recurrent immigration. Regarding spouses, a distinction was drawn between first-
and second-generation foreigners. For first-generation spouses, no
restrictions were imposed. By contrast, second-generation spouses
were generally excluded from family reunification, unless they had
reached the age of eighteen, the resident spouse had lived at least eight
years in the Federal Republic, and the marriage existed already for one
year. Interestingly, the negative formulation of this second-generation
restriction suggests toughness, whereas the actually stipulated conditions leave much space for family-building.

But the symbolic targeting of second-generation foreigners for
restrictive measures betrays the intention to draw the boundaries of

special moral obligations narrowly around the directly recruited guestworkers, while seeking to prevent historical turning into recurrent immigration. The federal government made this motivation explicit in its defence of the new family reunification policy before the Constitutional Court: 'Because of its recruitment of foreign workers the Federal Republic has accepted a special responsibility towards the recruited; but it has not obliged itself to accept a generation-spanning immigration of family members. The number of immigrating family members could be perpetually renewed by marriage and birth. The federal government does not see itself constitutionally obliged toward the children and grandchildren of recruited foreigners to accept family immigration that is exclusively determined by the personal decisions of the individuals, without consideration of the interests of the Federal Republic.'[33]

Far from settling the debate over family reunification, the new rules were only the beginning of new conflict along party-political and territorial lines. Regarding the first, the parliamentary opposition parties CDU/CSU found the government's policy insufficiently restrictive, launching one of the most inflammatory politicization campaigns in the history of German foreigner policy. The CDU/CSU cynically put out that family reunification was to occur, but only in the country of origin. In strong language, the party's parliamentary faction held the federal government responsible for the rising xenophobia and the 'unbearable political situation' of the day.[34] The march into a 'multi-nationality state' had to be stopped, because the Federal Republic was a 'national unity state' and 'part of a divided nation'. Accordingly, family reunification should not become a means of 'circumventing' the recruitment stop. Instead, an appropriate foreigner policy had to encourage the return migration of foreigners.

The conservative campaign against the SPD/FDP government's new family reunification rules culminated at a *Bundestag* debate in February 1982, where the opposition parties advocated a 'reasonable and humanitarian rotation system'.[35] As the parliamentary leader of the CDU, Alfred Dregger, pointed out, 'the return migration of foreigners had to be the rule' if the country was to remain 'open' to foreigners. Interestingly, this call for a rotation system was based on an argument about integration. In language that would be inconceivable in the United States, the CDU leader drew a discriminatory distinction between four foreigner groups, some good, some bad: German-speaking foreigners and European foreigners, both of which posed no integration problems; and Turks and, prospectively, Asians and

Africans,[36] who could not (and should not)[37] be assimilated. Because the latter formed the majority of current migration, rotation was the adequate response. The CDU hardliner's advocacy of return migration is interesting also in a second regard: it revokes the élite consensus of a special moral obligation toward the recruited guestworkers. 'To demand [the return migration of foreigners] is not immoral,' the CDU leader sternly declared; 'the recruited foreigners—not all of them have been recruited—certainly have followed only their own interest.' Dregger's equally hardline colleague, Eduard Spranger of the Bavarian CSU, brushed away 'humanitarian obligations' in even more drastic terms: 'It is a fact that [the foreigners] have come without being forced to come, in order to make a living here. It is also a fact that the Germans have a right that the federal government acts in their interest.' Such extreme positions have always been just that: extreme positions, with little impact on actual policies. But the fact that they were raised by leading politicians of mainstream parties indicates the brittleness of anti-populist norms in Germany, and the existence of challenges to a moderate and centrist foreigner policy.

A second line of conflict over family reunification was territorial. Because they did not have the character of binding law, the federal government rules on family reunification were implemented differently in different states (see Hailbronner, 1984: 195–8). Baden-Württemberg and Bavaria, advocating a tougher stance on second-generation marriages, introduced their three-year rule that was eventually found unconstitutional. At the other extreme, Bremen refused to lower from eighteen to sixteen years the maximum age of foreign children entitled to join their parents. Hesse, under the first Red-Green coalition government in 1984, pursued the most liberal policy of all, which included increasing the maximum age for foreign children to eighteen years and lowering the residence requirement for second-generation marriages from eight to five years. Also 'suitable housing' (a requirement for new residence permits) was differently interpreted in different states: Baden-Württemberg demanded twelve square-metres of living space for each family member, counting also the residence-entitled children living abroad; Bremen required only seven square-metres per member, not counting children abroad.

A reform of the Foreigner Law had been envisaged but perpetually postponed since the early 1980s. Underneath the divergent preferences for a more liberal or a more restrictive law, there was general agreement that the 'legal patchwork' of multiple, and often contradicting, administrative rules and decrees had to be streamlined and brought back under parliamentary control.[38] The reform effort switched to high gear under a restriction-minded CDU/FDP-led federal government, which had gained power in 1982. A first informal draft for a new Foreigner Law was issued by the Interior Ministry in September 1983. It included harsh measures, most notably a six-year age limit for the family immigration of children and a ban on marriage immigration for second-generation foreigners. In particular Interior Minister Friedrich Zimmermann's (CSU) crusade against the family immigration of children crossed the threshold of the morally acceptable.[39] 'No comparable country in Europe or North America,' said an outraged Commissioner for Foreigner Affairs, Lieselotte Funcke (FDP), 'would condone such a family-hostile [*familienfeindlich*] proposition.' Pointing at the moral impossibility of implementing this measure, her colleague Burkhart Hirsch (FDP) imagined 'with horror what would happen here if a child who overstayed a visit was forcibly separated from its parents and thrown out of the country'.[40] For the liberal leadership of the Free Democratic Party, headed by the party chair and Foreign Minister Hans-Dietrich Genscher himself, opposition to the Interior Minister's illiberal foreigner policy became a litmus test of party identity within the new coalition government. When the SPD parliamentary faction coolly launched a Great Inquiry on the Further Development of Foreigner Law in April 1984, in order to expose the severe coalition rift between CSU and FDP, Genscher blocked the Interior Ministry's written response, arguing that it lacked 'a liberal signature'.[41] The revised, final government response followed Genscher's line, announcing that no law would be passed to restrict the family immigration of children (see Meier-Braun, 1988: 47). In view of temporarily low immigration pressure,[42] Chancellor Kohl decided to shelve a reform of the Foreigner Law for four more years.

The second attempt to introduce a new Foreigner Law ended in equal embarrassment for the hardline Interior Minister. In February 1988, a 260-page draft for an ultra-restrictive new law leaked out to the public. It was the most stringent (but, as it turned out, intolerable) attempt so far to realize the 'no immigration' principle of German foreigner policy, and to historize the guestworker recruitment as a unique, non-recurrent event. The draft law was actually two laws, a generous Foreigner Integration Law that included various benefits and entitlements for the historical guestworker population, and a restrictive Foreigner Residence Law that denied a permanent-resident

status to all non-EU foreigners who had come later and under different provisions, such as refugees or students. In perfect correspondence
to the logic of German foreigner policy since the recruitment stop, the
draft law stated that the 'integration offer to the recruited foreign
workers is contingent upon treating [this recruitment] as a historically
unique, finite event'.[43] In turn, the purpose of the complementary
Foreigner Residence Law was characterized as 'preventing the permanent immigration of foreigners', strictly limiting the maximum stay of
these non-guestworker foreigners to eight years. Explicitly tying the
no-immigration maxim to the pecularities of German nationhood, the
draft justified its prevention of permanent immigration in reference to
the 'maintenance of national character', which was a 'historical obligation in light of the unresolved national question of the Germans'. As
a critic correctly summarized, Zimmermann's restrictive draft law
conceived 'of the foreigner as a "threat", from which national culture
must be protected. There is no consideration . . . of the interests of
foreigners' (Prantl, 1994: 70).

What had underlain the entire German policy approach toward foreigners since the guestworker period, could no longer be openly
stated, or even prolonged into the future, by the late 1980s. Even
within the CDU, especially the party's liberal Employee Section
(*Sozialausschüsse*), a new perception of the foreigner as 'partner' and
'co-citizen' had taken hold, which could not be reconciled with
Zimmermann's nationalist ruminations.[44] An unprecedentedly broad
coalition of political parties, charity organizations, unions, and
churches mobilized against the restrictive draft law of the Interior
Minister, busily convening and forging declarations at the Evangelical
Academy in Tutzing or the Catholic Academy in Stuttgart.[45] Even the
Catholic Bishops, who had so far stayed at a distance, jumped into the
fray, criticizing the 'narrow' pursuit of 'national interests' in foreigner
policy, and rejecting the concept of deterrence as 'socially unresponsi-
ble'.[46] Facing such broad public opposition, the draft law of the
Interior Minister had to be withdrawn.

If Interior Minister Zimmermann did everything wrong, his successor Wolfgang Schäuble (CDU) did everything right. The third, and
final, approach to a new Foreigner Law came under the heading of
'pragmatism' and 'deideologization'.[47] Worried by a new anti-
immigrant party, the *Republikaner*, that was gaining ground in recent
state and communal elections, the new and more liberal Interior
Minister decided to keep foreigner policy out of partisan politics. At
breathtaking speed, but from the start involving the FDP coalition

partner and even the pro-foreigner lobby of churches and charity organizations, Schäuble pushed his bill from first draft in September 1989 to final legislation in April 1990, just in time to keep the issue out of the federal election campaign of the autumn of 1990 (see Bade, 1994: 62–5). This was no small feat, considering the preceding eight years of repeatedly aborted reform efforts.

The new Foreigner Law, which went into effect in January 1991, is remarkable in several regards. As the CSU noticed in dismay, the 'not a country of immigration' formula cannot be found anywhere in the text of the new law. Also absent is the objective of encouraging the return migration of foreigners, which had been a key goal of foreigner policy since 1982. The law thus acknowledged that by 1990 almost 70 per cent of all foreigners had lived in Germany for ten years or more and that since 1970 1.5 million foreigners had been born in Germany. The past immigration could obviously not be undone, as the objective of return migration had falsely suggested. The new Foreigner Law is conceived in the spirit of replacing executive discretion by individual rights to be held against the executive. Above all, this meant putting into law the already existing administrative rules and legal constraints. For instance, according to the new law the issuing of unrestricted residence permits or the allowing of family immigration to children under sixteen was no longer at the discretion of the state; foreigners now had statutory residence and family rights, as long as certain conditions were fulfilled. The Foreigner Law thus essentially ratified what constitutional court rules had long established. But in several respects the law went beyond existing administrative and legal rules and practices. Regarding family reunification, the one-year waiting period for second-generation marriages, which had been found constitutional in 1987, was abolished. In addition, spouses and children were granted own residence rights, independently of the head of family. Finally, second- or third-generation foreigners who had temporarily returned to their home country were given the right of return. These measures indicate the independent workings of moral obligations, not just of legal constraints.

At the same time, the Foreigner Law of 1990 did not entail a 'fundamentally new foreigner policy' (Hailbronner, 1990: 57). It replicated the fundamental distinction between Germans and foreigners, however couched in a friendlier rhetoric of 'partnership'. It still conceived of the recruitment of guestworkers as a 'historically unique event', seeking to prevent the permanent immigration of non-EU nationals in the future (see Franz, 1990: 8). This implies, interestingly, a scheme for a new rotation system, in which the temporariness of new labour migration is explicitly inscribed and secured from the start. Obviously, the lesson of the guestworker period is: Never again! The new Foreigner Law thus stopped short of shifting to a self-conscious immigration policy, as had been demanded by the foreigner lobby.[48] But the new law bears little resemblance to its restrictive, aborted predecessors. Perhaps it contains as much liberalization as has been possible within the old framework of foreigner policy.

Recovering Sovereignty in Asylum Policy

Next to family reunification, asylum has been the second avenue of continued *de facto* immigration after the recruitment stop. If the guestworker-related foreigner policy had moved along a path of increasing liberalization and self-limited sovereignty, asylum policy moved into the opposite direction of increasing restrictionism and recovered sovereignty. This opposite movement must be seen in the context of uniquely impaired state sovereignty in asylum policy. Alone in the world, the German constitution provides a subjective right for political refugees to be granted asylum. Article 16 of the Basic Law stipulates: 'People who are politically persecuted enjoy the right of asylum.' In Germany, the right of asylum is not, as everywhere else, the right of the state to grant asylum, to be held against the persecuting state (see Goodwin-Gill, 1983), but the right of the persecuted individual to be held against the receiving state. This is a unique limit on state sovereignty, with unique implications. It invalidates the sovereign right of the state to deny access to its territory: every non-national claiming, however spuriously, to be politically persecuted enjoys the right of entry and the full arsenal of legal-constitutional protection, including access to the Constitutional Court.[49] Germany was the only state in the world that granted not only its own nationals, but literally the whole world a right of entry. The 'quick and dirty' border-screening, practised by all other states in the age of mass asylum-seeking (see Martin, 1988), has not been an option here. The constitutional right of asylum made Germany Europe's, if not the world's, prime target for the 'asylum strategy of immigration' (Teitelbaum, 1984: 77). Germany's asylum debate thus revolves around protecting, or abolishing, this vestige of German exceptionalism. Ironically, only European integration would eventually allow Germany to recover its sovereignty in asylum policy.[50]

Germany's unique asylum law has been a response to its negative Nazi past. The fathers of the Basic Law, many of them exiled during the Nazi regime, conceived of an asylum law that went far beyond existing international law as a conscious act of redemption and atonement. As Carlo Schmid famously defended Article 16 in 1948, 'the granting of asylum is always a question of generosity and if you want to be generous, you must take the risk of being mistaken in a particular case' (quoted in Wolken, 1988: 24). As a 'confessional right', the constitutional right of asylum depended on 'the continued presence of the [Nazi] experience' (Rottmann, 1984: 344). Accordingly, asylum advocates elevated Article 16 into a quasi-sacred taboo: 'The promise of the constitutional right of Article 16 . . . must remain untouched.'[51] On the other hand, one of the earliest advocates of abolishing Article 16 considered himself 'part of a generation that is free of personal guilt', pointing out the mundane need for the state to get out of its self-made asylum trap: 'We can't have our asylum law dictated by our guilt for the past.'[52] Because it was tied up with deeply divided views about national identity, the German asylum debate was more polarized and emotional-led than elsewhere. And only the time-bound weakening of the Nazi presence ('normalization' some would say) allowed the infringement of the tabooed 'confessional right' at all.

German asylum policy has revolved around two separate axes of conflict, a territorial axis and a political axis. The territorial axis has been dominant during a first round of conflict, from the late 1970s to the mid-1980s, in which the constitutional right of asylum remained largely unquestioned. In this phase, municipalities and *Länder* governments, which are legally responsible for providing housing and social welfare benefits for asylum-seekers, have unitedly pushed for more restrictive legislation through the second federal legislative chamber, the *Bundesrat*. There was initially great variation among the *Länder* in the treatment of asylum-seekers, which largely corresponded to their different stances in foreigner policy. The southern *Länder* of Bavaria and Baden-Württemberg, conservative but also vulnerable to south-to-north migrations, spearheaded measures of deterrence, such as herding asylum-seekers in camps, providing in-kind benefits only, imposing work-bans, and being quicker to deport rejected asylum applicants. The northern *Länder* of Lower Saxony and North Rhine-Westphalia and the city-states of Bremen and Hamburg, liberal but also more insulated, initially shied away from such negative measures. But the ensuing intra-German north–south pull of asylum-seekers forced the gentler north into a 'deterrence competition' (Münch, 1992: 140) that eventually flattened such differences.

Tellingly, a *Land* chief, Oskar Lafontaine (SPD) of the Saarland, stung by a local episode of fierce popular opposition to Romanian refugees, was one of the first major politicians to openly question the constitutional right of asylum.[53] But his quick silencing by the Social-Democratic party leadership indicates that this second round of the German asylum debate, which focused on Article 16 of the Basic Law, was made of different cloth. In this second round of conflict, the political Left vs. Right axis, as defined above all by different stances toward the national past, was dominant: the Left arguing that the humanitarian obligations stemming from the Nazi past made Article 16 sacrosanct; the Right arguing that no such obligations existed, and that in the interest of political stability Article 16 had to be abolished.

Before the debate about Article 16 started in earnest, the first round of asylum conflict was about neutralizing the constitutional asylum right through tightened legal procedures and measures of social deterrence.[54] This led to a curious disjuncture between a uniquely liberal asylum law and a harsh deterrence regime that a 1983 UNHCR report found equally 'unique in Europe' (Wolken, 1988: 60). Such deterrence must be seen in the context of Germany's zero-immigration policy after the oil crisis. After the recruitment stop in 1973, asylum was the only legal avenue available for non-family entries. Immediately after the guestworker stop, the number of asylum applications began to multiply.[55] The lifting of a general work-ban in 1975 (in order to ease the financial burdens of municipalities and states) and the equal distribution, since early 1974, of asylum applicants to the *Länder*, which made the industrial centres of the Ruhr and Rhine/Main accessible for the new migrants, amounted to additional invitations to pursue the asylum strategy of immigration. When the number of new asylum-seekers passed the 100,000 mark for the first time in 1980, more than half of them were Turks—also the biggest group of guestworkers in Germany. This led to obvious inconsistencies: new Turks arriving on the asylum ticket were granted automatic work permits, while Turks arriving under the family-reunification ticket had to wait several years before they were allowed to work.[56]

There is ample evidence that the notion of 'bogus asylum-seekers' (*Scheinasylanten*), which was the focus of the first society-wide debate over asylum in 1980, was not the invention of vitriolic right-wingers—even though the CDU did everything to politicize the issue, much like it did in the case of foreigner policy.[57] In the early 1980s, Turkish newspapers reprinted the German government form required to claim asylum, and a market developed in South Asia (especially Pakistan) for 'package tours' that included one-way air fare and legal instruction on how to apply for asylum upon arrival (see Teitelbaum, 1984: 79). Before the infamous *Asyl-Schleuse* (asylum gate) of East Berlin was closed in 1986, the East German Interflug airline advertised their *Schlepperflüge* in Pakistani newspapers: 'Take the fast and comfortable route to Germany. With regular bus service to West Berlin.'[58] Once an asylum applicant had arrived, the protective review procedures mandated by the Basic Law (the so-called 'legal protection guarantee' of Article 19) would virtually guarantee that he could stay. After a negative decision by the Federal Office for Foreign Refugees in the Bavarian Zirndorf, three administrative court instances were at his disposition, including the Federal Administrative Court, plus the possibility to call the Federal Constitutional Court; if that was to no avail, a deportation order from the Foreigner Office of the respective *Land* could be contested through no less than two administrative and three juridical appeal instances. Finally, the whole procedure could be repeated through filing one, two, or more 'follow-up application(s)' (*Folgeantrag*) (Münch, 1992: 58 f.).[59] In the early 1980s, this process could stretch out over eight or more years—long enough to rule out deportation for humanitarian reasons.

Between 1978 and 1991, no less than eight federal laws were passed to shorten the legal procedures and curtail the social incentives of asylum-seeking. Streamlining the legal process amounted to squaring a circle defined by the demanding requirements of constitutional law. Once the possibility of administrative appeal to the Federal Refugee Office was abolished, the administrative courts were flooded with asylum cases, creating a backlog that further lengthened the procedures and attracted new claimants in a vicious circle. In the first half of the 1980s, 80 per cent of all cases before the Federal Administrative Court were asylum cases, because most asylum-seekers (meanwhile helped by a rather shady branch of the legal profession)[60] showed no hesitation in exhausting the full repertory of legal protection.[61] The introduction of a fast-track procedure for 'obviously unfounded' asylum claims in the Asylum Procedures Law of 1982, which limited but did not abolish administrative court review, amounted to a first significant tightening of the applicants' recognition practice (Münch, 1992: 98).

The Asylum Procedures Law of 1982, which introduced a distinct legal framework for the processing of asylum claims, had two important implications. First, it put on a legal basis the social deterrence measures then practised *ad hoc* by some *Länder*; secondly, it removed from the asylum recognition process the subjective refugee concept of the Geneva Convention, and allowed only the narrower, objective refugee concept of the Basic Law.[62] With regard to the first, the stress on social deterrence in German asylum policy is a direct function of the constitutional impossibility of 'dirty' border-screening. But the equally dirty encampment, in-kind provision, and barring from work of asylum-seekers had negative consequences for all involved parties. For the municipalities and *Länder*, which had pushed for such measures in order to minimize the number of asylum-seekers within their jurisdictions, they further increased their financial load. This, in turn, fuelled their aversion to accepting their legal share of asylum-seekers. Beginning with Frankfurt in 1980, major cities declared total 'reception stops' for asylum-seekers, and the struggle of smaller villages and towns against having asylum camps erected on their territory became legion. For the asylum-seekers, encampment and forced idleness meant serious distress. A Caritas report about the conditions in a south-west German asylum camp found its sad inmates struck by 'instability, depressions, total apathy, persecution mania, psychosomatic diseases, aggression against other persons, things and auto-aggression, . . . [and] suicidal intentions', concluding that 'after several months or even years of encampment asylum-seekers find it very difficult to lead a normal life again'.[63] But most importantly, the creation of enclaves of idle, foreign-looking asylum-seekers living on social welfare reinforced the public image of the parasitic 'bogus asylum-seeker' and provided easy targets for public hostility. Social deterrence thus laid the grounds for the violent outbursts of xenophobia that would sweep the country a few years later.

Secondly, the Asylum Procedures Law made the narrow concept of persecution, as laid down in the Basic Law, the exclusive basis for the determination of refugee status. There has always been a tension, if not confusion, between the Geneva Convention and Article 16 in German asylum practice. Initially, Article 16 had been altogether 'forgotten' (Wolken, 1988: 32) and asylum claims were processed according to Article 1 of the Geneva Convention. Only the Foreigner Law of 1965 introduced a uniform procedure for both Constitution and Convention refugees. The 1982 Asylum Procedures Law, finally, dropped the category of Convention refugee, because the Constitutional notion of 'political persecution' was deemed to encompass also Convention-refugee status (Marx, 1992: 153). The law-makers overlooked that the Convention concept of persecution stresses the subjective element of fear, while the Constitution concept stresses the objective element of actual political persecution. Accordingly, federal courts adopted an extremely restrictive concept of objective persecution, similar to the 'clear probability' doctrine that US courts were just about to abandon. The asylum-seeker now had to prove the clear 'intention' of persecution on the part of the persecutor, and she had to prove that the act of persecution was targeted on one of her 'inalienable attributes' (opinion, religion, race, nationality, or membership of a particular group). Based on a narrow concept of objective persecution, even the proven victims of torture would no longer be automatically recognized as refugees. The concept of objective persecution has allowed federal courts to reject close to 95 per cent of all asylum-claims since the mid-1980s. Hyper-restrictive asylum-granting had to further incense a public that wondered why they were all here if they were all denied. But such restrictiveness distorts the overall picture. A large part of those denied full asylum status were still admitted as *de facto* refugees, according to the so-called 'small asylum' of the Foreigner Law (which approximates the non-refoulement obligation under international law).[64]

The arsenal of legal fast-tracking and social deterrence was exhausted when, from the late 1980s on, the number of new asylum applicants began to rise dramatically—103,076 in 1988, 121,318 in 1989, 193,063 in 1990, 256,112 in 1991, reaching the exorbitant level of 438,191 in 1992 (German Interior Ministry, 1993: 106 f.).[65] By then, the Federal Republic was receiving 60 to 70 per cent of all refugees in Western Europe, in 1992 even a staggering 80 per cent. This is when Article 16 itself came under attack.[66] One of the last liberal defence lines was a paradoxical one: rigorous deportations.[67] Germany was indeed a deportation-laggard. Only 1 to 2 per cent of denied asylum applicants were eventually deported. But this is no accident, because state violence against foreigners had sad precedents in Germany—deportation is 'continuation of Nazi politics by other means,' said a Gypsy asylum activist.[68] Conservative asylum critics took a different line: the problem was not a deficit of deportations; the problem was automatic territorial access. The problem was Article 16, which amounted to a self-imposed abandonment of state sovereignty. It is no small irony that the threat of Chancellor Kohl, issued at the height of the German asylum crisis in November 1992, to seal the porous borders by emergency decree would eventually push the Social Democrats toward accepting a change of the Basic Law[69]—'Sovereign is', Carl Schmitt (1934: 11) said famously, 'who decides about the emergency'.

Helmut Quaritsch (1985: 21) had an early foreboding that the 'loss of sovereignty' entailed by Article 16 could leave the state vulnerable to severe 'domestic unrest'. In fact, the unprecedented increase of asylum claims in the late 1980s and early 1990s triggered the most serious domestic crisis the Federal Republic had ever gone through. The situation was aggravated by the fact that, parallel to the new asylum-seekers (who were now predominantly from the civil war zones of postcommunist South-Eastern Europe), ethnic Germans from the Soviet Union, Poland, and Romania arrived in large numbers—close to a million between 1988 and 1990 (German Interior Ministry, 1993: 123). In addition, the breakdown of East Germany entailed a third movement of *Übersiedler*, with a peak of 340,000 in 1990. Taken together, the Federal Republic had to absorb three million new migrants between 1989 and 1992, almost twice as many as the American immigrant nation took in during the 1920s—no small thing for a country that was 'not a country of immigration'. Particularly the parallel inflow of ethnic Germans, who were granted automatic citizenship according to Article 116 of the Basic Law, and of asylum-seekers created insidious distinctions. 'The coming home of Germans ... has priority over the reception of foreigners,' wrote an influential columnist.[70] Because ethnic Germans and asylum-seekers competed for the same scarce resources, the welcoming of ethnic Germans implied the restricting of the right of asylum. In turn, Social Democrats and Greens favoured the dropping of Article 116, that anachronistic relic of *völkisch* nationhood, and the introduction of American-style immigration quotas, in which the ethnic Germans would be just another immigrant group.

While the politicians and intellectual élites became locked in a polarized and inconclusive debate about who should be prioritized, society felt the full stress of the unprecedented migrations. In a country with a housing shortage of three million units, there was simply no room to accommodate the new arrivals. Ramshackle container units were erected at the outskirts of almost every town or city, and mayors confiscated everything from gymnasiums, town halls, club halls, and vacant state-owned housing, even windowless air-raid shelters, to fulfill their quota obligations. At one point, the SPD-governed city-state of Bremen simply refused to accept any more asylum applications by Poles and Romanians (whose recognition rate was zero): 'I don't have any more housing to offer', the Lord Mayor declared flatly.[71] But the most fateful aggravation of societal stress was implied in a harmless-looking clause of the reunification treaty of October 1991, which allotted 20 per cent of new asylum-seekers to the new eastern *Länder*. This was in the spirit of burden-sharing, but culpably oblivious of a depressed society that had just escaped from two subsequent dictatorships and did not know how to deal with brown skin. Hoyerswerda and Rostock-Lichtenhagen, where the local population cheered on the violent attacks of skinheads and neo-Nazis on asylum camps, were the beginning of the worst wave of xenophobic violence that Germany had seen since the end of the Third Reich, leaving more than forty people dead. The spectre of Weimar, the first German democracy destroyed by extremist violence, loomed above the reunified country.[72] But the violent excesses of fringe groups, which were condemned by most, diverted attention from the real societal stress caused by uncontrolled immigration. A 1992 survey showed that three-quarters of Germans were then demanding drastic action to contain the asylum-flow, including the long-tabooed change of the Basic Law.[73]

Whose state is it? This key question of asylum policy was never far from the surface during the German asylum crisis. The defenders of Article 16 saw the state in the first place obliged to human-rights principles, and only secondarily to the people who constituted it. A leader of the Social Democrats resisted becoming 'the instrument . . . of popular sentiment', warning that 'domestic considerations must not influence asylum policy'.[74] This delicate slighting of democracy in favour of human rights is combined with the view that there is an inherent link between asylum and immigration.[75] Fusing both motives, Pro Asyl, an asylum-rights organization, declared that the alternative was between 'walling-in ourselves' or 'sharing our wealth' (quoted in Bade, 1994: 139). This conveys a defeatist-cum-moralist attitude toward asylum-based immigration as in principle uncontrollable and retributive of global injustice. A Green asylum advocate flatly stated that 'the issue is not if we *want* immigration but how we *manage* it', adding that 'the population of this country will have to get used to the fact of permanent immigration'.[76] By contrast, conservative critics of Article 16, not without complacency, saw themselves as acting on a popular mandate: 'My responsibility as politician is to optimize the conditions for the people who live here. It is not my duty to treat all problems in the world equally.'[77] Conservative asylum critics upheld the division of the world into sovereign states, each accountable to its own citizens first: 'Every state . . . has to serve its own citizens first, and only secondarily the rest of the world. . .Germany cannot become everyone's country.'[78]

Bullied by the street and by frenzied conservative campaigning, the SPD's final giving in to constitutional change could still draw upon one face-saving demand of the day: the European harmonization of asylum policy.[79] Since the European Union was obviously unwilling to go the German way,[80] Germany had to follow Europe. The Social Democratic initial stance to 'adjust' Article 16 only *after* Europe had agreed upon 'humane' asylum standards was hollow. Germany's neighbours profited from the status quo and showed no sign of accommodating German demands for substantive burden-sharing and supranational co-ordination, not to mention that 'humane' standards would never see the light of day.[81] Constrained by its national constitution, Germany could only conditionally participate in the Dublin and Schengen treaties, which stipulate that one Union state has to process an asylum case vicariously for the others. Article 16 of the German Basic Law prohibited this procedure, commanding instead that asylum-seekers rejected in France or Britain would get a second chance in Germany. One of the reasons for little Euro-enthusiasm among other member states in asylum policy was that they could 'dump' their rejected applicants on Germany, while Germany was constitutionally prohibited from responding in kind. Germany was indeed, to put it in the words of Interior Minister Schäuble, the 'reserve asylum country of Europe'. The Interior Minister's ingenious Euro-solution of the German asylum crisis turned the spit around: 'If we change our constitution, we would profit from the fact that we are surrounded by neighbours who can protect asylum-seekers from persecution . . . Then *we*, and not the others, would profit from our geographical location. Then our European neighbours, and not only we, would quickly want to find a joint solution.'[82]

The so-called 'asylum-compromise' between government and opposition (excluding the Greens), which provided the required two-thirds parliamentary majority for a change of the constitution, avoided hardline demands for a complete dropping of Article 16.[83] But the insertion of proviso clauses now enabled the state to do what it could not do before: to reject apparently fraudulent asylum-seekers at its borders (see Renner, 1993). The amended Article 16 restricts access to territory and to the constitutional asylum process through two inter-related clauses: first, asylum-seekers arriving through 'safe third states' (which include Poland and the Czech Republic) are by definition excluded from the asylum process and are denied entry or subjected to immediate deportation; secondly, asylum-seekers from 'safe countries of origin' are considered not politically persecuted and face an accelerated recognition procedure that generally ends in a rejection of their claims as 'obviously unfounded'. The cordon is sealed through the statutory 'airport regulation', which subjects asylum-seekers arriving by air from safe countries of origin or without valid passports to a quick recognition procedure in extraterritorial airport space, *before* they have legally entered the Federal Republic. In essence, only asylum-seekers arriving by air or sea with valid papers and without debilitating third-country stops from countries of certified persecution are still entitled to claim the constitutional right of asylum. As a critic put it sarcastically, 'the right of asylum still exists—but not the refugees entitled to use it' (Prantl, 1994: 96).

What the same critic denounced as the 'most momentous political failure in the history of the Federal Republic' (ibid. 100), helped solve Germany's biggest political crisis since World War II. Refugees continue to arrive, but in numbers considered commensurate with the country's capabilities—around 125,000 in 1994 and 1995, which is 70 per cent less than in 1992. More importantly perhaps, the recognition rate has gone up to 25 per cent, indicating a return to more efficient and 'just' screening.[84] Related or not, right-wing violence against foreigners has passed its peak.[85] Certainly, the German recovery of border control has created new follow-up problems. First, the creation of buffer zones and the 'farming out' of refugee acceptance is now being copied by Germany's eastern neighbours, and the resulting chain deportations could entail the undermining of non-refoulement obligations. Secondly, curtailing legal entry has created the new problem of illegal immigration, which—given Germany's open land borders—may be inherently difficult to contain. Thirdly, more rigidly practised deportations have become continued issues of contention, gripping the country's moral conscience. And fourthly, the Federal Constitutional Court has repeatedly stayed generic deportation orders, insisting on the constitutional principle of 'single-case examination' (*Einzelfallprüfung*). But, in its landmark decision of May 1996, the Court has found the asylum compromise constitutional. In the end, Germany has only adjusted its asylum law to the international standard. If this adjustment has appeared drastic and deviated from its usually incremental policy style, it is because an essential function of sovereignty, control of territorial access, has had to be recovered from a unique impairment.[86]

After Unity: Toward an Immigration Policy?

With national reunification and the end of communism, the 'not a country of immigration' maxim, which had guided German policy towards foreigners since the guestworker period, has lost its rationale. This is because the peculiarity of an incomplete, vicarious nation-state for all Germans in the communist diaspora is no more.[87] In a nutshell, Germany is no longer like Israel. Contrary to current diagnoses of German nationalism reborn, there are signs of increasing denational-ization—at least in foreigner policy, which is cautiously undergoing a transformation toward an explicit immigration policy.

On the eve of reunification, the full scale of (West) Germany's self-definition as a homeland of the dispersed German diaspora east of the Elbe became apparent. By 1989, the Federal Republic had absorbed about 14 million German refugees from the east, against whom the 4.5 million settled foreigners appear paltry. The massive exit of ethnic Germans from Eastern Europe and the Soviet Union since the late 1980s, which occurred exactly parallel to the dramatic increase of asylum-seekers, made plainly visible that Germany preferred some immigrants over others. 'We should not see [their] arrival as a burden, but as a chance, not only for them, but also for us. Their favourable age structure helps improve the relation between the old and the young generation considerably. This will have a noticeably positive effect on the long-term developments of the labour market and the social security system.'[88] These words by a leading CDU politician could have been equally applied to the young labour migrants who continued to arrive on the family reunification and asylum tickets; but they were reserved for ethnic migrants who classified as 'Germans', and there-fore were not seen as 'immigrants' at all. On the opposite side, for-eigner and refugee advocates mischievously classified the returning ethnic Germans, many of whom had suffered bitterly for the crimes of the Nazi regime, as regular 'immigrants' who did not deserve priority treatment. As a member of the Greens put it cunningly, 'resettlers [*Aussiedler*] are immigrants and refugees, independently of their ori-gins; the division [*Spaltung*] of immigrants into different nationalities cannot be justified with democratic arguments'.[89]

What may appear as an obscure struggle over classifications, was a struggle over the soul of Germany: ethnic and *Volk*-centred, as in the discourse of *Aussiedler* advocates; or civic and post-national, as in the discourse of 'immigrant' advocates. Underneath these polarized discourses, however, there were cracks in the exceptional status of ethnic resettlers, which opened up a window of opportunity for an explicit immigration policy. First, society responded rather unfavourably to the foreign-looking and, often, foreign-speaking migrants, some of whom had acquired their 'Germanness' in obscure and opportunistic ways and now received generous social benefits that even exceeded those for ordinary Germans.[90] On the political level, successive legislations have chipped away the priority status of ethnic Germans—such as the Integration Adjustment Law of 1989, which reduced the social benefits for *Aussiedler* (especially those that exceeded the benefits for domestic Germans), and the Resettler Reception Law of 1990, which forced would-be resettlers to file their applications from abroad.

Most importantly, the legal category of 'expulsion pressure' (*Vertreibungsdruck*), which distinguished German-origin individuals in, say, the Soviet Union from those in the United States, came under fire. Already in 1976, the Federal Administrative Court called 'very questionable' the wide application of this formula to the descendants of expellees, for whom such pressure no longer existed (Delfs, 1993: 6). But with the crumbling of communist regimes in Eastern Europe and the Soviet Union, the 'expulsion pressure' formula, which qualified an individual for preferred immigration status, had lost any justification. This is acknowledged in the Law on Removing the Consequences of the War (*Kriegsfolgenbereinigungsgesetz*) of 1992. According to this law, the existence of expulsion pressure, that is, of repression endured for one's Germanness, is no longer automatically assumed, but has to be credibly demonstrated by the respective individual—except for ethnic Germans from the former Soviet Union.[91] In addition, this law has limited the right to claim the status of *Aussiedler* to persons born before 1 January 1993 (the date of the law's going into effect). This is a momentous provision, because it has in principle closed the prioritized immigration of ethnic Germans (see Ronge, 1995: 15). Finally, the law imposed a limit of 225,000 ethnic Germans to be allowed in every year, which makes the intake of ethnic Germans appear much like regular immigration. After phasing out the privileged *Aussiedler* category, while approximating the reception of *Aussiedler* to quota immigration, a window of opportunity has opened up to transform an ethnic-priority into a general immigration policy.

Closing ethnic-priority immigration was part of the asylum compromise, and certainly a concession by the German-friendly CDU to the foreigner-friendly SPD. This asylum compromise was indeed a 'comprehensive migration compromise' (Bade, 1994: 123), in which the government promised to 'examine the possibilities of limiting and steering inmigration [*Zuwanderung*] on the national and international levels'.[92] This was a cryptic formulation for a willingness to rethink the basis of an increasingly anachronistic foreigner policy, and to explore the possibility of an encompassing immigration policy that fused considerations of asylum-granting, ethnic-priority immigration, and—most important for the SPD—a quota-based new-seed immigration. As of today, no substantial achievement has been made in this direction. But after the burden of unredeemed nationhood is no longer, and the problem of homeland-oriented German diasporas is in principle resolved, there has been a recognizable mellowing of the compulsive 'no immigration country' maxim, even within the CDU.

Already during the negotiations over the asylum compromise, the CDU had come close to accept a 'controlled, small inmigration quota' (*Zuwanderungsquote*) in exchange for the SPD's agreement to changing Article 16 of the Basic Law.[93] Ever since, the calls for a comprehensive 'immigration law' (*Einwanderungsgesetz*) have gained ground.[94] In the autumn of 1993, the FDP chair and Foreign Minister Klaus Kinkel has argued in public that for demographic reasons alone such an immigration law was necessary. At that time, the CDU still rejected an immigration law, arguing that as long as the migrations commanded by Articles 6, 16, and 116 of the Basic Law (that is, by family reunification, asylum granting, and ethnic resettling, respectively) exceeded the need for new migrants, any discussion about migration quotas had to be a 'phantom discussion': 'Under these conditions the goal of a reasonable and responsible policy can only be the limitation and steering, but not the stimulation of additional migration.'[95]

By this time the different positions in Germany's immigration debate had narrowed down to a cryptic distinction between 'inmigration' (*Zuwanderung*) and 'immigration' (*Einwanderung*). This was still a distinction of principle. *Zuwanderung*, the term preferred by restrictionists, means unwanted immigration that is tolerated for constitutional and moral-political reasons. *Einwanderung*, by contrast, connotes actively solicited, wanted immigration. Critics of a self-conscious 'immigration' policy and law have so far correctly pointed out that such a framework is foreign to European nation-states, which—in contrast to the transoceanic new settler nations—have never pursued active policies to populate unsettled lands. But once the inevitability, even necessity, of inmigration is acknowledged, the difference between *Zuwanderung* and *Einwanderung* is one of words only, and it is bound to disappear. Tellingly, Johannes Gerster (CDU), who had denounced the discussion over an immigration law in 1993 as a 'phantom discussion', supported an immigration law in 1996.[96] Most prominently, the German President Roman Herzog (CDU), in the 1970s the Interior Minister of foreigner-unfriendly Baden-Württemberg, is now campaigning for 'an active immigration policy', in order to increase the size of the working population and thus save Germany's pension system.[97] Most spectacularly perhaps, Heinrich Lummer (CDU), who had opted for repatriating foreigners in the early 1980s, has recently discovered that immigration laws are always laws to limit immigration, and that quotas are devised according to interests of state: 'Our interest, for instance, cannot be to let in primarily Muslims. About such questions of limiting inmigration a discussion is needed. Then an immigration law can make sense. It must not be an instrument to increase the number of migrants, but to reduce it to a lower level.'[98]

What's in a name? The more relaxed attitude to the previously shunned notion of immigration indicates a fundamental change of mind, one that became possible after the national question had been settled. It is still an open question if an explicit immigration policy is desirable, or even possible within the European Union. Kay Hailbronner has pointed out that the room for manœuvre beyond the existing flows of inmigration is exceedingly small, and that a German option for an immigration policy would be a curious outlier within a European Union that does not want immigration: 'A special German road towards a "country of immigration" will not come about, because of the legal constraints of the European Union.'[99] But, in turn, the 'not a country of immigration' formula has receded from public discourse, and chances are that it will recede even further in the future. The conditions under which it once made sense no longer exist.

This chapter investigated why immigration to Germany continued after the recruitment stop of 1973, despite official declarations that Germany was 'not a country of immigration'. The logic of a guest-worker regime, encapsulated in Germany's Foreigner Law, did not envisage the permanent stay of migrant workers, stipulating instead the priority of German 'state interests' over the interests of migrants. Migrant rights, especially the right to stay, were pushed through by independent courts, invoking the extensive human-rights catalogue of the Basic Law. Once the permanent-residence right of guestworkers was secured, family unification was one avenue along which immigration continued after the oil crisis. Family reunification was not only backed by the Basic Law, but by an emergent moral élite consensus to deal humanely with the recruited guestworkers. This I showed in the failure of a massive campaign in the 1980s to stop family unification, which was sealed by a liberalized new Foreigner Law in 1990. Asylum has been a second avenue of continued immigration after the oil crisis. I have discussed the long and tortured debate over Article 16 of the Basic Law, which provided the subjective right of asylum. In atonement for the Nazi past, the constitutional right of asylum amounted to a self-abdication of state sovereignty, making Germany the world's major asylum-granting country. As in the US case, cracks in German state control over entry and stay are home-made, resulting from strong constitutional protections for aliens, a national history that has discredited the very idea of sovereignty, and moral élite obligations toward particular immigrant groups.

4

The Zero-Immigration Country: Great Britain

However differently effected, expansiveness characterized the German and American approaches to immigration. This could not be said about Great Britain. On the contrary, Britain stands out as the Western world's foremost 'would-be zero immigration country' (Layton-Henry, 1994), displaying an exceptionally strong and unrelenting hand in bringing immigration down to the 'inescapable minimum'.[1] Between 1951 and 1961, the heyday of New Commonwealth immigration, Britain's net migration balance was barely positive; between 1961 and 1981 emigration outweighed immigration by more than one million (see Layton-Henry, 1992: 2). While obviously having a different capacity to act on it, Britain's aversion to immigration resembles Germany's. But this similarity is rooted in diametrically opposed nation-state problematiques. Germany rejected immigration because of political boundaries too narrow to encompass the nation: immigration threatened the historical mandate of (West) Germany to be the homeland of all Germans in the communist diaspora. By contrast, Britain rejected immigration because of political boundaries wider than the nation: its immigrants were formal co-nationals without substantive ties of belonging, capitalizing on political boundaries that had too expansively and indistinctly been drawn as the boundaries of empire.

The logic of British immigration policy is thus determined by the devolution of empire. Immigration policy has essentially been about restricting the entry and settlement of the former subjects of empire. As Gary Freeman (1979: 38) put it, 'one may interpret much of postwar immigration policy in Britain as an attempt to remove rights of citizenship too generously extended during the colonial period'. Accordingly, the peculiarity of British immigration policy is that it is directed not against aliens, but against formal co-nationals. One citizenship, in the form of equal British subjectship, has been the prize a democratic nation has paid for acquiring something profoundly non-democratic and non-national: an empire. This was solemnly, if already counterfactually, reaffirmed in the British Nationality Act of 1948, which invested some 800,000,000 subjects of the crumbling empire, inhabiting a quarter of the earth's land surface, with the equal right of entry and settlement in Britain. Once the subjects of empire began to act on their right, thus unexpectedly reversing the direction of four centuries of colonial settlement, it was no question that the illusion of empire had to go. Immigration policy meant preventing the outer reaches of empire from moving toward the centre.

The legacy of empire has afflicted British immigration policy with the enduring curse of racial discrimination. Immigration policy is usually premissed on a meaningful concept of citizenship, which divides the world into those who belong and those who do not, and in which legal status overlaps with identity. In absence of a meaningful concept of citizenship, British immigration policy had to operate on a proxy. This proxy has been race. A former Home Secretary, Reginald Maudling, credibly expressed the dilemma of an immigration policy that could not select on the basis of citizenship: 'While one talked always and rightly about the need to avoid discrimination between black and white it is a simple fact of human nature that for the British people there is a great difference between Australians and New Zealanders, for example, who come of British stock, and people from Africa, the Caribbean and the Indian sub-continent who were equally subjects of the Queen and entitled to total equality before the law when established here, but who in appearance, habits, religion and culture, were totally different from us' (quoted in J. M. Evans, 1983: 21). This statement comprises the two key objectives of British immigration policy: restrict immigration from the New Commonwealth, and enable the return migration of British settlers from the Old and New Commonwealths. Both objectives converge on race: keep out the coloured subjects of empire, toward whom there were no ties of belonging; embrace the descendants of British settlers, who mostly happened to be white.

It is difficult to determine if the racial preference implicit in this dual objective is one of intention or effect only. While the dynamics of instituting immigration controls was undeniably one of racial conflict, the actual statutes were only indirectly racially discriminatory. The logic of British immigration policy was to carve out the historical British homeland nation from the vast empire, and to subject the rest to immigration control. That the nation was predominantly white, while large sections of the empire were non-white, is the root cause of racial bias in British immigration policy. This bias inextricably fuses intention and effect, because immigration policy could not but exclude mostly non-whites. Short of retaining an illusory open-door stance, it is difficult to imagine any British immigration policy that would not have become subject to the charge of racial discrimination.

It follows that postwar immigration to Britain, which largely originated from New Commonwealth countries, was essentially unwanted immigration. This is expressed in the widely noted (and deplored) absence of economic considerations in British immigration policy (Freeman, 1979: ch. 6; Spencer, 1994). In contrast with Germany or France, the first oil crisis marks no turning-point in Britain. Primary New Commonwealth immigration had effectively been halted before 1973, and for entirely political reasons. If Britain had acquired its colonial empire in a fit of absentmindedness, its initial approach to postcolonial immigration was strikingly similar.[2] This immigration was at best passively tolerated by élites who stuck too long to the illusion of empire on which the sun never set. A hostile public, aggrieved by the most dramatic secular decline a modern nation had ever gone through, shook the élites out of their complacency. As if to compensate for their initial inattention, successive governments have henceforth clung to the stern imperative that New Commonwealth immigration had to be stopped. A sense of obligation, even guilt, toward its postcolonial immigrants has not been absent among British élites, and it was channelled into the buildup of a liberal race-relations regime. But the distinct lack of generosity and tight control mentality of British immigration policy is perhaps not unrelated to the fact that the immigration it is dealing with has at no point been actively solicited or wanted.[3]

Accordingly, British immigration policy cannot be understood within the framework of client politics. Its demiurge is not the receivers of concentrated benefits, such as employers or ethnic groups, but the bearers of diffuse costs: a public that has been overwhelmingly and immovably hostile to coloured immigration (see Studlar, 1974). This is expressed in the official assertion, endlessly and almost ritualistically repeated, that firm immigration control is necessary for 'improving community relations'.[4] The peculiarly 'lexicographic' ordering of immigration control and race relations (Favell, 1995: 99) amounts to admitting that the animus of British immigration policy is public hostility to coloured immigration. Smethwick in 1964, when an unknown Tory candidate sacked a safe Labour seat on a blatantly anti-immigrant ticket, was a traumatic key event in this regard, which has 'sunk deeply into the minds of the political élite' (Studlar, 1980). The latter drew two lessons from it: never to tinker with the public's no-immigration mandate, and to prevent the eruption of racial hostility by anticipatory, ever vigilant immigration controls; and to remove this sensitive issue from the realm of partisan politics. There has been an élite consensus over the basic contours of immigration and race-relations policy (see Freeman, 1979; Messina, 1989), whose best indicators are the noisy protestations whenever the 'race card' is played in British politics.

If, for different reasons, Britain shared with Germany a penchant for zero-immigration, the question arises why she has been so much better at realizing it. One reason is docile courts and the lack of constitutional protections for immigrants. A legal-constitutional system protective of immigrant interests has been the key to Germany's expansiveness toward immigrants, undermining the zero-immigration intentions circulating in the political system. In Britain, there has been little blockading of the political branches of government by recalcitrant courts. Sovereignty is firmly and unequivocally invested in Parliament, which knows no constitutional limits to its law-making powers. In immigration policy, this institutional arrangement entails a dualism of extreme legislative openness and executive closure, which is detrimental to the interests of immigrants. Parliamentary openness in the formulation of immigration policy keeps law-makers within the confines of a pervasively restrictionist public opinion. Once a policy has been decided upon, there is executive closure in its implementation, with the Home Office firmly and uncontestedly in charge.

J. A. G. Griffith (1979) has eloquently defended Britain's 'political constitution', in which the political process is unhampered by abstract legal rules: 'Law is not and cannot be a substitute for politics . . . [Written constitutions] merely pass political decisions out of the hands of politicians and into the hands of judges . . . I believe firmly that political decisions should be taken by politicians. In a society like ours this means by people who are removable' (p. 16). Pragmatism, aversion to fixed first principles, and balanced empirical reasoning have characterized British democracy for centuries, and they have served the cause of liberty well. But if the boundaries of the political community are at stake, as in immigration policy, the unprincipled British way becomes problematic: the 'ins' can now dispose of the 'outs' at will. Ian Macdonald, the doyen of British immigration lawyers, is right: 'The notion of parliamentary sovereignty may sound proper

enough when the judges explain that their job is merely to interpret
and apply the law passed by the legislature; but the ultimate sanction
of electoral accountability is of little utility if the laws are directed
against a vulnerable and electorally insignificant minority. There are,
bluntly, few votes for conceding administrative justice to immigrants,
and possibly quite a few more in "tougher" measures. To whom then
can immigrants look for protection of fundamental standards of fair
dealing?' (Macdonald and Blake, 1991: pp. v–vi). In the United States
and Germany, immigrants could turn to assertive courts backed by
written constitutions. In Britain, which does not have a written constitution, there could not be a comparable legal empowerment of
immigrants. This partially explains the greater effectiveness of British
immigration controls.

Who Belongs? The Dilemma of British Immigration Policy

Surveying the development of British immigration policy, one discov-
ers two major themes. First, this is a policy driven and dictated by
public hostility to coloured immigration. As Gary Freeman (1979:
316) correctly noted, the political élites acted 'out of real fears of the
ugly mood of the British people'. Following, rather than leading, the
public did not come lightly in a polity as thoroughly subscribed to
antipopulist norms as the British. Knowing that liberalism is not
democracy, J. A. G. Griffith (1979: 3) celebrated that Britain had
stayed clear of that 'one bit of nonsense . . . that sovereignty resides in
the people'. The disdain for populism was perhaps even stronger
among conservative Tories. Accordingly, both major parties were
reluctant to get drawn into the muddy waters of immigration (sc.
'race') control, and they were jointly inclined to remove the issue from
the political agenda.

Secondly, once it was realized that immigration control could not be
avoided, there was no clear criterion of membership on which it could
operate. Who are the British? At first, the multiple nations of the
English, Scots, and Welsh united by religion and war, against the
Roman papacy and Catholic France; then the builders of an oceanic
empire, the liberal civilizers immortalized in Kipling's 'White Man's
Burden' (see Colley, 1992). If the second 'Whig-imperialist' Britain
was Britain, as David Marquand (1995) suggestively maintains, the
devolution of empire had to pose a serious problem of identity.
Immigration policy both suffered from and aggravated the problem of

identity, demolishing the Whig-imperialist illusion in excluding certain subjects of empire, while having no alternative model of membership and community to build upon. Nevertheless forced to define who belongs, British immigration policy resorted to birth and ancestry, thus introducing an ethnic marker that had so far been absent from the definition of Britishness. That the ethnic marker was, in effect, also a racial marker between whites and non-whites is the root cause of the charge of racial discrimination, from which British immigration policy could never quite liberate itself.

When the first black immigrants arrived aboard the *Empire Windrush* in June 1948, the Cabinet Economic Policy Committee drily noted that these were 'private persons travelling at their own expense', and thus could not be stopped. But the committee urged the responsible Colonial Office to '[prevent] the occurrence of similar incidents' in the future (quoted in Paul, 1992: 457). The entire British immigration experience is encapsulated in this response to the first 492 Jamaicans landing on its shore. No one had asked them to come; they were perfectly free to come; more of them were too many of them. Strangely, while the memory of the war fought by civilized Britain against racist Germany was still fresh, never was racial discourse more openly, almost innocently, expressed than in the earliest encounter with black immigrants. In the face of a severe labour shortage, the Royal Commission on Population recommended in 1949 to recruit some 140,000 young immigrants, but only if they were 'of good human stock and . . . not prevented by their religion or race from intermarrying with the host population and becoming merged in it' (ibid. 463). The Ministry of Labour likewise 'rule[d] out any question of a concerted plan to bring West Indian colonial workers here', pointing out the serious 'social implications' that the introduction of 'other races' into the labour force would have (ibid. 460). While rejecting any concerted effort to recruit black immigrants, Britain engaged in its one and only active immigration policy in the postwar period, luring some 350,000 European Volunteer Workers (EVWs)—mostly Poles and other Europeans 'displaced' by the war—into the country (see Miles and Kay, 1990). They were welcome, and not just as German-style guestworkers. As a civil servant in the Ministry of Labour explained, the EVW's 'are coming definitely for permanent settlement here with a view to their intermarrying and complete absorption into our own working population' (in Paul, 1992: 464). Aliens being preferred to fellow subjects of the Crown—never was the disjunction between formal membership status and identity more obvious.

While the black immigrants were unwelcome, the Labour government responded with a 'policy of inaction' (Dean, 1987: 305), hoping that the influx would die away without its intervention. Indicative of where the winds of change were blowing from, a group of Labour back-benchers wrote to the Prime Minister after the arrival of the *Windrush*: 'An influx of coloured people domiciled here is likely to impair the harmony, strength and cohesion of our public and social life and to cause discord and unhappiness among all concerned' (quoted in Carter *et al.*, 1993: 56). Prime Minister Attlee's response was similarly indicative of the dominant élite thinking at the time: 'It is traditional that British subjects . . . of whatever race and colour . . . should be freely accessible to the UK. The tradition . . . is not to be lightly discarded . . . It would be fiercely resented in the Colonies themselves and it would be a great mistake to take any action which would tend to weaken the loyalty and goodwill of the Colonies to Great Britain' (quoted in Dean, 1987: 316). The empire was still a reality, and the government actively supported the out-migration of some 760,000 Britons between 1946 and 1951 to keep it British.

But before the winds of change would start to blow from within, they originated from the independence drives of the colonies and old dominions. When Canada devised its own immigration and citizenship laws in 1946 and India acquired its independence in 1947, Britain was forced to reconceive the meaning of membership in the empire. This was accomplished with the British Nationality Act of 1948, an emphatic reaffirmation of the unity of empire, in which the maintenance of non-national subjectship, defined by allegiance to the Crown, was consciously held against the nationalisms of the periphery. In refusing to devise a concept of national citizenship, the British Nationality Act created the core dilemma for all immigration laws and policies that followed: not to dispose of a clear criterion of belonging. Following the model of Canada, Britain instituted a separate 'citizenship of the United Kingdom and Colonies' as a gateway to 'British subjectship'. There was consensus between the Conservative and Labour Parties not to restrict free movement within the realm of empire, now democratically refashioned as the British Commonwealth of Nations. As the Tory Sir Maxwell Fyfe said during the second reading of the British Nationality Bill, 'we must maintain our great metropolitan tradition of hospitality to everyone from every part of our Empire'.[5] But there was dispute, first, over the feasibility of one-membership status for the UK and colonies, and—once this was settled—over labelling this inclusive membership 'citizenship', rather than 'subjectship'. Labour, somewhat hopefully, defended the notion of citizenship, because this would 'give the coloured races of the Empire the idea that . . . they are the equals of people in this country'.[6] Tories, perhaps covering their distaste for a republican concept, pointed out that 'citizenship', with its connotation of homogeneity and commonly shared rights and duties, was 'inappropriate to the immense variety of people, with the immense varieties of status of forms of Government, and civic rights and responsibilities, which are included in the group [i.e. United Kingdom and colonies] which the Home Secretary has chosen for them'.[7] Tories thus rightly anticipated that a citizenship including both 'head-hunters of Borneo (and) noble Lords'[8] had to be devoid of any meaning. Such an empty and over-inclusive notion of citizenship invited insidious sub-classifications once immigration control would appear on the agenda.

Immigration was definitely not on the agenda in 1948. As a Tory described the élite opinion of the time, 'we thought that there would be a free trade in citizens, that people would come and go, and that there would not be much of an overall balance in one direction or the other'.[9] The age of innocence came to an end with the 1958 race riots in Nottingham and Notting Hill, when 'illiberal opinion' (Deakin, 1968: 38)—transmitted into Parliament primarily by Conservative back-bench pressure, especially from the industrial Midlands—took the lead. In 1961, the number of new immigrants from New Commonwealth countries crossed the 100,000 mark for the first time, and the total intake since 1956 was over half a million. This was perceived as a problem for both external and internal reasons. Externally, the parallel race unrest in the United States created the not unreasonable fear that Britain was importing 'a colour problem approaching that of the United States'.[10] Internally, black immigration became especially problematic because of 'clotting', its spatial concentration in 'smallish areas of poor housing and high unemployment'.[11]

Striking about the early calls for restricting New Commonwealth immigration is their apologetic tone, which suggests that the political élites were pushed into something they did not like. Tory Home Secretary Butler confessed his 'great reluctance' when bringing in his 1961 Bill, characterizing the latter as only temporary, still more liberal than the general alien restrictions, and intent on controlling, rather than prohibiting, New Commonwealth immigration.[12] The Bill, which made new admissions dependent on largely skill- and need-based employment vouchers, was ostensibly a labour-market measure, but one that made no sense in the context of a full employment economy. In public, the Home Secretary declared that 'the Bill is drafted so that there is no racial discrimination',[13] but a cabinet memorandum reveals him admitting that 'its aim is primarily social and its restrictive effect is intended to, and would in fact, operate on coloured people almost exclusively'.[14] Both statements are not necessarily contradictory. The wording of the Bill is not racially discriminatory, while its effect certainly is. At the same time, it would be naïve to assume that this effect was not intended.

These quibbles revealed the British immigration-control dilemma: if controls were imposed, they had to be directed against the major source of immigration, which happened to be the non-white New Commonwealth. But no legitimate concept of citizenship was available on which such controls could operate. As a proxy for meaningful citizenship, the Commonwealth Immigrants Act of 1962, like all the legislations that followed, revolved around the notion of belonging, i.e. birth and ancestry. As Home Secretary Butler famously declared, 'except from control [are] persons who in common parlance belong to the United Kingdom'.[15] Belonging was then defined by birth in the UK and the holding of passports issued by the UK Government.[16] This took care of only one of the two main objectives of British immigration policy: to exclude those without sufficient ties of belonging, which happened to be the non-white periphery of the empire. The second objective of prioritizing the descendants of British settlers, particularly in the Old Dominions, was realized only later on.

In his powerful rejection of 'this miserable, shameful, shabby Bill', Labour leader Hugh Gaitskell rightly identified its motif as 'fear of racial disorder and friction'. Attacking the political élite's kowtow to illiberal opinion, Gaitskell exclaimed: 'I do not believe it to be our duty merely to follow what we are convinced are wrong and dangerous views.'[17] But characterizing New Commonwealth immigration as 'wanted' immigration was stretching the truth, as was his naïve theory that immigration would follow the 'movement of unfilled vacancies', and thus die away on its own. Six years later, it was a Labour government that did exactly what Gaitskell had denounced so eloquently: fall to the pressure of illiberal opinion. In the history of British immigration policy, the Commonwealth Immigrants Act of 1968, rushed through Parliament in just two days in an atmosphere of outright panic, stands out as the most blatant example of a policy dictated by public hostility toward coloured immigrants. Trying to make it more palatable for liberal opinion, Home Secretary James Callaghan strangely repackaged the illiberal dictate as a 'sense of fair play': 'We must trust the instinctive sense of fair play of the British people. Our policy . . . must be acceptable to them and to their sense of fair play.'[18] Looking back at this darkest hour of British immigration policy, a Labour MP from the Midlands, 'where racialism is a powerful force', was less reluctant to denounce his own support for the second immigrants bill as 'appalling violation of our deepest principles' (quoted in J. M. Evans, 1983: 95).

The Commonwealth Immigrants Act of 1968 took away the right of entry from 200,000 East African Asians with UK government passports, who had become the victims of the Africanization drive in post-independence Kenya. Britain thus came close to violating one of the fundamental norms of the international state system: the obligation of states to accept their own nationals. Such violation could be barely averted through the introduction of a special voucher scheme, which allowed the government to argue that its objective was not exclusion, but the forming of an 'orderly queue' commensurate with the country's limited capacity to absorb immigrants.[19] But there was no camouflaging that the government had broken its pledge to accept these—*de facto* stateless—British Asians if the need should arise.[20] Reginald Maudling, who had been involved in the independence negotiations on behalf of the Colonial Office, was clear about the pledge: 'There is no doubt about the rights which these people possess. When they were given these rights, it was our intention that they should be able to come to this country when they wanted to do. We knew it at the time. They knew it, and in many cases they have acted and taken decisions on this knowledge.' But breaking the pledge was justified by avoiding the social consequences of coloured immigration: 'Equally, there is no doubt about the problem which can, and will, be created if the rate of immigration goes ahead too rapidly . . . This clearly is a racial problem [that] arises quite simply from the arrival in this country of many people of wholly alien cultures, habits and outlook.'[21]

The exclusion of East African Asians was accomplished by extending immigration control to UK passport-holders without 'substantial connection' with the UK. 'Substantial connection' was not only birth in the UK—the core of Lord Butler's definition of 'belonging', but alternatively a parental or grandparental connection with the UK. This widened the scope of belongers to the descendants of certain categories of British settlers (i.e. those with UK and colonies citizenship), while excluding UK government passport-holders without ancestral connection to the UK. Home Secretary Callaghan defended this redefinition of belonging as 'geographical, not racial': 'Those who, or whose fathers or fathers' fathers, were born, naturalised, adopted, or registered in the United Kingdom, will be exempted [from immigration control] whatever their race.'[22] This was not inaccurate. And as a Tory defender of the grandfather clause pointed out, 'all the great nations of the earth have what the Jews call a Diaspora', and to recognize 'some special and residual obligation towards them' could not possibly be racial discrimination.[23]

In the first major indictment of British immigration policy by European institutions, the European Commission on Human Rights took a different view. Britain had wisely not signed the immigration-related Fourth Protocol to the European Convention on Human Rights, which stipulates that 'no one shall be deprived of the right to enter the territory of the State of which he is a national', and thus deemed itself beyond the pale of possible indictment on Convention grounds. While the Commission admitted that the Convention as such did not guarantee a right of entry, it still concluded that other treaty rights may be violated by immigration measures. In particular, the Commission found it 'established that the 1968 Act had racial motives and that it covered a racial group'.[24] In excluding formal citizens on these grounds, Britain had reduced them to the status of 'second-class citizens' with equal duties but lesser rights. This constituted 'degrading treatment' on the basis of race, in violation of Article 3 of the European Convention. Interestingly, the Commission took the Home Secretary's submission that the Act was in the interest of 'racial harmony' as one piece of evidence of the Act's racial motivation. This was certainly a positive and not a negative motive, but one that indeed was at odds with the claim that geography, not race, was driving the cuts (see Thornberry, 1980: 141). Even if it maintained a neutral façade and only belatedly introduced what other countries (including all Commonwealth countries) had long had: restrictions on entry, British immigration policy was still tainted by its empirical origins, the fear of racial disharmony. In the end, it cannot be denied that the exclusion of East African Asians had entailed the creation of 'second-class' citizenship on the grounds of race, as charged by the Commission. The lesson had to be that without a safe basis of citizenship the curse of racism could not be shed.

This lesson went unheeded in the Immigration Act of 1971, until today the main legal basis of British immigration policy. The Act followed upon the Tories' election pledge to halt 'large-scale permanent immigration' to Britain. The reluctance of previous governments to follow illiberal opinion had by now been replaced by the routine disposition to treat immigration policy as 'secondary' to 'that basic problem [of community relations]', as Tory Home Secretary Reginald Maudling put it.[25] Following the logic of the European Commission verdict on the 1968 Act, this fixation alone would qualify as racially discriminatory. The 1971 Act was the first immigration act to deal jointly with aliens and Commonwealth citizens, and it thus completed the development of assimilating Commonwealth citizens to aliens, already the rationale of previous legislation. This included the replacement of employment vouchers by the more rigid work-permit requirement already in place for aliens, greater deportation powers of the state, and a rockier transition path from temporary to permanent settlement.

Skirting the problem of citizenship, the Immigration Act introduced the notion of patriality to determine who had the 'right of abode' and thus was exempt from immigration control. Building on the concept of substantive connection in the 1968 Act, patrials were all citizens of the United Kingdom and colonies born in or with an ancestral connection to the UK, citizens who had settled for at least five years, and—this was a novelty—any Commonwealth citizen with a parent or grandparent in the UK. The last clause finally realized the second objective of British immigration policy, first intimated in the grandfather clause of 1968, to prioritize the re-migration of British settlers. As Reginald Maudling defended it, this was not a racial concept but in recognition of the 'family connection' with the British diaspora abroad.[26]

In removing the anomalous distinction between the control of aliens and of Commonwealth citizens, the Immigration Act moved Britain closer toward having a 'normal' immigration policy. But the Act also heightened the peculiar British disjunction of immigration and citizenship law, in distinguishing between citizens with and without the right to enter, rather than drawing this line between aliens and citizens as is 'normally' the case.

To realign citizenship and immigration law was the purpose of the British Nationality Act of 1981. While passed by a Tory government, the Act's rationale and architecture were first laid out in a Labour government Green Paper of 1977. In the postimperial era, the all-embracing citizenship stipulated by the British Nationality Act of 1948 no longer made sense. As the Green Paper put it, 'our present citizenship of the United Kingdom and Colonies . . . does not identify those who belong to this country and have the right to enter and live here freely; in consequence it prevents the United Kingdom from basing its

immigration policies on citizenship' (Home Office, 1977: 4). Its denial
of entry and settlement rights to formal co-nationals had made Britain
vulnerable to the charge of human-rights and international-law violations, as in the European Commission's *East African Asians* case.
Thatcher's Secretary of State in the Home Office put it in simpler
terms: 'We have got finally to dispose of the lingering notion that
Britain is somehow a haven for all those countries we once ruled'
(quoted in Blake 1982: 182).

Ostensibly an act about nationality, not immigration, any nationality reform in Britain had to be driven by the logic of immigration law
and policy, and thus perpetuate the spell that it had set out to exorcize.
This is most evident in the act's key provision, the breaking up of the
composite 'citizenship of the United Kingdom and Colonies' into
three separate citizenships: British Citizenship, British Dependent
Territory Citizenship, and British Overseas Citizenship. British citizenship incorporated and replaced the old notion of patriality, conferring the right of abode. Importantly, the category of Commonwealth
patrials, decried by many as racist, was phased out. While softened by
generous transition rules (former patrials retained the right of abode
over their lifetime), this meant in principle the end of ethnic priority
immigration for the descendants of British settlers. The two other citizenships, which comprise the non-patrials of old, are 'citizenship'
only in name, because they are not related to a state-like entity and do
not confer a right of abode anywhere.[27] But the government acknowledged certain 'moral and constitutional responsibilities' to the members of its former and existing colonies—which would soon become
relevant in the case of Hong Kong.[28] No clean slate could be had
through legislative fiat, and the shadow of empire continues to hover
over British citizenship law. Understandably, because it would lead
the reform *ad absurdum*, the government refused the category of
British national as an umbrella for the three citizenships, arguing also
that this 'would . . . raise expectations which . . . could not be realized'
(quoted in White and Hampson, 1982: 9). But the old umbrella notion
of Commonwealth citizen was strangely retained, and some legal
commentators have pointed out that under international law the
British dependent territory and overseas citizens are still nationals
with legitimate entry and protection claims (J. M. Evans, 1983: 75;
A. C. Evans, 1983: 95).

The influence of immigration concerns on the redefinition of citizenship is also visible in the partial abolishment of *jus soli*, the single
most contested aspect of the 1981 British Nationality Act. Originally

a feudal principle to make the product of the soil the property of the lord, *jus soli* had conferred automatic citizenship on all persons born in the UK, and thus had helped to integrate new immigrants. But now it stood in the way of both the ethnic redefinition of Britishness via 'belonging' and effective immigration control. Regarding the former, the government argued that in an age of intensified movement and communication the mere accident of birth on territory should not confer the precious good of citizenship: 'It is increasingly the case that children are born while their parents are here temporarily. The present arrangements lead to significant numbers of people acquiring the right of abode here although they have no real ties with this country.'[29] But the true animus of restricting *jus soli* was effective immigration control. Once endowed with citizen children, non-citizen parents who had entered illegally or overstayed might be more difficult to deport. As the House of Commons Standing Committee put it maliciously, 'one of the various international courts whose jurisdiction we have accepted . . . might find . . . that it was wrong to remove the parents of a patrial child' (quoted in Blake, 1982: 185). The possibility that domestic courts might protect family rights was obviously ruled out from the start. Both ethnic-membership and immigration-control considerations led to a restricted *jus soli* law, according to which only children born to parents with British citizenship or settled in the UK could become British citizens at birth.

Enoch Powell celebrated the 1981 British Nationality Act as finally declaring Britain a nation.[30] This is misguided. The exigencies of immigration continue to 'wag the nationality tail' (Macdonald and Blake, 1991: 2). The British citizenship created in 1981 confers only one right, the right of abode, and thus is little more than a transposition of immigration law. Even political rights, like the right to vote, are still attached to the common law concept of British subject. As a legal observer notes, the nationality reform aroused little public interest, and it did not spark a debate over the meaning of Britishness in a postimperial age (Blake, 1982: 179). Such evasiveness may be faithful to the general lack of debate on principle and purpose in British public life. But the question of who belongs still lingers, and the dilemma of British immigration policy remains unresolved.

Dividing Families: Britain's Firm Hand on Secondary Immigration

With the 1971 Immigration Act, primary immigration had been brought under control, if not stopped. The last category of work-permit for unskilled workers was abolished in 1975, limiting new primary entries to the indispensable functionaries of the global economy (Macdonald and Blake, 1991: 16). Accordingly, the focus of British immigration policy shifted to the control of secondary immigration, that is, family reunification. Generally, states have full discretion to accept or reject primary immigrants; this makes them wanted immigrants. However, regarding secondary immigrants, state discretion is limited. States do not want secondary immigrants; they have to accept them in recognition of the family rights of their wanted, primary immigrants. This recognition of the family rights of primary immigrants has a legal and a moral component. In the case of Germany, a constitution protecting elementary family rights and an élite consensus about special obligations towards the recruited guestworkers narrowed the possibilities of clamping down on secondary immigration.

The British state has been less affected by such legal and moral constraints. Legally, there is no constitution protecting family rights, and it is at the discretion of Parliament to hand out, or withdraw, statutory rights for individuals, immigrants included. The one family right for immigrants so granted, Section 1(5) of the 1971 Immigrants Act, which allowed the pre-1973 New Commonwealth immigrants to bring in their wives and children at will, was simply slashed once it came into the way of firm immigration control.[31] Regarding moral constraints, already the primary immigrants were unwanted, at best they were tolerated. Accordingly, there was a lesser sense of special obligation towards them among the élites—the brief and noiseless slashing of Section 1(5) in the 1988 Immigration Act proves exactly that. In addition, the weaker moral constraints that existed found no territorial and political space to be expressed. Regarding territorial space, the system of entry clearance allowed the drama of denied family reunion to be conveniently displaced overseas, to the British embassies and High Commissions in Dhaka, Islamabad, or Bombay—far away from the controlling sight of liberal opinion. Regarding political space, the unitary British state did not provide any point of entry for immigrant-friendly dissent, such as a German-style Liberal (FDP) coalition party or Red-Green state government. The one immigrant-friendly force: the Labour Party, was perpetually tainted by its past bowing to illiberal opinion. As a result of weaker legal and moral constraints, British policy on secondary immigration took an opposite direction from German policy, embracing, rather than rejecting, drastic solutions.

British policy on secondary immigration moved away from the public arena of parliamentary law-making into a half-world of executive closure, where state discretion was almost complete. Tellingly, there has been no change in statutory immigration law from 1971 to 1988, and immigration largely disappeared from the public agenda. But there has been a flurry of changes in the so-called immigration rules, the real body of British immigration law and policy. The Immigration Act only defines who is subject to immigration control; the immigration rules provide the substantive criteria, terms and conditions for admission. The legal status of these rules is unclear. Lord Denning influentially characterized them as 'not rules of law' but 'rules of practice' laid down for the guidance of immigration and entry clearance officers (in Bevan, 1986: 14). While they are subject to parliamentary approval, the rules are authored by the Home Secretary, who is free to make or unmake them according to the exigencies of the moment. As non-legislated 'rules of practice' the immigration rules do not even bind the Home Secretary and his executive machinery, thus epitomizing the reign of absolute state discretion in British immigration policy. The immigration rules have been the perfectly flexible and adaptable tool for the 'loophole-closing' and 'fine-tuning' that characterized British immigration policy in its post-statutory phase.[32]

Next to executive closure, the presumption of 'bogus' has been a second characteristic of British policy on secondary immigration. In this mindset, primary immigration was stopped, and would-be immigrants, especially from poor and insecure parts of the world where the 'pressure to emigrate' was high, were trying to pass as entitled family members of settled immigrants.[33] Accordingly, the focus had to be on distinguishing 'genuine' from 'bogus' immigrants. A Government White Paper of 1978 put it this way: 'The prevention and detection of attempted evasion and abuse of the control, where it is shown to exist, is one of the main features of the Government's immigrant policy . . . It is a regrettable though inevitable consequence of the need to prevent abuse that some genuine applicants suffer inconvenience' (quoted in CRE, 1985: 9). Remarkably, the need to detect evasion outweighs the interests of genuine applicants. This is the price coolly paid for the sake of effective immigration control: 'If one accepts that there should be immigration control, one has to accept that the individual's desires cannot be overriding.'[34]

The bogus presumption is the logical outcome of an immigration policy that from the start had been a negative policy of keeping out unwanted immigrants. But, applied to secondary immigration, it also reflected real difficulties in handling immigration pressure from a distant, economically backward and culturally different part of the world. Secondary immigration pressure largely originated from the Indian subcontinent, and here from relatively small 'catchment areas'—Gujerat and Punjab in India, Kashmir and Punjab in Pakistan, and Sylhet in Bangladesh (see CRE, 1985: 157). This reflects different migration patterns of Afro-Caribbean and South Asian immigrants, Britain's two main New Commonwealth immigrant groups. In contrast to Caribbean immigrants, who had arrived as entire families, immigrants from the Indian subcontinent had at first been single men, who only later sought reunion with wives and children. Indian subcontinental immigration pressures were themselves differentiated according to the time of primary entry. By the mid-1980s, secondary immigration pressure was lowest from India, whose primary immigrants had arrived earliest, and it was highest—and most problematic because of extreme poverty levels, both at home and in the UK—from Bangladesh, whose primary immigration had peaked only in the early 1970s. Against the backdrop of long-established migration networks from Third-World areas plagued by overpopulation, underdevelopment, and political instability, it was rational to assume that secondary was really a means for primary entry, and to devise policies that effectively filtered out entrants by deception.

However, once the imperative of 'preventing evasion' and 'abuse of controls' had been erected, it became almost impossible to operate against family structures that were radically different from the Euro-American model of the nuclear family. From the British perspective, controlling family reunification from South Asia meant a descent into a strange and exotic world of child brides, polygamy, arranged marriage, and *talaq* divorces. In fact, British common law has proved astonishingly flexible in recognizing and incorporating such foreign family customs (see Poulter, 1986). But how, for example, to distinguish between 'genuine' marriage and 'bogus' marriage in the case of arranged marriage, which continues to be the dominant marriage custom even among second-generation Asian immigrants in Britain? As interview protocols and secret instruction materials reveal, British immigration and entrance clearance officers became practising anthropologists, with an astounding knowledge of local customs in areas where the 'pressure to emigrate' was high.[35] But cultural incompatibility further reinforced the control imperative, in a vicious circle of uncertainty and increased vigilance, up to a point which the Commission for Racial Equality has branded as 'excessive' attention to the detection and prevention of bogus immigration (CRE, 1985: 12).

The system of entry clearance, introduced in 1969 as a 'humane' and effective way of relieving congestion at the ports of entry (see Bevan, 1986: 165), exterritorialized the processing of family reunification to the Indian subcontinent. Each applicant for settlement had to first convince a local entry-clearance officer of the legitimacy of her claim. This was a formidable hurdle to take for many, which included stressful and repeated long journeys to the British outposts in New Delhi, Islamabad, or Dhaka, where applicants were subjected to prolonged and tortuous interviews (see Sondhi, 1987: ch. 2). While originally created for purely administrative convenience and purportedly neutral on applicant rights, the entry-clearance system developed into an unofficial quota system that allowed drastic reduction of the rate of entry.[36] One year after its introduction, the entry-clearance system helped cut in half the number of admitted wives and children, from 47,000 in 1968 to 26,000 in 1970 (J. M. Evans, 1983: 128). As a result of systematic understaffing, significant queues built up. In the first quarter of 1985, the average waiting time for a first interview was 14 months in New Delhi, 11.5 months in Islamabad, and 23 months in Dhaka (House of Commons, 1986, ii. 90).[37] The entry clearance system was also a convenient way of displacing the painful refusal of family immigrants. Between 1977 and 1983, 21.1 per cent of the women and 38.5 per cent of the children applying for family reunification were refused, which amounts to a considerable combined refusal rate of one-third (CRE, 1985: 19). Overseas entry-clearance officers thus became the masters of the fate of numerous transnational British families.[38]

At face value, the range of entitled family immigrants is similar in Britain and Germany: relatively unrestricted entry for the nuclear family of spouses and children, and sharply reduced entry rights for extended family; in addition, Section 1(5) of the 1971 Immigrants Act, which prioritized the wives and children of pre-1973 primary immigrants, resembled Germany's special obligation toward its first-generation guestworkers. But there are three important differences in the handling of family reunification in Britain: the lack of constitutional family rights, which greatly increased the executive scope of controlling secondary immigration;[39] the greater effort to cross-check

the identity of applicant wives and children, in order to detect and prevent deception; and, most strikingly, an ultra-restrictive regime for
husbands and fiancés, who were either flatly denied entry or subjected
to a special 'primary purpose' test to rule out that their marriage was
concocted to achieve immigration to Britain.

Regarding wives and children, the focus of entry-clearance procedures was on verifying their identity and status. This was no mere
chicanery, but reflective of objective difficulties in establishing the
validity of claims. In the rural Indian subcontinent the documentation
of births, marriages, even deaths, is fragmentary and unreliable, if it
exists at all. Since British immigration authorities request such documentation, a whole industry of producing fraudulent documents has
sprung up. A local guidance for entry-clearance officers in Dhaka
describes the situation in Sylhet: 'It is an extremely simple matter in
Sylhet to obtain documents which are to all intents and purposes genuine, but contain fraudulent information. A marriage registrar, for
example, will often draw up a certificate at someone's dictate, officially
sign and seal it, and insert it at the appropriate place in its records.
Birth certificates, death certificates, and even passports are issued with
minimum of investigation' (quoted in CRE, 1985: 30). The only
reliable documentation being land deeds, it is no wonder that entry-
clearance officers never treated documents as conclusive. Instead, they
came to rely almost exclusively on interviews, in which applicants are
asked to provide so-called family trees, which are cross-checked for
inconsistencies against parallel statements of relatives, or—in the case
of lingering doubt—followed up by village visits.

An altogether different control regime was imposed on husbands
and fiancés, who were either entirely barred from entry or subjected
to a severe test, not of identity, but of intention. From the early 1970s
to the mid-1980s, when secondary immigration became a dominant
concern, the rules on husbands and fiancés underwent no less than five
changes, some of them volte-face (Grant, 1987: 39). This has been the
most volatile and fiercely contested issue in British policy on secondary immigration. There are at least three reasons for this. First, and
most importantly, husbands were male immigrants, thus blurring the
line between secondary and primary immigration. Husbands were
perceived as covert primary immigrants, crowding an already strained
labour market, whose protection had been precisely the reason for
closing down primary immigration by the late 1960s. As Minister of
State Charles Waddington put it, 'It would be absurd if, having tightened up the work-permit system to prevent young men coming here

and going on to the labour market, we were to allow these same young men to come here by using marriage as a device' (quoted in House of Commons, 1986, ii. 108).

Secondly, getting tough on husbands rested on a lingering presumption in British law and customs that the wife should be where the husband as head of family was, and not vice versa. Shadow Home Secretary William Whitelaw admitted this quite frankly: 'Abode of the husband in marriage should normally be viewed as the natural place of residence.'[40] Asymmetrical treatment of wives and husbands was only the most drastic example of an immigration law shot through with sex inequalities, allowing unmarried girls over 18 to immigrate, but not boys, allowing in widows at any age, but not widowers, stipulating that au pairs must be girls, and allowing pre-1973 male (but not female) immigrants to be freely joined by their spouses and children. When the pattern of secondary immigration gradually shifted from the wives and children of primary male immigrants to the fiancé(e)s and spouses of those who had grown up in the United Kingdom (see House of Commons, 1986, i. p. vi), the range of clamping down on this source of new immigration was limited by Section 1(5) of the 1971 Immigration Act, which granted unrestricted marriage rights to all settled male immigrants born before 1 January 1973—barely teenagers in the mid-1980s. Accordingly, the immigration pressure originating from Britain's own second-generation immigrants could be defeated at the domestic female, but not male, front.

There was a third, more subdued, but forever present justification for keeping husbands out. It was tradition in Muslim culture that wives would move to the residence of their husbands. In giving in to an arranged marriage (which most of the immigration marriages were), young British Muslim women evidently professed their adherence to traditional Muslim culture. Asking these women to join their prospective husbands in Bangladesh or Pakistan was the logical next step. This was also a mischievous way of using multiculturalism for purposes of immigration control. Its reasoning was hypocritical, because it was driven by an obvious (if never admitted) animus against arranged marriage, while positively invoking its principles at the same time. When the 'primary purpose' rule advanced as the chief means of keeping husbands out, immigrant foes used the patrilocal norm to expose all arranged marriage as bogus. A Tory back-bencher, in a debate over immigration rules in 1982, put it this way: 'It is the custom on the Indian subcontinent for the woman to live in the husband's home town . . . If [she] seek[s] an arranged marriage with someone outside

this country and wish[es] to bring [him] into this country, by definition that must be for purposes of immigration.'[41]

In a fine demonstration of bipartisan consensus in British immigration policy, it was a Labour government which first conceived the idea
of keeping husbands out. Just having completed the 1968 Commonwealth Immigrants Act, Home Secretary James Callaghan discovered
that 'marriage is being used by many young men of working age as a
means of entering, working and settling in this country. This abuse of
the concession is inconsistent with the general scheme of Commonwealth immigration control' (quoted in Dummett and Nicol, 1990:
206). The 'concession' referred to is a provision in earlier instructions
to immigration officers to normally admit husbands and fiancés,
although their status was not defined in statutory immigration law
(ibid. 207). The logic is clear: immigrants did not have rights; at best
they might profit from concessions made to them by a benevolent
government. But the following first-time exclusion of foreign husbands was so sweeping that all British women, including white patrial
women, were prevented from bringing in foreign husbands. In 1974,
Roy Jenkins, Home Secretary of a new Labour government, after
some hesitation, allowed husbands back in, convinced of 'the stark and
unacceptable nature of the discrimination' (quoted in Bevan, 1986:
247). For the next three years, all women settled in Britain could be
freely joined by their spouses and fiancés. But in 1977, pressured by a
press campaign against illegal immigration racketeering and 'brides for
purchase', the same Labour government tightened the screw again,
introducing a provision against 'marriages of convenience' and imposing on foreign husbands (but not wives) a probationary period of
twelve months to ensure that the marriage was genuine. This created a
first wedge between immigration and family law, because for the
latter, ceremony and certificate were conclusive, whereas the former
screened for the 'right' motivation. The door had been opened for
intrusive questioning and subjective discretion on the part of immigration officials, which would become more fully expressed under the
reign of the 'primary purpose' rule.

The war on foreign husbands started in earnest under the new Tory
government of Mrs Thatcher. During the election campaign, the aspiring Prime Minister had expressed her often-quoted concern that
Britain was being 'rather swamped by people with a different culture'
(quoted in Layton-Henry, 1992: 184), and the Tory 1979 election manifesto included a high-priority pledge to combat the swamping by
excluding foreign husbands: 'We shall end the concession introduced

Thatcher cuts husbands

by the Labour government in 1974 to husbands and male fiancés.'[42] Indeed, after Jenkins's dropping of the first husbands ban the number of admitted foreign husbands had increased from 277 in 1974 to 3,005 in 1978 (Sachdeva, 1993: 64). It did not matter that the various rule changes on husbands instituted in the first half of the 1980s all occurred against a record decline of new immigration, especially from the New Commonwealth and Pakistan.[43] Here was a 'loophole' that had to be closed, and once the husbands ban had been elevated to an election pledge there was no tinkering with a popular mandate. One of the first measures of the new government was the introduction, in 1980, of new immigration rules that barred foreign husbands and fiancés from settlement in Britain. As the Minister of State explained the measure in the House of Commons, 'We have a particular aim—to cut back on primary male immigration' (quoted in Thornberry, 1980: 146).

But this was no simple return to the first husbands ban under Callaghan. The new rules were both more lenient and more restrictive: more lenient toward white patrial women, because, under pressure, the government exempted from the ban the husbands and fiancés of UK citizens born or with a grandparent born in the UK; and more restrictive, because this exemption was granted only at the price of new safeguards. The husbands and fiancés joining eligible UK women now had to prove, first, that the 'primary purpose' of their marriage was not immigration, secondly, that they intended to live together permanently with their wives, and, thirdly, in an obvious slap at arranged marriages, that the parties had met before. These safeguards were insignificant at first, because the majority of New Commonwealth husbands were already excluded by the female birth and ancestry clause. Indeed, the applications by New Commonwealth husbands and fiancés promptly fell from 3,660 in 1979 to just 820 in 1980 (Sachdeva, 1993: 68). Three thousand more or less immigrants per year was the meagre stake in the husbands war, but in that business of loophole-closing there was no rest until the balance was down to zero.

husbands now had to prove 3 things.

Reflecting the absence of domestic legal-political remedies, the critique of the husbands ban was from the start formulated in terms of its international implications. As Lord Scarman feared, the new immigration rules 'will tarnish our national reputation among the free democracies of the world.'[44] Indeed, the government had to be fully aware that the husbands ban in the 1980 immigration rules was in breach of Britain's legal international obligations, especially regarding the European Convention on Human Rights.[45] This was no mere moral

prob with new rules

obligation, but one that in case of a negative European Court rule could be legally enforced in Britain. When the European Commission on Human Rights accepted for review the cases of three migrant wives affected by the husband rule, the British government responded with a prophylactic rule change, which opened up round two in the husbands war. As laid out in a White Paper of October 1982, henceforth all female British citizens, irrespective of birth or ancestry, would be allowed to be joined by their husbands and fiancés. Interestingly, this rule change was framed as an adjustment to the British Nationality Act, rather than pressure from abroad, which was ostentatiously ignored throughout. As Home Secretary William Whitelaw justified the liberalization of immigration rules in the House of Commons, after the creation of a British citizenship 'in line with those who belong to Britain' it would be wrong to make invidious subdistinctions according to birth or ancestry.[46] This could not be the end of the matter, because settled immigrant women (in contrast to men) still remained separated from their husbands. Section 1(5) of the 1971 Immigration Act, and the government's repeated pledge to honour the family rights of pre-1973 male immigrants, stood in the way of closing the husbands war—at least as long as the government wanted to maintain its firm hand on secondary immigration and not throw out privileges left and right.[47]

This second round in the husbands war was fought under the banner of a Tory back-bench rebellion, which demonstrated the extraordinarily narrow range for generous solutions to British immigration dilemmas. 'If we give way here,' howled the back-benchers against the proposed softening of the husbands ban, 'we would be allowing again a source of primary immigration which has just been stopped'.[48] To placate the rebels, the government flanked its partial sex equalization with tougher safeguards. Most importantly, the burden of proof in the primary-purpose test was shifted to the applicant.[49] Only now could the primary-purpose rule unfold its venomous powers, providing the government with the perfect tool to close the loophole that had opened up at the sex equalization front. But even that failed to move the rebels. In December 1982, the government was given its first serious parliamentary defeat, and Home Secretary Whitelaw was pushed to the edge of resignation, when over fifty Tory rebels joined Labour to reject the new immigration rules. 'What stuck in our throat was the reversal of the manifesto commitment,' a rebel said, 'it is a question of honour'.[50] This was an interesting way of injecting morality into the British immigration debate. Mollifying its back-benchers, whose rebellion cracked in February 1983, the government pointed out that never since 1962 had immigration been so low, and that the figures were particularly small regarding husbands and fiancés.[51] This was true, but why then this war on husbands?

Round three of the husbands war opened up in Strasbourg. In May 1985, the European Court of Human Rights ruled in *Abdulaziz, Cabales and Balkandali* that the 1980 immigration rules were discriminatory on the ground of sex, in violation of Article 14 taken together with Article 8. The court rejected the British government view that sexual discrimination was justified by its interest in protecting the labour market, which was allegedly more heavily burdened by male than by female immigrants. After chastising Britain for its antique conception of women as housekeepers, the Court went on to argue that 'the difference that may nevertheless exist between the respective impact of men and of women on the domestic labour market is [not] sufficiently important to justify the difference of treatment'.[52] This rule let off Britain lightly, because the plaintiffs's parallel charge of discrimination on the grounds of race and birth was dismissed.[53] Moreover, the court refused to construe a right of family reunion out of Article 8 alone, reaffirming that 'a State has the right to control the entry of non-nationals into its territory,' and opining that family reunion could as well take place in 'their husbands' home'.[54] This meant that the primary-purpose rule, which Britain's policy on secondary immigration increasingly came to rely on, could remain.

However lenient, the Strasbourg rule forced the government to remove the last trace of sex discrimination from its immigration rules. As Secretary of State Leon Brittan reckoned in the House of Commons, the government faced two choices.[55] The first choice was between 'narrowing' or 'widening' the husbands rule: bar settled immigrant men from bringing in their wives and fiancées, or permit settled immigrant wives to bring in their husbands and fiancés. 'Narrowing' would imply dishonouring the government commitment to the family rights of settled immigrant men, enshrined in Section 1(5) of the 1971 Immigration Act. Accordingly, the government opted for 'widening'. But in this case, the additional intake of about 2,000 more immigrant husbands per year had to be offset by new safeguards. This preset the government's second choice between 'abandoning' or 'extending' its marriage tests. To drop the tests currently applied to husbands only 'would be to go back on our firm commitment to strict immigration control'.[56] But if the tests were to be kept, the mandate of the Strasbourg rule was to apply them equally to men and women.

Brittan concluded his sharp logical exercise: 'We cannot expect the European Court to endorse . . . the continuation of giving wives preferential treatment by not making them subject to the same requirements.'[57] And such equality of misery cut both ways. Because the existing immigration rules required that post-1973 male immigrants had to demonstrate adequate funds and accommodation for their newly admitted wives, the logic of the Strasbourg rule forced the imposition of the same maintenance requirement on newly admitted husbands. While a Labour front-bencher railed against the government's 'spiteful and vindictive course',[58] one cannot but admire the cleverness of turning a European Court indictment into a means of even firmer immigration control.

As sharp as it appeared, the Home Secretary's logic was faulty. The commitment to Section 1(5), which motivated his choice of 'widening' the husbands rule, was undermined by his second choice of 'extending' the safeguards. As long as Section 1(5) was in force, the marriage tests, including the primary purpose rule, could not be used on pre-1973 settled immigrant men. If safeguards were to be maintained, the logic of the Strasbourg rule implied the removal of this privilege. Accordingly, even the one piece of generosity in the government's response to the Strasbourg rule was a chimera.[59]

Because Section 1(5), which finally stood in the way of full sex equality in British policy on secondary immigration, had the status of a statutory right, it could be removed only through a change of law. This was achieved in the 1988 Immigration Act, the first change of immigration law in seventeen years. Happening without much noise or protestation, the removal of Section 1(5) was a most extraordinary event. This was the only family right that had existed in British immigration law. It had created a stir already during the debate over the 1971 Immigration Act, when wide-spread protests, including from the House of Lords, forced the government to elevate this family right from the brittle status of discretionary rule to the solid status of statutory right. Successive governments had reaffirmed their commitment to honour this right. But all rights are relative in British law, as its painless removal by a simple parliamentary majority epitomizes. In dropping Section 1(5), the government also abandoned the one moral commitment it had undertaken *vis-à-vis* its primary New Commonwealth immigrants.[60] Now there was no limit any longer to the power of firm immigration control.

The removal of Section 1(5) had immediate victims. Bangladeshis, the last to arrive before New Commonwealth immigration was stopped in the 1960s, and poorer than most Asians, had so far hesitated to bring their families. Now they could be prevented from doing this by the generalized tough maintenance and accommodation requirements.[61] As Ian Macdonald pointed out, the erosion of family rights caught the Bangladeshis in a 'classic catch-22' situation: 'Until the family arrive, the husband in the UK will be unable to obtain council or other accommodation large enough to house his family. So they won't be able to come.'[62] But this was not all. Section 1(5) had so far protected the great majority of Britons, white patrials, from the marriage tests. Now they were subject to them too. The immigration tail came to wag the vast non-immigrant rest. In a telling dissonance, Section 7 of the 1988 Immigration Act exempted European Union nationals from the leave-to-enter requirement, in due compliance with the freedom of movement mandate of the Treaty of Rome. Simultaneously restricting the rights of British citizens and expanding the rights of European Union nationals epitomized the strange consequence of Britain's firm immigration policy. As Roy Hattersley correctly pointed out in his House of Commons outburst against that 'most tawdry little measure', it was now easier for a Frenchman living in Britain to bring in his American wife than it was for a British citizen to do the same.[63]

While the exclusion of husbands was gone, the primary-purpose rule reigned supreme. This was a logical outcome, because the marriage tests had originally been introduced to counteract the ever-widening exemptions from the husband ban. The ironic result of the Strasbourg rule was to broaden the war on husbands into a general war on all immigrant marriages.[64] The main weapon in this war was no longer objective exclusion on grounds of sex and citizenship, but subjective exclusion on grounds of intention. This became possible with the 1983 shift in the marriage test's burden of proof to the applicant, which activated the exclusion power of the primary-purpose rule. In a validation of Coleman's 'hydraulic analogy', this enthronment of the primary-purpose rule exactly compensated for the liberalization of the husbands rule. In 1982, the total refusal rate of foreign husbands was 47 per cent, of which 82 per cent were rejected on objective grounds (most notably the wife's citizenship). In 1983, the total refusal rate was still at 47 per cent. But now 73 per cent of those refused were refused on primary-purpose grounds. By 1984, the primary-purpose rule even accounted for 87 per cent of all refused applications (House of Commons, 1986, ii. 109).

The primary-purpose rule encapsulates the essence of British immigration law and policy: unfettered state discretion. The primary-purpose rule, as its very name indicates, presumes the existence of bogus applications, and leaves it to the applicant to prove the contrary, putting the latter into the no-win position of disproving a negative intention. And immigration officers are asked to measure what cannot be measured: intention. Because immigration officers are nevertheless forced to make a decision, a second set of 'hidden' immigration rules has been built up to inform such decisions. One of these secret instructions recognizes that there are 'no absolute criteria' on which a decision can be based, and that 'if there is no clear evidence either way . . . [an applicant] should no longer be given the benefit of the doubt' (quoted in CRE, 1985: 64).[65] The most questionable component of the subjective science of intention-measuring is the separate consideration of the genuineness of marriage, which can be quasi-objectively assessed by the actual intention and practice of living together, and of primary-purpose proper, for which there is no such indicator.[66] Splitting both components apart means that perfectly genuine marriages can still fail the primary-purpose test.

The primary-purpose rule puts applicants into a catch-22 situation, because the very application can be taken as evidence that the principal reason of the marriage is immigration to Britain. Gerald Kaufman of the Labour Party phrased the dilemma this way: 'How does one prove that one's application is not intended to achieve admission, when the success of one's application will, of course, result in one's admission?'[67] Especially in the case of arranged marriages, where it was unlikely that affection would cancel out instrumental motivation, the primary-purpose rule was an almost foolproof tool of exclusion.

In response to the high refusal rate of marriage immigration on primary-purpose grounds, a huge amount of case-law has accumulated.[68] Initially, judges showed sympathy for the plight of immigrants. In *Arun Kumar* (1986), Lord Donaldson denounced the catch-22 of taking an application for settlement as evidence that the primary purpose of marriage was immigration: 'If . . . the wife is already settled here, . . . it is idle for her to marry a man who does not wish to obtain admission to the United Kingdom. Yet it is fatally easy to treat his admission as evidence that this is the primary purpose of the marriage' (quoted in Scannell, 1992: 3). In addition, courts argued that the parties' demonstrated intention to live together permanently as man and wife after marriage (the 'genuineness' of marriage) should be taken as evidence that the primary purpose had not been immigration—thus fusing the two criteria of primary purpose and intention to cohabit that the Home Office's Immigration Rules from 1980 onwards had torn apart. The high-water mark of this liberal approach has been the High Court decision in *Matwander Singh* (1987), which argued that 'it will always be important when considering . . . marriage to obtain admission and . . . marriage to bind oneself for life to a particular person, to bear in mind, the enormity . . . and corresponding improbability of undertaking the latter to secure the former' (quoted in Scannell, 1992: 3).

But the counterpoint to such liberalism was the precedence-setting High Court and Court of Appeal decisions in *Vinod Bhatia* (1985). If there had been any doubt, *Bhatia* hammered down where the burden of proof rested: on the applicant, and that the demonstrated intention to cohabit did not yet prove that the primary purpose was not immigration. More than that, given that one was dealing 'with a situation where marriages might be arranged by parents for the purpose of securing the entry of the intended bridegroom into the UK', the presumption of the primary-purpose rule was always deception, that is, marriage concocted for immigration, unless and until the applicant proved the contrary.[69]

Seeking to reconcile these divergent court rules, the Court of Appeal, in its combined review of *Hoque and Singh* (1988), developed a catalogue of ten 'propositions of law' that were to be applied by immigration officers in marriage cases. While taking up some liberal tenets of earlier case-law, *Hoque and Singh* stipulated that the genuineness of marriage could not prejudge its primary purpose, and that 'in the end, it must be left to entry-clearance officers to decide how they do their work' (in Sachdeva, 1993: 142). This was a blank cheque for executive discretion. And it was the position reiterated in the decidedly illiberal bulk of later case-law.[70]

The primary-purpose rule is only the most drastic example of a wide policy repertory of keeping immigrant families divided.[71] Legal observers suggest that the primary-purpose rule has passed its zenith, the mechanism of exclusion shifting to tougher financial support and accommodation requirements.[72] Wherever the ball may roll next, Britain has played such a firm hand on secondary immigration that its family rights are now significantly below the European Union standard. This has been exposed by the European Court of Justice rule on *Surinder Singh* (1992).[73] The court held that a British national returning from employment in a member state of the European Union has the unconditional right to be accompanied by her husband, whatever his nationality. This follows from Article 52 of the EEC Treaty, which prohibits restrictions on the freedom of movement. Accordingly, a British citizen has more family rights under European Union law than under domestic law. To be sure, such protection by EU law only applies to the few mobile border-crossers; the reign of domestic law over the immobile rest remains untouched. As is sometimes misunderstood, the *Singh* rule is no indictment of the primary purpose rule, under whose weight British family rights have sunk below the European standard. But it creates the paradoxical situation that a British citizen moving around in Europe is exempted from the primary purpose rule. Accordingly, there is now the generic possibility of circumventing Britain's harsh immigration law by the European route. It is unlikely that this paradox will prevail. Britain's firm hand on secondary immigration may have to loosen a little.[74]

Always Firm: British Asylum Policy

Britain has a proud tradition of receiving refugees, which long precedes the 1951 Geneva Convention. In fact, the word 'refugee' was first used for the French Huguenots who found refuge in England from Catholic persecution after the revocation of the Edict of Nantes in 1685. In the age of mass asylum-seeking, this tradition fell victim to the zero-immigration imperative that quickly and unreservedly seized asylum policy. Just when secondary family immigration had been brought down to a trickle in the mid-1980s, asylum emerged as a potential new floodgate of primary immigration. Clearly, here was another 'loophole' that had to be closed. Britain was uniquely well prepared to do this. No recalcitrant judiciary stood in the way of an iron-handed executive redeploying its formidable arsenal of immigration controls at the asylum front.

Accordingly, a key characteristic of British asylum policy is its rhetorical and structural conflation with immigration policy. When the arrival of Tamils in 1985 signalled Britain's entry into the age of mass asylum-seeking, the colour-couched control mentality of immigration policy instantly took hold of the new asylum field.[75] Home Secretary Douglas Hurd even applied the government's old immigration policy slogan to its new asylum policy: 'firm but fair'.[76] The cleavages and discursive metaphors of immigration policy became exactly mirrored in asylum policy: asylum advocates calling racist the government's assumption that most refugees were economic migrants, and the government defending its get-tough approach toward asylum-seekers as in the interest of firm immigration control and good race relations (see Kaye, 1994). In a demonstration of this, the government defended the first explicit asylum legislation in 1992 as 'strengthen-[ing] our system of controlling entry and excluding people not entitled to be here. Good race relations are heavily dependent on strict immigration control'.[77]

But the conflation of asylum and immigration policy was not only rhetorical. Until the passing of the Asylum and Immigration Appeals Act in 1993, there was no separate asylum law. Asylum was processed according to the Immigration Act of 1971 and the non-statutory Immigration Rules (see Macdonald and Blake, 1991: ch. 12). This meant that the shortcomings of immigration law and practice were *ipso facto* shortcomings of asylum determination: the lack of an in-country appeal procedure for would-be entrants rejected at the border, which entailed the generic possibility of refoulement (see Goodwin-Gill, 1978: 119);[78] and the unchecked discretion of the executive to detain and deport immigrants and asylum-seekers alike. About the immigration officers a Law Lord had this to say: 'They cannot be expected to know or apply the [European] Convention [on Human Rights]. They must go simply by the Immigration Rules laid down by the Secretary of State and not by the Convention' (quoted in Storey, 1994: 123). Since the Aliens Restriction Acts of 1914 and 1919, asylum has been the uncontested *refugium* of the Home Office (Macdonald and Blake, 1991: 302). The self-abdication of the judiciary was reaffirmed in the 1985 landmark asylum case of *Bugdaycay*. Here the High Court argued that the judiciary had absolutely no say in the determination of refugee status, because Parliament had decided that *all* questions of entry and stay (including asylum) should be determined by an immigration officer and the Secretary of State, respectively: 'There was no basis on which any jurisdiction in the High Court could be found to determine the question whether a person was a refugee or should be granted asylum.'[79]

Reviewing British asylum policy, one is struck by its inclination to make maximal fuss over minimal numbers. From 1980 to 1988, Britain received less than 38,000 asylum applications, the annual numbers rarely exceeding the 5,000 mark (Amnesty International, 1991: 4). This made Britain the country with the lowest per capita, and the second lowest nominal, refugee intake in Europe (Ruff, 1989: 485). The low numbers are partially the result of quick footwork in externalizing refugee streams, which took full advantage of Britain's geographical insulation. The most important of these has been a tight and instantly imposed visa regime. In an application of the 'pressure to emigrate' doctrine, every incipient refugee stream was quickly countered by a new visa requirement: Sri Lanka in 1985; India, Pakistan, Nigeria, Ghana, and Bangladesh in 1986; Turkey in June 1989; Somalia in July 1990; and ex-Yugoslavia in November 1992, among others. Fast legislation backed up these administrative measures. The Carriers' Liability Act of 1987, which imposed a fine of £1,000 sterling for each passenger carried to Britain's ports without valid passport and visa, effectively farmed out the burden of immigration control to shipping and airline personnel. The administrative and legislative externalization of refugee streams was sealed by the geopolitical advocacy of keeping refugees in their home countries, which made Britain recognize the fledgling states of Kurdistan and Bosnia as a substitute for accepting their refugees (Cohen, 1994: 98).

The resulting low numbers have allowed Britain to reject initially relatively few asylum-applicants: still in 1989, 30 per cent were granted refugee status, 60 per cent were granted 'exceptional leave to remain' (*de facto* refugee status), and only 10 per cent were rejected (Amnesty International, 1991: 4). But in a strange counterbalance to a mild recognition practice behind the scenes, the front of the stage was occupied by a few highly publicized deportation cases, some of which entailed proven violations of Britain's international non-refoulement obligation. They may have been few, but they pointed to the crux of British asylum policy: the lack of effective in-country appeal procedures, and the quasi-absolute power of the executive in asylum determination.

Tamils have played a sad major part in such deportation cases. As an asylum advocate put it, '[the Tamils] were . . . typical of the very people that immigration law had been keeping out for decades. They were black, they were young men, they were from the Indian subcontinent'.[80] There was an instant reflex to brand the Tamils, who began arriving in larger numbers in 1985, as 'economic migrants' or 'bogus' refugees. Not without reason, because they came from the region where the 'pressure to emigrate' was highest and that was accordingly targeted by the government to strike at family-based immigration: the Indian subcontinent. Getting tough on Tamils was indeed determined by the need for consistency with tight immigration controls: 'queue jumping' was no abstraction where the Home Office had erected huge administrative hurdles for family reunification from Bangladesh or India. In a way, the logic of immigration control exerted assimilatory pressure on asylum policy.[81] A hastily imposed visa requirement for Sri Lankans, the first ever for a Commonwealth country, was a first measure of realigning asylum admissions with immigration control; precedent-setting deportations were the second.

The two major deportation cases involving Tamils were of radically opposite nature, and they epitomize the whole ambiguity of the asylum phenomenon, not only in Britain. The first case involved an ethnic Sinhalese supporting the Tamil cause, Viraj Mendis, who was forcibly removed to Sri Lanka in 1989 after having spent two years in church asylum. This most politicized deportation case of all is a classic case of 'boot-strapping' (Teitelbaum, 1984: 80 ff.), the *post factum* creation of asylum causes. An ex-student who had overstayed for eleven years, Mendis had applied for asylum in order to avoid a deportation order. A failed 'bogus' marriage with a British citizen on his record, Mendis's political engagement intensified just when his resident status in Britain became endangered. Even the UNHCR did not support his case. As a *Guardian* commentator wrote sarcastically, 'He had failed his exams, his marriage to an Englishwoman was a sham, and most of all he had developed political views for the sake of convenience. All in all, you mused, he would make an ideal Tory MP'.[82] Far from this, Mendis became a cause célèbre for Britain's race-relations Left, particularly the Socialist Workers Party and Revolutionary Communist Group (RCG), which supported him in a two-year long, country-wide campaign that included 24-hour vigils at his church shelter, regular demonstrations and signature drives, and a Labour-initiated committee of inquiry at the Commons. But for the Home Office the shy yet determined Sinhalese represented that typical example of 'law-dodger masquerading as genuine refugee',[83] and it went after him with a vehemence that bordered on revengefulness. In Mendis, the government vindicated the central motive of its asylum policy: no mercy for 'bogus refugees'. After thirteen years on British soil (ten years are normally sufficient to be granted permanent resident status), Mendis was surprised one morning by a police squad that showed no scruples in demolishing church doors, and he was thrown into the next plane to Colombo. What most liberal states would not have done for humanitarian reasons, the British showed no hesitation to do.[84]

The second Tamil deportation case is diametrically opposed, because it involved the refoulement of genuine refugees. In February 1988, the Home Office expelled five Tamil asylum-seekers, who had arrived without entry clearance on various dates in 1987. The lack of proper visas excluded them from using the in-country appeals system—appeal they could, but only from back home! Their only remedy: a toothless judicial review, could assess the procedural correctness, but not the substantial merits of the case. On these limited grounds, the House of Lords eventually upheld the Home Office's deportation order (see Blake, 1988). Characteristically denounced by a Tory MP as 'liars, cheats, and queue jumpers', three of the five deported Tamils subsequently endured torture and severe maltreatment by Sinhalese police and soldiers.[85] An immigration appeals adjudicator decided in their out-of-country appeal that all five were entitled to political asylum, ordering the Home Office to bring them back to Britain 'with the minimum delay' (see Blake, 1990). For Amnesty International, this was the first conclusive evidence that Britain was breaching the UN convention, pointing out the 'pressing need' for statutory appeal rights *within* Britain.[86]

The Tamil refoulement was only the beginning of a series of deportation blunders that are without parallel in the Western world. A High Court review found that twenty-three Turkish Kurds were 'unlawfully' deported in mid-1989.[87] Three of them, who had not even been allowed to leave the aeroplane at Heathrow, had to endure prolonged torture in police custody after their return. The government's 'street fighting approach' (Burgess, 1991: 50) came to a head in the case of 'M', a Zairean asylum-seeker who was deported in May 1991 (and has since disappeared and is presumed dead), in direct contravention of a court order granting interim relief and a stay of deportation. Ignoring a court injunction was common practice by an aloof executive that deemed itself protected by traditional 'Crown immunity'. Enshrined in the Crown Proceedings Act of 1947, the doctrine of Crown immunity held that officers of the Crown were not subject to administrative law remedies, such as injunctions and specific performance (Ward, 1994: 195 f.). But in *M* v. *Home Office*, which was hailed by constitutional lawyers as one of the most important court cases in the last 200 years (Wade, 1992: 1275), the Court of Appeal, and subsequently the House of Lords, decided differently. In dramatic terms, Lord Templeman argued in the Court of Appeals: 'If upheld, [the argument of crown immunity would] establish the proposition that the executive obey the law as a matter of grace and not as a matter of necessity, a proposition which would reverse the result of the Civil War.'[88] Accordingly, the court found the Home Secretary guilty of 'contempt of court'. This was a novelty in British legal history, which signals a transition from the traditional 'trust and co-operation' relationship between judiciary and executive to a 'mandatory model of judicial review' (Harlow, 1994: 620).

It is important to point out that the growing impatience of British judges with a high-handed executive has European roots. In

Factortame No.2, the European Court of Justice had for the first time instructed British courts to grant interim coercive relief against the government in matters of European law. As Lord Donaldson pointed out in *M v. Home Office*, this created the 'anomalous' situation that the government could be indicted for breaches of European law, but not for breaches of domestic law (Ward, 1994: 200). *M v. Home Office* removed this anomaly by applying the more demanding European standards of individual-rights protection to British domestic law.

Indicative of the weight of the European challenge was the one liberalizing measure in the 1993 Asylum and Immigration Appeals Act: the granting of an in-country right of appeal for all asylum-seekers, which was in anticipation of a European Court indictment.[89] But this was more than offset by two restrictive features of the new act: the removal of the right to appeal for refused short-term visitors and students, and the introduction of a 'fast-track' procedure for 'manifestly unfounded' asylum claims (see Randall, 1994). Giving a right to asylum-seekers while taking an established right away from another group subject to immigration controls highlights Britain's structural conflation of asylum and immigration policy. Had the bill's (rather rocky) career started in 1991 as an exclusive 'asylum bill', its final incarnation in 1993 was largely criticized as an 'anti-black family' measure that further curtailed the family reunion rights of Britain's settled immigrants.[90] The original backdrop of the 1993 Act, which for the first time established a statutory framework for the determination of asylum claims, was a sharp rise in the number of new asylum seekers: 11,635 in 1989, 22,000 in 1990, and 44,840 in 1991—a tenfold increase since 1988 (BRC, 1992: 2). This was still a trickle compared with other Western states, but enough to push the British government into action.

The Asylum Act also demonstrates that in certain regards Europe was not a challenge to, but of help to Britain's firm asylum policy. The Act's core provisions: fingerprinting of applicants, stiffened carrier sanctions, and 'fast-tracking' of 'manifestly unfounded' applications (which include applications by people arriving from 'safe third countries' and applications based on forged or destroyed documents), are identical with the emergent European Union asylum policy, and designed to obviate a future European adjustment of Britain's national policy.[91] In fact, Britain, while jealously protecting its sovereignty on immigration from encroachment by European Union institutions, has been an enthusiastic leader of the intergovernmental Trevi Group of EU immigration ministers, in whose secrecy the new British-cum-European asylum policy has been put together. If Fortress Europe is being built on the foundation of its lowest common denominator, it is the Fortress Britain turned inside out.

The Asylum Act's fast processing of 'manifestly unfounded' asylum claims has led to an unprecedented decline of Britain's refugee recognition rate. The rate of refused asylum applications leaped from 16 per cent in 1993 to 75 per cent in 1994, most of the refused facing involuntary repatriation.[92] Those not deported immediately, are increasingly housed in prison-like detention centres. Arbitrary detention of asylum-seekers has been standard practice since the first arrival of Tamils a decade earlier. But after the new Asylum Act, detentions acquired a new quality, the number of detainees doubling from 300 in 1993 to over 600 in 1994. In Campsfield House, Britain's newest and largest Immigration Detention Centre near Oxford, detained asylum-seekers felt 'treated like prisoners', initiating a wave of hunger strikes and riots that affected other detention centres throughout the country.[93] While defended as in the interest of 'good race relations' (Home Secretary Kenneth Baker), the Asylum and Immigration Act's impact on black family life was no less negative. On Christmas Eve 1993, immigration officers detained a whole planeload of Jamaican visitors; they had come to see their relatives, but eventually saw iron bars at Campsfield House, before being summarily returned to Kingston. This was possible because appeal rights for refused visitors no longer existed. What shocked the British public and caused a diplomatic row with Jamaica, was stoically defended by a Tory MP: 'The Government has every right to send back anybody it wants.'[94] Such has been the British approach to immigration and asylum policy alike.[95]

The Challenge of Europe

Both the German and British approaches to immigration have outlived the historical contexts in which they had emerged and they were attuned to, the guestworker era and decolonization, respectively. But whereas German foreigner policy is currently undergoing a fundamental reconsideration, British immigration policy is thoroughly entrenched, with 'no argument on fundamental policy' (Dummett and Nicol, 1990: 253). At the same time, both policies face the challenge of an emergent European Union immigration regime, but in diametrically opposite directions. The new enthusiasm in Germany over an explicit immigration policy is nudged by a European Union that does not want immigration and that has no philosophical problems with pre-reunification Germany's 'not a country of immigration' formula. By contrast, the European challenge to British immigration policy is not a restrictive but liberalizing one, bringing into question the very bases of this policy: tight border controls and executive discretion over the fate of immigrants.

Britain's geography has favoured a system of immigration control that is centred on rigorous checks at the points of entry. As in the United States, border-centred immigration control has minimized the need for internal controls, and Britain is now one of only two countries in Europe without a mandatory ID-card scheme. The situation is the reverse in continental Europe, where uncontrollable land borders have favoured elaborate systems of domestic supervision. Now the dismantling of internal frontiers, as mandated by the Single European Act, is imposing continental ways on Britain. No wonder she balks at this, Euro-friendly Labour politicians no less than Euro-sceptic Tories. Farcical compromise attempts, such as the 'Bangemann-wave' (where EU passengers would merely hold up their unopened passports without being stopped), only underline that there is no third way.[96] Britain continues to insist that for the sake of illegal immigration, terrorism, and drug control, internal border controls are to be maintained. However, having signed the Treaty on European Union, whose Clause 8a mandates the making of 'an area without internal frontiers in which the free movement of goods, persons, services and capital is ensured', Britain cannot win this battle, unless she withdraws from Europe.

The material stakes in the battle over border control are surprisingly low. In 1990, British immigration officers denied entry to only 19,000 of 50 million passengers, most of whom had arrived on flights from non-EU countries (which will continue to be controlled).[97] Almost half of the 15 million foreigners in the EU, which Britain refuses to lose control of, are EU nationals living in another EU country and Britain's own New Commonwealth immigrants; the other half, which includes the huge immigrant populations of France or Germany, have few incentives to move to a country whose standard of living has sunk below the European average. But the symbolic stakes are high. The essence of British immigration philosophy: keep them out, refugees no less than rabies, is at risk. More than that, the demon of race conflict that had driven British immigration policy since its inception might finally have its way: 'The moment the public gain the impression that we aren't totally in control of entry across our borders,' speculates a Tory MP, 'nasty things will happen with race relations'.[98] Far beyond immigration, the crumbling of old certainties, from the monarchy to the integrity of the multinational state, has left the border, so clearly marked as the line that separates the land from the sea, as the one certainty that must and will not go.

A second European challenge is not just logistical, but goes to the heart of immigration law and the relationship between individual and the state. Britain now has two separate systems of immigration law, one attuned to the empire that enshrines the absolute supremacy of the state over the individual, and a second, European system that is based on the opposite principle of liberating the individual from mobility restrictions by member states. This has led to the paradox that EU-nationals have more immigration rights in Britain than domestic citizens. In the long run, the adaptation pressure is upwards, not downwards. With the exception of the 1951 Geneva Convention on Refugees, Britain has not domestically incorporated any of the major international human rights conventions and treaties, and even refused to ratify those that came in the way of firm immigration controls.[99] But in two crucial exceptions this obtrusiveness does not matter much. The European Convention on Human Rights, set up by the Council of Europe after the horror of a continent destroyed in war and the Nazi crimes against humanity, is one of the few international treaties that are legally binding, with a commission and a court to ensure compliance. European Union Law has even shed the character of international law, and a big part of it is directly applicable in member states and creates rights for individuals.

The message from *East African Asians* to *M* v. *Home Office* is clear. Through the European Convention of Human Rights and EU law, continental-style human-rights protections and judicial politics have silently invaded domestic immigration law and practice. This is more benign than rabies, because it protects the individual from the vagaries of parliamentary-cum-executive sovereignty. Under the influence of Europe, the calls for a domestic bill of rights have gained ground, if only to help Britain shed her reputation as Europe's worst human rights offender, and national courts are cautiously venturing into the new grounds of judicial review.[100] Its entrenchment is deceptive, because nothing less than a fundamental reorientation of British immigration law and policy is bound to happen, from unlimited state discretion toward the rule of law and human rights protection. Firmness may suffer, but British liberty will win.

This chapter showed that the state sometimes classified as 'weak' if compared with continental Europe's 'strong' states has displayed an exceptionally strong hand in immigration policy. The principle of parliamentary sovereignty and common law restraints have neutralized the courts as effective opponents of the executive, resulting in Home Office absolutism in immigration policy. But the notion of immigration policy is misleading, because Britain never had proactively engaged in the recruitment of foreigners; all it had was a *laissez-passer* regime for nominal subjects of the Crown. This proved tremendously controversial for coloured migrants from the New Commonwealth, whose barring from entry and settlement has been the logic of British immigration policy. This chapter concentrated on the harsh measures of the executive to bring even family unification and asylum-granting down to a trickle. Both immigration and asylum pressures originated mostly from the Indian subcontinent, which reinforced a peculiar conflation of immigration control and asylum policy. In the British case, human-rights constraints on state sovereignty are indeed external, as the recurrent citations of Britain to European courts demonstrate. But they have (so far) been ineffective in loosening up Europe's tightest zero-immigration regime.

PART II

Multicultural Integration

Introduction to Part II

The comparison of immigrant integration is a good deal messier than the comparison of immigration control. Whereas 'control' dealt mainly with state policies and their determinants and implications, 'integration' touches on a multiplicity of economic, social, and cultural dimensions beyond the narrowly political one, including the forms of self-organization and ethnic identity of immigrants. I also have to concede that control and integration are not as unrelated as their analytical division here might suggest. Restricting access to formal membership or welfare benefits, as in the negative integration policies currently being forged in the United States, may be in the service of more effective immigration control. Or generous integration offers to historically particular immigrant groups may be legitimate props for the shift to zero-immigration policies—this has certainly been the European experience. By the same token, a key difference in the handling of immigrant integration is the propensity of European states to devise explicit integration policies, while in the United States this process has been left to the economy and society. This reflects the relative novelty and incompatibility of immigration with nationhood in Europe, and its relative entrenchment and compatibility with traditional nation-building in the United States.

This crucial difference in mind, the following comparison focuses on the political opportunity structures that have channelled the integration of migrants. Leaving out equally important economic, social, or demographic aspects of integration, this is a limited perspective. But it follows from our interest in the relationship between immigration and the membership component of nation-states, citizenship.

The two opposite poles in the recent literature on immigration and citizenship, Brubakerian citizenship traditionalism and Soysalian membership postnationalism, may serve as preliminary guides to our comparison of immigrant integration. What would we expect to find in light of these theories? Citizenship traditionalism, which stresses the inertia and ultra-stability of national citizenship traditions, would predict uniform pressure to mould new members in shape of the old, and a distaste for tolerating new membership forms and identities that deviate from national citizenship. By contrast, membership post-nationalism, which postulates the rise of the same model of universal personhood across states, would predict a weakening of nationally particular citizenship models and the institutional stabilization of similar denizenship forms and new identities across states.

To anticipate the main result of the following three chapters, what we find instead is an extreme variety of outcomes that defies both citizenship traditionalism and membership postnationalism. Perhaps a general theory of immigration and citizenship is impossible: one cannot say more about it than what one finds in specific contexts and constellations. Accordingly, the following chapters have a moderate aim. They compare the particular membership conceptions in place at the point of new immigration, and seek to capture the different ways in which the immigration experience reconfirmed or transformed these membership conceptions. The local explanations provided in these chapters still have general implications. Against citizenship traditionalism, they reveal the malleability of citizenship in liberal states; against membership postnationalism, they show that national citizenship remains indispensable for integrating immigrants.

In the United States, citizenship as a legal category is 'thin citizenship' (Heller, 1997: 26–7), easy to acquire if certain residence conditions are fulfilled, and conferring few privileges beyond those already granted to legal permanent residents. This is not because of global human-rights discourse inventing a new form of non-citizen membership. Rather, in a society cherishing markets over the state and the open border over bounded community, entry and residence have always been more meaningful than citizenship. Accordingly, the American Constitution and legal order make personhood and residence, rather than citizenship, protected categories. A formal citizenship was only introduced with the 14th Amendment in 1868, with a specific purpose in mind: the enfranchisement of black slaves (see Bickel, 1975; Ueda, 1982). Because of its elasticity and low acquisition threshold, American citizenship as a legal status has generally not been challenged or modified by post-1965 immigration.

Instead, American citizenship as an identity has come under fire. Post-1965 immigrants, predominantly from Latin America and Asia, arrive in a political environment that classifies them as racial minorities, and thus locks them into a corporate category between individual and citizen. Previously, immigrants had carried with them an ethnicity, which was a material resource of adaptation first and a symbolic identity option later. Such ethnicity was reconcilable with the ethnically anonymous, political concept of American citizenship and nationhood. Race is different. Its content is not a positive heritage (however modified) transplanted into the new society, but the negative experience of oppression at the hands of the receiving society. Its direction is not integration into a (white) majority deemed oppressive, but restitution for harm and public existence as a protected, separate group. It is important to stress that racial minority status for non-European immigrants is not a deliberate policy of immigrant integration, but a non-intended consequence of compensating the historical victims of American nation-building. Thus, 'Hispanic' immigrants today (whatever their ultimate origins) are compensated for the nineteenth century colonization of the American South-West; 'Asian' immigrants today are compensated for their past exclusion under a racist immigration and citizenship regime (which is an irony, because Asians were allowed to enter in significant numbers exactly after the removal of the old regime). Some commentators have responded to the immigration-fuelled proliferation of ethnoracial groups with alarm: it undermines common citizenship and leads to the fragmenting of the American nation.[1] This alarm is mistaken. The race discourse is domestic élite discourse, especially in higher education. It is not necessarily shared by the immigrants themselves, for whom, now as before, ethnicity functions as a pivotal resource of adaptation to the new society.

The German case of immigrant integration is diametrically opposed to the American case. The baseline of the German integration problematique is a 'thick' concept of citizenship, which is genealogical rather than territorial, and thus normally closed to non-nationals. Accordingly, postwar immigration has put huge pressure on citizenship as a legal status, toward facilitating its acquisition by long-settled and later-generation immigrants. In turn, there has been less debate about the ethnicity or race of immigrants, partly because there were few non-white immigrants, and partly because these are concepts delegitimized by recent German history.

For long, the integration of guestworkers in Germany was characterized by the co-existence of traditional ethnic citizenship, closed to foreigners, and of postnational membership, in which the universal human-rights provisions in the Basic Law endowed settled foreigners with most of the rights and privileges that Germans enjoy. These were two sides of the same coin: postnational membership allowed the maintainance of ethnic citizenship, which survived after its delegitimization by Nazism only indirectly, as the homeland obligations of the Federal Republic to the ethnic German diaspora imprisoned by communism.

National reunification has brought to an end the temporary coexistence of ethnic citizenship and postnational membership. With the demise of an ethnic diaspora to redeem, there is no longer a rationale for maintaining ethnic citizenship. In addition, the wave of xenophobic violence in post-reunification Germany has thrown the problem of integrating third-generation immigrants into sharp relief, exerting pressure on a descent-based citizenship regime that keeps even the children of those foreigners who were themselves born in Germany outside the national community. Pulled by a legal citizenship regime that has lost its historical legitimacy, and pushed by the problem of integrating young third-generation foreigners, Germany is now moving from an ethnic toward a civic-territorial citizenship regime. Few have noticed that the introduction of as-of-right naturalization in the early 1990s has done away with assimilation as a requirement for citizenship acquisition, making the German naturalization process even more liberal than the American one (which is still based on an assimilation test). In addition, the introduction of *jus soli* citizenship for third-generation immigrants enjoys overwhelming public and political support, and seems to be only temporarily blocked by the dwindling rearguard defenders of the status quo.

Finally, Great Britain shows an altogether different relationship between immigration and citizenship. Until 1981, Britain had no national citizenship at all, but only a 'thin', pre-national concept of subjectship, defined as allegiance to the Crown, which included Borneo cannibals and noble Lords alike. In addition, Britain dealt with immigrants who had the same legal status as the native population. Britain had two separate citizenship debates in response to its New Commonwealth immigration. One was related to the problem of immigration control (as discussed in Chapter 4), and culminated in the making of the British Nationality Act of 1981. The Act consolidated the already existing restrictions on New Commonwealth immigration by introducing the legal status of British citizen that alone conferred the right of abode in the UK. Note that this belated introduction of national citizenship narrowed the circle of those entitled to belong, and that its partial introduction of *jus sanguinis* ethnicized a previously civic definition of political membership. Britain thus moved in the exactly opposite direction as Germany had done, which widened the circle of those entitled to citizenship and moved from ethnic to civic criteria of membership.

However, citizenship was also the idiom of integrating New Commonwealth immigrants. Remember that these immigrants arrived as quasi-citizens, with full civil and political rights. The next logical step was to give them social rights as well. This was supported by the fact that the arrival of the immigrants coincided with the building of a national welfare state, and Marshallian citizenship universalism was the idiom of the day. The logic of this welfare state was provision on the basis of individual need, rather than group status. This meant avoiding treating immigrants as a group. Colour-blindness or 'racial inexplicitness' (Kirp, 1979) has been the initial British approach to immigrant integration—also in a conscious attempt to avoid the parallel American move toward racial explicitness.

Marshallian citizenship universalism has always uneasily coexisted with acknowledging the racial difference of postcolonial immigrants. After all, the British integration regime became known as a 'race relations' regime. Accordingly, a precarious balance between citizenship universalism and racial-group particularism came to characterize British immigrant integration. Over time, this balance tipped toward racial group particularism, stopping short, however, of granting group rights to immigrants. Why did group particularism grow stronger? First, it was always there, from the imperial legacy of indirect rule to the tradition of multi-ethnic nationhood. Secondly, group particularism was fostered by race activists, who sought to implement elements of the American 'black power' model at the level of local government. Thirdly, group particularism became institutionally recognized after the race riots in the early 1980s, which fed a sense of urgency on the part of political élites to do more to integrate anomic second-generation immigrants.

Looking at the three cases combined, we see an extreme variety of immigration-citizenship linkages that cannot be pressed into the corset of either citizenship traditionalism or membership postnationalism. Britain and the United States never had strong concepts of national citizenship to exert closure functions. By the same token, they do not have postnational membership to replace or relativize outworn national citizenship. Britain even used the immigration challenge to create what it did not have before, national citizenship. The schemes of citizenship traditionalism and membership postnationalism have a certain relevance for the German case, but in ways not reconcilable with their own assumptions. Citizenship traditionalism and postnational membership have co-existed there for a while, one conditioning the other, instead of being in a relationship of partial substitution as predicted by postnational membership analysts. And the content of persisting national citizenship has not remained stable over time, as predicted by citizenship traditionalists, but has undergone change, from ethnic to civic-territorial.

There is, however, one strong generalization to make. All three have been instances of multicultural integration, which shuns the assimilation of immigrants. This corresponds to the logic of liberal states, which have learned to accommodate a plurality of cultures, immigrant or non-immigrant based. The following three chapters provide ample evidence that 'multicultural citizenship' (Kymlicka, 1995*a*) is not an abstract demand of philosopher or activist; it is a reality in liberal states. But as these chapters will also demonstrate, the communality of multicultural integration is couched in distinct national colours: compensation for historical oppression in the United States, liberal *laissez-faire* in Britain, and counter-programme to a historically incriminated nation-state in Germany. In this sense, even multicultural integration is unmistakably national integration.

'Race' Attacks the Melting-Pot: The United States

The United States has never had public policies and institutions specifically designed to integrate immigrants, leaving this process to the self-regulating forces of economy and society.[1] There also has never been agreement about the meaning of integration. In response to the late nineteenth-century immigration from Southern and Eastern Europe, two competing models of integration emerged. One stipulated the abandonment of the immigrant's ancestral ways and the acceptance of a new American identity. It was canonized in Israel Zangwill's notion of America as 'the great Melting-Pot where all the races of Europe are melting and re-forming' (in Gordon, 1964: 120). While in line with America's founding myth of a non-ethnic, politically constituted new nation, the melting-pot model has always been sociologically naïve. In theory, it stipulated the bi-directional adjustment of immigrants and receiving society. In reality, it meant the uni-directional assimilation of immigrants into an already established Anglo-American culture. At the height of World War I, the assimilationist bent of the melting-pot model found its expression in a hysterical Americanization campaign, directed particularly against the culturally assertive and politically suspicious immigrants of German origins. In response to the ensuing ethnicization of American national identity, a number of liberal intellectuals formulated a counter-model of integration, commonly referred to as 'cultural pluralism'.[2] It stipulated the maintenance of immigrant ethnicity, conceiving of the United States as a 'federation of nationalities' (Kallen, 1915) or—somewhat paradoxically—an 'international nation' (Bourne, 1916). Through defending the ethnicity of immigrants, cultural pluralists sought to vindicate the originally non-ethnic, political meaning of American nationhood, which had been lost in the assimilationist transmutation of the melting-pot model.

The conflict between melting-pot assimilationists and cultural pluralists betrays a fundamental uncertainty about the meaning of

American nationhood, and about the role ethnicity plays in it. Originally, as Philip Gleason (1980: 31) put it, American identity was conceived in 'abstract ideological terms', and was devoid of ethnic connotations. It could not be otherwise, because the anti-British colonialists had no language, religion, or common culture to rely on for a separate national identity. Accordingly, the United States defined itself as a nation by commitment to the anti-monarchic principles of liberty, equality, and consent-based government. But over time, the original ideological quality, newness, and future-orientation of American nationality had to take on quasi-ethnic contours, acquiring itself the 'grandfather effect' in which Horace Kallen had seen the spring of resilient immigrant ethnicity. As Philip Gleason (ibid. 56) says, 'American nationality became more a reality and less a project for the future simply because of the accumulation of lived experience by people who thought of themselves as Americans'. More importantly, in confrontation with non-Protestant, non-Anglo immigrants, the ethnic contours of the Protestant, English-speaking Anglo-Saxon core culture could not but become visible, and be held as assimilatory norm against the newcomers. Here lies the origin of the various nativist campaigns that have regularly accompanied major immigration waves (see Higham, 1955). However, it is important to stress that the ethnicization of American identity, to which cultural pluralists critically reacted, has been inconsistent with its civic core. Philip Gleason (1980: 56) clarifies: 'In establishing American nationality on the basis of abstract social and political ideas, Protestant Americans of British background had in fact committed the nation to a principle that made it inconsistent to erect particularist ethnic criteria into tests of true Americanism.' Accordingly, the meaning of American is 'ethnically anonymous' (Walzer, 1990), amenable to be accompanied by the cultural diversity imported by immigration. Ethnicity is not something the immigrant meets as an external barrier to (and norm of) integration, but as something she carries from home (however modified, or even created, in the receiving society) and that is reconcilable with the acquisition of a new, political American identity.

The debate over melting-pot assimilation versus cultural pluralism has always been a sterile one, because it was led in abstraction from the empirical processes and outcomes of immigrant integration. In a suggestive survey, Nathan Glazer (1954: 169) found that 'the course of immigrant assimilation in America is not linear', but dependent upon the national origins, conditions of settlement, and the generational evolution of immigrants. Moreover, due to the absence of a statist integration regime, ethnicity has been a pivotal resource of immigrant integration. William I. Thomas and Florian Znaniecki (1984) have famously elaborated this in the case of Polish immigrants, in which ethnic self-organization in the form of boarding-houses, mutual benefit societies, parishes, and parochial schools has protected the rural newcomers from the 'complete wildness' of urban America: 'It is this Polish-American society, not American society, that constitutes the social milieu into which the immigrant who comes from Poland becomes incorporated and to whose standards and institutions he must adapt himself' (p. 240). The ethnic group smoothed the adaptation to the new society. Paradoxically, assimilation occurred through ethnic group formation. In his epic history of immigrant America, Oscar Handlin (1951: 166) describes this paradox: 'Becoming an American meant . . . not the simple conformity to a previous pattern, but the adjustment to a new situation. In the process the immigrants became more rather than less conscious of their own peculiarities. As the immediate environment called forth the succession of fresh institutions and novel modes of behavior, the immigrants found themselves progressively separated as groups.'

For the descendants of European immigrants, ethnicity eventually thinned down to 'symbolic ethnicity' (Gans, 1979). In the absence of systematic discrimination, ethnicity was drained of its instrumental interest component, and took on exclusively expressive, identity-related functions.[3] The logic of symbolic ethnicity was first captured in Marcus Hansen's early observation that the third generation of immigrants tried to remember what the second, over-adjusting immigrant generation had tried to forget.[4] Symbolic ethnicity is voluntary, costless, and situationally invoked; it does not even require functioning groups, networks, or a practised culture (Gans, 1979: 12). In her excellent portrait of third- and fourth-generation white Catholic ethnics in two American suburbs, Mary Waters (1990) depicted them as 'choosing' identities, the choices often inconsistent with an individual's majority ancestry, and even changing over time and across context.[5] Why has symbolic ethnicity been so resilient? First, according to Waters (ibid., ch. 7), it provides a 'costless community' that reconciles two opposite strands of American culture: the quest for community and individualism. But secondly, symbolic ethnicity feeds the idea that *all* ethnicity is symbolic, costless, and voluntary, and thus functions as a 'subtle reinforcement of racism' (p. 164). Waters further argues that not all ethnicity is symbolic: 'The social and political consequences of being Asian or Hispanic or black are *not* symbolic for the most part, or voluntary. They are real and often hurtful' (p. 156). The racism charge obscures that race has also been a source of opportunities, and thus a matter of choice, for Asian or Hispanic immigrants.

The Resurgence of Race

Since the new immigration regime was created in 1965, the United States has undergone probably the largest immigration wave in its history. Between 1971 and 1993, over 15.5 million new legal immigrants arrived. Adding the unknown number of illegal immigrants, the absolute number of new immigrants may well outstrip the 18.6 million immigrants received between 1901 and 1930 (Massey, 1995: 634). Whereas almost 80 per cent of the older immigrants were European, about 84 per cent of post-1971 immigrants came from Latin America (49.6 per cent) and Asia (34.5 per cent). Independently of the heated ideological debate now raging over the assimilability of the recent Third-World immigrants, the sheer demography of contemporary immigration suggests that the European experience is a poor model for the latter's incorporation. As Douglas Massey (1995) points out, there are at least three structural differences between both immigration waves. First, contemporary immigration is an ongoing process, with no end in sight. There is unlikely to be anything like the 40-year hiatus between 1930 and 1970, when in a period of quasi-zero immigration the immigrants from South and Eastern Europe quietly succumbed to the assimilatory forces of American economy and society. Ethnicity is being constantly refurbished by new arrivals, shifting the balance toward the language and culture of the sending society. Secondly, today's immigrants meet a highly stratified society with huge income inequality and segmented labour markets, thus finding the main pathway of assimilation blocked: upward mobility. And thirdly, the national origins and places of settlement of today's newcomers are more concentrated than ever, creating large foreign-language and cultural enclaves in a few, but highly visible parts of the United States.[6]

A perhaps even more important difference between European and non-European immigration is the resurgence of race as a positive group-marker. In the restrictionist movement that led to the national origins regime in place between 1929 and 1965, race had figured as a negative device to exclude allegedly inferior non-Anglo-Saxon immigrants. Borrowing its conceptual arsenal from the then fashionable discipline of eugenics, the restrictionist case was a case for maintaining the 'racial homogeneity' of the social body, which was seen as threatened by the mixing of the Anglo-Saxon core with 'inferior races' from the southern periphery of Europe and elsewhere.[7] Interestingly, the prolongation of the national-origins system in the McCarren–Walter Act of 1952 was no longer defended in openly racial terms, but as a prudential measure of maintaining a long-accustomed institution that had brought stability to American society (see Divine, 1957: ch. 9). The victory over Nazism had come in between, forever outlawing the recourse to biological racialism in a liberal state.

The single most important effect of postwar anti-colonialism on Western politics was to re-evaluate race as a legitimate category of group identification. Frantz Fanon (1963: 39 f.) grimly depicted the colonial world as a 'world divided into compartments, . . . inhabited by two different species', in which the black race was not just exploited by the white settlers, but robbed of its dignity and culture. Accordingly, separation rather than integration had to be the direction for oppressed racial groups. Anti-colonialism first entered Western politics on the platform of the American civil-rights movement. At first, this was a movement for civic inclusion; under the impact of anti-colonialism, it refashioned itself as a movement for racial separation. Refuting Gunnar Myrdal's (1944) old manifesto for civic inclusion, the authors of *Black Power* state: 'There is no "American dilemma" because black people in this country form a colony, and it is not in the interest of the colonial power to liberate them' (Ture and Hamilton, 1992: 5). This manifesto for black power shows the close linkage between domestic and Third-World liberation: '. . . Black Power means that black people see themselves as part of a new force, sometimes called the "Third World"; that we see our struggle as closely related to liberation struggles around the world' (ibid., p. xix). 'Integration', that goal shared in the immigration context by melting-pot assimilationists and cultural pluralists alike, is consequently rejected as 'a subterfuge for the maintenance of white supremacy' (ibid. 54). Rather than integration, black power stipulates a 'total revamping of . . . society' (ibid. 60 f.). In his afterword for the 1992 edition of *Black Power*, Charles Hamilton belittles the new strategy as mere 'self-help': 'Wasn't this the way other groups had made it in society?' (ibid. 298). This parallel obscures the fundamentally different logics of ethnic and race politics.

In fact, the advocates of the race paradigm have been keen to reject what Robert Blauner (1972: 2) called the 'immigrant analogy', that is, 'the assumption . . . that there are no essential long-term differences . . . between the third world or racial minorities and the European ethnic groups'. Instead, Blauner proposed a new perspective of 'internal colonialism' for racial minorities. This perspective depicts the minorities' entry into society as forced rather than voluntary, and sees the latter subjected to an economy of unfree labour and a culture of 'white Westerners' that systematically destroys the values and beliefs of the colonized. Along with this 'Third-World perspective' (Blauner) goes a fundamental re-evaluation of the American experience. In Gunnar Myrdal's (1944) epic of black liberation, slavery and its segregationist legacy were seen as aberrations from the 'American creed' of liberty and equality, and the blacks' best weapon was to mobilize these American ideals against their shameful violation in reality. From the anti-Whiggish Third-World perspective, 'racism' is not an aberration from American ideals, but at the very core of the American experience. In their influential treatise on *Racial Formation in the United States*, Michael Omi and Howard Winant (1986: 1) put it this way: 'The hallmark of this [American] history has been racism, not the abstract ethos of equality, and while racial minority groups have been treated differently, all can bear witness to the tragic consequences of racial oppression . . . The examples are familiar: Native Americans faced genocide, blacks were subjected to racial slavery, Mexicans were invaded and colonized, and Asians faced exclusion.' And once it is there, racism will never go away: 'Race will *always* be at the center of the American experience' (p. 6). If this is the case, contemporary African, Mexican, and Asian immigrants are also subject to the ineradicable legacies of slavery, conquest, and exclusion, and are forever denied the assimilatory trajectory of ethnic Europeans.

Eager to avoid any biological connotation of race, proponents of the race paradigm stress that race, no less than ethnicity, is 'socially constructed'. If both are created rather than innate, how does race differ from ethnicity? Essentially, ethnicity is depicted as voluntary, whereas race is involuntary. The content of race is oppression. As Yen Le Espiritu (1992: 5) characterizes the nature of 'Asian American panethnicity', it implies 'calling attention . . . to the coercively imposed (rather than voluntary) nature of ethnicity.' However, the notion of 'calling attention' betrays that an act of will, that is, choice, is involved in the making of racial no less than in the making of ethnic identity. Accordingly, the histories of the Brown, Yellow, and Red Power movements following upon the model of Black Power are unfailingly histories of 'consciousness-raising' and willed conversion, histories of 'reject[ing] ethnic identity in favor of a more radical racial identity' (Omi and Winant, 1986: 20). This contradicts the stipulated imposition and involuntariness of racial (as against ethnic) markers. Structurally equivalent to the Marxist class paradigm, the race paradigm stipulates one fundamentally inegalitarian principle underlying the organization of society (race in lieu of class),[8] accessible to a truth-depicting theory with a practical mission, emancipation—the one difference being that class is destined to be abolished, whereas a positive race identity will stay even after the sting of oppression has been pulled.

The race paradigm obviously modifies the meaning of immigrant integration, which had previously stood in a normative (if empirically mute) tension between melting-pot assimilation and cultural pluralism. The retention of culture makes the race paradigm similar to cultural pluralism. But two differences stand out. Cultural pluralists have always stipulated the overall goal of integration under the umbrella of positively valued nationhood—they perceived their vision as authentically American. The anti-Whig perspective of the race paradigm, according to which the United States is an inherently 'racial state', 'despotic for much of its history' (Omi and Winant, 1986: 76), forbids such integration, and 'American' figures as a code word for 'white supremacy' (Almaguer, 1996). Secondly, cultural pluralists conceived of the composite groups making up American society as cultural, rather than political entities—group distinctions would not pervade the realm of the state and remain 'legally invisible' (Gordon, 1964: 4). The race paradigm calls for the official recognition of 'minority' group status, and retributive action by the state. This has occurred under the name of affirmative action.

Affirmative Action

If the resurgence of race were limited to the realm of militant movements and eccentric academia, one might be inclined to take no further notice of it. But its enshrinement in modern civil-rights law and official state practices has made race a 'hard' institutional fact, which provides incentives for Third-World immigrants to identify and mobilize on these grounds. Ironically, the institutionalization of race is the unintended effect of getting rid of race-based discrimination. In its original intention, modern civil-rights law, with its dual pillars of the Civil Rights Act of 1964 and the Voting Rights Act of 1965, was inspired by Judge Harlan's famous dissent in *Plessy* v. *Ferguson* that 'our Constitution is color-blind', sacking the Supreme Court's 'separate but equal' doctrine that had condemned the descendants of black slaves to second-class citizenship, particularly in the American South. Any segregation and discrimination on the ground of 'race, color, religion, or national origin' in the use of public facilities, provision of public services, employment, education, and voting was henceforth outlawed, and the federal state was endowed with the necessary powers to bring even the recalcitrant South into line.

Two transmutations of civil-rights law made the latter an enduringly contested thing: its reorientation from equal opportunity to equal results, and its expansion to 'minorities' other than black, including immigrant-based minorities. The first transmutation is commonly referred to as 'affirmative action'. The word first appeared in President Kennedy's Executive Order No. 10925 of March 1961, which required government contractors to 'take affirmative action to ensure that applicants are employed, and employees are treated during their employment, without regard to their race, creed, color, or national origin' (in Mills, 1994: 5). The meaning of 'affirmative action' was nowhere defined. But it originally meant little more than traditional non-discrimination plus, perhaps, some proactive efforts of advertising or seeking out sources of minority employment. In fact, during the Congressional debates leading to the Civil Rights Act of 1964, the introduction of fixed numerical quotas of minority hiring was widely debated, and almost unanimously rejected—even by the leading civil-rights organizations. 'The argument for compensatory racial quotas flew in the face of an overwhelming consensus of American opinion,' writes the foremost chronicler of the evolution of civil-rights law (Graham, 1990: 109). To accommodate Southern conservatives, the heavily embattled Title VII of the Act (which covered non-discrimination in private employment) contained a section that explicitly outlawed quotas: 'Nothing contained in this title shall be interpreted to require any employer . . . to grant preferential treatment to any individual or to any group because of the race, color, religion, sex, or national origin of such individual or group . . .' (in Glazer, 1987: 44).[9] Federal court rules and executive orders eventually undermined Congressional intention. By 1970, a staff of the Equal Employment Opportunity Commission (a regulatory agency created to supervise and implement Title VII) could say: 'The anti-preferential provisions are a big zero, a nothing, a nullity. They don't mean anything at all to us' (ibid. 53).

The shift from equal opportunity to equal result, first defended in President Lyndon Johnson's often-quoted Howard University commencement speech of June 1965,[10] occurred above all in the arcane arena of implementing the civil-rights laws. The agencies charged with implementing the civil-rights laws found it time-consuming and cumbersome to demonstrate the actual intent of discrimination in individual cases. They soon faced huge case backlogs, and there was an obvious need for more enforcement powers. As John Skrentny (1996*a*) showed in the case of the Equal Employment Opportunity Commission, no conscious pressure by civil-rights groups, but the sheer difficulties of implementation pushed regulatory agencies into the statistical result-oriented direction, which released them from the difficult task of proving discriminatory intent. Inspired by the social engineering fantasies of the time, and pressured by the black urban ghettos exploding just when the colour-blind civil-rights reforms had come to their successful conclusion, the agencies simply wanted a method that 'worked', and the statistical result approach promised just that.

Affirmative action entails the attribution of special benefits and privileges on the basis of ascriptive group membership. This is an astonishing deviation from the American individual-rights tradition. But if the lack of parity between a minority group's population share and its representation in the employed workforce, higher education, or the political system was seen as an indication of 'institutional' discrimination, the mandate was to preferentially recruit, admit, or elect members of this group until statistical parity was reached. In the official reading, this recognition of group rights was to be only temporary. Judge Blackmun expressed the paradoxical motif in his dissent in the Supreme Court's *Bakke* case of 1978: 'To get beyond racism, we must first take account of race.' But Daniel Moynihan recognized the self-perpetuating, expansive dynamics of affirmative action: 'Once this process gets legitimated, there is no stopping it' (in Graham, 1990: 458).

Expansion to Immigrant Groups

If affirmative action is based on a logic of group rights, the question arises who should count as a 'minority' group subject to its provisions. There is no doubt that the crafters of the original Civil Rights and Voting Right Acts had only the descendants of black slaves in mind. In fact, if no notable resistance arose to the result-oriented shift of civil-rights law, it was because it was seen as compensation for the past injustice done to blacks and as a necessary tool to lift them out of their deplorable political and socioeconomic situation today. But the colour-blind logic of civil-rights law did not *name* its main addressee—instead, it spoke abstractly of 'citizens', 'individuals', or 'persons' who were to be protected from discrimination on the ground of 'race, color, religion, or national origin'. Ironically, this group-indifferent formulation became the inroad for groups other than black to claim minority status.

Much like the turning from equal opportunity to equal result, the determination of the minority groups to be covered by affirmative action occurred in the arcane arena of government bureaucracy. Since 1977, the Statistical Directive 15 of the Office of Management and Budget (OMB), which controls the racial and ethnic categories on all federal forms and statistics, has acknowledged four racial groups in the United States: White, American Indian or Alaskan Native, Asian or Pacific Islander, and Black; in addition, the OMB directive breaks down ethnicity into Hispanic Origin and Not of Hispanic Origin. From these categories, which are present on everything from school enrolment to job application and, of course, the US Census forms, comes the information to monitor and enforce civil-rights law. Through sheer administrative fiat, the minority pantheon has come to encompass not just Blacks, but also American Indians, Asians, and Hispanics. Why and how federal authorities settled on just these four ethnoracial minorities, is not known. 'I have yet to learn who decided, and on what basis, which ethnic minorities were candidates for affirmative action on their behalf,' writes a government statistics expert (Lowry, 1982: 49).[11]

Certainly, there was prima-facie justification to bring also American Indians, Asians, and Hispanics under the umbrella of civil-rights law, because all had suffered discrimination in the process of American nation-building. American Indians had been the victims of genocide; Asian immigrants had been the subject of racial exclusion, as in the Chinese Exclusion Act of 1882 and the internment of Japanese-Americans during World War II; and the Hispanics in the South-West had been forcibly incorporated after the Mexican–American War of 1848. But 'historical accident' (Skerry, 1989: 88) would have it that two of the groups classified as protected classes under civil-rights law, Asians and Hispanics, would also form the vast majority of post-1965 immigrants, who could not look back at a history of discrimination at the hand of Euro-America. If Oscar Handlin (1951: 273) had celebrated the immigrant as an individual *tout court*, 'apart from place and station', and the stuff out of which this new nation was made, the affirmative-action context transformed even those who had come to America by individual choice into members of long-entrenched, domestically oppressed racial groups, not unlike American blacks.

The evolution of the Voting Rights Act of 1965 epitomizes the self-perpetuating thrust of affirmative action, and its expansion to immigrant-based ethnoracial groups other than blacks. The Act's original goal was the enfranchisement of blacks in the South, who had been deprived of their right to vote through literacy tests, poll taxes, and outright intimidation and violence. But the act named no group; instead it protected all citizens denied the right to vote on account of 'race or color'. This was the inroad for the first national campaign of Mexican-Americans to amend civil-rights law in their favour. In the debate leading to the 1975 amendment of the act, the Mexican-American Legal Defense Fund (MALDEF) successfully argued that English-language ballots had as equally a discriminatory effect on 'language minorities' as literacy tests had had on blacks in the South. Accordingly, the 1975 amendment extended the coverage of the Voting Right Act to 375 jurisdictions outside the South, in which more than 5 per cent of voting-age citizens were from a language minority group. These jurisdictions were required to print ballots in the native language, and—most importantly—they were now subject to federal preclearance. For MALDEF, the federal supervision of elections was essential to achieve a redrawing of district lines that minimized vote dilution. This meant the creation of 'majority minority' districts, in which the numerical weight of a minority group guaranteed that one from their ranks would be elected into office. MALDEF's purpose was fully realized only in the next amendment of the Voting Rights Act in 1982. It allowed minority voters nationwide to challenge any method of election, whenever instituted, on the ground of a discriminatory result rather than intention. A 'discriminatory result' existed if minority voters had 'less opportunity than other members of the electorate to participate in the political process and to elect representatives of their choice' (in Thernstrom, 1987: 304). The 1982 amendment of the Voting Rights Act applied the result-oriented logic of affirmative action to the political process, replacing the classic principle of the territorial representation of abstract citizens by a new principle of group representation based on race or language.

What had started as a regional effort to root out black disenfranchisement in the South, has profoundly transformed the political geography of the entire United States. Traditional at-large voting and multi-member districts are at the point of disappearing, due to the legislative mandate to create smaller single-member, majority minority districts whenever demographically possible. This has greatly increased the number of black and Hispanic elected representatives at all levels of government. But packing the largest possible number of minority citizens into at times bizarrely shaped districts, has 'whitened' the other districts, making Republican Party victories more likely and feeding the idea that white majority representatives are no longer responsible for minority interests.[12] 'This is a dangerous game for any minority to play,' says Linda Chavez (1992: 86).

Counting and Classifying

Affirmative action in employment, education, and voting has politicized the process of counting and classifying the population. An ethnic group's partaking in the benefits of affirmative action depends, first, on being officially classified within one of the 'big four' ethnoracial minority categories, and, secondly, on their numerical size. The Federal Census, once a remote and technical backwater of demographers and statisticians, is now a highly political stake in group struggle. In the old days of colour-blindness, the American Civil Liberties Union (ACLU) had tried to get 'race' deleted from the 1960 Census schedule, and local jurisdictions eradicated ethnic and race identifications from employment and college applications (Petersen, 1987: 195). In the affirmative-action era, the Hispanic National Council of La Raza has (so far unsuccessfully) lobbied the Federal Bureau of Census to be considered a race, not just an ethnic group; the National Coalition for an Accurate Count of Asian Pacific Americans wants Cambodians and Laotians added to the nine nationalities already listed under the racial heading 'Asian and Pacific Islanders'; and the Arab American Institute would like to see persons from the Middle East— now counted as white—under a separate, protected category of their own (Wright, 1994: 47). Indian Americans, entirely a product of post-1965 immigration, successfully lobbied the Census Bureau to be reclassified from 'white/Caucasian' to 'Asian Indian' in the 1980 Census questionnaire (Fisher, 1978: 280). This has led to the curious result that a group whose average educational and occupational attainments exceed those of white Americans qualifies for affirmative action benefits, such as 'minority set-asides' from the Small Business Administration (LaNoue and Sullivan, 1994: 450–2). Aware of the absence of past discrimination, Indian Americans defended their campaign for minority status as a 'prophylactic measure' for future immigrants arriving under family reunification, who were likely to lack the high professional profile of the first generation admitted on the occupational ticket (Fisher, 1978: 281).

The 1980 Census was the first to bear the mark of minority group mobilization (see Anderson, 1988: ch. 9). The major bone of contention was a disproportionate minority undercount in the 1970 census. This was nothing new, because of the technical problems of recording the poor, illiterate, or clandestine, who happen to be disproportionally members of minority groups. In fact, due to improved statistical techniques the undercount of blacks in the 1970 Census (6.5 per cent) had been the lowest since 1940 (Skerry, 1992: 22). But when in the affirmative-action era federal benefits came to depend on a minority group's relative population share, *any* undercount was impermissible. In addition, ethnic activists attacked either the lack of categories for their constituencies (such as the Taiwanese Club of America opposing the umbrella label 'Chinese'), or the use of categories in which their constituencies did not recognize themselves (a problem especially for the 'Hispanic', 'Spanish-origin', or 'Latino' population and their various national components) (Lowry, 1982: 49 f.). In response to such criticisms, the Census Bureau formed three advisory committees for the Black, Hispanic, and Asian populations in the preparation of the 1980 Census. Each committee, staffed more with ethnic activists than with demographers and statisticians, pushed for measures to increase the count of its constituents, or to make its constituents more visible on the census form. The results are readily visible on the 1980 Census questionnaire. The impact of Asian lobbying can be seen in the 'color or race' question on the all-important short census form for 100 per cent enumeration. Next to the categories White, Black or Negro, and Indian (American), the race question lists nine categories for Asian respondents (Japanese, Chinese, Filipino, Korean, Vietnamese, Asian Indian, Hawaiian, Guamanian, and Samoan). The result is a bizarre hotchpotch of racial, national, and territorial distinctions on different levels of classification, some entries not being mutually exclusive. The 'origin or descent' query on the short form must be considered the chief triumph of lobbying by Hispanics, who had demanded to be counted via ethnic self-identification rather than objective surname, language, or birthplace entries as in previous censuses (see Choldin, 1986). The origin/descent question asks every respondent to answer, 'Is this person of Spanish/Hispanic origin or descent?', with No or Yes (the latter broken down into 'Mexican, Mexican-American, Chicano' [as one category], Puerto Rican, Cuban, or 'other Spanish/Hispanic'). In contrast to the race question, the origin/descent question offers options that are logically complete. But it is designed to maximize the Hispanic entries—a respondent whose lineage, however remotely, includes any individual born in one of the named or unnamed countries, is encouraged to identify herself as Hispanic. As Ira Lowry (1982: 53) assesses the politicized 1980 Census, 'the [Census] Bureau's success in balancing the claims of constituencies was achieved at the expense of its fundamental mission—gathering valid and reliable information about the population of the United States.'

From Discrimination to Diversity

Expanding the minority pantheon from blacks to other ethnoracial groups, constituted by immigration rather than internal colonialism à la Blauner, increasingly hollowed out the main rationale of affirmative action to be the remedy for past discrimination. As affirmative action comprised more groups and grew into a permanent, rather than temporary, institution, there was need for a new justification. This was found in the notion of diversity. It first took hold in the sphere of higher education, and was formulated in the opinion of Justice Powell in the Supreme Court case *Regents of the University of California* v. *Bakke* (1978). In this most famous of all legal affirmative-action cases, a rejected white applicant for medical school had sued the University of California for race-based discrimination. Its medical school on the Davis campus then practised a separate admissions programme for blacks, Chicanos, Asians, and Native Americans, which led to the admission of minority candidates with significantly lower academic credentials than Bakke's. A sharply divided Supreme Court declared that the Davis programme was illegal and ordered Bakke admitted on equal protection grounds. But the decisive-swing opinion of Justice Powell also stated that as a means of reaching 'educational diversity' universities could take race into account as 'a plus' factor (among others) that sometimes 'tips the balance' in an applicant's favour (quoted in Eastland, 1996: 67). According to Powell, the use of race as an admission criterion was justified by the university's First Amendment freedom to make judgements about its educational mission; one such legitimate judgement was that selecting a racially diverse student body would promote academic excellence through enabling a wider and more robust exchange of ideas.

Bakke not only sanctioned the practice of preferential minority admission flourishing throughout the next two decades especially at American élite universities. More than that, it provided an entirely new rationale for affirmative action, even outside the sphere of education.[13] The latter was no longer remedial action for past injustice, but a forward-looking device for integrating an increasingly diverse society (Foster, 1993: 107). Moreover, the reference to diversity allowed the justification of affirmative action as the permanent, rather than temporary, institution that it had factually developed into. But the diversity rationale had a catch: it did not determine which differences should matter and when, and in removing the sting of past discrimination it robbed affirmative action of its moral force. In the diversity paradigm, whites figured as just a group competing with other groups. The diversity paradigm thus espoused a dangerous relativism that might become an inroad for doing away with affirmative action *in toto*. This relativism was already visible in Judge Powell's opinion in *Bakke*, in which racial diversity was put on a par with geographic, cultural, and other sources of diversity, all equally valid to promote the 'robust exchange of ideas'. Moreover, Powell depicted the United States as a 'nation of minorities' in which the parts either whites or blacks had played were symmetric, and in which all groups had had to fight discrimination at one point: 'During the dormancy of the Equal Protection clause, the United States had become a nation of minorities. Each had to struggle . . . to overcome the prejudices not of a monolithic majority, but of a "majority" composed of various minority groups of whom it was said . . . that a shared characteristic was a willingness to disadvantage other groups . . .' (in Natapoff, 1995: 1070). The symmetric 'nation of minorities', in which also whites were but a minority, could (and eventually would) be turned into an argument against race-based preferences.

Ongoing mass immigration is in fact transforming the United States into a nation of minorities, at least demographically speaking. If current trends continue, the minority share of the US population is projected to increase from 25 per cent in 1990 to 47 per cent in 2050, making the non-Hispanic whites a near-minority.[14] In 1992, the combined population of the four ethnoracial minority groups was estimated at 64.3 million. If they constituted an independent country, it would be the 13th largest in the world—larger than Great Britain, France, or Italy (O'Hare, 1992: 9). Moreover, over 75 per cent of all immigrants having arrived since the mid-1960s belonged to one of the 'big four' minority groups, reshuffling the relative weight of individual minority groups (ibid. 13). If blacks constituted 96 per cent of the minority population in 1960, their share was down to 50 per cent by 1990; by 2010, Hispanics are expected to surpass blacks in number and become America's largest minority group. According to the US Bureau of the Census, Asians grew by a phenomenal 123.5 per cent between 1980 and 1992, amounting to a total of 8 million people in 1992; Hispanics were second with a 65.3 per cent increase in the same period, with a total of 24 million in 1992. By contrast, blacks increased by only 16.4 per cent, and non-Hispanic whites by a meagre 5.5 per cent (ibid. 10).

Mass minority immigration is bound to have negative consequences for affirmative action. In the following, I will discuss three of them: growing interracial conflict over scarce minority spoils; an increasingly exclusionary effect on whites, which is feeding the current backlash against affirmative action; and multiracial mixing and related claims-making that has cast into doubt the whole edifice of race-based classifications and preferences.

Inter-Minority Conflict

Civil-rights law and discourse, centring around remedial action by whites toward blacks, is ill-prepared to articulate and accommodate inter-minority group conflict over scarce affirmative-action benefits. Blacks, who are vastly overrepresented in public-sector employment (not least the civil-rights industry itself), are bound to lose if other minority groups, like Hispanics, act on the logic of proportionality and insist on their fair share in minority spoils, which is steadily increasing through ongoing immigration.[15] From the very beginning, black leaders have resisted the entry of Hispanics into civil-rights politics. When Hispanics vied for inclusion in the 1975 Voting Rights Act extension, this was vigorously opposed by the National Association for the Advancement of Coloured People (NAACP), the major black civil-rights organization. Its leader exclaimed that 'Blacks were dying for the right to vote when you people (Hispanics) couldn't decide whether you were Caucasians.'[16] On the opposite side, the Hispanic leadership has criticized the 'Black dominance of the civil rights agenda', even claiming that the black-dominated system of civil rights enforcement 'discriminates against Hispanics at all levels' (Kamasaki and Yzaguirre, 1991: 18 and 9, respectively). As La Raza leader Charles Kamasaki sees it, 'the behavior of African-Americans towards Hispanics . . . appears to reflect a power relationship rather than a value relationship.'[17] This is a cryptic way of saying that blacks now use civil-rights rhetorics for their own narrow interests, and, by implication, that the torch of genuine civil-rights advocacy has been passed on to Hispanics.

Inter-minority conflict between blacks and Hispanics is especially visible in political redistricting. The large size and interspersed settlement patterns of both groups in some metropolitan areas increasingly pits them against each other in a zero-sum competition over the creation of majority minority districts. In the most dramatic case so far, blacks and Hispanics fought each other all the way up to the Supreme Court over a 1992 Florida House and Senate redistricting plan that allegedly diluted the strength of either group in Dade County, the Miami metropolitan area. The district court initially acknowledged the vote-dilution claims of both groups, but faced the dilemma that the remedies for blacks and Hispanics were mutually exclusive: the creation of a majority Hispanic Senate district would be at the cost of black voting strength, and vice versa. Unable to balance the competing interests of both minority groups, the court held that no remedy for this particular situation existed, leaving the original plan unchanged and declaring that 'these political questions' are best resolved by the legislature (in Ramirez, 1995: 970). The court was obviously unwilling to investigate 'the question . . . whether the Hispanic community has been harmed the same way the black community has', as a black state legislator demanded.[18] Nor was the court moved by another black legislator's claim that Hispanics, who constitute a majority of the population in Miami, should not be considered a minority protected by the Voting Rights Act.[19] The conflict took on an additional twist through the fact that 'Hispanics' in this case were Cuban exiles, the Republican-leaning élite rather than an oppressed minority in Miami. This exposed a core dilemma of affirmative action, whose generic ethnoracial categories often comprise privileged subgroups. 'The Cubans have ridden on the backs of Mexicans and Puerto Ricans to claim privileges which, as the only middle-class emigres of any size . . . in this country, they don't need,' says a state senator supporting the black cause. As *Johnson* v. *De Grandy* (1994), the Florida conflict eventually reached the Supreme Court. However, in contrast to the district court, the Supreme Court ruled that Florida's reapportionment plan had not violated the Voting Rights Act. The court thus skirted the tricky remedial problem raised by the case: how to decide between two equally viable, but mutually exclusive minority claims?

An altogether different inter-minority rift has emerged around Asian-Americans, who are about to opt out of the affirmative action coalition in higher education. Many élite universities now practise negative quotas against high-performing Asian applicants, truthful to the affirmative-action logic of statistical parity between population and enrolment share, but painfully reminiscent of the Jewish quota once in place at the prestigious East Coast universities. The Asian-American dilemma is most visible in the much-publicized conflict over the admissions procedure at San Francisco's Lowell High School. This is the only public school in San Francisco's Unified School District (SFUSD) with highly selective admission and a reputation for academic excellence. In response to an anti-race segregation suit filed by the black NAACP, a 1983 'consent decree' determined that each school in the district had to enrol students from at least four out of nine specified ethnoracial groups, further stipulating that no group may constitute more than 40 per cent of total enrolment. Courts have allowed such open quotas in school desegregation, because (in contrast to employment or higher education) public education is not considered a scarce good, and public schools are treated as interchangeable (Dong, 1995: 1035). At Lowell, the quota regime entailed higher admission standards for Chinese than for white students, in order to limit their enrolment to the 40 per cent cap. Over the opposition of NAACP, a group of Chinese parents subsequently sued the San Francisco school district for denying their children equal access to education on the basis of race, denouncing the consent decree as 'affirmative action for whites'. The suit raises the paradox that race-conscious remedies may hurt some minority groups, who then opt for a colour-blind stance. But the polemical notion of 'affirmative action for whites' betrays the staying power of minority rhetoric. A clever lawyer recommended to the Chinese plaintiffs to treat Lowell High School as an institution of higher learning, which would allow them to denounce the racial cap as an impermissible set-aside under *Bakke*; and to argue further that even for a 'racial minority' no longer in need of preferential treatment, any treatment worse than that afforded whites would violate the equal-protection principle (Dong, 1995: 1056). This amounts to eating the cake and having it too: asking for preferential minority treatment while rejecting the principle of race-based preferences.

Backlash

The case of Lowell High School is grist to the mill of the current backlash against affirmative action. Affirmative action has never been popular, not because of a racist animus against its beneficiaries, but because of a strong and persistent dislike for the underlying race-conscious policy agenda.[20] Since Gallup started surveying public opinion on preferential treatment in employment and higher education in 1977, vast majorities of Americans across race and party lines have objected to this, and this opposition has grown over the years (Skrentny, 1996*b*: 4 f.). Accordingly, the truly interesting question is not why affirmative action has recently come under heavy attack, but why such an unpopular policy could last as long as it did.

An increasingly conservative Supreme Court initiated the backlash. Overall, the legal retreat from affirmative action is based upon the spectre of a Balkanized society with multiplying minority claims. More than that, the immigration-based marginalization of whites is indirectly used to construe whites as a 'minority' in need of equal protection from the vicissitudes of race politics. Eleven years after *Bakke*, the Supreme Court invoked a rather darkened version of Judge Powell's 'nation of minorities' to strike down a municipal minority set-aside for construction contracts, up to then one of the commonest forms of affirmative action at all levels of government. The stake in *City of Richmond* v. *J. R. Croson Co.* (1989) was a set-aside programme passed by the black-led city council of Richmond, Virginia, in 1983, which required prime contractors with the city to subcontract at least 30 per cent of the project value to 'minority business enterprises'. Even though Richmond's non-black minorities constituted less than 2 per cent of the (predominantly black) city population, the designated minority groups were the usual 'big four' (Blacks, Hispanic, Asian, American Indians) plus Eskimos and Aleuts—the latter being just three and two persons, respectively, according to the 1980 Census (Eastland, 1996: 214). In the majority opinion, Justice O'Connor wrote: 'To accept Richmond's claim that past societal discrimination alone can serve as the basis for rigid racial preferences would be to open the door to competing claims for "remedial relief" for every disadvantaged group. The dream of a Nation of equal citizens in a society where race is irrelevant to personal opportunity and achievement would be lost in a mosaic of shifting preferences based on inherently unmeasurable claims of past wrongs' (in Natapoff, 1995: 1073). This reasoning would have been difficult to conceive in 1964, when the race conflict was one between white and black only; it reflects the inflation of minority claims in immigrant America. *Croson* is significant because it reinterprets the equal-protection clause in strictly colour-blind terms. Until the advent of affirmative action, the equal-protection clause had subjected all racial classifications to 'strict scrutiny', rendering them unconstitutional unless 'narrowly tailored' to achieve a 'compelling state interest'. In the era of affirmative action, racial preferences sponsored by government were mellowed down to 'benign racial classifications', subject only to a more relaxed standard of 'intermediate scrutiny'. First appearing in Justice Brennan's minority opinion in *Bakke*, this view became official court doctrine in *Metro Broadcasting*. It implied a 'groupist' interpretation of the equal-protection clause—the latter did not protect individuals of *any* race, but only of 'disadvantaged groups'.[21] *Croson* put an end to this. *All* racial classifications were inherently suspicious, and subject to the demanding standard of strict scrutiny, as they had been before the arrival of affirmative action. This meant that more than a vague reference to 'past societal discrimination' was needed to justify racial preferences: the latter were 'strictly reserved for remedial settings', which had to be assessed case-by-case. In the absence of such individual scrutiny, Richmond's generic set-aside was 'simple racial politics' (O'Connor). This was a not so subtle reference to the fact that five of the nine members of Richmond city council were black. It carried the 'nation of minorities' imagery to its logical conclusion: where they formed the numerical minority, whites also were the potential victims of racial exclusion.

The Supreme Court's retreat from affirmative action culminated in its decision *Adarand Construction* v. *Pena* (1995), whose essence is to hold the federal government to the same standard of strict scrutiny in making race-based preferences as local and state governments. *Adarand* thus applied the logic of *Croson* to the federal level, while overruling *Metro Broadcasting* that had granted Congress (as co-equal branch of government) the liberty to use race as a benign classification, subject to a more relaxed standard of intermediate scrutiny. The plaintiff in *Adarand* was the white owner of a construction firm, who claimed that his losing-out against a higher-bidding Hispanic-owned company on a federal highway project in Colorado was reverse discrimination. While the non-Hispanic bid was the lower, a federal bonus scheme for subcontracting to minority firms provided a rational incentive for the main contractor to go for the higher but minority bid. The high court returned the case to the lower courts, which had earlier approved the minority subcontracting under the intermediate scrutiny standard. 'All racial classifications, imposed by whatever Federal, state, or local governmental actor, must be analyzed by a reviewing court under strict scrutiny,' Justice O'Connor wrote in the majority opinion.[22] *Adarand* follows the reasoning of *Croson* that whites also could suffer racial discrimination, and that the equal protection clause was there to help them, because the former protected individuals, not groups. While living up to the ideal of colour-blindness, *Adarand* may be subjected to the charge of 'cruel formalism' (Horwitz, 1993: 107) that had already been raised against the Court's previous restrictions on affirmative action. This charge is eloquently expressed in Justice Stevens' dissenting opinion: 'There is no moral or constitutional equivalence between a policy that is designed to perpetuate a caste system and one that seeks to eradicate racial subordination.'[23] Adarand thus touched upon the irresolvable conflict underlying the affirmative-action debate, its supporters saying that law and policy could not be ignorant of race as a social fact, its critics responding that enshrining it legally perpetuates, rather than eradicates, racial division.

The Supreme Court's decisions from *Croson* to *Adarand* have narrowed, but not closed, the door for racial preferences. In *Adarand* the Court conceded the 'unhappy persistence of racial discrimination against minorities', which government is 'not disqualified' from acting against.[24] Accordingly, the fate of affirmative action is ultimately to be decided in the political arena. Already the Republican capture of both Congressional chambers in the 1994 elections had forced the Clinton administration to review the 160 racial preference programmes in place at the federal level alone. After *Adarand*, federal programmes must be justified by evidence of particularized discrimination in a specific sector rather than by a general assumption of 'racism' or 'sexism'. Also the wings of the diversity rationale, which had swung widely beyond the field of higher education after *Bakke*, have been clipped. 'Diversity would not be justified if you're talking about the manufacturing of widgets', quibbled a senior official of the Justice Department.[25]

In the context of ethnic animosities proliferating worldwide, it is field-day for political entrepreneurs to capitalize on society's distaste for subsidizing racial distinctions. As in the anti-immigration campaign, California is leading the way. In July 1995, Republican Governor Pete Wilson moved the Regents of the University of California (the flagship of affirmative-action in higher education) to abolish racial and sexual preferences in the admission of students and the recruitment of faculty and staff. In November 1996, a well-orchestrated Civil Rights Initiative convinced a majority of Californians to vote for its Proposition 209, which deliberately mimics the colour-blind language of the 1964 Civil

Rights Act: 'The state shall not discriminate against, or grant preferential treatment to, any individual or group on the basis of race, sex, color, ethnicity, or national origin in the operation of public employment, public education, or public contracting' (in Eastland, 1996: 166 f.). As in the anti-immigration campaign, it is no accident that California is leading the way. In 1995, 42 per cent of the state's population was Latino, Asian, or black. If one adds women to this, 73 per cent of all Californians are theoretically entitled to some form of affirmative action (ibid. 167). Minorities are indeed the majority here, and nowhere has affirmative action shot so much beyond its original goal to help out American blacks. The sheer entrenchment of affirmative action may ensure that it will stay, under a new name perhaps. After Proposition 209, the city of San Jose simply renamed its affirmative-action department as 'office of equality assurance'.[26]

Mixed Race

A third challenge to affirmative action arises from a group that considers itself outside the 'ethnoracial pentagon'.[27] Since the Supreme Court struck down the last anti-miscegenation laws in 1967, the number of interracial marriages has vastly increased. If the 1970 census counted less than 400,000 interracial couples, there were 1.5 million of them in 1990. In the same period, the number of children living in interracial families has quadrupled, from less than half a million to two million.[28] These multiracial children have no place in the ethnoracial pentagon. 'When I received my 1990 census form, I realized that there was no race category for my children,' laments a white woman married to a black man (in Wright, 1994: 47). From such dissonances has sprung an increasingly organized multiracial constituency, whose major cause is official recognition through a 'mixed-race' category in the federal census to be held in the year 2000.

The mixed-race movement poses a paradox. On the one hand, its identity concerns feed upon and reinforce the logic of racial distinction, which is evident in the quest to be considered a separate group on a par with the established ethnoracial groups. Accordingly, a mixed-race advocate warned that the non-recognition by government 'would result in cultural genocide' (Gilanshah, 1993: 197). On the other hand, the logic of mixed race undermines the whole edifice of racial classifications. It is estimated that more than three-quarters of American blacks have some white or Indian ancestry (Ramirez, 1995: 964). This would make them potentially 'mixed race' if the option is provided.

Thus it is not surprising that the demand for a 'mixed-race' category has drawn fire from the major ethnic and civil-rights groups of the ethnoracial pentagon: it threatens to deplete their numbers and subsequent affirmative action benefits. 'There's no concern on any of these [mixed-race] people's part about the effect on policy—it's just a subjective feeling that their identity needs to be stroked,' complains a defender of the status quo (in Wright, 1994: 47).

Most importantly, the mixed-race movement has cast a long shadow across the way the government administers race—with or without an official 'mixed-race' category. There is a disturbing dichotomy between the importance of race classifications to civil rights law and policy and the 'fundamental indeterminacy' of race as a social construct, with little empirical or scientific basis (Ford, 1994: 1231). Partially as a result of ethnic lobbying, all post-1960 censuses have relied on ethnic and racial self-identification. This is in line with our contemporary understanding of race as a social construct devoid of a biological basis. But the self-identification technique raises the problem of the manipulation of entries for reaping minority benefits.[29] Rejecting the claim of minority-group depletion through a new mixed-race category, a mixed-race advocate only half-joked that her constituency would know 'to check the right box to get the goodies' (Wright, 1994: 47). Moreover, the enforcement of anti-discrimination law in employment combines self-reported census data with employer-provided records of the ethnoracial and gender composition of the workforce, with the census data determining the objective benchmark of workforce availability and the employer data indicating how many of an available minority group were actually hired. Not only do both schemes operate with different classifications;[30] the reliance on employer identification also introduces a second source of manipulating entries according to an interest. As muddled and confused as the process of racial categorization seems to be, it is perhaps necessarily so in a liberal state. An objective categorization by a Ministry of Race Classification would certainly be incompatible with liberal (that is, still colour-blind) norms. As Christopher Ford (1994: 1283 f.) concludes his analysis of administering race in the United States, 'race classification is a type of necessary decisionmaking that is *most conveniently* done in the shadows, so as to allow us more easily to pretend it really isn't happening.'

Multiculturalism in Education

Paradoxically, explicit multiculturalism arose long after race had become a hard institutional fact in law and politics. Whereas in 1981 the words 'multiculturalism' and 'multicultural' appeared in only 40 articles in all major American newspapers, in 1992 they appeared in 2,000 articles (Bernstein, 1995: 4). Accordingly, multicultural claims-making flourished exactly when the use of racial distinctions became increasingly questioned in the legal and political spheres. This dissonance has contributed to the extraordinary heat and polemics surrounding American multiculturalism, which has so far escaped the cool gaze of disengaged analysis.[31] But polemics is not only added on, but intrinsic to multiculturalism. Multiculturalism everywhere presents itself as the oppositional movement that it no longer is, if it has ever been. At least in the sphere of education, multiculturalism is the new orthodoxy. The 1991 social studies curriculum for New York public schools takes as undisputed premiss that 'previous ideals of assimilation' have run their course: 'The various peoples who make up . . . this multicultural nation [are] unwilling to give up or celebrate in private that with which they have previously been identified, [and] they insist that their participation be recognized, and that their knowledge and perspectives be treated with parity' (New York State Social Studies Review, 1991: p. vii).

Multicultural curricula, speech codes, and norms of behaviour are often justified in reference to a diversifying immigrant society. Multiculturalism then appears as a contemporary version of Kallenian cultural pluralism. Such a view obscures the centrality of race and the anti-colonial impulse in multiculturalism. Much like affirmative action, multiculturalism is at first a proposal to solve the race problem, and it has only subsequently been adopted by claims-making immigrant groups. Its most extreme form is the advocacy of an Afrocentric curriculum, which denies the possibility of a shared culture of nationhood: 'There is no common American culture as is claimed by the defenders of the status quo. There is a hegemonic culture to be sure, pushed as if it were a common culture' (Asante, 1992: 308).

Certainly, there is also a mellower 'pluralistic multiculturalism' that wishes to achieve 'a richer common culture' (Ravitch, 1992: 276). As Nathan Glazer (1997) observed, there are only multiculturalists now, some closer to traditional cultural pluralism, others more influenced by the race paradigm. Accordingly, the old debate between melting-pot assimilationists and cultural pluralists has been recast as a debate between cultural pluralists (the new, quasi-assimilationist conservatives) and the radical advocates of the race paradigm.

More than the old debate, which had yielded an Americanization campaign with deep imprints on society, the new debate is one behind the walls of academia. Richard Bernstein (1995: 162) noted the irony that, precisely after the emergence of a world culture made up of American images, immigrants are exoticized as carriers of difference, and he concluded: 'It is the American élites already in place who have lost their collective will to require, as a price of admission to the benefits of American life, the acceptance of a common culture, a price that the immigrants are perfectly willing to pay.' Immigrants are at best 'junior partners' (Glazer, 1991: 19) in multiculturalism, which is largely a domestic élite phenomenon. Nevertheless, there are sites where élite multiculturalism touches upon the integration of immigrants. I will briefly discuss two of them: bilingual education and the school and college curriculum.

Bilingual Education

Among the few explicit policies to help integrating immigrants in the United States are federally mandated programmes for bilingual education. As the irony would have it, this rare integration policy amounts to federal subsidies for the retention of the immigrant's language and culture of origin. The mostly implicit and silent transformation of bilingual education from a measure of English language acquisition to one of cultural maintainance repeats the general trend in civil-rights law and politics, which started colour-blind and ended up colour-conscious. In line with the remedial logic of civil rights, bilingual education was not originally proposed for immigrants qua immigrants. Rather, the sponsor of the 1968 Bilingual Education Act, Texan Senator Ralph Yarborough, had in mind only Mexican-Americans in the South-West, because they 'had our culture superimposed on them' instead of arriving voluntarily (in Ravitch, 1983: 271). While this group restriction had to be dropped to secure the passing of the bill, Hispanics have always remained the main addressees, as well as claimants, of bilingual education programmes. In the 1967 Congressional hearings to the bilingualism bill, one can even observe Hispanics in their first major piracy of Black Power's race paradigm (see Thernstrom, 1980). Hispanic activists argued that their children's high drop-out rate in school was due to the denial of their native culture. A Puerto Rican spokesman branded as the 'psychic cost of the melting-pot' the high degree of 'mental and emotional illness' among language minority children, whose subjection to English would force upon them a 'negative self-image' (in Ravitch, 1983: 272). Accordingly, education in the native tongue was seen as necessary to acquire positive 'self-esteem'. Such anti-colonial reasoning had wide resonance at the time, as indicated in the parallel Kerner Commission's attribution of ghetto unrest to 'white racism'. However strange the theory to bolster bilingual education, it was equally clear that the latter's original purpose was 'just to try to make those children fully literate in English', as Senator Yarborough put it (in Citrin, 1990: 98).

The further development of bilingual education mirrors the phenomenal growth and entrenchment of the civil-rights sector. The 1974 amendment of the Bilingual Education Act, pushed through by a Democratic Congress against a weak Republican administration mired in the Watergate scandal, eliminated the poverty clause that had limited the law's reach to poor children. Whereas the earlier act had not specified the method to achieve English proficiency, the 1974 amendment explicitly recommends 'bilingual practices'.[32] And in stressing the importance of nourishing an immigrant child's 'cultural heritage', the new act established the 'bilingual-bicultural' linkage that has henceforth become the signature of bilingual education. But only a Supreme Court rule, *Lau v. Nichols* (1974), transformed bilingual education from an experimental option into a statutory right on behalf of the immigrant child, according to Title VI of the Civil Rights Act.[33] If a language minority was beyond a certain size (twenty students per district), local school districts were now mandated to offer remedial language instruction. While the Court had not specified any particular educational approach, the so-called 'Lau remedies' issued by the Office of Civil Rights to comply with the ruling did so: bilingual education that emphasized instruction in the native language and culture. In sum, by 1976 federal directives had transformed bilingual education from a compensatory and voluntary option into a comprehensive and mandatory programme including all language minorities, regardless of socioeconomic background (San Miguel, 1984: 510).

Abigail Thernstrom (1980: 15) characterized the grim review of the Bilingual Education Act in 1978 as 'the morning after'. A federally commissioned four-year study of 11,500 Hispanic students had come to negative results: most of the children drafted into bilingual education did not need to learn English; those who needed to did not in fact learn English; and the segregation into special classes further alienated minority children from the mainstream. Sheer entrenchment of the 'bilingual bureaucracy' (Porter, 1990) prevented a fundamental reconsideration at this critical moment. By now there existed an Office of Bilingual Education within the Federal Office of Education, and funding had increased from a meagre $7.5 million spread over 76 projects in 1969 to a considerable $135 million spread over 565 projects for 70 language groups in 1978 (Thernstrom, 1980: 14 f.). The controversy over bilingual education, variously denounced as 'affirmative ethnicity' or 'jobs program' for Spanish teachers (in San Miguel, 1984: 511–13), continues unabated today. In New York City, the controversy came full circle by the growing opposition of Hispanic parents to the mandatory enrolment of their 'limited English proficient' children in bilingual classes. By 1995, almost one-fifth of the city's one million public school students were in bilingual education programmes, at an annual cost of over $300 million. In autumn 1995, a group of Hispanic parents filed suit against a result of earlier Hispanic lobbying: the automatic testing of all children with Hispanic surnames for proficiency in English. Once championed by ethnic activists, this practice was now rejected as 'discriminatory', because it funnelled poorly performing children into bilingual programmes, if the parents wanted it or not.[34] There they languished for up to six years, against the law that had established a maximum of three years, and they often ended up illiterate in either language. A Hispanic leader of the Bushwick Parents Association in Brooklyn, which filed the suit, professes: 'Yes, I am proud of my Hispanic heritage, and I want my children and grandchildren to speak Spanish. But if bilingual classes leave a child illiterate in two languages, something is wrong.'[35]

Overall, such intra-Hispanic opposition to bilingual education has remained the exception. A more visible opposition gathered around an 'official English' movement, which perceived bilingualism as an affront to national unity. Since 1983, a well-funded organization called US English has lobbied legislatures and initiated public referendums to declare English the official language of the United States, and to phase out most bilingual programmes and government services. While failing to achieve an English Language Amendment to the federal Constitution in 1983, US English has been highly successful at the state and local levels. By 1987, twelve states (including California) had introduced official language statutes or constitutional amendments.[36] Despite enjoying overwhelming public support,[37] the effect of official language declarations has remained 'almost entirely symbolic' (Citrin, 1990: 101), because either bureaucracies have not acted on these (vaguely formulated) declarations, or courts have stalled their implementation on equal protection grounds. Attacked by their opponents as nativist or racist, an interesting feature of the official English movement is its attempt to avoid precisely such rhetoric, if perhaps only on tactical grounds.[38] After succeeding at the polls, the chairman of the California English Campaign stated that 'Californians, at the private level of the home and church can and should remain multilingual and multicultural.'[39] This indicates that cultural pluralism, the liberal fringe opposition to the melting-pot orthodoxy at the turn of this century, has now gone mainstream. Interestingly, US English has avoided fusing its language campaign with a call to restrict immigration, fearing that this combination would smack of 'old nativism' (Crawford, 1992: 153).[40] Its current chairman is a smooth-talking immigrant from Chile, who could present himself to the American public with a striking introduction: 'Why A Hispanic Heads An Organization Called US English'.[41]

Curriculum Battles

'Hey-hey, ho-ho, Western culture's got to go!', Stanford University students shouted in their 1988 campaign against the mandatory Western-civilization course, which shifted a long-standing campaign to 'diversify' the American college curriculum into high gear. A characteristic feature of such diversity campaigns is their running into open doors. By July 1991, 48 per cent of America's four-year colleges had a 'multicultural education requirement'—meaning that it was not just optional but mandatory for students to explore the 'diversity of our constituent cultural traditions', as the University of California at Berkeley denotes the purpose of its American Cultures Breadth Requirement (in Bernstein, 1995: 295).[42] Universities, particularly the very best, have been champions of multiculturalism, even *avant la lettre*: establishing ethnic and women's studies programmes since the late 1960s; recruiting minority students according to their population share since the 1970s; diversifying the curriculum and enforced recruiting of minority faculty since the 1980s. Multiculturalism has become the mainstream in American higher education, and frictions arise only from the uneven speed of implementing its various components.

Most leaders of the ethnic (immigrant) organizations interviewed by the author in 1994 depicted themselves 'reborn' as ethnic or racial persons at college or university. Asked where she had discovered her ethnic roots, Angela Oh, the eloquent voice of Korean-Americans after the Los Angeles riots of 1992, has a quick response: 'My discovery was in college, I guess . . . The racial features you know as a child, you know that. But you become conscious of it only later. Thankfully there are professors in the universities who begin to open these doors and make you see.'[43] The Berkeley Diversity Project of 1991, a research effort to examine how undergraduate students experience 'the new ethnic and racial diversity' at the University of California's Berkeley campus, described this personal conversion (with Omi and Winant, 1986) as 'racialization', 'a development where social relations that were formerly defined in terms of factors other than race come to be defined in racial terms' (Diversity Project, 1991: 44). The authors of the Diversity Project noticed that racialization, especially of Latinos and Latinas, did not begin at High School, so that among the difficult 'identity issues' the latter had to deal with at Berkeley was 'their inability to speak Spanish, their fair appearance, and . . . a confusing tension between cultural assimilation to the dominant white society and pressure from peers at Cal to adopt a Chicano/Latino identity' (ibid. 32). The authors further noticed that many of the interviewed Asian-American students did not identify with the label 'Asian-American', and that 'several talked about having to *learn what it means to be Asian-American*' (ibid. 23). This is exactly what these students are likely to learn at multicultural Berkeley.

The creation of multicultural curricula in American public schools touches not only upon a small élite segment but American society at large. As the 'great equalizer' (Horace Mann) and 'opportunity to escape from the limitations of the social group in which [one] was born' (John Dewey), the public school has been America's classic instrument of nation-building.[44] Multiculturalism is turning public schools into instruments of ethnoracial consciousness building. Interestingly, one can observe here the same spiralling logic of explicit multiculturalism trumping multiculturalism *avant la lettre* that had already characterized the campus debate. This is because there is no internal stopping-point in multiculturalism's endeavour to multiply perspectives or articulate previously muted 'voices', and in its urge to unravel the omnivorous powers exerted by 'dominant culture'. Take the examples of New York and California, America's pacesetters of a multicultural public school curriculum.

In June 1991, the New York State Department of Education issued new guidelines to reform the history and social studies curriculum for some 2.5 million pupils at the state's public schools, entitled *One*

Nation, Many Peoples: A Declaration of Cultural Interdependence (New York State Social Studies Review, 1991). Education commissioner Thomas Sobol stated in a letter to the Board of Regents that the purpose was to establish a social studies curriculum 'more "multicultural" than that now in existence'.[45] Indeed, New York had been a pioneer of multicultural education for twenty years. As recently as 1987, the state had radically overhauled the way history was taught: a new two-years Global Studies programme had cut back the history of Western Europe from a full year to one quarter of the second year, and equal time was allotted to seven major world regions, including Africa and Latin America. Already the pre-1991 curriculum was spiked with eccentric wisdom, such as grounding the US Constitution equally in European enlightenment thought and the political system of the Iroquois Indians (see Ravitch, 1992: 285 f.). In 1989, a Task Force on Minorities, immediately appointed by the incoming Sobol, indicted an already impeccably multicultural curriculum as permeated by 'deepseated pathologies of racial hatred' and 'white nationalism' (ibid. 291). Co-written by the controversial black educator Leonard Jeffries, who had become known for dividing the world into black 'sun people' and white 'ice people', the 1989 Task Force report (misleadingly entitled *A Curriculum of Inclusion*) demanded a history curriculum that would ensure that 'children from Native American, Puerto Rican/Latino, Asian-American, and African-American cultures will have higher self-esteem and self-respect, while children from European cultures will have a less arrogant perspective of being part of the group that has "done it all" ' (ibid. 292). *One Nation, Many Peoples*, the 1991 follow-up to the 1989 Task Force report, actually avoided such extremist rhetoric, and the accompanying Sobol circular stressed what was 'NOT recommended': 'trashing the traditions of the West', 'an Afrocentric curriculum', or 'ethnic cheerleading and separatism' (among others).[46] The more centrist final recommendations, which the Board of Regents officially endorsed in July 1991, were limited to excising 'insensitive language' (such as saying 'enslaved persons' instead of 'slaves', in order to 'call forth the essential humanity of those enslaved') and cultivating 'multiple perspectives' (such as celebrating Thanksgiving and Columbus Day not 'without examining other perspectives than those of Europeans, such as the perspectives of Native Americans').[47] Harmless stuff indeed, and Nathan Glazer, the eminent critic of 'affirmative discrimination' and member of the curriculum review committee, used the occasion to come out 'in defense of multiculturalism' (Glazer, 1991).

Like New York, California has been a pioneer in multiculturalism. But here the upheaval was not about a public school curriculum going too far, but about one not going far enough. The politics of curriculum and text books is potentially more intense in California, because this is one of twenty-eight states where the education department centrally selects appropriate textbooks, and—after public hearings—makes them mandatory for local school districts.[48] In 1987, the California State Board of Education adopted a new history and social studies framework, which introduced world history and social studies into the earliest grades and demanded that the public schools 'accurately portray the cultural and racial diversity of our society'—emphasizing, however, the 'centrality of Western civilizations as the source of American political institutions, laws and ideology'.[49] Little noticed in the beginning, the new curriculum caught attention only when a new textbook series written on this basis was introduced four years later. Co-authored by Gary Nash, a noted UCLA historian and left-liberal proponent of multiculturalism, the new textbooks went to 'amusing lengths to achieve political correctness', as a *New York Times* journalist found,[50] and they included a considerable eighty pages on African history for 12-year-olds. But they did not go far enough, according to the fierce opposition in a number of school districts. At a raucous public hearing in San Francisco, a Black Studies professor attacked the books for distorting black history, 'so Europe could be celebrated', and an American Indian Studies professor disliked the 'reductionist' depiction of 'our sun dance and medicine dance'.[51] The thrust of these critiques is clear: the new textbooks had not abdicated the 'idea of common democratic principles', and they refused to make 'everything . . . race, gender or class', as the state superintendent for education defended the books.[52]

Most California school districts eventually accepted the new textbooks. Among the notable exceptions was the Oakland Unified School District, where the four black members of the seven-member school board voted against the books, overriding the positive recommendation of the district's teachers and administrators.[53] Ninety-one per cent of Oakland's students are minority, including 57 per cent blacks, and the dropout rate is a soaring 35 per cent. 'These books did very little for those children . . . Their self-esteem is way down,' says a black board member. As a result, Oakland had to make do without any textbooks at all, putting its classrooms in chaos for a while.[54] Other school districts, such as Detroit, Atlanta, and Washington, DC, went one step further in establishing Afrocentric curricula, in which the 'self-esteem' of black pupils is bolstered by therapeutic history.[55] Some black educators have even turned away from the goal of racially integrated schools, and advocate all-black schools.[56] In re-embracing the doctrine of 'separate but equal', which the Supreme Court had outlawed in its famous *Brown* v. *Board of Education* ruling in 1954, multiculturalism has brought the civil-rights revolution to full circle.

Ethnicity: Elite and on the Ground

Panethnicity of Elites

Affirmative action and multiculturalism have conditioned the incorporation of the large bulk of post-1965 immigrants in ethnoracial terms, as 'Hispanics' and 'Asians'. In contrast to the American-made 'Italian patriots' of earlier days, whose reference point was a real nation (Glazer, 1954: 167), 'Hispanic' and 'Asian' are artificial categories that lack a national referent; they have no meaning beyond the American domestic sphere. In this sense, 'Hispanic' and 'Asian' denote a pure form of 'emergent ethnicity' (Yancey *et al.*, 1976), produced by the structural positioning of immigrant groups in the receiving society, rather than transplanted cultural heritage. Felix Padilla (1985) showed in the example of making 'Latinos' out of Mexican-Americans and Puerto Ricans in Chicago that only the seeking of affirmative action benefits provided the common ground for panethnic organizing: 'Latinismo is political ethnicity, a manipulative device for the pursuit of collective . . . interests in society' (p. 163). This political ethnicity has two minimal characteristics: it is negatively defined, and it is only indirectly linked to contemporary immigration. The content of political ethnicity is discrimination first experienced in a pre-immigration context, such as the nineteenth-century colonization of (some) Hispanics and racial exclusion of (some) Asians, which is then generalized across time and national groups.

Because their content is generalized discrimination, 'Asian' and 'Hispanic' are racial markers, modelled along the experience of American blacks. 'The term Asian-American arose out of the racist discourse that constructs Asians as a homogeneous group,' argues the author of *Asian American Panethnicity* (Espiritu, 1992: 6). This is slightly misleading, because the term Asian-American has originated in the anti-racist discourse of the campus-based Third World movement, and later became fixed in the administrative discourse of affirmative action. It would be inconsistent with the stipulated construct-edness of group boundaries and identities to ground the latter in a quasi-ontological racism of society. In fact, the phenomenal growth of the Asian-American population from under one million in 1965 to over seven million by 1990 is precisely due to the removal of racism in the immigration system. Accordingly, not external racism, but the reinterpretation of ethnic experience in terms of race is the origin of 'Asian-American'. A scholar-activist's statement that 'the notion of an Asian-American identity seemed to be emerging when I was a fresh-man at Berkeley' (Ong Hing, 1994: 169) has to be taken at face value. Of course, this does not mean that racism is a figment of the anti-racist imagination.[57] But this imagination extrapolates racist events and episodes into the group- and society-defining experience, also because there is nothing else that Chinese-, Japanese-, or Korean-Americans have in common. Among the components of this negative 'history of exploitation, oppression, and discrimination' (Espiritu, 1992: 17) are keeping awake the memory of 'Oriental' exclusion, dramatizing the resurgence of racially motivated 'hate crimes',[58] and destroying the patronizing notion of model minority.[59] The identity created by this exercise has little in common with immigrant ethnicity. As Yen Le Espiritu (1992: 50) points out correctly, pan-Asianism is 'the ideology of native-born, American-educated, and middle-class Asians' that 'barely touch[es] the Asian ethnic enclaves'. The Asian ethnic enclaves, such as the Vietnamese refugee community, identify along national origin rather than racial status lines (see Kibria, 1993: 171).

The making of an Hispanic identity involves a similar reinterpreta-tion of ethnic as racial history. The turn to a racial identity is even more visible here, because there is a rich history of pre-1960s organizing especially by Mexican-Americans, who initially tried to avoid what they later would try to achieve: racial-minority status. 'Reserve your citizenship and preserve it; honor your country, maintain its tradition in the spirit of its citizens, and embody yourself into its culture and civilization,' says the 1929 Code of the League of United Latin American Citizens (LULAC), the oldest Mexican-American civil-rights organization (in Garcia, 1989: 25). Led by assimilation-minded lower middle-class professionals and businessmen, LULAC restricted its membership to US citizens, and declared English as its official lan-guage. LULAC's purpose of developing within their members the 'purest and most perfect type of a true and loyal citizen of the United States of America' (ibid. 31) implied a restrictionist stance on immi-gration. LULAC opposed the Bracero guestworker programme, and supported the drastic Operation Wetback as legitimate means to combat the 'fearful problem', illegal immigration from Mexico (ibid. 52). In the summary of Mario Garcia (1989: 59), Mexican-American organizing in the pre-civil-rights era was carried by an 'idealistic faith in the ability of the American system to reform itself'.

This faith was shattered in the 1960s, when LULAC underwent a 'minoritization' along the black power model. The Mexican-American equivalent to black power was to adopt a Chicano identity.[60] It revolved around recovering the pre-colonial legacy of Aztlan, the presumed ancestral homeland of Aztecs, and thus, of Mexicans, which had been surrendered to the United States after the Mexican–American War of 1848. As Chicanos, Mexican-Americans were colonized people, who had to fight for self-control rather than integration: 'We will not integrate into this gringo society', proclaimed a 1960s Chicano activist (in Gutierrez, 1995: 187). Chicanismo entailed a redrawing of group boundaries in which immigration and citizenship status were irrelevant. Chicanos were a 'people without borders', one for which even the 'Mexican' national referent was lastly irrelevant. The Los Angeles-based Chicano leader Bert Corona declares: 'Our unity has to include not only Chicanos born here, but also those who come from Mexico and Central and South America with documents and those who come . . . without' (ibid. 192).

Radical Chicanismo is nowhere alive today, except on a few college campuses in southern California. But its redrawing of group boundaries has gone mainstream. Whereas pre-1960s LULAC admitted as members only US citizens, today's Mexican-American Legal Defense and Educational Fund (MALDEF) protects 'the civil and constitutional rights of *all Hispanics* in the United States, whether they are legal, undocumented, or US citizens'.[61] Shifting from a restrictionist to a pro-immigration stance is not only due to Hispanic panethnicity, but a rational adaptation to the proportional logic of affirmative action, according to which minority benefits depend on a group's population share.[62]

MALDEF epitomizes the way Hispanic interests are organized in the American polity today. Explicitly modelled on the black NAACP's Legal Defense Fund, MALDEF was set up in 1968, 'top down', by a grant of the liberal Ford Foundation.[63] While speaking on behalf of Hispanics, MALDEF is thus not accountable to their constituencies. An exclusively litigation-oriented organization without a rank-and-file membership, MALDEF has been instrumental in having Hispanics partake of civil-rights law protection and affirmative-action benefits. All legal steps in constructing a Hispanic minority bear the strong imprint of MALDEF—the 1975 and 1982 amendments of the Voting Rights Act that made Hispanics a protected 'language minority'; the Supreme Court's *Lau* v. *Nichols* (1974) and *Plyler* v. *Doe* (1982) landmark rules, which secured bilingual education and free public schools for immigrant children, independent of their legal status; and court-imposed majority minority districts, which greatly increased the electoral representation of Hispanics at all levels of the American polity.[64]

Conservative critics have scorned Hispanic organizations like MALDEF or the National Council of La Raza[65] for being ethnic power-brokers without community ties, and for fashioning Hispanics as a racial minority rather than an ethnic-immigrant group (e.g. Chavez, 1991; Skerry, 1993). While this catches an important factual aspect of contemporary ethnic politics in the United States, the normative tone is mistaken. MALDEF and La Raza only respond to a political opportunity structure in which ethnic claims are more effectively raised as racial-minority claims.

Here it is important to point to a notable difference of ethnic claims-making in academia and the organizing world. The secluded world of ethnic-studies programmes and humanity departments is prone to generate rampant multiculturalism, with all-out attacks on the old melting-pot ideal and pedantic quibbles such as if 'Hispanics' are better called 'Latinos' (for the latter, see Calderon, 1992). In the world of organizing, the cross-pressures of compromise-making and coalition-building prevent such extremes. When naïvely asked to take a stance on the notion of melting-pot, MALDEF's chief Washington lobbyist was utterly flabbergasted: ' "Melting-pot"? MALDEF has no position on "melting-pot" [*laughs*]. Melting-pot? If that means that the rights of the Latino community are the same as the rights of everybody else, it's okay with me. I have no problem with it. *There is no effort to set up a distinct, separate system, or to isolate the Latino community* ... All our efforts have been to assimilate, and to bring down barriers to that assimilation, to bring down barriers to access to education, employment, politics and the political process—which is fundamental to the rights of being a citizen.'[66] For this entirely credible lobbyist, who also refused to call the US 'racist' but instead held it 'the best country in the world to live in', Hispanics today pursue exactly what Jews, Italians, Irish, or Poles pursued eighty years earlier—the only difference being the Civil Rights Act of 1964, which has fundamentally altered the means of ethnic politics.

Ethnicity on the Ground

There is a deep gulf separating the panethnic élites from their ethnic-immigrant constituencies. Ethnicity on the ground means a continued clinging of immigrants to national-origins identification, even into the second generation, and optimistic views that contradict the racial pessimism of the élites. Take the case of Hispanics, who are closer to blacks than to non-Hispanic whites or Asians on most socioeconomic indices. The Latino National Political Survey of 1989/90 found that only relatively small shares of Hispanics adopt panethnic labels. Among first-generation immigrants, a bare 14 per cent of Mexicans, 13 per cent of Puerto Ricans, and 12 per cent of Cubans identified themselves panethnically.[67] Panethnic identification increases in the second generation to 28 per cent of Mexicans, 19 per cent of Puerto Ricans, and 20 per cent of Cubans. But there is a parallel trend toward an unhyphenated 'American' identity among second-generation immigrants: 10 per cent of Mexican, 21 per cent of Puerto Rican, and a staggering 39 per cent of Cuban second-generation immigrants prefer to call themselves simply 'Americans'. Next to being lukewarm panethnics, Hispanic immigrants share a pragmatic and optimistic outlook. Portes and Bach's (1985) longitudinal study of recent immigrants from Mexico and Cuba found 'high levels of satisfaction' among both groupings, and a general denial that racial discrimination was taking place—characteristically, the perception of discrimination grew over time, especially with greater education, knowledge of English, and 'modernity' of immigrants (ibid. 296). Similarly, in the 1989/90 Latino National Political Survey the overwhelming majority of immigrants took stances directly opposite to those of the Hispanic leadership: agreeing that there were 'too many immigrants', stressing the importance of learning English, preferring (with the exception of Puerto Ricans) to be taught American rather than ethnic homeland history, describing themselves as politically moderate to conservative, and showing a lack of interest in most Hispanic groups, leaders, or causes. A co-researcher of the Latino Survey concludes: 'The implication is that there is a growing gulf between the Latino leadership and the community.'[68]

For today's Asian and Latin American no less than for yesterday's European immigrants, ethnicity functions as a pivotal resource of adjusting to the new society. And for those who do not dispose of protective ethnicity, 'assimilation' may take on a radically new meaning. According to classic theories of immigrant integration (e.g. Park, 1950:

ch. 10), there was a 'straight line' from exclusion in the beginning to assimilation at the end, mediated by the ethnic cushion. Today, the meaning of assimilation is not necessarily positive, but in an entirely different sense than conveyed by multicultural critics. Mary Waters (1994) has demonstrated that for second-generation black immigrants from the Caribbean 'assimilation' may mean adopting the anomic ways of the American black underclass. The children of black immigrants face a fundamental choice: to maintain the ethnic-origin identification of their parents, or to adopt the racial identity that the host society holds ready for them, that is, to become 'black American'. Assimilation in today's pluralistic society and culture may mean that the youngsters who do resist the assimilatory pressure of their urban peers and stick to their parents' ethnic-origin identity are better off than those who do not. Under conditions of 'segmented assimilation' (Portes and Rumbaut, 1996: ch. 7), to adopt an American identity is more a threat than a promise, because it may lock the immigrant child into the self-destructive culture of the ghetto. Mary Waters (1994: 809) has captured the mischiefs of becoming American in this statement of an 'assimilated' second-generation West Indian: 'My feelings are more like blacks than theirs [West Indians]. I am lazy. I am really lazy and my parents are always making comments and things about how I am lazy. They are always like, in Trinidad you could not be this lazy. In Trinidad you would have to keep working.'[69]

Cubans in Miami are an extreme case of using immigrant ethnicity for socioeconomic advancement. Like Japanese and Jewish immigrants in earlier days, the Cuban refugees of the Castro regime have built a tight ethnic enclave, in which the ethnic community delivers everything from labour, capital, and customers to the immaterial resources of trust and identification (see Portes and Bach, 1985: ch. 6).[70] By 1977, the Miami area was home to half of the forty largest Hispanic firms in the United States and to the largest bank, and there was one firm for every twenty-seven Cuban-born (Portes and Stepick, 1993: 135). By 1987, the aggregate receipts of Hispanic firms in Miami were at $3.8 billion, outshining the $400 million Hispanic receipts in Los Angeles, despite the latter's vastly bigger Hispanic population (ibid. 146). The secret of Cuban success was a strong sense of 'us-ness' created by the joint experience of political defeat and exile. More than any other immigrant group, Cubans would buy from other Cubans, hand out loans based on nothing else but 'character' (in effect, Cuban nationality), and hire preferably co-nationals. This paid off for Cuban newcomers. Portes and Stepick found that the single most significant predictor in self-employment among Cubans in 1979 was employment in a Cuban-owned firm three years earlier.

The Cuban-led transformation of Miami from sleepy retirement home to bustling metropolis went along with making the city more bicultural and bilingual than any other in the United States, and it is no accident that the national English-Only movement was born here. However, the disgruntled natives overlook that they are dealing with fierce American patriots at the same time. Indeed, Cuban ethnicity is not made of resentment, but goes along with a more positive American identification than among any other immigrant group. The local radio station WQBA, *La Cubanisima* (The Most Cuban), greets its listeners every day with a pledge to America: 'It's noontime. Let us give thanks to God for living in a country of full liberty and democracy' (ibid. 139). This vignette is supported by hard survey evidence. In a comparison of five second-geneneration nationalities (Portes and Rumbaut, 1996: 258 f.), the descendants of the Cuban enclave were also the ones most likely to self-identify as 'American' (33.1 per cent) or 'hyphenated American' (59.3), and both panethnic and national-origin identifications were practically absent (with 3.5 per cent each).

Alas, ethnicity is not always positive, and it may work to the detriment of some immigrant groups. The formation of supportive immigrant ethnicity is dependent both upon the conditions of entry into the United States and the orientations of immigrants. As Sarah Mahler (1995) has shown in her riveting portrait of Salvadorian and Peruvian illegal immigrants on Long Island, under conditions of illegality immigrants are prone to take advantage of their co-ethnics. Instead of an ethnic niche, Mahler found only exploitation by co-ethnics: 'Finding their greatest opportunity for socioeconomic mobility within their ethnic group, [immigrants] learn how to squeeze profits out of their communities as informal entrepreneurs providing services and products to coethnics' (ibid. 216). The propensity for ethnic self-exploitation among Mahler's subjects was additionally fed by their retention of homeland ties, which locked them into two competing sets of allegiances in the sending and the receiving society: 'Because immigrants are asked to provide mutual assistance to disparate groups of people in different countries, they may not engage in reciprocal relations in the same way that they did in their homelands' (ibid. 99). The emergence of 'transnational' migrant communities, which some scholars have celebrated as avant-gardes of multiple and border-transcending identities in a postnational world,[71] may thus be more liability than resource for immigrants.[72]

This chapter showed 'race' in an unorthodox light, less as a form of discrimination (that it certainly is) than as a source of opportunities. In the civil-rights era, ethnic leaders have incentives to model their immigrant constituencies as victimized clients of the state, and to clamour for affirmative-action privileges: preferential college admission, government jobs and business contracts, and political representation in majority minority districts. 'Hispanics' and 'Asians' have originally been administrative categories, without correspondence to collective identities. Multiculturalism in education may be understood as attempts to breathe life into these categories, as the panethnic production of Hispanics and Asians. This implies a conscious racialization of ethnic boundaries (what else do 'Asians' have in common?), drawing a Fanonesque line between racial minorities and the white majority. From this perspective, the idea of common citizenship and nationhood disappears. However, contrary to scare scenarios of 'Balkanization', multicultural élite discourse should not be mistaken for the common immigrant's unwillingness to integrate, for which there is little evidence. On the ground, ethnicity functions much as it always did, as a source of adjusting to the new society.

6

From Postnational Membership to Citizenship: Germany

The case of immigrant integration in Germany casts doubt on both Soysal's diagnosis of postnational membership and Brubaker's insistence on the ultrastability of national citizenship traditions. For long, (West) Germany's approach to integrating its *de facto* immigrants followed strictly Soysalian lines: keep them as foreigners and deny them citizenship, also in order to ensure that 'guestworkers' would stay just that; but give them full civil, social, perhaps even political rights. Eventually, however, the limitations of postnational integration had to become apparent. Postnational membership is well-suited for the first generation of *de facto* immigrants, who stick to the—often deceptive—idea of returning home one day. It is ill-suited for second- and third-generation immigrants, who may enjoy (almost) equal rights but are forever kept separate and stigmatizable as 'foreigners'. The tragic wave of zenophobic violence of the early 1990s ratified the failure of postnational immigrant integration in Germany. 'Think of ten-year-old Yeliz Asslan,' said President Weizsäcker in commemoration of two Turkish girls and their mother murdered by arsonists in Mölln. 'She was born among us and had never lived anywhere else. In our press, however, we read only about "three Turks".'[1]

The painful recognition that citizenship mattered had to go along with its redefinition. Moving away from postnational membership à la Soysal could not mean embracing traditional ethnocultural citizenship, as diagnosed by Brubaker. In fact, both models had coexisted up to this point, one conditioning the other: endowing foreigners with equal rights enabled maintaining the limitation of citizenship to ethnic Germans. On the other hand, easing the access of foreigners to citizenship through as-of-right naturalization, *jus soli*, or the acceptance of double citizenship had to entail a civic-territorial redefinition of the traditional German model of ethno-genealogical citizenship. Germany's slow and tortured turn from postnational to national immigrant integration thus carries a double message. First, immigration does not render obsolete national citizenship, as postnational membership analysts would have it. Secondly, and contrary to Brubaker's diagnosis of long-entrenched models of nationhood determining citizenship laws and policies, immigration may trigger a redefinition of citizenship, in departure from traditional models of nationhood.

The German differs from the American case of immigrant integration in at least two respects. First, the alien–citizen distinction, unproblematic in the United States, became heavily embattled in Germany, with shifting emphases on which direction to take: secure the status of alien, or ease the transition to citizenship. Further besieged by the problem of unredeemed national unity, Germany had to bear the full brunt of a non-immigrant nation facing the altogether new phenomenon of immigration, and it had to become embroiled in a foundational debate about the legal and cultural meanings of membership and citizenship. Secondly, while there was confusion about which direction to take, there was a clear sense that the integration of immigrants could not be left to society; it had to be a matter for the state. If the story of immigrant integration in the United States was largely one of immigrants adjusting to the opportunity structures of polity and society, the story of immigrant integration in Germany is largely one of domestic élites struggling vicariously about the very meaning and implications of 'immigration', with the immigrants themselves only marginally and passively involved.

The initial trend toward postnational immigrant integration was less the result of grand design than of muddling through. But it still appears as the adequate response to the vexed problem of nationhood in postwar Germany. Nationhood was at once delegitimized as a political ordering principle, and transposed to the question of denied unity. Thus, membership in a tainted nation could not be expected to be adopted by immigrants, nor was it made accessible to them. The delegitimation of nationhood was forcefully expressed by Karl Jaspers in the early years of the Federal Republic: 'The history of the nation-state has come to an end. What we, as a great nation, can teach to ourselves and to the world is the deep insight into the world situation today: that the principle of the nation-state is the disaster [*Unheil*] of Europe and of all continents' (in Mommsen, 1990: 63 f.). Representative for many, political scientist Dieter Oberndörfer (1993) carried this motif into the immigration debate, juxtaposing the 'open republic', based on universal human rights and friendly to newcomers, and the particularistic 'nation-state', against which immigration itself might deliver the *coup de grâce*. There was no question that immigrants could not be expected to become members (that is, 'citizens') of this antiquated, if not incriminated political thing, the nation-state.

On the other hand, immigrants were not entitled to become members of the divided nation, because this would undermine the self-definition of the Federal Republic as the provisional, incomplete state of all Germans, mandated to achieve national unity. A conservative legal scholar argued that, for the sake of unity, immigrants had to be kept out of the national community: 'The Federal Republic has not been conceived of as a country of immigration or as a multinational state. Rather she has been created by the German people for the German people, as a state with the mandate of reunification, in which all powers derive from the German people' (Uhlitz, 1986: 145). The most pertinent expression of the unity mandate, and of the concomitant ethnocultural closure of citizenship, has been the construct of an all-German citizenship, embracing all ethnic Germans under communism, which was based on the legal fiction that for the purposes of citizenship law the old Reich was still in existence (Hailbronner, 1989: 73).

The tension between creedal postnationalism and perpetuated ethnocultural nationhood has been legally embodied in the German constitution, the Basic Law. It's Preamble, which the German Constitutional Court has found not only politically meaningful but legally binding, celebrates postnationalism in the new Republic's mission to 'strive for world peace in a united Europe', but reaffirms ethnocultural nationhood in the mandate to 'complete the unity and freedom of Germany in free self-determination' (see Döhring, 1979).[2] Accordingly, the constitution has been flexible, or ambivalent, enough to justify both keeping immigrants out of the national community and embracing them as equal members of a postnational republic.

Strikingly, in both nationally exclusive and postnationally inclusive perspectives immigrants are not expected to assimilate. The rejection of assimilation is the one continuity in the unprincipled, wavering German approach to immigrant integration. Characteristically, the newly elected Kohl government, while propounding a more restrictive foreigner policy than the one pursued under its Social Democratic predecessor, still held to a mellow concept of integration: 'Integration does not mean giving up one's own identity, but aims at a relaxed co-existence between foreigners and Germans' (in Uhlitz, 1986: 144). For advocates of national closure, assimilation was both impossible and undesirable, because it rested on the strange belief that the state could mould its citizens, French-style, and, if it occurred on a grand scale, it threatened to destroy the ethnocultural texture of the nation. This attitude is enshrined in the German naturalization rules, according to which the adoption of German citizenship was always exceptional and contingent upon a magic transformation of the applicant into a quasi-ethnic German *before* being granted the formal membership status.[3] For postnationalists, assimilation was both undesirable and unnecessary, because it violated the dignity of the individual and was rendered obsolete by a constitution that protected the liberty of the person (independently of citizenship status) from encroachment by the state.[4] From the joint distaste for assimilation follows a peculiar blurring of ideological lines in the German debate on immigrant integration. For instance, a conservative opponent of facilitating the naturalization of foreigners would advocate 'national minority rights' for (Turkish) immigrants (Quaritsch, 1981: 78); and a liberal advocate of local voting rights for foreigners would reject as unconstitutional 'forced integration' the education of second-generation immigrants in regular German classes, thus defending the Bavarian Model of mother-tongue education, whose main purpose had been the return migration of the guestworkers (Schwerdtfeger, 1980: A99). On top of such strange alliances, the few immigrant voices in the integration debate demanded 'equal co-existence between the immigrants residing in the Federal Republic and the German population,'[5] which is equally premissed on keeping immigrants and Germans apart. In this motley front of not burdening foreigners with national membership, not wanting them as fellow-nationals, or—on the part of immigrants—not wanting to give up established national allegiances, a crucial dimension of immigrant integration, the transformation of aliens into citizens, faded from view.

Elements of Postnational Integration

In her comparison of national models of immigrant integration, Dominique Schnapper (1994) noted that the economic rather than national identity of the Bonn Republic conditioned an economic mode of integrating immigrants, in which the nationality of the latter was irrelevant. Here it is useful to illuminate the spirit in which the first guestworkers were received. When in late 1964 the one millionth guestworker was welcomed in festive atmosphere at Cologne's railway station, a representative of the Federal Employers'

Association acknowledged that 'the successes of the West German economy would not have been possible without the help of the guest-workers.'[6] On the same occasion, the Federal Minister of Labour even celebrated the guestworkers as harbingers of a Europe beyond nation-states, because they had brought about 'the unification of Europe and the rapprochement between persons of highly diverse backgrounds and cultures in a spirit of friendship' (in Herbert, 1990: 213). These statements convey the world as a big economy-plus-peace bazaar. In the view from Bonn, national markers no longer mattered. If one adds the rechannelling of national discourse to the problem of divided Germany, there was a strong cultural predisposition to integrate guest-workers without tinkering with their nationality.

Once the cultural disposition was there, the Basic Law's protection of citizenship-transcending universal human rights provided the hard legal basis for postnational immigrant integration (see Chapter 3). Albert Bleckmann (1980: 694) even found that the automatism of the Basic Law obliterated the 'choice between a system that approximates foreigners to citizens and dispenses with an inclusive citizenship policy, and a system that, on the contrary, differentiates strongly between citizens and foreigners and legally protects the latter through an inclusive citizenship policy'. Accordingly, under the sway of the Basic Law's human-rights universalism the German solution to immigrant integration was 'the full inlander equality of foreigners', who in fact became 'Germans in the sense of residence and domicile' (ibid.).

However, the idea of equal rights for foreign residents is no invention of the Basic Law. It reflects the territoriality principle of the modern welfare state, which has constitutional rank according to Article 20 of the Basic Law.[7] The welfare state is nationality-blind; only residence in the territory matters. As Kay Hailbronner (1992: 79) circumscribes the principle of nationality-blind welfare state inclusion, 'the basic rules of social justice prohibit the differentiation within a solidary community of the insured according to nationality'. In residual areas, such as social benefits not grounded in own contributions or access to the labour market, initially legitimate nationality discrimination becomes illegitimate with increasing length of residence. If, in 1989, 3.5 million foreigners (out of a total of 4.5 million) had lived longer than eight years in the Federal Republic, they enjoyed most of the social and labour market rights that Germans enjoyed.

A third, and increasingly important, legal source of postnational immigrant integration has been European Union law. According to the free movement clause of the Treaty of Rome, the 1.3 million foreign EU nationals living in the Federal Republic in 1989 had a privileged legal status, if compared with third-state nationals: they were not subject to the Foreigner Law. Nationality-based discriminations against EU nationals are prohibited in principle, not just with increasing length of residence. EU nationals may take residence in Germany as they see fit, they enjoy equal access to the labour market, they can fully import or export social entitlements gained in any member state,[8] and—as stipulated by the Maastricht Treaty—they are even allowed to vote in local elections. For Italian, Spanish, or Greek guestworkers the acquisition of German citizenship, and thus any other but a postnational mode of immigrant integration, would not just be redundant; it would be contrary to the idea of European unification. In addition, European Union law has spread from EU nationals to third-state nationals. The European Court of Justice increasingly applies the prohibition of nationality-based discrimination to the 1.5 million Turks living in Germany, invoking the three-decade-old EU Association Treaty with Turkey (Rittstieg and Rowe, 1992: 25). But more than legal, the pull of Europe is moral. Every new privilege for EU immigrants raises the question why non-EU immigrants should not have it too. For example, the granting of local voting rights for EU nationals has revived the old demand that all resident foreigners should be entitled to vote in local elections. The call not to distinguish between 'first-' and 'second-class' foreigners is legally and politically confused, because it ignores the inevitability of boundaries even in a united Europe; but it is still morally compelling. In sum, the process of Europeanization has drawn even non-European immigrants into the suction of postnational integration.

Postnational immigrant integration has been framed by a peculiarly German brand of multiculturalism. In contrast to American multiculturalism, which consisted of claims by excluded minority groups for recognition or even privileged treatment, German multiculturalism is an attack on the principle of the nation-state.[9] This attack proceeds in two steps. In a first step, 'multiculturalism' figures as the description of a society in which immigration has taken place. 'Germany is a country of immigration', and therefore a 'multicultural society', says a publication of the Federal Commissioner for Foreigner Affairs (Schmalz-Jacobsen *et al.*, 1993). In a second step, the description of a society diversified by immigration is transformed into the normative claim that the nation could no longer be the legitimizing principle of the state. Accordingly, the Federal Commissioner demands the 'overcoming of national thinking', and the putting of 'postnational republican community feeling' in its place (ibid. 305 and 298, respectively).[10] How the boundaries of a postnation state are to be drawn, and what name it should carry, most advocates of multiculturalism do not say. Dieter Oberndörfer (1993), whose 'open republic' is of course 'multicultural', is among the few to spell out the implication: his Goodbye to the nation-state is the Hello to the 'republican world confederation' (p. 129). No wonder that multiculturalism *à l'allemand* has few friends in the Federal Ministry of the Interior. A civil servant in the Interior Ministry correctly identifies German multiculturalism as the quest for the equal co-existence of domestic and immigrant cultures, and he finds the idea wanting (Schiffer, 1992). Certainly, immigrants were free to hold to their cultural identity; but they had to respect what sedentary groups had always expected of newcomers: 'When in Rome, do as the Romans do'.

Except in a few experiments of 'intercultural education',[11] German multiculturalism has rarely been more than rhetoric. However, its influence is visible in three legislative proposals, all of them unsuccessful, but epitomizing the logic of postnational immigrant integration. The first is the proposal, raised repeatedly by the Green Party, for a 'residence law' (*Niederlassungsgesetz*). The Greens have always been the true children of the postnational Bonn Republic. Their proposal for a residence law, first introduced in 1984, carries the logic of postnational immigrant integration to its ultimate. Under the fanfare of 'equal rights for all who live here permanently' (The Greens, 1990: 4), the residence law would exempt from the jurisdiction of the Foreigner Law those foreigners who have legally resided in the Federal Republic for at least five years, and thus give them all the rights that Germans have, including political rights. This sounds innocuous, but has momentous implications. The residence law would reintroduce the old Prussian *Wohnsitzprinzip* (residence principle), which had tied state membership to mere residence in the territory. All aspiring nation-states, like Prussia in 1842, had replaced the residence principle by the more demanding principles of *jus soli* or *jus sanguinis*, reflecting that modern states were not just territorial but membership organizations (see Hailbronner and Renner, 1991: 4). The residence law would revoke this transformation; its postnationalism is also prenationalism. The draft bill still reads like a catalogue of existing administrative and legal practice (see The Greens, 1990: 72–7). Most of the rights the proposed law wished to grant *de jure* were already in place *de facto*, or they would be instituted soon. Under the new law, resident foreigners could no longer be deported—but the legal barriers to deportations were high already, even in the cases of crime, unemployment, and welfare dependency; resident foreigners would receive the same social benefits as Germans—as if there were severe discriminations in this area; finally, family members would receive an independent residence right, and resident foreigners temporarily returning to their home countries would have a right to return (*Wiederkehroption*)—both measures were realized in the 1990 Foreigner Law. Where the resident law really goes beyond existing practice is granting full political rights to resident foreigners, and giving them a right to double citizenship. Only, one may ask, what is the point of acquiring German citizenship if all its goodies are already included in residentship? In his rejection of the Green proposal, the Federal Minister of the Interior argued correctly that a residence law would perpetuate the foreigner status over generations, and 'create permanent national minorities' (ibid. 84). However, this was no less hypocritical than the Green proposal, because the existing policy of postnational immigrant integration had exactly the same result.

If the effect of postnational immigrant integration is to create national minorities, an obvious consequence is to give them legal protection. This is the aim of a proposed anti-discrimination law, which would proscribe nationality-based private discrimination in education, employment, housing, and the service sector.[12] A more radical proposal has been to include an article on minority protection in the constitution. This would be in breach of the Basic Law's individual-rights philosophy.[13] Of the two postwar Germanys, only communist East Germany had elevated minority protection to constitutional rank, targeting the traditional Sorb minority living near the Polish border. The Unity Treaty of 1990 opened up the possibility of transporting minority protection into the all-German Basic Law (see Franke and Hofmann, 1992). This was uncontroversial for the Sorbs, Danes, and Frisians, all national minorities with long-established language and regional autonomy rights.[14] But a new demand was to enlarge the range of minority protection from national to 'cultural' minorities, most notably the non-EU immigrants in western Germany. According to international law, minority protection is contingent on citizenship in the protecting state. The novelty of 'cultural' minority protection was to include non-citizens also. Torn between a CDU/CSU (particularly in the eastern *Länder*) resisting the inclusion of non-citizen immigrants, and a (western) pro-immigrant lobby in SPD and the Greens in favour of this inclusion, the Federal Commission for Constitutional Reform suggested a compromise formula in 1994: 'The state recognizes the identity of ethnic, cultural, and linguistic minorities.' Inclusion of the word 'cultural' attests to the success of the pro-immigrant lobby. But as a mere recognition clause, the proposed article would fall back behind international law and national constitutions that proactively 'protected' rather than passively 'recognized' minority groups. However weakened through compromise, minority protection in the German context would mean keeping minority groups and majority society apart, allowing the latter to remain unaffected by immigration. It is thus not far-fetched to denigrate the campaign for minority protection as a hidden prolongation of '*völkisch* thinking'.[15]

The logic of postnational immigrant integration is to endow foreign residents with full civil and social rights, but to deny them political rights. This was no residual of *völkisch* thinking, but reflective of the French connection of democracy and nationhood. However, once the civil and social equality of immigrants had been achieved, the next logical step was to tackle the political front—the Green proposal for a residence law was the most radical expression of this logic. The foreigner councils (*Ausländerbeiräte*) or foreigner parliaments instituted at the local level gave the immigrants some 'influence', perhaps, but no decision-making powers (see Bommes, 1991). Already by 1975, SPD and FDP therefore advocated local voting rights for foreigners.[16] In 1980, the 53rd National Lawyers' Meeting (*Juristentag*) in Berlin joined this campaign, arguing that the right to vote in local elections was a necessary step to 'realize the constitutional principle of democracy' (Deutscher Juristentag, 1980: L289). The campaign drew further support when neighbouring countries such as the Netherlands, following the early example of Sweden, introduced local voting rights for foreigners in the early 1980s.

In 1989, Social-Democratic Schleswig-Holstein and Hamburg finally introduced local alien suffrage by means of simple legislation. Both schemes were rather different. Schleswig-Holstein granted local suffrage only to citizens of countries with a similar right already in place, on the basis of reciprocity; this meant local voting rights for 5,500 Danes, Irish, Norwegians, Dutch, Swedes, and Swiss citizens living in the Federal Republic for at least five years. Hamburg, more boldly, enfranchised all foreigners who had resided in the Federal Republic for at least eight years, thus opening the door to local district elections for 150,000 foreigners then living in the city-state. Predictably, the Federal Minister of the Interior, CSU-hardliner Friedrich Zimmermann, howled that an 'assault on the Constitution' had taken place.[17] The CDU/CSU faction in the *Bundestag*, pressurized by the electoral successes of the right-wing *Republikaner* at the time, and the state of Bavaria quickly called upon the Federal Constitutional Court in Karlsruhe to pass a final verdict. In the plaintiffs' view, Hamburg and Schleswig-Holstein were only 'test-drilling' for the 'real cut'—indeed, Berlin, Bremen, and North Rhine-Westphalia were waiting in the wings to enfranchise their immigrants; and once foreigners could vote locally, why not in state and federal elections also?[18]

The German debate over alien suffrage was a foundational debate over the meaning of membership and citizenship in the nation-state.[19] More specifically, it was a battle over the two conflicting principles of 'democratic' and national stateness enshrined in the Basic Law. The first conceived of the Federal Republic as an open state devoted to human rights, peace, and the unity of Europe; the second perpetuated ethnocultural closure through the unity mandate. Both principles suggested different interpretations of fundamental constitutional tenets. For a defender of the national principle, Article 20(2) of the Basic Law: 'All state authority emanates from the people', meant that only Germans were entitled to vote (e.g. Isensee, 1987); for a defender of the democratic principle, the same article meant that state legitimacy had to derive bottom-up, from society, rather than top-down, from God or from princes (e.g. Zuleeg, 1989). To be sure, the separation of democracy and nationhood appeared as such only for the defenders of the alien suffrage, who skilfully deployed the historical delegitimation of German nationhood to make their case.[20]

Next to the pragmatic argument that alien suffrage was good for integrating immigrants, suffrage advocates advanced two principled arguments: first, alien suffrage was commanded by the democracy principle of the Basic Law; and secondly, local government was different in kind from state and federal government, allowing foreigners to be part of the former. At heart, the advocates of alien suffrage were true multiculturalists, viewing it as a means of decoupling democracy from the nation. Manfred Zuleeg (1987), for instance, conceded that democracy 'may have' arisen historically within the nation-state; but he saw no reason why this marriage should last forever, reminding his (presumably forgetful) audience 'that the concept of the nation-state had conjured up two world-wars' (p. 158). In a slightly different version of this argument, Zuleeg (1980) admitted that there was no doubt that the creators of the Basic Law had only 'Germans' in mind when they stipulated that 'all state authority emanates from the people'. But now a new situation had arisen in which foreigners also were part of the 'community of destiny' that constituted the people (*Volk*) according to the Basic Law. Most importantly, however, the democracy principle, equally enshrined in the Basic Law, commanded that those 'affected' (*betroffen*) by the rule of the state should be part of the state: 'The constitutional principle of democracy commands that an individual should partake of the power that is exerted over him or her' (Zuleeg, 1980: 430). There is obvious confusion here between grounding alien suffrage in a redefined nation, or grounding it in democracy as such, divorced from any nation. Because even a French-style civic nation would allow only its 'citizens' to be part of the business of rule, Zuleeg's redefinition of *Volk* in a French direction seems merely rhetorical; the thrust of his argument is to liberate democracy from the principle of any bounded community. If 'affectedness' by the state is the only presupposition for constituting the state, the distinction between citizens and aliens is moot, and one is left with an undifferentiated concept of humankind, floating between the jurisdictions of states. However feasible a subject of democracy 'humankind' may be, the advocates of alien suffrage smelled the chance to make a larger point here.

A second, more technical, line of defending alien suffrage argued that local government was not part of the state, and thus not bound by the Basic Law's diction that 'all state authority emanates from the people'. As Gunther Schwerdtfeger (1980: A107–11) influentially argued, the 'people' according to Article 20(2) of the Basic Law was clearly the 'German people'—accordingly, there was no point in redefining the people or even arguing that democracy could do without it. But, in a constitutional sense, local government (*Gemeinde*) was separate from the state; historically, the *Gemeinde* had even defended society *against* the monarchical state. This is expressed in Article 28(2) of the Basic Law, according to which local governments had the right to 'determine all affairs of the local community [*örtliche Gemeinschaft*] under their own responsibility'. If the local community was not part of the state, one could argue next that membership in the *Volk* was not a prerequisite for determining local affairs. Foreigners could be part of the local community, as much as they were part of universities, trade unions, or professional associations—all of which had long allowed foreigners to vote or run for office in their limited spheres.

'Who are the People? This is the Question'—this is how Josef Isensee, the prominent constitutional lawyer and consultant of the federal government in the suffrage debate, introduced his case against alien suffrage.[21] But this was not so much a German case, along *völk-isch* lines, as a critic wrongly suggested (Weiler, 1995: 9); rather, it was a French-style case that democracy could not exist in a vacuum, but was dependent on a bounded collectivity. Since the French Revolution, the carrier of democracy has been the nation. And this nation must carry a name, in this case 'German'. Opponents of alien suffrage were at first plain nationalists, defenders of the French connection of democracy and nationhood. They were *völkisch* nationalists only by implication, because membership in the German nation happened to proceed along ethnic lines. However, membership in the nation was, strictly speaking, not the issue in the suffrage debate, only if some non-members were *also* entitled to some democratic privileges usually reserved to members. In that regard, not 'who are the people', but 'are only the people (as the German version of the nation) entitled to vote locally', should be seen as the central issue of the alien suffrage debate.

In any case, Isensee—and, following him, the Federal Constitutional Court—only responded to the argument of some suffrage advocates that the Basic Law's failure to say '*German* people' in Article 20(2) left open the possibility that foreigners might be included. If that were the case, the implication of 'all state authority emanates from the people' would be that foreigners could vote not only in local, but also in state and federal elections. This again would imply that the Federal Republic was not conceived as a (however incomplete) nation-state at all, but as an open republic with free-floating members.[22] An absurd assumption indeed, but the one made by some suffrage advocates, and adopted by their opponents as the beast to beat. This was not difficult. Albert Bleckmann (1988) showed that the nation-state principle was indeed prescribed by the Basic Law: the Preamble's unity mandate and the reservation of some rights to Germans (especially the political rights of free assembly, association, and resistance to autocracy) leave no doubt about this. As Manfred Birkenheier (1976: 31) added, the Basic Law's rationale for not saying '*German* people' in Article 20(2) was not to include potentially everyone in the business of rule, but a bow to federalism: the latter required that the source of legitimate *Land* government had to be the *Land* people, and not the federal (that is, 'German') people. Once it was established that the 'people' in Article 20 was the 'German' people, it followed from the homogeneity principle of Article 28(1) that the people had to be the same at all horizontal levels of the state—local, *Land*, and federal.[23]

In applying the homogeneity principle, suffrage opponents also had to refute the notion that local government was not part of the state, and thus not subject to the exigencies of popular sovereignty. This was no difficult task either. As again Birkenheier (ibid. 108) pointed out, the dualism of state and society, and the conception of local government as the place of societal self-determination against the state, belongs to the nineteenth century. In the modern interventionist welfare state, it was impossible to draw any sharp line between state and society. Local government now functioned as part of state administration (according to the principle of *Auftragsverwaltung*), and thus had to be legitimized by the state-constituting people.[24] This precluded construing local government along the functional spheres of professional associations or trade unions, in which foreigners were fully included.

Not content with proving that the Basic Law had not loosened the tie of nationhood and democracy, suffrage foes further sought to show that it made sense to maintain this tie, constitutionally prescribed or not. Josef Isensee (1987: 301 f.) argued that it was in the nature of state membership to tie an individual 'inescapably' (*unentrinnbar*) to the fate of the state association; accordingly, only proper state members, that is, citizens, should be entitled to determine the affairs of the state. Alien suffrage would create two classes of active citizens (*Aktivbürger*), one of which could escape the effects of their decisions by returning to their state of origin, and thus enjoy 'freedom without responsibility' (ibid. 302). In short, alien suffrage would take away the last major privilege of citizenship: the right to vote, and devalue the latter by leaving only duties, not rights, as its distinguishing mark.

Finally, suffrage foes questioned what suffrage advocates took for granted: that alien suffrage was an appropriate measure of immigrant integration. As again Isensee (ibid. 304) pointed out, granting suffrage for the sake of achieving social policy goals would be abusing an elementary political right. Helmut Quaritsch (1983) argued similarly that suffrage was an attribute of the public *citoyen*, not the private *bourgeois*: 'It would be . . . a privatistic misunderstanding of suffrage, and would denature representative democracy, if suffrage were granted to satisfy group interests' (p. 12). Empirically, under the condition of persistent homeland-orientation of even long-settled guestworkers, alien suffrage might turn the domestic electoral arena into a platform of foreign homeland politics. This was no phantom of xenophobes. Even the liberal Kühn Memorandum had recommended only active, not passive local suffrage to aliens.[25] Kühn defended this precaution as follows: 'Passive suffrage might lead to new parties of, say, Yugoslav communists or Turkish nationalists. Croats would fight against communists, socialist against nationalist Turks. We don't want to have these conflicts fought out here [in Germany]' (in Quaritsch, 1981: 51). Burkhart Hirsch, the leading foreigner advocate in the FDP, had a similar fear, which even led him to reject alien suffrage as a whole: 'I cannot imagine that a Greek in local government would care about the needs of the Turks.'[26]

The Constitutional Court's final verdict against alien suffrage avoided any principled reflection on the nature of democracy and nationhood, which had characterized the passionate legal-political debate throughout the 1980s. Instead, the court resorted to the formal argument that the 'people' in Article 20(2) had to be the 'German' people; taken together with the homogeneity principle of Article 28(2), this interpretation of 'people' implied that German citizenship was a prerequisite for electoral participation at *all* levels of the state, including the local level. Passed just four weeks after German reunification, the court verdict was almost apologetic in tone. After all, defensive nationalism had now lost its function. Considering the pending Maastricht clause on local voting rights for EU nationals, the Court conceded that a constitutional change might make this possible. This occurred without much noise in December 1992. Most significantly, the Court lauded the concern of suffrage advocates to enfranchise the millions of *de facto* immigrants in Germany, who were locked out of the political process. But the Court concluded: 'The only possible response to this situation is a reform of citizenship law, . . . to make it easier to acquire German citizenship.'[27] The Court thus anticipated a fundamental change of direction in the German debate on immigrant integration.

Toward National Integration: Foreigners Into Citizens

Barbara John, Berlin's respected Foreigner Commissioner, was one of the first to realize the limits of postnational immigrant integration. According to Mrs John, the quest for 'special group status' for foreigners was 'socially divisive': '[The foreigner] is tied to the Federal Republic only through his or her interest to collect from this society as many group rights as possible' (John, 1985: 6). On the other hand, discontented and resentful parts of the majority society were provided with obvious scapegoats. Ever since the wave of xenophobic violence in the 1990s, the failure to make foreigners citizens has been recognized as the most serious deficit of postnational immigrant integration. But sheer demography pointed in the same direction. As a third generation of immigrants, born to foreign parents who had themselves been born or grown up in Germany, was growing up without citizenship, the prospect of a self-perpetuating minority forever locked out of majority society appeared ever more threatening.[28] Furthermore, the limits of postnational immigrant integration became openly visible with the massive arrival, since the late 1980s, of ethnic Germans from Eastern Europe and the former Soviet Union. Now you had the grotesque dissonance of *de facto* foreigners automatically classified as Germans and of *de facto* Germans still classified as foreigners.

However, the foreign Germans were also messengers of fundamental change. With the breakdown of communism and national reunification, the rationale for keeping foreigners out of the national community of Germans has disappeared. For the first time since the end of the war, the Germans have been free to rethink the meaning of membership in the nation-state—no more unity mandate or homeland responsibilities can come in the way of reforming its antique citizenship regime. And considering that not even a decade has passed since the Eastern European revolutions, the pace of change has been breathtaking. The introduction of as-of-right naturalization in 1992 has swept away cultural assimilation and state discretion as barriers to citizenship acquisition. Few have noticed it, but Germany is now refashioning itself as a civic nation *à la française*. As Berlin's perceptive Foreigner Commissioner envisages the cultural impact of making foreigners citizens, it 'would necessarily lead to a new form of German identity'.[29] A second-generation Turkish-German intellectual strikes a similar, Rushdie-esque chord that had so far been absent in the German debate on immigrant integration: 'What matters is an enlargement of the notion of Germanness. The Turk belongs as a German element to Germany and not as a Turkish (element). Only so can it change, enter into [new] symbioses, and give birth to a hybrid culture. Turkish language, literature, music, symbols, mosques—all that would be a natural part of a manifold culture in Germany' (Senocak, 1993: 11). An effusive, perhaps too optimistic vision, but one that could not exist without allowing Turks to enter into the national community.

Before reunification, a liberal foreigner-rights regime had co-existed with an ultra-restrictive citizenship regime. As Kay Hailbronner (1989: 79) outlined this nexus, in a situation where permanent residents without citizenship, outside the political sphere, had nearly the same rights as citizens, 'it seems reasonable to make the few privileges of citizenship contingent on a serious and enduring commitment to the new polity'. Pre-unity Germany's restrictive citizenship regime is a confluence of maintaining the *jus sanguinis*-based Citizenship Law of 1913 and conceiving of the Federal Republic as an incomplete nation-state, whose unity—short of being political—could only be cultural (Bleckmann, 1990: 1399). More by accident than by design, the maintenance of the Wilhelminian Citizenship Law allowed the Federal Republic to do two things at the same time: claim that its citizenship law was not West German but all-German law; and maintain this fiction across the generations through the law's core tenet of attributing citizenship purely by descent, without any element of attribution by birth on territory. While the Basic Law is silent on how to define and attribute citizenship, its Preamble and Article 116(1) indirectly prescribe either an assimilationist, and thus a restrictive, or a descent-based citizenship regime.[30] Otherwise the unity mandate of the Preamble and the diasporic obligations to ethnic Germans according to Article 116(1) could not realistically be maintained.

The Naturalization Rules (*Einbürgerungsrichtlinien*), passed under a Social-Democratic government in 1977, give a chilling insight into a regime that, in principle, refused to make foreigners citizens. Not only do the rules enshrine the philosophy that 'the Federal Republic is not a country of immigration', and thus not intent on 'deliberately increasing the number of German citizens through naturalization'.[31] They also prescribe absolute state discretion in naturalizing foreigners, even if all the formal prerequisites (like ten years residence) have been met by the applicant; and they make the granting of citizenship contingent upon the cultural assimilation of the applicant. Regarding state discretion, the rules stipulate that 'the granting of German citizenship can only be considered if there is a public interest in [it] . . . The personal wishes and economic interests of the applicant cannot be decisive', adding that 'in the German legal system resident aliens enjoy far-reaching rights and liberties anyway'. Regarding the assimilation requirement, naturalization is contingent on the applicant's 'free and permanent orientation [*Hinwendung*] to Germany', which could be assessed by his or her 'basic attitude to German culture'.[32] This does not only imply an 'orientation to the German state', as Zuleeg (1987: 190) erroneously claims, but to the 'German people' as well. It implies what the political élites of all shades have untiringly reiterated they would *not* demand of the immigrants—their cultural assimilation. Such assimilation cannot be formally derived from the existence of certain prerequisites, such as length of residence; it has to be assessed case by case. For instance, for validating the 'integrity' of the applicant it was not enough to check her criminal record; in addition, an individual 'examination . . . of the life course and the personality' of the applicant was necessary.[33] In practice, this meant intrusive home visits and questioning of neighbours by vigilant naturalization officers, who—to put it bluntly—read an applicant's 'orientation to Germany' from her preference for flowered wallpaper and cabbage or from her good standing with card-carrying Germans.[34] Kay Hailbronner (1989) is certainly right that the admission into the political community of the nation-state cannot itself be a matter of democracy, and that it is legitimate for nation-states to make full citizenship conditional 'on some degree of cultural assimilation' (ibid. 72). This sounds good, but on paper only. A closer examination of pre-unity Germany's naturalization practice would surely reveal a violation of the liberal philosophy that the Federal Republic was *also* based upon.

In the context of an assimilationist citizenship regime, it is no wonder that foreigners showed little enthusiasm for acquiring German citizenship. Until the late 1980s, the absolute number of discretionary naturalizations was around 14,000 a year; if one considers that one-third of them occurred under the eased conditions of marriage-based naturalization, the annual number drops even below 10,000. This amounts to a naturalization rate of under one-half per cent of those entitled to naturalize—the lowest naturalization rate in Europe (see Schmidt Hornstein, 1995: 112 f.).

Before it would become obsolete with national reunification, (West) Germany's restrictive citizenship regime had already suffered some cracks.[35] The opening salvo was the Kühn Memorandum's demand for an optional right to naturalize for second-generation foreigners. It became dormant under the conservative Kohl government, which at first saw no need for a more friendly citizenship policy. But even the conservatives mellowed soon. In response to the SPD's Great Inquiry on Foreigner Policy of 1984, the Federal Ministry of the Interior admitted that 'no state can accept that a numerically significant part of the population remains permanently outside the national community', and he came out in favour of a more generous naturalization procedure for second- and third-generation immigrants.[36] Six more years had to pass before the promise was realized. The reformed Foreigner Law of 1990, issued shortly before the Unity Treaty was signed, marks the first real advance toward a more liberal citizenship regime. The new law introduced the so-called 'as a general rule' naturalization for first-generation immigrants with at least fifteen years of residence, and for second- and third-generation immigrants who had stayed at least eight years in the Federal Republic.[37] Such 'as a general rule' naturalization was not 'as of right' naturalization; but naturalization could only be denied in exceptional cases (see Neuman, 1995: 29). In addition, the new Foreigner Law lowered the previously prohibitive costs of naturalization to a symbolic lump sum of DM100. Finally, it inflicted a first blow to a hitherto sacrosanct tenet of German citizenship law: the divestiture of prior nationality, by granting exceptions if this condition was impossible or extremely difficult to meet for the applicant.

An even more far-reaching change of German citizenship law and policy occurred in the context of the Asylum Compromise of December 1992, in which the SPD traded its submission to a more restrictive asylum law for more liberalization on the citizenship front. The two concessions wrung out of the CDU government looked innocent enough: first, eliminating the 31 December 1995 deadline for citizenship requests by first-generation immigrants, thus converting a transitional provision directed at foreigners who had arrived in Germany before 1980 into a permanent provision for all foreigners after fifteen years residence; and, secondly, eliminating the remaining discretion to deny naturalization through turning 'as a general rule' into 'as of right' naturalizations. The second concession has fundamental ramifications, which few have as yet realized. The two core principles of the Naturalization Rules: absolute state discretion and cultural assimilation as precondition for citizenship, are no longer. Assimilation is simply deduced from the applicant's length of residence; it is no longer examined, case by case, on the basis of his or her economic situation, cultural orientation, and crime record. This means that 'assimilation' is effectively void as a criterion for being granted citizenship. Membership in the German nation-state is no longer premissed on being part of the ethnocultural nation. This allows two interpretations: first, that state and nation are effectively decoupled, because membership in the latter is no longer a precondition for membership in the former; or, secondly, that the meaning of German nationhood is itself undergoing transformation, because it can no longer be defined in ethnic terms, but now will have to routinely include and absorb non-German entrants. Including the factor of time, both interpretations are really one. If the nation qua ethnocultural nation is no longer the basis of the German state, this does not mean that the latter is becoming a non-national state. Rather, it means that, over time, German nationhood will have to be defined more along civic-territorial than exclusively ethno-genealogical lines.

The right of naturalization has fundamentally transformed the German citizenship regime: citizenship for foreigners is no longer the exception, but the rule. In theory, at least. There is one more hurdle to take before it can become reality: the current government's stubborn rejection of double citizenship. Only if double citizenship is accepted, not as a good in itself but as an inevitable bad, can elements of *jus soli* loosen up Germany's descent-based citizenship regime, the only pure *jus sanguinis* regime among Europe's major immigration countries. This is all the more important because the continued reluctance of entitled foreigners to naturalize seems to be due to their attachment, sentimental or instrumental, to their old citizenship.[38] But for the rearguard defenders of ethnocultural nationhood, forbidding dual citizenship is the last straw to grasp, and they will not cede it lightly. Erwin Marschewski, one of the CDU's fiercest opponents of citizenship reform, reiterates the orthodox view: 'Granting citizenship cannot be an instrument of integrating foreign residents. Instead, naturalization requires that the integration of the respective foreigner has already occurred. A foreigner who wants to acquire German citizenship must commit himself to our national community. Tolerating double citizenship would further the formation of permanent national minorities.'[39] Citizenship as the final point, rather than a means, of integration, and the imperative not to divide one's loyalties between two national communities—these are the thin residuals of ethnocultural nationhood today.

Since a Germanic exaltation of the nation as a community of destiny would be inopportune in the late twentieth century, most defenders of undivided citizenship hide behind an international agreement, the European Council's Convention on the Reduction of Multiple Nationality, passed in May 1963. In addition, there is domestic legal backing in terms of the Federal Constitutional Court's so-called '*Übel* Doctrine', according to which dual or multiple nationality is 'an evil [*Übel*] that should be avoided or eliminated if possible in the interest of states as well as in the interest of the affected citizen' (in Neuman, 1995: 45). While good to know that the Constitutional Court worries about the interest of citizens, the rigid objection to multiple citizenship is hollow on at least three accounts. First, it is notoriously misunderstood that the European Council Convention does not require the receiving state to check and tilt an applicant's other nationalities; rather, the Convention urges the sending state to release emigrants from their old citizenship (see Renner, 1994). This is why all European immigrant countries, except Germany, have tolerated double citizen-

ship, without violating the European Council Convention.⁴⁰
Secondly, the 'evils' generated by multiple citizenship have already
been controlled, or are in principle controllable, by international law.
For instance, the pre-war Hague Convention solves the problem of
loyalty conflicts by stipulating that military service and diplomatic
protection are due to or owed by the state in which an individual
actually resides, thus leaving the other citizenship ˉdormant
(Wollenschläger and Schraml, 1994: 228).

Finally, double citizenship is so common a practice already, even in
Germany, that one wonders why no state has as yet collapsed—if the
former were as 'evil' as its critics say. In the cases of ethnic Germans,
children of bi-national parents, and children born to German parents
in *jus soli* countries, double citizenship is routinely accepted. Of
almost 670,000 naturalizations between 1975 and 1990, some 430,000
entailed double citizenship—for ethnic Germans.⁴¹ But even among
the discretionary naturalizations of resident foreigners at least one-
third result in double citizenship (Hoffmann, 1994: 262). This is
because German authorities are increasingly generous in allowing
exceptions if the applicant faces undue hardship—such as military service as a precondition for being released from Turkish citizenship.
Berlin, which has long insisted on making its immigrants citizens,
accepts the Turkish embassy's permission to naturalize, but does not
check if an applicant actually divests herself of the old citizenship.⁴²
Also on the Turkish side there have been important changes. In 1995
Turkey removed all restrictions on acquiring or inheriting property
for her former citizens, deleting the biggest material incentive for
Turks to stay Turkish. In addition, after being lobbied by a leader of
Turkish immigrants in Germany, the Turkish government now permits its released citizens to reacquire Turkish citizenship instantly.⁴³
As a result, most Turkish applicants for German citizenship divest
themselves of their old citizenship only temporarily, for the sake of
satisfying German authorities. No wonder, that the naturalization rate
of Turks has gone up significantly in the fast few years: 12,915 in 1993,
19,500 in 1994, 31,578 in 1995.⁴⁴ A recent survey found 'an almost
dramatic increase' in the intention to naturalize among Turks
(Mehrländer *et al.*, 1996: 455). Whereas in 1985 only 7 per cent of
Turkish residents had intended to naturalize, in 1995 over 26 per cent
did so (ibid. 413). Most importantly, among the 46.7 per cent of
Turkish respondents still refusing to naturalize in 1995, the large
majority simply wanted to retain their national identity; practically
no one mentioned legal obstacles as a reason. In fact, these obstacles

factually no longer exist. The 'evil' of double citizenship has long turned from an obstacle into a—however reluctantly—tolerated side-effect of naturalization.

The groundswell for a reform of citizenship law turned into a mighty wave in the early 1990s, in the wake of the gruesome violence against undifferentiated 'foreigners', long-settled immigrants no less than recent asylum-seekers. For the first time, the quest for formally recognizing double citizenship was no longer a Red-Green élite affair, but a grassrooots movement—one million signatures were collected on its behalf in the summer of 1993. After the murders of Solingen, even the Turkish government joined the campaign. The frantic search for measures to stop the rage provided an opening for questioning the orthodoxy that citizenship could only be the 'final point', not the 'means', of immigrant integration. The Federal Minister of Justice, Mrs Leutheusser (FDP), now argued that double citizenship 'could be both integrative and consciousness-raising, and thus be a tool against aggression and xenophobia'.[45] Even among the Christian Democrats, the front against double citizenship was breaking apart. Horst Eylmann, the chairman of the parliamentary committee on judicial affairs, still a hardliner in the asylum debate, now attacked 'the myth of the one and indivisible citizenship'.[46] Johannes Gerster, a proponent of the 1990 Foreigner Law, did not go quite so far. But he still found it 'intolerable' to put someone who wants to naturalize before the alternative of acquiring German citizenship or losing property rights in his or her country of origin, and he recommended acceptance of double citizenship in such cases—but not in principle.[47] Finally, Chancellor Kohl himself, addressing the *Bundestag* shortly after Solingen, called for a 'reform of citizenship law', while warning against 'idolizing the nation'.[48]

At this stage, a further reform of citizenship law could not but tackle the antiquated core of the German citizenship regime, the attribution of citizenship via *jus sanguinis*. It is sometimes overlooked that all continental European citizenship regimes are *jus sanguinis* regimes. However, Germany has been the only immigrant-receiving country not to complement the rule of blood with the rule of territory, *jus soli*. The unresolved national question is responsible for this, but also the fear—shared across party and ideological lines—of 'Germanizing' foreigners against their will. The Social Democrats were the first to break the taboo in 1986, calling for birthright citizenship for third-generation immigrants. As in a similar SPD proposal of 1993, such third-generation *jus soli* came with the right of parents to reject the offer. After all, no one was to be 'lured or pushed' into German citizenship (Blumenwitz, 1993: 152). However, considering the empirical reticence of first- and even second-generation foreigners to naturalize, it is increasingly recognized that decoupling citizenship acquisition from parental veto is the whole point of *jus soli*. A prominent legal scholar of Greek origins calms the weak German nerves: '[The children] themselves must decide if they want to keep their German citizenship or if they would rather give it up. Calling this "imposed citizenship" or "forced Germanization" is ridiculous.'[49]

The crux of *jus soli* is to institutionalize double citizenship. In fact, the existence of double citizenship is not due to the laxity of liberal states; it is the inevitable result of the co-existence of *jus sanguinis* and *jus soli* rules both within states and in the state system (Renner, 1994: 871). The first cautious government proposal to institute *jus soli* tried to eat the cake and have it too, attribute citizenship territorially and avoid double citizenship. The so-called 'children's citizenship' (*Kinderstaatszugehörigkeit*) was the CDU/CSU's attempt to live up to its 1994 coalition agreement with the liberal FDP, which envisaged an encompassing reform of citizenship law. A *Staatszugehörigkeit* rather than a *Staatsan*gehörigkeit (nationality), this is an untranslatable thing, a provisional quasi-nationality not known in international law. It would not come automatically, but only if the parents applied for it before the child's twelfth birthday; and it would expire on the child's nineteenth birthday, if the child did not divest itself of its other nationalities. Not a true nationality, this novelty in international law would not shield the child from the clutches of foreigner law, such as—in the extreme case—deportation. And, as Gerald Neuman (1995: 55) pointed out, 'it is not clear why parents who decline to naturalize would choose it for their children.' The deputy leader of the CDU/CSU parliamentary group admitted that this quasi-nationality was unnecessary indeed, because a right to naturalize already existed. But it was good as a 'psychological' device.[50]

What is interesting about the *Kinderstaatszugehörigkeit* is not its muddled conception, but the fact that the federal government has broken the ground for an entirely new citizenship regime. Even within the CDU, the inconclusive quasi-nationality was subjected to a scathing critique, and more far-reaching *jus soli* proposals were launched immediately. Johannes Gerster, who had still rejected *jus soli* as 'forced Germanization' in 1993, came out for automatic birthright citizenship in 1994, under the condition that at majority age an individual had to decide for one citizenship only.[51] Gerster is not alone in his party. He is supported by an assertive group of young *Bundestag* deputies, who have no mercy for the 'abstruse' *Kinderstaatszugehörigkeit* and deem themselves supported by the Chancellor himself.[52] For Wolfgang Schäuble, the chairman of the CDU parliamentary group and architect of the 1990 Foreigner Law, it would not be 'the end of the world' to reconceive the quasi-nationality as full nationality—in German language, it amounts to as little as replacing the *zu* in *Kinderstaats-zugehörigkeit* with *an*.[53] Two letters only, but still a difference of principle! As the obstinate opponents of double citizenship correctly see, once German citizenship had been granted at birth, it would be practically impossible to take it away later.

A CDU reform advocate noted that the continued rejection of double citizenship is 'hard to explain in rational terms'.[54] However, in this rejection hangs the whole legacy of ethnocultural nationhood. One cannot expect it to disappear without a fight. Its chances are nevertheless slim. There is now a numerical majority in the *Bundestag* to introduce *jus soli* for third-generation immigrants, and thus for an entirely new citizenship regime. The SPD and the Greens have repeatedly introduced such bills in the past few years, only to embarrass a liberal FDP that would like to join, but is bullied by its conservative coalition partner not to (see Blumenwitz, 1994: 246). Essentially, only the Bavarian CSU and parochial parts of the CDU stand in the way of doing away with the last pillar of Germany's antiquated citizenship regime. Robbed of any substantive argument since reunification, the reform opponents' barren agenda is electoral: 'I know my voters well,' said one of the opponents, perhaps thinking to himself that making foreigners citizens was not likely to bolster the pool of CSU voters.[55]

Immigrant Ethnicity in Germany: The Case of the Turks

Considering the unanimous rejection of assimilating her immigrants, one might expect Germany to be a fertile ground for ethnic self-organization. This is not so. A second-generation Turkish community organizer deplored the lack of an 'ethnic infrastructure' among Turks in Germany: 'There are no own newspapers, significant educational institutions, schools, foundations, or (communal) childcare, health, or old age organizations' (Uzun, 1993: 57). Not to mention that Turkish immigrants do not have an effective political organization to represent their interests before the German public or in the political process. This lack of an ethnic infrastructure is not so much the result of legal obstacles. According to the Basic Law, foreigners enjoy all the political rights that are human rights, such as freedom of information, opinion, and coalition. In addition, some of the political rights constitutionally reserved for Germans, such as the freedom of assembly and forming associations, are granted to foreigners by means of statutory law (Cryns, 1988: 39). Rather than legal, the obstacles to ethnic self-organizing have been social. On the push-side, guestworkers lacked the initiative and capacity to embellish a situation deemed only temporary. On the pull-side, a developed welfare state obviated the need for ethnic self-organization. Regarding the push side, a prominent foreigner advocate looks back at two decades of failed attempts to organize foreigners politically: 'With the exception of a tiny politically conscious élite, there was simply no political interest among the migrant population.'[56] Regarding the pull side, the delivery of essential services by host-society institutions kept foreigners in the status of passive clients, rather than active participants. Ethnic self-organization was not only prevented in fact, but abhorred in principle. 'Ethnicization' figured as a negative term for discrimination and reactive self-isolation of migrants.[57] A German sociologist well-versed in the positive valuation of immigrant ethnicity in the United States notes its bad reputation in Germany: 'There is a [pseudo-]progressive consensus . . . that equates the development of ethnic institutions in our country with the formation of ghettos and the prevention of social integration' (Elwert, 1982: 717).

Vicarious Immigrant Organization

In lieu of ethnic self-organization, 'German *Helfer*' have vicariously represented immigrant interests (Leuninger, 1984: 155). The informal Foreigner Lobby (*Ausländerlobby*), which emerged in the 1980s as an increasingly effective liberalizer of the federal government's foreigner policy, did not include foreigners. Its three main constituents were churches, charity organizations, and unions. If immigrants qua immigrants wanted to have an impact on public policy, they had to pass through these host-society institutions. Here they would experience that the German *Helfer* led 'a discourse about the migrants and not a dialogue with them' (Radtke, 1994: 35). This could not be otherwise, because the *Helfer* had to pursue the interests of the organizations that employed them. The *Helfer*, even if they followed the educational mandate to 'make the immigrants capable of representing their own interests',[58] could not but perpetuate their marginalization.

The German context both fed ethnic immigrant identities and undermined their political capacity. The paradox of simultaneous production and destruction of immigrant ethnicity is evident in the example of charity organizations. Since the early 1960s, para-public charity organizations had taken over the social care of the guestworker population. This was in line with historical precedent and with the structure of Germany's welfare system. Already in the nineteenth century, church-related charity organizations had attended to the Italian and Polish *Fremdarbeiter* (Thränhardt, 1983: 62). In the Federal Republic, the state acted on the subsidiarity principle of welfare provision, delegating the care of marginal groups to the major charity organizations (Heinze and Olk, 1981). These organizations vicariously represented the interests of their constituencies. The latter were clients rather than members, chosen rather than choosing, and inevitably instrumentalized for the pursuit of organizational interests. The guestworkers were no exception to this. In an informal agreement sanctioned by the state (which provided the funds), Germany's three big charity organizations distributed the guestworker population among themselves. The Catholic Church's Caritas took over the guestworkers from Italy, Spain, and Portugal; the Protestant Churches' *Diakonisches Werk* got the Greeks; and the non-church-related *Arbeiterwohlfahrt* (AWO) became responsible for Turks, Moroccans, and Tunisians. Interestingly, the Yugoslav guestworkers were divided between the Catholic Croats, who were taken over by Caritas, and the non-Catholic rest, for whom AWO accepted responsibility.

This categorization and division of the guestworker population is not as obvious as it seems. Instead of classifying the latter according to national origin, one could have done so on the basis of function (work, education, or leisure), generation, or occupation (see Radtke, 1990: 29 f.). In fact, when second generation immigrants emerged as the main target of integration policy in the late 1970s, the established national-origin classification of the guestworker population proved a major obstacle to this (Schwarz, 1992: 11). However, the self-interest of the charity organizations conditioned a carving up of the guestworkers according to religion and language. As the case of the Yugoslavs—who were split up in the diaspora before they fell apart at home—shows, religion figured above national origins—the Catholic organization taking fellow Catholics, the Protestant organization taking the fellow (even if Orthodox) Christians, and the only non-religious organizations taking the sizeable Muslim rest. If religion figured as a matter of principle, language was a pragmatic choice, because it minimized the costs of communicating with a foreign-language clientele. Except for the poor Yugoslavs, the combination of religion and language entailed a carving up of guestworkers according to their national origins. It would be naïve to assume that guestworkers arrived without national identities at hand. But the institutions of the receiving society evidently reinforced these identities: 'Migrants were turned into representatives of their national cultures' (Radtke, 1994: 34). From here it was no big leap to conceive of a migrant-receiving society as 'multicultural', and it is not by accident that it was churches and charity organizations who introduced this term in the early 1980s.[59]

By the early 1990s, the charity organizations had established about 600 local foreigner bureaus, staffed by 850 social workers—most of them foreigners themselves (German Interior Ministry, 1993: 19). Next to becoming a works councillor (*Betriebsrat*) or union official, to become a social worker was often the peak of an employment career for first-generation guestworkers (see Thränhardt, 1983: 63–5). Social workers formed an élite among the guestworker population, who were only matched by foreign students, teachers, and works councillors. The social workers, responsible for everything from legal advice, the translation of documents, to marriage and youth counselling, acquired a powerful mediating position between the socially illiterate guestworkers and their host society. Mostly employed by a distant *Land* church, and not by the municipality in which they operated, social workers were difficult to control, and even more so because of the language barrier. They were destined to take on leadership roles for their respective national groups, with a heavy dose of Mediterranean clientelism. Because the social workers often fused several functions, their foreign clients did not know in which function to approach them: 'The foreigner does not know if help is exercised in the function of social counsellor—then without payment, in the function of priest—then against a small donation, or in the function of private translator—who, of course, may expect to be paid for his or her service' (Stratmann, 1984: 23). Due to this lack of transparency and control, social workers came to consider their respective fellow-nationals as 'their' turf. Local examples abound where recalcitrant social workers have sought to prevent the formation of elected foreigner councils, which appeared as a threat to their representation monopoly (e.g. ibid. 24).

The charity organizations fed ethnicity through their mode of carving up the foreign clientele. But they also undermined the political articulation of this ethnicity. This was through their sheer existence, which kept immigrants as passive clients. And it was through their active opposition to ethnic self-organization, which not only threatened the organizations' legitimacy but would deprive them of a considerable source of income.[60] The charity organizations farmed out to foreigners only the leisure and cultural sector, under the condition that politics was kept out and no membership fees were raised (Thränhardt, 1983: 65–7). Any non-licensed activity was guarded with jealous eyes. The *Arbeiterwohlfahrt*, while notionally committed to spare young foreigners the fate of assimilation, still rejected the formation of ethnic structures as 'inimical to integration' (Schwarz, 1992: 97). Caritas was likewise committed to 'furthering the autonomy of foreigners', but also feared that under the mantle of ethnic self-organization 'a political control . . . by foreign governments' would occur (ibid. 98). And *Diakonisches Werk* acknowledged the 'important support' by self-organizations, but warned against having its 'professional and differentiated work' replaced by volunteers (ibid. 99). Only in Berlin, where an unorthodox CDU Senate looked for ways of devolving an oversized welfare state, the warning went unheeded. Since the mid-1980s, the Senate's Social Ministry redirected its monies for integrating foreign children and youth into the ethnic self-help sector, simply because this was cheaper, if not necessarily more effective.[61] In the exceptional case of Berlin, the state thus helped create what was otherwise abhorred: an ethnic (Turkish) infrastructure.

Ethnic Self-Organization

The German approach to immigrant ethnicity has been paradoxical. In the context of a postnational integration regime, the guestworkers were not to be robbed of their national and cultural identities. But a negative reading of ethnicity as discriminatory and isolationist 'ethnicization' demanded the articulation of guestworker interests within host-society institutions. Topping the paradox, these host-society institutions tended to reinforce the national-origins identifications of guestworkers, while working against their political expression. In a liberal state, ethnic self-organization did nevertheless occur. It tended toward replicating the culture and politics of the homeland.

Turks, Germany's biggest foreigner group with 1.9 million residents in 1993, are an extreme case of transplanted homeland politics.[62] In fact, who wants to understand the bewildering variety of Turkish ethnic politics in Germany is well advised to take a course in Turkish national politics first. Turkish community life in Germany reflects the fate of modern Turkey, this secular offshoot of a Muslim empire, an unstable democracy torn between violent left- and right-wing extremism (which has provoked three military interventions since 1960), and plagued by Islamic fundamentalism and Kurdish separatism in the 1990s. To speak about Turkish 'self'-organizations is actually misleading, because the largest Turkish diaspora in Europe (and in one of Europe's most liberal states at that) provided an ideal target of recruitment and field of operation for Turkish political parties banned at home or seeking to strengthen themselves abroad.

Throughout the 1970s, the leftist spectrum was dominated by replicas of communist parties that were illegal in Turkey, such as the moderately popular FIDEF, which tried hard to hide its steering by the Moscow-oriented Turkish Communist Party (exiled in East Berlin), and a plethora of Maoist splinter groups. FIDEF defined itself as 'the mass organization of Turkish workers in the Federal Republic and Westberlin',[63] but with 9,000 members in 1978 it certainly fell short of this claim (Özcan, 1989: 238, 250). Leftist organizations like FIDEF were mostly run by students or exiled intellectuals, who stood at some distance from their rural, undereducated fellow-nationals.[64] Their internationalist ideology made them prone to address host-society concerns, such as offering German language classes, legal counselling, and joining in the campaign for local voting rights.

This could not be said about the rightist spectrum, which was dominated by camouflage organizations of parties on the rise in Turkey.[65] The most important of these was the Nationalistic Movement Party (MHP), which operated in Germany under various names, such as National Ideas Association, Islamic Association, or Turkish Community. When its leader Türkes, a retired colonel, was vice-prime minister in two Nationalistic Front coalitions under the conservative Demirel in the 1970s, he deployed scores of right-wing consular officials, teachers and imams into the Federal Republic, and built up his infamous youth organization, the Grey Wolves, to combat rival communists. After the socialist government takeover by Ecevit in 1978, many persecuted MHP activists moved to Germany—on the asylum-ticket! Here they forged a Europe-wide front organization against Ecevit, the Turk Federation (ADUETDF), with 33,000 members in 1979 (ibid. 184). While trumpeting that it was in favour of a 'free and democratic society' the Turk Federation's first leader happened to be involved in the attempted murder of the Pope, for which he was arrested and extradited to Italy in 1982. As renegades revealed, the Turk Federation operated with two separate statutes, a front statute adjusted to the host-society and a secret one imported from Turkey; and it had two separate membership lists, with an inner circle of armed activists involved in international heroin- and arms-trafficking. While not without support in certain conservative circles in Germany, these nationalists did little to integrate Turks in Germany. The Turk Federation demanded the opening of Turkish schools and kindergartens in Germany, while parroting the multicultural vision of 'the Turkish and German peoples [living together] in acceptance of the other's culture and in mutual understanding and good harmony' (ibid. 188).

It is right to object that the dispositions of the extremist fringes are not to be mistaken for the dispositions of the majority of Turks in Germany. But the evidence abounds that the extreme homeland-orientation of organized Turks is shared by ordinary Turks. In fact, the insulation of the German national community is perfectly complemented by the insulation of its Turkish counterpart, and the German disgust for assimilation is mirrored in the stubborn unwillingness of Turks to assimilate.[66] This insulation and unwillingness to assimilate is certainly *also* a response to discrimination.[67] But its self-induced component cannot be overlooked. Consider the peculiar migration history of Turks to Germany. The bulk of Turkish migration occurred rapidly and in clusters of chain migration, which discouraged a gradual adjustment to the receiving society. Whereas the first Turkish guestworkers were skilled and from urban areas in western Turkey, by the early 1970s the majority of new arrivals were unskilled and from rural eastern Turkey. The latter arrived via chain migration, which transplanted whole village networks into the German diaspora (Gitmez and Wilpert, 1987: 96). Not so much nationalism, but traditionalism kept these rural Turks separate. Through chain migration, migrating Turks never actually left their traditional village world, with its patriarchal family structures and stiff sanctions against 'stepping outside'. As Gitmez and Wilpert (ibid.) found in their excellent ethnography of Turks in Berlin, the Turks arriving through chain migration tended to live with and restrict contact to people from the same village. Most importantly, there was a wide pattern of arranged marriage with cousins from the village of origin. The reluctance to intermarry was not only toward Germans; Sunni Muslims could not conceive of marrying Alevites,[68] and vice versa; migrants from one village would not marry a person from another village; etc. (ibid. 97). Especially for first-generation Turkish guestworkers, German society, with its temptations of premarital sex, loose family ties, and lax morality, was the

Sodom from which their offspring were to be protected. A Turkish father explains his difficulties: 'Actually, Germany is not of value to a Turkish child . . . You're not even allowed to hit your children here . . . Of course we should not become like Germans. We have our own customs that we have learned from our parents; we cannot just throw these customs away . . .' (in Wilpert, 1988: 101).

Islamization

Islam has helped to bolster these customs. A first-generation Turkish guestworker explains: 'Islam makes it possible to maintain a piece of home. Religion is one of the few supports, something one can be proud of.'[69] Since the early 1970s, Islam has undergone meteoric growth among Turks in Germany. While there were three Islamic parishes in 1969/70, there were 1,500 of them in 1990 (Gür, 1993: 16). According to the 1987 census, over half of the 1.7 million Muslims in Germany were practising their religion, that is, attending a mosque at least occasionally (Amiraux, 1996: 37 f.). Organized Turkish Islam in Germany has been shaped by two factors. First, the secular Turkish government has long ignored the religious needs of its emigrant diaspora, thus creating an opening for a plethora of radical Islamic sects, many of which were banned and persecuted in Turkey for openly propagating the aim of an Islamic state. Secondly, the notorious blossom of these sects, the Quran schools, which were attended by about half of all Turkish school-age children by the early 1980s, could flourish because German schools have generally failed to offer religous instruction to Muslim children.

Given the considerable reach of organized Islam, its ideology and practices merit further inspection.[70] It is safe to say that the various branches of organized Islam do not advocate a merging of Turkish immigrants with the receiving society. On the contrary, there is a trend toward an institutionally complete parallel society. Consider the three most important Islamic organizations in Germany. The Islamic Cultural Centres, founded 1973 in Cologne and comprising 18,000 formal members in 1980, are a branch of the Süleymanci movement, which is illegal in Turkey. The religious leader Süleymanci had been an opponent of the secular state during the days of Kemal Atatürk, advocating an Islamic state based on the Sharia. Süleymanci's German imams stick to the orthodox division of the world into the House of Islam and the House of War, which shall not be mixed: 'It is not permitted that a believing (Muslim) becomes friend with a non-believer. Quran orders this explicitly. Who nevertheless does it, is not only committing a sin, but . . . has broken with his God' (in Binswanger and Sipahioglu, 1988: 56). This means that assimilation is out of the question. Frankfurt's imam explains: 'We are against Germanization and alienization [*Fremdmacherei*]. We must lead our lives according to our rights, laws, traditions, and our faith' (ibid.).

By far the most influential of the Islamic sects has been Milli Görüs, the German affiliate of former Turkish Minister President Erbakan's Refah Party. 'Milli Görüs' means 'National Perspective', according to Erbakan one of the three possible ways to look at the world: the left-ist, the liberal, and the national. While more adept than the other sects in hiding its fundamentalist creed, and recently even presenting itself as close to the Green Party,[71] Milli Görüs is not different from the rest. Its leaders consider Germany no less than Turkey as the House of War, and most of its mosques bear the word 'Conqueror' in their names. One of Milli Görüs's most reviled figures is the 'Christian missionary', who is lurking around every corner to lead Muslims from the right path: 'They [the Christian missionaries] are agents and spies. They can appear as doctors, as nurses, as wise teachers, as union officials, but all of them are enemies of Islam' (ibid. 96). Mohammad Abdullah (1993: 17), after busily presenting Milli Görüs as a model of a moderate, dialogue-oriented Islam, qualifies the meaning of 'dialogue': 'Traditional Islam considers dialogue as part of the proselytizing duty [*dawa*] of all Muslims, not as the religious conversation among equal partners.' Increasing its membership to 26,000 after the successes of the Refah Party in Turkey, Milli Görüs has learned from the Muslim organizations in Algeria or Egypt to recruit youngsters through a wide menu of social activities, beyond religious service. Milli Görüs has perfected the trend toward a Muslim parallel society, offering edu-cation and computer courses, sports and cultural activities, not to mention that about one-sixth of Turkish grocery stores are owned by the organization.[72]

Having left the field to the radical sects for all too long, Turkish State Islam made its belated entry in the early 1980s, quickly drawing about half of the practising Muslims to its side.[73] The Turkish Islamic Union (DITIB), founded in 1982 in Cologne, is the German branch of Ankara's Directorate of Religious Affairs (Diyanet), whose state-employed imams administer the official laicistic and nationalistic Islam of Turkey. German state authorities tend to take DITIB as the legitimate representative of Turkish Islam (see Amiraux, 1998: 24). However, many fundamentalist sect leaders in Germany had once been employees of the Diyanet in Turkey, before the latter was purged by the military in 1980. In addition, Diyanet employees, at home and abroad, receive stipends from the Saudi Arabian World Muslim League, which propagates the ideal of an Islamic world state (see Binswanger, 1990: 84). In fact, the State Islam's ideology is not different from the sects'. In DITIB's Handbook for the Guestworker (1984), the host society is reduced to a world of hostile 'Christian missionaries', against whom Muslims have to be on guard: 'The Christian world has always been the unremitting persecutor of Islam' (in Binswanger and Sipahioglu, 1988: 83). A German imam instructs his parish: 'You have a holy duty. In a foreign society you have to make sure that the coming generations will remain Turkish and Muslim' (ibid. 85).

It is important to stress that only 25,000 of the 1.8 million Turks residing in Germany in 1993 were believed to be religious or nationalist extremists.[74] But it also cannot be ignored that about half of the Turkish immigrant population is reached by the kind of organized Islam discussed above. Interestingly, while instructing their followers to stay separate, the Turkish imams are keenly aware of the favourable environment for Islam in Germany. One even praised 'the hospitality' Islamists enjoyed in the Federal Republic, certainly with an eye at the rougher environs of Turkey.[75] Now that the big Islamic organizations have accommodated themselves to the 'permanent presence' of Muslim immigrants in Germany (Abdullah, 1993: 24), their attempt is to further institutionalize their religion in Germany. As of the mid-1990s, there was only one officially recognized Islamic primary school in Germany (Amiraux, 1996: 44). Since the early 1980s, there have been repeated attempts by various Islamic umbrella organizations to be recognized as a 'body of public law' (*Körperschaft des öffentlichen Rechts*), which would put Islam on a par with the Catholic and Protestant Churches, and allow the former to collect taxes from their members and to provide mandatory Islamic instruction in the state schools. Some German state authorities (outside Bavaria) are friendly to this endeavour, because it would draw the religious supervision of Turkish youngsters out of the hands of obscure imams. But the lack of a hierarchical church structure and of an established clergy in Islam makes it impossible for the state to decide which of the rivaling Islamic organizations can legitimately speak for the Muslims (see Thomae-Venske, 1988: 83).

After Solingen

The xenophobic violence in the early 1990s has been a watershed event in the development of Turkish immigrant ethnicity. It has catalyzed two opposite trends, one toward pragmatism and host-society orientation among a new type of professionalized self-organization, and a second toward diasporic renationalization and anomic protest culture, particularly among young third-generation immigrants. In his government declaration after the arson murders in Solingen, Chancellor Kohl mentioned that among the immigrant population there were some 88,000 entrepreneurs with non-family employees, and that all foreigners combined had paid DM90 billion in taxes and social security deductions in 1992: 'This is decisively more than they have cost the state.'[76] The spectre of Islamization has obscured the emergence of a Turkish middle-class, with 37,000 entrepreneurs employing some 125,000 workers (half of them German), 1,000 doctors, 4,000 teachers, 12,000 university students, and 22,000 high school (*Gymnasium*) students.[77] At DM3,650 per month in 1993, the average net household income of Turks was about the same as that of Germans.[78] In addition, the average savings quota of Turkish households has plunged from 45 per cent to just 16 per cent, which is just above the German mark, and less than 15 per cent of Turkish income is now being remitted to Turkey—a 50 per cent reduction since the 1970s. This is the backdrop to a new type of Turkish self-organization in Germany: business and professional associations.[79]

The European Association of Turkish Academics (EATA) epitomizes this new type of pragmatic and host-society-oriented self-organization. The young leader of its Berlin-based German branch scorns the left-wing politicos of bygone times, who 'sit in the café the whole day, talk only about Turkey, smoke five packages of Marlboro, and pretend to save the home country in this way—this is not my thing.'[80] Operating from a spacious office in one of western Berlin's pricier neighbourhoods, this smooth-talking, smartly dressed man had picked up the idea of a Turkish lobby when studying at the American University in Washington, DC and working as an aid in Congress. He characterizes EATA as a 'product of the second generation', which combines 'the pragmatism of the nineties, German work mentality, and Turkish heart'.[81] Interestingly, Ertugrul Uzun had discovered EATA while working three months for the Turkish Industrial and Business Association in Istanbul. 'There was an article in the newspaper about EATA, a European-wide Turkish organization in the

making. And then I read the word "lobby". It was the first time that
the Turkish second generation had started to build a lobby! I looked
them up immediately . . . When I entered their meeting room, I saw 50
to 60 young people, typical *Deutschländer*. I thought "they are the
ones".'[82] EATA's importance is not so much its feeble membership
base of 500, but its mindset. For Uzun the Left–Right distinction is
irrelevant, and he characterizes EATA as 'issue-oriented, not ideological'. This includes a distaste for the 'ethno-idealization' of the
German Left, which denies that every society has a 'normative culture'
that newcomers have to adjust to. Instead of counting on minority status for Turks, Uzun feels that Turks have to organize themselves 'in
the first as German citizens'. However, he realizes that becoming
German is not as easy as becoming American: 'We are dealing with a
nation that has a broken identity. How can one identify with it?'
Speculating about his political future, Uzun considers joining a
German political party: 'But I can tell you, it would be a conservative
party . . . This is also because the CDU is friendly toward Turkey.'

The example of EATA and its smart young leader is not unique.
There has emerged a host-society-oriented, German-educated Turkish
intelligentsia. For novelist and essayist Zafer Senocak, who had come
to Germany as an eight-year-old boy in 1970, there never was an alternative to 'orient oneself to Germany and become an immigrant'.[83] He
writes exclusively in German, 'also because I don't write well in
Turkish'. Having acquired German (double) citizenship in 1993,
Senocak sees immigration as a chance for the Germans to relieve themselves of their historical burdens: 'Because there are Germans now
who have nothing to do with German history, German memory is
bound to change over time . . . If one looks into the future in a unified
Germany, immigration will be more a relief than a burden. Alas, no
one sees it this way.'[84]

In the world of organizing, a significant post-Solingen trend has
been to 'correct the image of Turks' by forging a cross-party political
organization of Turks in Germany, oriented to the host society rather
than the homeland.[85] In fact, never had Turks more painfully experienced being 'Turks' than when they became targets of violence, and it
was high time to act on this marker—independently of one's religious
or political creed. Much like ordinary Croatians discovered their
Croatianness after being pulled into a bloody war,[86] ordinary Turkish
immigrants became conscious of their Turkishness after being
offended and mutilated on these grounds. A second-generation
Turkish female student, who otherwise refused to be 'reduced to the

status of a passive carrier of culture', discovered after Solingen that 'I was really a Turk, even though I had nothing, almost nothing to do with Turkey' (in Schmidt Hornstein, 1995: 46). However, the Turkish Community in Germany, founded by long-time Turkish immigrant advocate Hakki Kestin in December 1995, soon experienced that the Turkish marker was a most problematic one to build a political organization upon. If German xenophobia forged the unity of Turks in Germany, parallel events in Turkey were tearing this unity apart. In the course of the protracted war of Turkey against Kurdish separatists in the region bordering Iraq, and after bloody programs by fundamentalist Muslims against Alevites in Turkey, the sizeable sections of Kurds and Alevites among the 'Turkish' immigrants in Germany suddenly discovered, and began to act on, their difference.[87] Accordingly, leaders of the Kurdish and Alevite immigrant communities took offence at the Turkish Community's claim to represent 'the German residents of Turkish origins'—'Turkish' now had an ethnic connotation that it did not have before. At the same time, the minority leaders denounced the organization's initiator Keskin as defender of the 'Kemalist' Turkish state élite.[88]

As the difficult start of the Turkish Community demonstrates, the pragmatic turn to host-society concerns was undercut by the homeland-based fracturing of Turks in Germany. In fact, Turkish immigrant ethnicity has taken a second development after Solingen, toward diasporic renationalization and anomic protest. This has come in many shades: as the fights between Turkish Grey Wolves and Maoist *Dev Sol* activists in the streets of Solingen, the farcical rebirth of a long-dead cleavage line; as the Kurdish terror organization PKK's opening of a 'second front' in Germany, which has made the old spectre of Germany becoming a stage for foreign nationality battles a bloody reality;[89] and as the rise of street gangs, rap, and ghetto culture among disillusioned third-generation Turks. Mixing a heady brew of young Turks turning to street violence, drugs, and— of course—Islamic fundamentalism, Germany's leading news magazine even flatly declared that 'the integration of foreigners has failed'.[90]

This is nonsense. But there are new forms of subcultural withdrawal and anomic assertiveness among third-generation immigrants. When the Wall came down, immigrant metropoles such as Berlin saw something new: ethnic street gangs. In response to attacks by neo-Nazist Skinheads, young Turks have resorted to self-defence. By 1990, there were about thirty Turkish street gangs in Berlin, such as the

36-ers (named after Berlin-Kreuzberg's zip code), the Tegel Fighters, or the Black Panthers.[91] They responded to the Skins' '*Kanaken* chasing' with their own 'bald-head chasing', seeking to create a 'Nazi-free space' where the Skins had tried to make a '*Kanaken*-free space'. The space metaphor is not accidental. These young Turks defend a territory they had considered their own, but now see invaded not only by Skins but 'Easterners' in general, with genealogical claims to Germanness. A sixteen-year old Tegel Fighter complains: 'And suddenly these Easterners arrive and have more rights than I have, only because they are Germans.'[92] Against this putative invasion the young ethno-fighters set up territorial defence. A member of Berlin's 36-ers street gang declares: 'You know, we are guys from Kreuzberg. Let's put it this way: Kreuzberg is our's. We are in charge here.'[93] In Berlin, the Turkish ethno-gangs have entered into a strange alliance with black-hooded German anarchists, the so-called *Autonome*, who celebrate their Turkish peers' 'orientation to supermarkets and *Faschos*' as rectification of the 'unjust distribution of property in this society'.[94] Since 1990, this means ritual havoc on 3 October, Germany's Unity Day, with 'Germany, We Have Enough' banners, smashed shop windows, and the like.

In the case of Berlin, a trickle of 7,000 third-generation Turks are estimated to be active in street gangs.[95] But the culture of the ghetto has spread beyond this small enclave. Similar to the black ghetto culture in the United States, there is now a Turkish ghetto culture in Germany. The revaluation of 'nigger' in black rap music corresponds to the revaluation of '*Kanaken*' in Turkish rap, which has invented a new hybrid '*Kanak Sprak*' (Kanak language).[96] In Turkish ghetto culture, the assertion of Turkishness is no nostalgic clinging to a homeland one has never seen, but the turning of the stigma into a matter of pride, much like American Blackness. '*Türksun*, You Are A Turk . . . In Germany . . . Understand that, Don't forget that!' goes a song-line of the Turkish-German rap band, Cartel.[97] This culture of the ghetto is not limited to the ghetto. EATA's polyglot leader likes it too: 'Even though we work with Germans, we have our own Turkish subculture. There is even a Turkish discotheque [in Berlin]. That is, a Turkish culture. We talk Turkish, my friends are Turkish.'[98] And he looks with a bit of envy at third-generation teenagers, who proudly carry badges with Turkey's half moon and star: 'They are fully integrated here [in Germany], and much more self-confident than I had been at twenty. This old self-denial is no longer. They carry a half moon and star. Not as a religious symbol, but as an ethnic symbol.'

However, playful ghetto aesthetics co-exists uneasily with a more worrying trend toward nationalist and religious withdrawal among third-generation Turks. So far it was a widely shared assumption that Islamization was mostly a phenomenon of first-generation immigrants.[99] This assumption is mistaken. A recent survey of Turkish third-generation immigrants revealed an astonishing degree of nationalist and religious attitudes (Heitmeyer *et al.*, 1997). Fifty-seven per cent of the interviewed youngsters agreed with the Turk-Federation slogan: 'Turkdom is our body, our soul is Islam. A body without a soul is a corpse' (ibid. 111). Even 65.9 per cent agreed to the following statement: 'Every [Muslim] must know that the religions of other nations are nul and void, and that their members are non-believers. Islam is the only right religion' (ibid. 123). In addition, close to half of the interviewees felt 'well' or 'partially' represented by the nationalist Grey Wolves (of the Turk Federation) or by Milli Görüs (ibid. 141). Far from being in conflict with their traditionalist parents, two-thirds of the young Turks surveyed did agree with their family education, and espoused 'authoritarian-patriarchical' norms and values (ibid. 151). As these findings suggest, the integration of Turkish immigrants remains unfinished business.

This chapter has shown the limits of integrating immigrants without making them citizens. Non-citizen status is especially problematic for second- and third-generation immigrants, who are thus exposed as stigmatizable minorities. Accordingly, the German integration debate moved from earlier campaigns for local voting rights for foreigners (which left their non-citizen status untouched) to demands for territorial citizenship, which includes the toleration of double citizenship. This has been a long and difficult transition, because the 'Germanization' of foreigners had originally been rejected by Left and Right alike. As European integration proceeds, the problem of integrating immigrants has largely reduced itself to the integration of Turks. Our case-study of Turkish immigrant ethnicity showed a bifurcation between increasing pragmatism and host-society orientation, on the one hand, and subcultural withdrawal and Islamization, on the other, which makes the future of Turkish immigrant integration difficult to gauge.

Between Citizenship and Race: Great Britain

If postwar immigration led to a widening of citizenship in Germany, it led to its narrowing in Great Britain. As we saw in Chapter 4, British citizenship reforms were not meant to help integrate immigrants, as in Germany, but to keep them out. However, it would be wrong to conclude that citizenship was irrelevant to the British debate on immigrant integration. In fact, the British case shows in the extreme citizenship's dual nature to be 'externally exclusive' and 'internally inclusive' (Brubaker, 1992: ch. 2), making it deployable for purposes of immigration control *and* immigrant integration. On the control side, the legacy of empire had left Britain devoid of a national citizenship, in which identity would coincide with formal nationality. Consequently, the devolution of empire meant adjusting an over-inclusive nationality to an exclusive identity based on 'blood and culture' (Paul, 1997: 26). However, the British debate on immigrant integration also occurred in the idiom of citizenship, now understood in the Marshallian sense as progressively expanding equal rights. The Marshallian citizenship idiom is visible, for instance, in the Labour government's influential 1965 White Paper *Immigration from the Commonwealth*, which stipulated that it could be 'no question of allowing . . . [the commonwealth immigrants] to be regarded as second-class citizens' (p. 10).

The 1965 White Paper also took for granted that the United Kingdom was 'already a multi-racial society' (ibid.). The factual recognition of a multiracial society and the normative vision of Marshallian citizenship universalism point to a tension in the British approach to immigrant integration. Because the Commonwealth immigrants came as formal citizens, with equal civil and political rights, it was within the logic of Marshall's scheme to bestow on them the material conditions that made formal equality a reality, that is, securing them adequate housing, education, employment, and health care.[1] Accordingly, British immigrant integration was first and foremost welfare-state integration (see Jones, 1977). The needs-based universalism of modern British welfare provision, built in opposition to the 'shame' and 'stigma' inherent in the old poor laws, prohibited the carving out of particular, and thus stigmatizable, groups (see Titmuss, 1976: 114). Along these lines, the 1965 White Paper suggested that inadequate housing for immigrants should not be remedied through 'special treatment' for immigrants, but through 'a determined attack on the housing shortage generally'(p. 10). On the other hand, the mark of colour inevitably set the new immigrants apart. E. J. B. Rose's classic survey on New Commonwealth immigration even rejected the 'immigrant-host' framework, which would have put the new immigrants on a par with the Irish, Jewish, or Polish immigrants of old; instead, this self-declared 'Myrdal for Britain' opted for the 'factor of colour' as the guide to its analysis (Rose, 1969: 6). This was not a random choice. Note that the British regime for integrating immigrants presented itself from the start as a race relations regime, a regime for managing the relations between groups kept apart by the immutable mark of skin colour.

In particular French authors have been fond of identifying the 'minoritarian' logic of British immigrant integration, juxtaposing it to the norm of Republican assimilation in France (e.g. Schnapper, 1992: 108–13). This is at best a half-truth, for two reasons. First, as Patrick Weil and John Crowley (1994: 112) have seen, there is 'no common British myth, widely shared across the spectrum of political opinion'. Accordingly, integration policy has been driven more by pragmatism than by principle, and its direction has at times been severely contested. Secondly, the stress on group particularism ignores the countervailing citizenship universalism that has *also* been at work in Britain.

Nevertheless, Britain's readiness to acknowledge immigrants as ethnic minorities has deep historical roots. British nationhood has always comprised various ethnicities, with no intention of swallowing them. British nationhood was elastic, or indeterminate, enough to live with groups set apart by ethnicity or race. More concretely, the empire provided a pluralistic model for dealing with postimperial immigrants. If imperial France had tried to assimilate her colonies, imperial Britain had never had such pretensions. As Sir Ernest Barker (1951: 155) formulated the British approach to empire, 'the African native . . . had better be left an African, but aided to become a better African'. When the 'natives' moved from the periphery into the centre of empire, there was no presumption of their becoming 'British' or 'English' in any way. In conservative reading, assimilation was not possible. In Enoch Powell's malicious diction, 'the West Indian or Indian does not, by being born in England, become an Englishman. In law he becomes a United Kingdom citizen by birth; in fact he is still a West Indian or an Asian' (quoted in Paul, 1997: 178). In liberal reading, assimilation was not required. Home Secretary Roy Jenkins, champion of the mid-1960s 'liberal hour' of British race relations, argued that 'integration' could not mean 'the loss, by immigrants of their own national characteristics and culture', and he famously continued: 'I do not think that we need in this country a "melting-pot" . . . I define integration, therefore, not as a flattening process of assimilation but as equal opportunity, accompanied by cultural diversity, in an atmosphere of mutual tolerance' (quoted in Banton, 1985: 71). Jenkins's abdication of the melting-pot and Powell's 'little England' nationalism are not as opposite as they seem; they are based on the same premiss of keeping immigrants and domestic society apart. However, the liberal variant of group particularism eventually won the day over its parochial competitor. An élite-crafted, official multiculturalism became Britain's institutional solution to her New Commonwealth immigration.

While Britain and the United States are equally prone to address their immigrants as 'minorities', the meaning of minority is sharply different in both cases. The British identification of postwar immigration with coloured immigration suggested American blacks as a reference group, and thus the major *non*-immigrant minority in the United States. In fact, the development of British race-relations law and institutions has closely followed the American civil-rights model, with one important difference. US civil-rights law conceives of the descendants of black slaves as a historically discriminated-against group entitled to compensation. By contrast, British race-relations law has desisted from endowing black immigrants with privileged group status. E. J. B. Rose (1969) responded with a resounding 'No' to his question if there was a 'British dilemma' similar to the 'American dilemma' of race. As he pointed out, the descendants of Caribbean plantation slaves had come 'as immigrants', and because of their voluntary entry they were unlikely 'to be on the conscience of the country in the way that the Negro had for generations been on the conscience of Americans' (p. 4 f.). Unburdened by a legacy of domestic apartheid, Britain has firmly stood back from granting affirmative action privileges to her black immigrants. What immigrants qua minority could expect was not to be targeted as objects of racial discrimination, and to partake on equal terms in social citizenship—both to be achieved by strictly colour-blind means. The American strategy of taking account of race in order to get rid of it was rejected in Britain, initially at least.

Race Relations Law

Britain shares with Germany the propensity to not leave the integration of immigrants to society, but to make it a matter of state policy. However, the model to follow has been the American attempt to incorporate its major non-immigrant minority, the blacks. As indicated above, in this transatlantic transfer the American model underwent significant changes. First, what resulted in the United States from the pressure of a social movement, occurred in Britain as an anticipatory move by élites who were eager to *avoid* the explosive race dynamics of the United States. As Home Secretary Frank Soskice outlined the rationale of the first race-relations bill of 1965, 'it is far better to put this Bill on the Statute Book now, before social stresses and ill-will have the chance of corrupting and distorting our relationships'.[2] As a result, the smell of élite paternalism has always tainted British race relations law and institutions.

The paternalism charge is not groundless, especially if one considers a second difference between British race-relations and American civil-rights law. The spirit of British race-relations law is not the protection of individual rights, as in the American case, but the protection of public order. Consider Home Secretary Soskice's characterization of the 1965 race-relations bill: 'Basically, the Bill is concerned with public order. Overt acts of discrimination in public places, intensely wounding to the feelings of those against whom these acts are practised, . . . may disturb the peace.'[3] Accordingly, the offended individual is marginal to British race-relations law—initially not having the right to bring a discrimination charge before a court, receiving only token compensations for direct discrimination, or no compensation at all in the case of indirect discrimination. Informal reconciliation, rather than formal litigation, has been the preferred mode of settling race disputes, reflecting also the low profile and passiveness of Britain's common-law judiciary.

Finally, 'racial inexplicitness' (Kirp, 1979: 2) has been the guiding norm of British race-relations law and policy, in deliberate aversion to the American drift toward colour-consciousness and affirmative action. As indicated above, racial inexplicitness reflected the logic of the British welfare state project, in which an individual's entitlement to social service was decoupled from her social status. As Richard Titmuss, one of the intellectual architects of the British welfare state, describes this logic: 'It is not . . . an objective of social policy to build the identity of a person around some community with which he is associated' (quoted ibid. 59). Immigrants were thus enlisted in the postwar project of building a national (welfare) community through status-blind treatment.

Making immigrant issues local issues was one way of trying to achieve racial inexplicitness. The two main government programs to tackle racial disadvantage were local government programmes, and to be implemented by local authority as a matter of discretion rather than mandate. Section 11 of the 1966 Local Government Act, which paid local authorities for the staff expenses incurred from educating and servicing immigrants, went to great lengths to define these immigrants in non-racial terms, distributing its monies to local authorities with 'substantial numbers of immigrants from the Commonwealth whose *language* and *customs* differ from those of the community' (quoted in Young, 1983: 293). The second government programme targeting black immigrants, the Urban Programme of 1968, even avoided any group reference, and directed its funds to 'urban areas of general social need' (ibid. 289). Passed right after Enoch Powell's racially inflammatory 'River of Blood' speech,[4] everyone knew that this was an immigrant-related measure. But presenting the problem of immigrant poverty as a problem of distressed areas was a way of corresponding to the norm of racial inexplicitness.

Characteristically, the only government programme explicitly addressing immigrants qua groups, Section 11 of the Local Government Act, became unacceptable when a revised version of it was presented as a measure to help 'ethnic groups'. The Local Governments Grants (Ethnic Groups) Bill, which died after the Tory takeover in 1979, sought to remedy certain shortcomings of Section 11. Under the old act, only Commonwealth immigrants with less than ten years residence in the UK were entitled to its support. This was an anachronism when over 40 per cent of the immigrant population was born or had grown up in the UK, with a growing part of them of non-Commonwealth origins. Moreover, as the Labour-held Home Office defended the new bill in Parliament, the problem of racial discrimination was only incompletely captured by the circumstantial 'language' and 'custom' criteria.[5] The new bill would repair these deficiencies, targeting more broadly defined 'ethnic groups' experiencing a wider range of discrimination. For the Tory opponents such explicitness was anathema, finding fault with the claims proliferation, group separatism, and 'positive discrimination' entailed by the new bill.[6]

The three themes of élite anticipation, public order protection, and racial inexplicitness are constants in a race-relations law that has nevertheless undergone considerable modification over time. The first Race Relations Act of 1965 was narrow in scope, outlawing racial discrimination only in places of public resort, such as pubs or hotels. As harmless as it seems, the adoption of a law to further racial equality was still 'a radical departure from the traditional neutrality and passivity of our legal system' (Lester and Bindman, 1972: 15). The most important facet of this law was to make racial discrimination a civil rather than a criminal wrong, to be remedied by informal conciliation instead of formal legal procedure. Interestingly, this suited the opponents and proponents of race relations-law alike. Conservatives, who branded race-relations law as illicit state intrusion into civil society and attack on free speech, had rejected an earlier version of the bill for introducing 'criminal sanctions into a field more appropriate for conciliation'.[7] Liberals, who saw the 1965 Act as only the first step toward a more encompassing anti-discrimination law, feared that a criminal-law approach would establish overly high standards of proof and prohibit the extension of race-relations law to areas like housing and employment.

This extension occurred in the second Race Relations Act of 1968, which was meant to fill the most glaring deficits of the old law. A 1967 government-commissioned Political and Economic Planning (PEP) report had found widespread patterns of race discrimination in housing, employment, and insurance, which were entirely outside the scope of the 1965 Act.[8] Such discrimination was especially intolerable in the face of second-generation immigrants, who were 'not so much Asians or West Indians as coloured Britons, dressing and speaking much as we do, and looking for the same opportunities as the rest of us'.[9] The new focus on second-generation immigrants reinforced the Marshallian citizenship frame of British race-relations law and policy. Consider that Home Secretary James Callaghan introduced the second race-relations bill as part of the British 'struggle to achieve full citizenship': 'It would be a denial of our own history if, having won these freedoms [of full citizenship] for ourselves, we were now to exclude other groups who have come here to live as full citizens.'[10] By the same token, this was not a bill for a particular group but 'a Bill for the whole nation', whose purpose was to 'protect society as a whole' from race-based 'social disruption'.[11] This core theme of British race-relations law bore remembering in the immediate aftermath of Powell's River of Blood speech, which was a most inopportune moment for conferring new privileges on coloured immigrants. Accordingly, Callaghan played down the discontinuities, while highlighting the continuities of the new bill. A wide catalogue of exceptions watered down the prohibition of discrimination in employment and housing.[12] More importantly, the non-legal conciliation approach was left in place. As the Home Secretary stressed, 'the essential task of the [Race Relations] Board is to settle cases of discrimination by conciliation, and . . . it would be inconsistent with this to give the Board judicial authority or compulsory powers.'[13]

The creation of a new Commission for Racial Equality (CRE) with stronger investigation and enforcement powers was one of the rationales of the third Race Relations Act of 1976, which is still in force today. A new PEP report had revealed that, despite the 1968 Act, racial discrimination continued unabated, particularly in the employment area—the main target of the 1976 Act.[14] However, the 1976 Act was not so much a response to continuing racial discrimination as to an imbalance in the government policies against sexual and racial discrimination. The 1975 Sex Discrimination Act, itself designed to avoid the weaknesses of the 1968 Race Relations Act, had created an Equal Opportunity Commission with far-reaching subpoena powers and the right to issue legally binding non-discrimination notices. Moreover, the Sex Discrimination Act gave individuals the right of action in courts and Industrial Tribunals, on the basis of an enlarged concept of discrimination covering also incidents of indirect discrimination. Once these privileges had been granted to women, it was difficult to deny them to immigrants. In championing the Sex Discrimination Act, the Tory opposition was pre-empted from blocking similar legislation on race discrimination. As a result, the 1976 Race Relations Act passed with 'remarkable little opposition' (Sooben, 1990: 1).

The crucial novelty of the 1976 Race Relations Act was also to cover indirect discrimination, in conscious imitation of US practice.[15] Race-relations law now included two kinds of discrimination: direct discrimination, in which an individual treats another 'less favourably' on the grounds of 'colour, race, nationality or ethnic or national origins'; and indirect discrimination, in which a 'condition or requirement' is applied that does not allow persons of a particular race to comply with it equally, is not 'justifiable' on non-racial grounds, and works to the 'detriment' of these persons.[16] Defended by Home Secretary Roy

Jenkins as 'a broad and . . . realistic rather than a purely narrow and legalistic view of discrimination',[17] the notion of indirect discrimination corresponded exactly to the reinterpretation of American civil-rights law from equal opportunity to equal result, to be achieved by means of affirmative action. However, the Home Office took great pains to assure that affirmative action was *not* on its mind. Its *Guide to the Race Relations Act 1976* makes it clear that the act 'does not permit "reverse discrimination" ' and that 'it is unlawful to discriminate in favour of a particular racial group in recruitment or promotion on the grounds that members of that group have in the past suffered from adverse discrimination and should be given the chance to "catch up" ' (quoted in Sooben, 1990: 39).

In its firm repudiation of reverse discrimination, the 1976 Race Relations Act reaffirmed strict non-discrimination as the fundamental principle of British race-relations law. 'John Bull did not learn from Jim Crow', as David Kirp (1979: 119) put it. The 1976 Act only allowed certain 'exceptions' to the principle of non-discrimination, which became known as 'positive action' (see CRE, 1989). Sections 37 and 38 of the Race Relations Act permit employers to provide special job training for their underrepresented minority employees, and to place special job advertisements in the minority press. Section 5(2)(d) permits the priority hiring of minority workers if related to the nature of the job—say, the hiring of an Indian social worker to counsel the Indian immigrant community. Finally, Section 35 affords minority members access to facilities or services to meet their 'special needs' in education, training, or welfare—say, shelters for battered Asian women. In contrast to American affirmative action, British positive action is permissive rather than mandatory; an employer or local authority *may* engage in it, but is not required to do so. And in the all-important field of employment, some (reverse) discrimination may occur preceding, but never at the point of, selection or promotion. In its rationale, positive action is not, like affirmative action, a compensation for harm, but a 'consequentialist' tool for stabilizing the social order (see Edwards, 1987: 33).

The introduction of indirect discrimination in the 1976 Act nevertheless created a space for the language of group rights and for the result-oriented logic of achieving statistical parity between the races. Accordingly, some local authorities pushed positive toward affirmative action. For instance, London's Camden Council gave out this new employment policy in January 1978: 'If two people of equal ability but of different colour apply for a job, we will pick the coloured person because coloured people are so underrepresented at the moment' (quoted in Lustgarten, 1980: 26). This was plainly outside the 1976 Race Relations Act, and constituted unlawful discrimination. But under the strange name of 'equal opportunity policy',[18] it became widespread practice nevertheless, particularly in local councils held by radical factions of the Labour Party in urban immigrant districts.

Venturing the grey zone between positive and affirmative action became legitimate after the Brixton disorders in April 1981, the most serious race unrest in British history.[19] The government-commissioned Scarman report (1981) and a parallel House of Commons report on Racial Disadvantage (1981) located the causes of the riot in oppressive policing and the dismal social conditions of young second-generation immigrants. As the House of Commons report put it, 'far too many Asian and West Indian youngsters are unemployed, unskilled, unqualified and disenchanted and it is above all to this problem that Parliament and the nation must address themselves' (House of Commons, 1981: p. vii). The Scarman report displays an uneasy awareness that the old welfare universalism was insufficient to tackle the protracted problem of racial disadvantage: 'The ethnic minorities tend both to suffer the same problems as the rest of society, but more severely, and to have certain special problems of their own' (Scarman, 1981: 102). Accordingly, Lord Scarman recommended more 'positive action' measures in the areas of housing, education, and employment, and particularly a reform of Section 11 funding as originally envisaged in the aborted Ethnic Groups Bill.[20] The riot experience had evidently swept away the old distaste for privileged-group treatment: 'A policy of direct co-ordinated attack on racial disadvantage inevitably means that the ethnic minorities will enjoy for a time a positive discrimination in their favour. But it is a price worth paying if it accelerates the elimination of the unsettling factor of racial disadvantage from the social fabric of the United Kingdom' (ibid. 135).

The tackling of indirect discrimination is dependent on reliable statistical information about the ethnic-minority population, without which there would be no yardstick for employers and others to assess the need and measure the success of 'equal opportunity' policies (White Paper, 1988: 13). Until recently, such information has not been available in Great Britain. The House of Commons report *Racial Disadvantage* (1981) deplored that 'we know neither the total ethnic-minority population nor their true rate of unemployment' (p. ix). Interestingly, the government plan to put an ethnic-minority question into the 1981 national census had failed because of the opposition of ethnic-minority groups, who feared the abuse of data for purposes of immigration control. Before an ethnic-group question was finally included in the 1991 census, estimates for the ethnic-minority population were derived indirectly from 'country of birth' information of the head of households (Teague, 1993: 12). This was a most incomplete proxy for estimates of the ethnic-minority population, because it did not include a direct count of second-generation immigrants. Remedying this problem through inserting a question on parents' birthplace, as in the 1971 census, was no long-term solution either, because it had to leave out the increasing contingent of black and Asian children with parents born in Britain (Sillitoe and White, 1992: 142). If immigrant opposition to an ethnic-group question in the 1981 census gave way to unanimous support in the 1991 census, this was because in the meantime 'ethnic monitoring' had become standard practice, particularly at the local authority level. In the wake of the Brixton riots, central and local government introduced ethnic counts of their civil servants, and a number of private employers followed suit. A CRE official characterized ethnic monitoring as the 'great battle of the 1980s', and one that has been 'won'.[21] Now there existed a clear rationale for collecting ethnic origin-data, and suspicion about the abuse of such data faded away. With the introduction of an ethnic-minority question in the 1991 census, Britain is now—next to the Netherlands—the only country in Western Europe to recognize 'ethnic minorities' of immigrant origin in law and official statistics (Coleman and Salt, 1996: 17). Under the sway of combating indirect discrimination through positive action and 'equal opportunity' policies, Britain's precarious balance between social-citizenship universalism and racial-group particularism has shifted toward the latter pole.

No wonder that the Commission for Racial Equality's battle of the 1990s is to accomplish the half-step from positive to affirmative action. A model for this exists: the Fair Employment (Northern Ireland) Act of 1989. It legally requires employers to monitor their workforce by religion and to draw up detailed plans to achieve statistical parity between the major religious groups in the workforce, whose fulfillment is secured through the economic lever of 'contract compliance'. If the parallel to sex discrimination had once helped to improve race-relations law, why not now draw a parallel to religious discrimination? As the CRE put it, 'we believe that the kinds of obligations placed on employers to avoid discrimination on the ground of religion should be matched here by equivalent provisions on race'.[22] It is questionable if the formal analogy between race and religion holds, because (against

Enoch Powell's expectation) no comparable civil war has taken place between the races of the United Kingdom, which might move the government to the exceptional concession that the Northern Ireland Act surely is. Interestingly, the CRE denies that its advocated 'equality targets' have any resemblance to 'quotas'. But the difference is difficult to see. Note that the CRE's *Second Review of the Race Relations Act 1976* (1992) calls for legally binding 'goals and timetables' to check the achievement of 'equality of opportunity' in employment. The prospects for a race-relations act revised along these lines are weak.[23] But the sheer logic of recognizing indirect discrimination has drawn John Bull a bit into the orbit of Jim Crow.

Official Multiculturalism

As indicated in Roy Jenkins's famous abdication of the melting-pot in 1966, Britain turned against the idea of assimilating her immigrants earlier than any other country in the Western world. The Home Secretary's recognition of 'cultural diversity' coincided with the changing profile of immigrants, the earlier predominance of West Indians, who were socialized in British colonial culture and 'regarded England as their mother country' (Rose, 1969: 419), giving way to the predominance of South Asian immigrants, who considered Britain a foreign country and showed little inclination to abandon their indigenous language and culture. But, in contrast to the American and German cases, British multiculturalism sprang more from political élite anticipation than the pressure of society.

Official multiculturalism has multiple sources—the indirect rule of empire and the legacy of multi-ethnic nationhood, as indicated above, but also an empty concept of citizenship that imposes no assimilation requirements on new members and confers only one right, the right of abode in the UK. An often overlooked, but fundamental, source of multiculturalism *avant la lettre* has been the English common-law tradition. The spirit of common law is well captured in this statement by an English judge: 'England, it may be said, is not a country where everything is forbidden except what is expressly permitted; it is a country where everything is permitted except where it is expressly forbidden' (quoted in Poulter, 1990: 1). Guided by the unprincipled pragmatism of 'common sense, good manners and a reasonable tolerance' (Poulter, 1987: 594), the common-law judiciary has been remarkably tolerant of cultural pluralism, outlawing only morally 'repugnant' practices like polygamy, forced marriage, female circumcision, and some Muslim divorces. The flexibility of the common law is visible in its treatment of foreign marriage and divorce customs. Polygamous marriage and the marriage of minors, 'repugnant' from a Western view but common practice in Islamic countries, are valid in English law if the individual's 'domicile' is in a foreign country where such marriage is within the law.[24] Muslim *talaq* divorces, in which a Muslim husband may unilaterally repudiate and divorce his wife by simple oral pronouncement, are valid in English law if conducted overseas and with some element of formality.[25]

The flexible and pragmatic spirit of the common law has found statutory expression in exempting some ethnic minorities from some requirements of the law. Turbanned Sikhs, for instance, are exempted by the Employment Act 1989 from the Construction (Head Protection) Regulations of 1989, which make it compulsory for workers on construction sites to wear safety helmets. Parliament passed this law only to protect the 40,000 Sikhs working in the construction industry. Epitomizing the spirit of flexibility and pragmatism, the 1989 law holds Sikhs partly responsible for injuries received from not wearing a safety helmet, allowing only damage claims for injuries that would have been suffered even if the injured person had been wearing suitable head protection (Poulter, 1990: 103 f.). Similar examples of statutory exemption for ethnic minorities abound. The Motor-Cycle Crash Helmets (Religious Exemption) Act of 1976 exempts Sikhs from the duty of wearing helmets when riding motorcycles (according to the 1972 Road Traffic Act), provided they are wearing a turban. The Slaughterhouse Act 1974 and Slaughter of Poultry Act 1967 contain exemptions for Muslims and Jews from the legal duty of stunning animals before killing them, enabling them to comply with their religious laws and traditions. And, with an eye on the burial rites of Hindus and Sikhs, the Water Act of 1989 includes a provision for the scattering of human ashes and the sinking of corpses in tidal and estuary waters.

Many of the ethnic-minority protections that in Germany and the United States are grounded in constitutional human-rights guarantees have been achieved in Great Britain by unprincipled common law and flexible statute-making. Consider the key areas of education and employment. Here the 'indirect discrimination' clause of the 1976 Race Relations Act has helped to protect ethnic minority customs and practices. In *Mandla* v. *Dowell Lee* (1983), the House of Lords ruled against a headmaster who had refused to admit a Sikh boy as a pupil solely because he was wearing a turban and thus in violation of the official dress code. In this British 'turban affair' that never was, the Law Lords found the headmaster's refusal 'indirect discrimination' according to the 1976 Act—a notionally neutral measure having a disproportionally negative effect on an ethnic minority that was not 'justifiable' on non-racial grounds.[26] Remarkably, in a country that still forces its pupils to wear school uniforms, ethnic-minority children are generally free to wear their traditional religious dresses. Similar help from the 'indirect discrimination' clause came in the area of employment. Religiously prescribed beards, headgear, and time-outs for prayer and religious observance are no longer easily discriminated against in the name of safety, hygiene, or work schedules, especially since courts have applied the strict American test of 'objective necessity' to the discriminatory practices of employers (Poulter, 1990: 102 f.). The CRE's Code of Practice, a list of recommended non-discrimination practices for employers approved by Parliament in 1983,[27] suggests: 'Where employees have particular cultural and religious needs which conflict with existing work requirements, it is recommended that employers should consider whether it is reasonably practicable to vary or adapt these requirements to enable such needs to be met' (ibid. 105 f.). The Code mentions as protectable needs the observance of prayer times by Muslims, observance of religious holidays, the wearing of saris or shalwar trousers by Asian women, and, of course, the turban-wearing of Sikhs. With some ingenuity, ethnic-minority customs have mellowed the stiff protocol of British public life. For instance, Sikhs may be seen wearing blue turbans in the police force, blue and yellow turbans as traffic wardens, green turbans as tennis umpires and linesmen at Wimbledon, khaki turbans in the army, and white turbans in place of wigs as barristers and judges.

The main site of official multiculturalism is education, its main document being the government-commissioned report *Education for All* (Swann, 1985). David Kirp (1979) had taken schooling as the prime example for the 'racial inexplicitness' of British immigrant integration. Indeed, in the early 1960s education had aimed at the cultural assimilation of immigrants. A 1963 report of the Commonwealth Immigrant Advisory Council said that 'a national system cannot be expected to perpetuate the different values of immigrant groups' (in Rose, 1969: 266). The 1973 Select Committee on Race Relations and Immigration report *Education* was already uneasy about racial inexplicitness, doubting that the children of immigrants were 'immigrants' but still settling for the term 'for want of a better', and questioning the orthodox view that the situation of immigrant children was the same as that of all children in deprived areas—'special problems need special remedies'.[28] When it set up the 1979 committee under Anthony Rampton to study the problem of West Indian underachievement in schools, the government had all but abandoned racial inexplicitness, having no qualms about calling immigrant children 'ethnic minorities' and arguing that schools were to prepare 'all pupils for life in a society which is both multi-racial and culturally diverse'.[29] Multicultural curriculum reform and teacher training bloomed especially at the local level, and by 1983, 36 of 105 surveyed Local Education Authorities had written policy statements on multicultural education (Tomlinson, 1986: 193).

When Lord Swann replaced Anthony Rampton as chair of the Committee of Inquiry into the Education of Children from Ethnic Minority Groups, the committee's focus tacitly shifted from the problem of West Indian underachievement to the problem of integrating Asian pupils with distinct languages and cultures.[30] *Education for All* envisages Great Britain as a 'genuinely pluralist society, . . . both socially cohesive and culturally diverse' (p. 6), which avoids the twin dangers of 'full assimilation' and 'separatism'. It depicts individuals primarily as members of ethnic groups, and only secondarily as 'part of the wider national society' (p. 3). The task of state policy is not only tolerating but actively 'assisting the ethnic minority communities in maintaining their distinct ethnic identities' (p. 5). Cleverly, the report stresses that the 'pluralist ideal', while 'far from being realized', is no deviation from traditional Britishness, but in line with its pluralistic and 'dynamic and ever changing' nature (p. 7).

Citizenship universalism appears in *Education for All* only in an inverted way, as the claim of a pervasive 'racism' that has to be countered by multicultural education 'for all', black and white children alike. This was also a conscious break with the paternalist tradition of considering the integration of immigrants a problem of immigrants only. Inverted citizenship universalism goes along with a repudiation of colour-blindness in the classroom: 'We . . . regard "colour-blindness" . . . as potentially just as negative as a straightforward rejection of people with a different skin colour since both types of attitude seek to deny the validity of an important aspect of a person's identity' (p. 27). The report's broad indictment of racism and abandonment of the norm of racial inexplicitness certainly reflect the 'anti-racist' strategies thriving since the early 1980s in radical local Labour councils. The one difference is that in *Education for All* racism is not the vice of whites only: 'We firmly believe . . . that *all* forms of prejudice against groups of people on racial grounds are wrong' (p. 28).

Inverted citizenship universalism, according to which *all* schools and teachers, not only those in minority areas, had to be reached by multiculturalism, entailed a demand for central direction that conflicted with the traditional decentralization and local autonomy of the British education system. Not surprisingly, nationally uniform top-down multiculturalism à la Swann never came. But some receptive Local Education Authorities (LEAs), and of course mostly those in immigrant areas, eagerly picked up the report's recommendations, such as instituting a 'permeating' multicultural curriculum (which includes the teaching of science and mathematics 'in different cultures'),[31] in-service teacher preparation for a multicultural classroom (including Racism Awareness Training), and the 'equal opportunity' hiring of minority teachers. However, as I will show in the following section, at the local level official multiculturalism tended to be outflanked by more radical 'anti-racism'.

Local Race Politics

It is a truism that immigrant integration occurs first and foremost at the local level, the site of everyday life and of the concrete encounter with the host society. Britain differs from Germany and the United States in giving political form to local immigrant integration. This is a result of demography and statecraft alike. Demographically, Commonwealth immigrants are extremely spatially concentrated. According to the 1991 census, over 70 per cent of the three million members of 'ethnic minority groups', which account for 5.5 per cent of the British population, live in England's South-East and the West Midlands (Peach, 1996: 10). Here they are further concentrated in a few urban centres. Almost half of the British minority population (44.6 per cent) lives in Greater London. For some ethnic groups this concentration is even higher, as for Afro-Caribbeans (55 per cent of whom live in or near London) (Jones, 1996: 16). The uneven distribution of minority groups further increases at the district and ward levels. London boroughs such as Brent, Newham, or Tower Hamlets have ethnic minority shares of 44.8 per cent, 42.3 per cent, and 35.6 per cent, respectively (Peach, 1996: 14). Down at the ward level, 70 per cent of black and Asian immigrants and their descendants can be found in wards that contain less than 10 per cent of the population—

such as in Ealing's Northcote ward, which has a non-white ethnic population of 90 per cent. These urban minority pockets would become hothouses of local race politics in the 1980s.

However, local immigrant integration is also the result of statecraft. In Britain, local governments are 'key agents of the welfare state' (Stoker, 1991: 3), being responsible for—and autonomous in—the provision of education, housing, and a host of social and infrastructural services, and accounting for a quarter of total public expenditure in 1988–9. To the degree that immigrant integration was welfare state integration, its natural site was local government. In addition, Section 71 of the 1976 Race Relations Act imposed on local governments the double task of 'eliminat[ing] unlawful discrimination' and 'promot[ing] equal opportunity'. This made local government a highly coveted stake of race politics.

Community Relations Councils

Before local government would enter centre stage, local 'community relations councils' (CRCs) were main agents of immigrant integration. Ira Katznelson (1973: ch. 11) castigated them as 'racial buffers', 'quasi-colonial institutional structures to deal with the issues of race outside of the traditional political arenas' (p. 178).[32] In this conspiratorial view, CRCs—as epitome of the entire race-relations enterprise—helped contain the rise of an US-style civil-rights movement, while keeping the delicate race issue outside of mainstream politics. This exaggerates the degree of planning in the set-up of these councils, as well as their effectiveness—ethnic minority leaders tended to take these 'buffers' as what they appeared to be, and local governments gradually preferred direct over CRC-mediated contact with ethnic-minority groups (Messina, 1987).

The origin of CRCs are local voluntary organizations, which popped up spontaneously wherever there were new arrivals in need of basic aid and welfare services. A local volunteer characterized their purpose plainly as 'help[ing] the local coloured community to settle down as happily and as easily as possible' (in Hill and Issacharoff, 1971: 1). This was no small thing in the earliest phase of New Commonwealth immigration, when there was general confusion over where the responsibility for immigrant welfare rested—in the Colonial Office and central government, local governments, or even the Commonwealth governments (ibid. 4). The 1965 White Paper *Immigration from the Commonwealth* set out to bring these local voluntary efforts under state control, by means of financial incentives. The government offered a full-time paid official to each 'voluntary liaison committee', provided it satisfied three conditions: it consisted of a 'joint project' of immigrant and host community, had the 'full backing' of the local authorities, and was 'non-sectarian' and 'non-political' in outlook (White Paper, 1965: 16). This integration measure was paternalistic, depicting the local liaison committees as sites 'where the structure of British society can be explained to the immigrants' (ibid. 17); and it showed the British distaste for setting up a separate structure for immigrants, mandating the committees to 'help immigrants to use the ordinary facilities of social services provided for the whole community' (ibid.). An early critic branded the (mostly white-led) local committees as Uncle Tom factories, in which white society could mould the non-white immigrants in their image, and he lashed out against the whole race-relations enterprise: 'The dominant attitude to race relations is one of paternalism. Attention is invariably focused on the minority group: it is *they* who must be educated, improved, brought up to acceptable British specifications.'[33]

This criticism was fuelled by the fact that the state began to institutionalize the voluntary sector just when a US-style civil-rights movement seemed to be in the making—the Campaign Against Racial Discrimination (CARD). Founded in 1964 after a short visit by Martin Luther King in London, CARD was the only truly national and cross-group immigrant organization that Britain has ever seen, and it helped shape the first Race Relations Act of 1965 (see Heineman, 1972). When CARD broke apart over a rift between radical advocates of black power and a weakening liberal mainstream, Michael Dummett—the Oxford philosopher and strident immigrant advocate—held the government responsible for this. By providing financial incentives for (moderate) voluntary liaison committees to join the statist National Committee for Commonwealth Immigrants (NCCI), rather than CARD, government had killed the 'embryo civil rights movement', intent on 'keep[ing] the black community under control, not to give them a part in determining how things are run' (in Hill and Issacharoff, 1971: 30 f.).

However paternalistic their beginning, the Community Relations Councils (CRCs)[34] eventually changed from white-led 'welfare organizations' into 'representatives of the minorities' themselves (Banton, 1985: 116). By 1980, there were 104 CRCs with some 500 full-time paid staff (ibid. 101), too big a machine and employment site to be overlooked by race activists. For instance, the (Marxist) Indian

Workers Association (IWA), the oldest and most influential political organization of immigrants from India, decided in the early 1980s to join the previously despised Community Relations Councils.[35] While always tamed by the CRE's financial whip, the politicization of the CRCs did little to improve their reputation, in the view of immigrants and domestic society alike. Far from providing a platform for all ethnic minorities, the CRCs often became captured by a particular minority, turning them into sites of inter-minority strife (ibid. 104 f.).

The CRCs' demise as mediating bodies between immigrants and host society occurred in the wake of the 1981 racial unrests. The 1981 Home Affairs Committee report *Racial Disadvantage* encouraged local authorities 'to make every effort to make as much direct contact as possible with minorities and to rid themselves of the notion that the local CRC is or should be their sole spokesman' (p. xxxvi).[36] The CRCs now found themselves in direct competition with self-help groups for funding and legitimate minority representation. Even the Commission for Racial Equality (CRE) went over to fund self-help groups directly, which led a commentator to the prediction that the end of local CRCs was nigh.[37]

Anti-Racism

In the early 1980s the focus of local race politics shifted from the Community Relations Councils to local government itself. This was partially due to Section 71 of the 1976 Race Relations Act, reinforced by the post-1981 pressure to do more against racial discrimination. But equally important, after its national defeat in 1979 the Labour Party sought to entrench itself in local town halls. In opposition, Labour underwent a radicalization, moving away from its traditional working-class core to embrace the claims of ethnic groups, women, and homosexuals. Since the late 1970s, local Labour councils in London boroughs like Lambeth, Haringey, Camden, Brent and Newham waged aggressive 'race equality initiatives' (Ouseley, 1984: 133).[38] This included the formulation of equal opportunity policy statements and 'equality targets', to be implemented by positive action in name, but affirmative action in fact; the formation of race-relations committees and hiring of race-advisers; the adoption of codes of practice, and of compulsory 'anti-racist' training for staff; the direct consultation of local immigrant communities, which obviated the mediating role of the CRCs; and handing out generous grant aid to ethnic self-help initiatives.

Particularly in the employment domain, these race initiatives had impressive results. For instance, in Lambeth, which had started its race policy in 1978, the ethnic-minority share of council staff increased from under 10 per cent to 25 per cent in 1985 (Lansley *et al.*, 1989: 124); Hackney's ethnic minority share increased from 11.5 per cent in 1980 to 34.0 per cent in 1988 (Ouseley, 1990: 151 f.). This mattered because local authorities were often the largest local employers. Labour councils also were generous donors to the voluntary sector. Camden's grant aid to ethnic-minority groups increased from £164,000 in 1983/4 to £610,000 in 1987/8 (Mufti, 1988: 17). The Greater London Council, the most profligate spender of all, increased its funding of voluntary organizations from £6 million in 1981 to a stunning £50 million in 1984 (Lansley *et al.*, 1989: 55). Direct consultation meant that ethnic minorities were no longer side-tracked into irrelevant 'buffers', but were included in the government machinery. Camden Council's Race and Commmunity Relations Committee, for instance, comprised representatives of all major ethnic-minority groups in the borough, which were nominated by the respective group and then co-opted onto the committee (Prashar and Nicholas, 1986: ch. 2).

When it fell into Labour hands after the 1981 elections, the Greater London Council (GLC) became 'the flagship of municipal socialism' (Lansley *et al.*, 1989: 47). Its flamboyant leader Ken Livingstone vowed to 'use the council machinery as part of a political campaign both against the government and in defence of socialist policies'.[39] Created in 1964 by a Conservative government as a 'strategic' authority over the London boroughs, the GLC had no responsibility for most personal services like housing, education, and social services, which rested with the boroughs. But with 22,000 employees the GLC was one of London's largest employers, and Council leader Livingstone showed no hesitation to 'pension-off racists' and to divide up the employment spoils among his followers, US-machine style.[40] With one of the UK's largest council budgets in its hands, and without direct service responsibilities, the GLC was free to veer into the symbolic politics of war and peace, anti-racism, and gay and lesbian rights. At the race front, the GLC's aim was nothing less than 'total and complete racial equality in London' (GLC, 1983). An Ethnic Minorities Committee, chaired by the Council leader himself, was established in 1981 to implement Section 71 responsibilities, and all other committees (like the Police, Transport, or Housing Committees) were mandated to subject their policies to the test of race-equality impact statements. In addition, an Ethnic Minorities Unit was set up under a Principal Race Relations Adviser to 'shadow' the other GLC departments (like Finance, Personnel, or the Fire Brigade) for the race implications of their activities (Ouseley, 1990: 139). Under Livingstone's reign, the Victorian County Hall across the River Thames became the 'People's Palace'. The first two-year report of the Labour GLC (1983) lists no less than 170 ethnic-minority groups and projects supported with grants (including obscure entries like Rastafari Universal Zion, Mixi-Fren, or Vee Tee AY—The Voice). Under the slogan 'Working for London', the city was showered with ethnic festivals, free rock concerts, and political congregations of the anti-establishment kind; 1983 was Peace Year, 1984 was Anti-Racist Year, with London declared an Anti-Apartheid Zone.

The GLC's equivalent in the field of education, the Inner London Education Authority (ILEA), canonized the 'anti-racist' ideology guiding local race politics. Its programmatic paper *A Policy for Equality: Race* (ILEA, 1983) distinguishes between three approaches to race relations: assimilation, cultural diversity, and equality. Assimilation, no longer supported by anyone, had tried to adjust immigrants to the British way by colour-blind means; it was 'wrong' because it took non-white immigrants as the 'problem', and because of its 'racist' premiss of 'white cultural superiority'. Cultural diversity, the position taken by the government now, abandoned these presumptions; but it was still 'wrong' because it denied the 'structural aspects of racism' and the 'power relations between white and black people'. With equality, the third perspective, nothing was wrong. It targeted the 'central and pervasive influence of racism' that had been obscured by the ethnic bazaar of official multiculturalism. The equality perspective is assimilation inverted, in which 'whites' figure as the problem subject to correction; and, not unlike the old notion of 'coloured', the new label 'black' swallows the diversity of South Asian and Afro-Caribbean immigrants, but now as a fighting term for their 'common experience . . . of being victims of racism, and their common determination to oppose racism' (ibid. 4).

The annals of local anti-racism are not short on follies. In a 1986 campaign, the London borough of Brent found its schools 'permeated with racism overt and covert' (in Lansley *et al.*, 1989: 135), firing a popular headteacher and planning to deploy a small army of 180 race advisers to inculcate correct attitudes upon the rest.[41] In this 'nuttiest of left-wing councils', even the local museum staff was forced to undergo Racial Awareness Training.[42] Hackney, Haringey, and

Islington Councils put the nursery rhyme 'Baa Baa Black Sheep' on the index, Camden banned 'sunshine' as racially offensive, and a GLC personnel officer was accused of racism for referring to the internal grape-vine as 'jungle drums'.[43] Big Brother was watching you in the GLC's 'London Against Racism' campaign, which plastered the city with posters saying 'If you are not part of the solution, you are part of the problem'. Zealous renaming of streets and places provoked the ire of ordinary English people, who found their local habitats changed beyond recognition. South London's Brockwell Park became Zephania Mothopeng Park (the name of an imprisoned South African anti-apartheid leader), and East London's Hackney council dared to turn Britannia Walk into Shaheed-E-Azam Bhagot Singh Avenue (the name of an Indian independence fighter). 'If it wasn't so serious we'd all die laughing', wrote the tabloid *Sun*.[44]

Attack on Local Government

Tabloids eagerly picked up and amplified anti-racist follies. In response to Hackney's Bhagot Singh provocation the *Sun* sent 'Britannia to rule down our street'.[45] The liberal consensus that had so far supported British race relations threatened to break apart under the pincer movement of anti-racist militancy and an 'anti-antiracist' nationalism. In the stuffy pages of the *Salisbury Review*, conservative intellectuals sought to rescue the English (or, variously, British) nation from the anti-racist assault. For one of them, yes, the English were a race, which 'really stands proxy for that feeling for, loyalty to people of one's own kind', and rioting West Indians were *'structurally* likely to be at odds' with it, leaving only one solution: repatriation.[46] This was an extreme position, even among conservatives. A more moderate conservative found the liberal establishment's 'guilty rejection of its own cultural heritage' as the soil from which anti-racist demonology could blossom.[47] For a third conservative critic, the anti-racist provocation was an opportunity to question the entire framework of race relations, had it not, instead improving relations between the races, 'made each one of them more conscious of the ways in which it differs from the rest' (Lewis, 1988: 56).

On the political front, Tories who had long kept quiet about liberal race relations spoke out against town-hall 'totalitarianism', likening life in Brent or Lambeth to life in communist Poland or East Germany.[48] In fact, the parallel rise of Thatcherism and municipal socialism had to put both on a collision course. Since a direct attack on democratically legitimized local governments was impossible, Mrs Thatcher chose the indirect avenue of indicting their economic wastefulness. During the Thatcher reign, a flurry of legislation sought to impose market discipline on local government, making it less flexible to pursue equal-opportunity policies on race (see Stoker, 1991: 161–229). The 1980 Local Government, Planning and Land Act introduced centrally determined 'block grants', which replaced the old system of reimbursing local government on the basis of existing expenditure patterns. The 1982 Local Government Finance Act framed the block grants with ceilings on local spending, whose transgressing was penalized by the withholding of block grants. High spenders like the GLC and the ILEA now had to generate their entire revenue from local rates, without central government support. In addition, the 1982 Act abolished the right of local authorities to raise supplementary rates, which had been an obvious way of circumventing diminishing block grant income. Between 1981 and 1984, £713 million of block grant were 'held back' from local governments in England alone, and the proportion of local authority revenue expenditure provided by central government fell from 48.5 per cent in 1979/80 to 35.9 per cent in 1982/3 (ibid. 165). Local governments responded to this assault with a variety of measures, such as seeking redress in court, 'creative accounting', and—above all—raising the rates to be paid by local residents. To close also this escape route, the government passed the 1984 Rate Act, which gives the Secretary of State for the Environment the power to limit the rates of named authorities. In June 1984, the government published a list of 18 local authorities to be 'rate-capped' in the following year. Sixteen of them were Labour councils, including the champions of anti-racism: Brent, Camden, GLC, Hackney, Haringey, ILEA, Lambeth, and Islington. The rate offenders now sought backing in the local interest communities, such as ethnic-minority groups, who profited from high spending. In March 1985 their anti-rate-capping campaign galvanized a rally of 70,000 in London (ibid. 172). But this failed to stop the central-government offensive. The 1985 Local Government Act redeemed the Conservative manifesto pledge of 1983 to abolish the GLC and the six metropolitan counties, those 'wasteful and unnecessary tiers of government' (in O'Leary, 1987: 193 f.).[49]

Next to putting limits on spending, Thatcher sought to discipline local government through privatization. In perhaps the most popular of all Thatcherite reforms, the 1980 Housing Act gave council-house tenants the 'right-to-buy' their rented houses and flats for below-market prices. Millions of council tenants accepted the invitation. This reduced local authorities' use of council housing for equal opportunity policies. In addition, the introduction of compulsory 'competitive tendering' in the 1988 Local Government Act forced local authorities to contract-out in-house services that could be delivered for less money by private firms, such as refuse collection or street cleaning. Competitive tendering diminished council employment as an area of remedial race policies. In addition, the 1988 Act abolished 'non-commercial' contract conditions, such as 'contract compliance' that withheld government contracts from employers who did not hire sufficient numbers of minority-group members. A final measure to introduce market discipline into service delivery was the 1988 Education Reform Act. This act aimed at reducing the power of local education authorities, especially those pursuing 'multicultural' or even 'anti-racist' strategies, often against the wishes of parents. The Education Act allowed parents to send their children to the school of their choice, rather than the one commanded by the LEA on the basis of spatial proximity. In addition, parents were given the right to remove local schools from the local authority sector, and to make them free-standing 'Grant-Maintained Schools', funded directly by central government.[50] Finally, the introduction of a National Curriculum restricted the range of multicultural and anti-racist curriculum reform conducted by some LEAs.

Minority Entrenchment and Fragmentation

After the Tory assault, local governments no longer enjoy the independence and power they possessed during the heyday of anti-racism in the early 1980s. Nevertheless, ethnic-minority groups have become entrenched in the political system. After the end of the Thatcher decade, an annual gathering of the National Association of Race Equality Advisers noticed that 'new realism' had tempered the municipal socialism of old; but the meeting also consisted of 1,000 participants, all of them professionals paid to advise local governments on race matters.[51] In fact, by the early 1990s there were 1,370 race-relations officers in local government, plus an estimated 1,000 race officers in central government, housing associations, universities, and other organizations (Coleman and Salt, 1996: 11). In addition, there were about 300 elected local councillors from ethnic-minority groups, and a few were even council leaders (Goulbourne, 1992: 359).

The case of Birmingham shows that even off the noisy London tracks ethnic minorities have consolidated their presence in local government (see Solomos and Back, 1995). Whereas the classic pattern had been one of patronage, with ethnic-minority leaders backing white elected councillors in return for benefits and protection, by 1994 over twenty councillors in Birmingham (which is one-third of the ruling Labour group) were members of ethnic-minority groups. John Solomos and Les Back (1995: 201) conclude that 'black politicians (have become) an integral part of Birmingham's political system'. Birmingham pursued a 'sensible socialism' distinct from London's militant anti-racism. But its actual measures on race were quite similar. A Conservative administration had started the ethnic monitoring of the city's workforce in the early 1980s. A newly installed Labour council stepped up the race initiative in 1984 by creating a Race Relations and Equal Opportunities Committee, along with an administrative Race Relations Unit. Setting itself a 20 per cent minority employment target, the city (with 40,000 employees the region's largest employer) managed to increase its ethnic-minority workforce from 6.1 per cent in 1983 to 15.4 per cent in 1993 (ibid. 180).

Solomos and Back's Birmingham study makes a second interesting observation: the minority-groups' fragmentation into some 500 separate organizations, and their 'inability to overcome ethnic and cultural differences' (ibid. 200). While the authors remain faithful to the race-relations jargon of calling all ethnic-minority people 'black', Birmingham's blacks *an sich* were nowhere blacks *für sich*. In fact, nationwide survey evidence shows that even blacks *an sich* are at best a political fiction, justifying David Kirp's (1979: 118) caustic remark that UK blacks were 'a categorical artefact, rather like redheads'. Instead of a homogenous mass of blacks equally blocked in their advancement by racial discrimination, one can see a huge variety of ethnic trajectories.

The most recent ethnic-minority survey distinguishes between three clusters of ethnic groups, which performed rather differently on key indices like education and employment (Modood *et al.*, 1997: ch. 10). African-Asians and Chinese are Britain's most successful immigrants, even exceeding the average income, educational level, and self-employment rate of whites. At the opposite end, Pakistanis and Bangladeshis are Britain's worst-performing immigrants. Their male unemployment in 1994 was 2.5 times higher than white male unemployment. Pakistani and Bengali women of all age groups show extremely low levels of economic activity and English proficiency.

Both ethnic groups have among the worst housing in Britain, and 80 per cent of their households have an income below half the national average. In between these over- and under-performing clusters there is a middle cluster of Indians and Caribbeans, who show contradictory features.[52] Indian and Caribbean women have slightly higher average earnings from full-time work than white women. But Indian men and women combined were one-third more likely to be unemployed than whites in 1994, and Caribbeans had double the white unemployment rate. Caribbeans have the lowest self-employment rate of ethnic groups in Britain, whereas Indians have one of the highest—both, however, have higher financial returns from self-employment than whites.

In addition to inter-ethnic disparity, there is also considerable intra-ethnic variation in succeeding or not succeeding in Britain. Afro-Caribbean men, for instance, are more likely to be found in low-skilled jobs, while Afro-Caribbean women hold jobs equivalent to the jobs held by white women (Jones, 1996: 160).[53] And on some indices, like enrolment in higher education, all minorities combined are out-doing whites—ethnic minorities are more likely than whites to stay in education after the school-leaving age of 16 (ibid. 33). If one presumes that racial discrimination against non-whites affects all minority groups alike (ibid. 158), discrimination cannot explain the different patterns of minority success or failure. Modood *et al.* (1997: 347) even conclude: 'Those ethnic groups that had an above-average middle-class professional and business profile before migration seem to have been able to re-create that profile despite the occupational downgrading that all minority groups initially experienced.'

These inter- and intra-ethnic variations are irreconcilable with the umbrella label 'black' that had undergirded local race politics in the 1980s. In fact, political blackness helped to camouflage that Afro-Caribbeans had set the agenda of 'anti-racism', with their fixation on the state and white supremacy. Asian concerns, like the maintenance of religion and culture, have never had a prominent place on the anti-racist agenda (see Modood, 1994*a*: 867).[54] As Tariq Modood (1994*b*: 89) explicates the uneasiness of Asians about political blackness, 'they resist being defined by their mode of oppression and seek space and dignity for their mode of being.' In 1982, the Commission for Racial Equality, well aware that Asians disagreed, had categorized all minorities as 'black', because this was the 'conventional way now of regarding all those who suffer from the particular disadvantage related to colour' (quoted in Modood, Beishon, and Virdee, 1994: 104). In 1988,

Asian community leaders protested against the CRE's continued referral to Asians as 'blacks',[55] and the Commission ceased to recommend this category for purposes of ethnic monitoring. This was one year before the Rushdie affair would tear apart even 'Asian' unity, and bring to the fore a minority claim that was altogether irresolvable within the race-relations framework.

Not a Racial Group: Muslims

With the outlawing of indirect discrimination, the 1976 Race Relations Act acknowledged the legal existence of 'racial groups', thus moving away from the initial approach of citizenship universalism. Now it became imperative to carve out the boundaries of the racial groups protected by law. The Race Relations Act itself gives little help in this. Its Section 3(1) calls a 'racial group' any 'group of persons defined by reference to colour, race, nationality or ethnic or national origins'. Apart from raising the question how 'colour' might differ from 'race', this is a most peculiar definition of a racial group: it includes citizens of other countries and white English men and women with roots in the Celtic fringe or continental Europe. The race statute obviously leaves a wide margin of interpretation as to what is a racial group. [56]

The census and case-law were two ways of pinning down more precisely the boundaries of racial groups. Defining racial groups for the census was a difficult balancing act between constructing objective categories that captured relevant patterns of discrimination and disadvantage and acknowledging the subjective self-definition of groups. Since the limitations of birthplace information and the need for an explicit descent-question was recognized in the mid-1970s, the Office for Population Census and Surveys (OPCS) experimented with a wide variety of categories.[57] Interestingly, the government consistently preferred ethnic over race labels, which it saw tainted by 'discredited beliefs about the non-physical differences between racial types' (Sillitoe and White, 1992: 143). This is visible in the 1991 census, which disguises as an 'ethnic group question' its actual interest in finding out how 'whites' differ from the non-white rest—evidently a racial distinction. While the breakdown of the Asian immigrant population according to national origins (such as Indian, Pakistani, and Bangladeshi) proved uncontroversial, the categorization of Afro-Caribbeans became contested. Afro-Caribbeans resisted being categorized according to overseas ancestry (such as West Indian), and preferred the domestic umbrella labels 'black' or 'British black'. However, this would swallow the demographic and social differences between West Indian and African blacks. After intense negotiation with the affected minority groups, the 1991 census finally settled for six discrete 'ethnic group' categories: White, Black-Caribbean, Black-African, Black-Other, Indian, Pakistani, Bangladeshi, Chinese, and a seventh 'any other group' category. This mixture of racial and national-origin classifications is now the largely undisputed core of the British ethnic-minority universe.[58]

Case-law has dealt with the more difficult question when 'ethnic origins' qualified a group for entry into the racial-group pantheon. In *Mandla* v. *Dowell Lee* (1983), Lord Frazer delivered a widely followed guide of how to determine an ethnic-origins group.[59] He started from the premiss that a racial-protection claim by Sikhs could not be based on colour, race, nationality, or national origins, because in these respects Sikhs were not distinguishable from many other groups, especially those in the Punjab. Accordingly, the question of the racial groupness of Sikhs had to turn on their ethnic origins. To determine an ethnic-origins group, Lord Frazer distinguished between two 'essential' and a number of relevant but 'non-essential' characteristics. Essential is that a group has a 'long shared history' kept alive by memory and a 'cultural tradition' of its own. Among the relevant but non-essential characteristics are common geographical origin, language, literature, religion, or oppression. As Lord Templeman further specified in his concurring opinion, the fact that Sikhs were 'more than a religious sect, . . . almost a race and almost a nation' made them a racial group on the ethnic-origins ticket.[60] Following *Mandla*, courts granted similar racial-group status to gypsies, but not to Rastafarians. The Appeal Court argued in *Dawkins* v. *Crown Suppliers* (1993) that Rastafarians stood the test of 'cultural tradition', but not of 'shared history'—their sixty years existence were deemed too short to establish such a claim.[61]

The largest and most problematic group to be denied racial-group status are Muslims. This was affirmed in several industrial tribunal rules. In *Tariq* v. *Young* (1979), the Birmingham industrial tribunal decided that a Muslim employee who felt derogated by the company managers for his religious affiliation had no case under the Race Relations Act: 'We find Muslims are identified by their religion and not by their race or nationality or as being an ethnic group. It is similar in this respect to a person being of the Christian faith. They are found all over the world in the same way as Muslims are found.'[62]

Muslims were different in this regard from Sikhs, who qualified as an ethnic group by being linked to a specific territory. In *CRE* v. *Precision Engineering IT* (1991), the Sheffield industrial tribunal ruled similarly that an employer refusing to hire Muslims had not committed unlawful direct discrimination because Muslims were not a race: 'To discriminate against Muslims, appalling and inexcusable as it may be, is not to discriminate on racial grounds.'[63] But the tribunal found this employer guilty of indirect discrimination, because national-orgins groups with Muslim majorities were disproportionately affected by the job ban on Muslims. This meant that Pakistani and Bengali Muslims were only indirectly protected under the Race Relations Act, through the national-origins provision, while Chinese or Caribbean Muslims were not protected at all.

Muslims first appeared as a unified group at the national level in their opposition to Salman Rushdie's *Satanic Verses*. The Rushdie affair, which is sometimes put on a par with the French 'headscarf affair' to demonstrate the failure of integrating Muslim immigrants in Western Europe,[64] is actually an anomaly within the usually generous and noiseless processing of Muslim claims in Britain. While not protected by national race-relations law and remaining outsiders in a state that is still legally ruled by the Anglican Church, Muslim immigrants have been hugely successful at the local government level. In cities like Bradford and Birmingham, with Muslim populations of 60,000 and 100,000, respectively, Muslims have effectively used the local race-relations committees and council structures to realize some of their key demands, particularly regarding schooling, religious observance, and social service provision. Bradford, the only English town with a Muslim majority population, was also the first English town to elect an immigrant Muslim mayor in 1985, and by 1992 eleven city councillors were Muslims (Kepel, 1997: 117). The local Council for Mosques, set up with the help of a local government grant in 1981, served as powerful interlocutor for the city's Muslim population, even taking over some service functions usually reserved to local government. Through a dense network of overlapping membership and cooperation between Muslim councillors, Council for Mosque activists, and CRC functionaries, Muslims in Bradford have 'learned to participate in the local state' (Lewis, 1994: 207 f.). Muslim success is especially visible in the sphere of education. Since the early 1980s, Bradford's Local Education Authority installed prayer rooms for Muslim children, granted Muslim parents the right to withdraw girls over ten from mixed school activities, tolerated extended vacations in

South Asia, provided *halal* food in schools, and allowed Muslim girls to wear traditional dress in school. Similar concessions can be observed in Birmingham, England's second Muslim stronghold, where the Muslim Liaison Committee negotiated with local authority an extensive catalogue of 'Guidelines on meeting the religious and cultural needs of Muslim pupils', which included the introduction of a 'multi-faith' syllabus, vegetarian menus in schools, and liberal dress codes (see Joly, 1995: 109).

Against this backdrop, the strident posture of Muslims in the Rushdie affair attests to the success, rather than failure, of British-style immigrant integration, and it may be read as an attempt to achieve nationally what had already been achieved locally. By the same token, the Rushdie affair made visible that British-style immigrant integration went along with a disturbing degree of ethnic assertiveness. As M. Anwar (1994: 23) observed in his survey on young Muslims in Britain, 'as a community and as individuals most have not become acculturated'.

It is important to point out that the religious identification of South-Asian immigrants in Muslim terms is a late and improbable development, given their extreme division along ethnic, clan, and sectarian lines.[65] Moreover, the emergent Muslim identity only reinforced a disposition for group closure and separation that has deeper cultural and social-structural roots. E. J. B. Rose's survey of first-generation immigrants from Pakistan, who provide the largest proportion of British Muslims,[66] found them 'as a people apart' (Rose, 1969: 448), organized along patrilinear village-kin groupings (*baridari*). Whereas West Indians migrated as individuals, Pakistanis did so as members of *baridaris*, with close kin pooling money to send one male member abroad, and the migrant sponsoring other relatives in turn. These *baridaris* kept controlling the individual in the diaspora, especially through the norm of arranged in-group (preferentially, first-cousin) marriage.[67] Interestingly, religion did not matter much in the early days, when Pakistani immigrants were predominantly male and return-oriented. According to E. J. B. Rose, there was 'very little religious observance among male Pakistanis; few said their prayers; few houses contained a copy of the Koran. Attendance at the mosque was very rare' (p. 446 f.). This changed with the onset of family reunification after the first Commonwealth Immigrants Act; now religious observance served as stabilizer of reconstituted family units. In her interesting study of the small Pakistani community in Oxford, Alison Shaw (1994: 36) argued that religious identification replaced the 'myth of return' as 'an effective way for migrants to maintain and control their distinctive culture and social structure'.

However, the Muslim label is no less fictitious than calling South-Asian immigrants Asians, Pakistanis, or Bangladeshis. The revaluation of religious identity and practices in the wake of family reunification went along with replicating the sectarian divisions of Muslims on the Indian subcontinent. There is a sequence from fusion, when one mosque in a particular locale was sufficient for the religious needs of all nominal Muslims, to fission, with each sect, caste, or ethnic group establishing their own place of prayer. Far from being political or even fundamentalist in orientation, as one might falsely conclude from the Rushdie affair, the various sects that make up British Islam are actually apolitical and moderate. Most of them had emerged after the British deposition of the Muslim Moghul dynasty in 1857, such as the orthodox-scriptural Deobandis and the populist-mystical Barelvis (who are the majority of British Muslims). These were sects specializing in the maintainance of Islam under non-Muslim rule, and they were thus tailor-made to be transferred from the Indian into the British diaspora. Tariq Modood (1990: 152) thus rightly asked how these accommodationist and pragmatic sects could be portrayed, in the wake of the Rushdie affair, as a 'radical assault upon British values, a threat to the state and an enemy to good race relations'.

But with the Rushdie affair a world-wide politicized Islam, particularly of Middle Eastern provenance, entered the British scene, casting aside old sectarian and national-origins divisions in favour of a unified and more militant Muslim identity. The Rushdie affair is only incompletely understood in domestic terms; it must be seen in the context of a transnationally operating Islamic movement. Consider the bewildering succession of places in which the Rushdie affair unfolded. Its first round occurred in far-away India, where outraged Muslims quickly achieved a legal ban of the book. Through the Jama'at-i Islami, a political sect advocating an Islamic state and operating both on the Indian subcontinent and in Britain, the campaign was carried to Britain. Jama'at-i's British arm, the Islamic Foundation in Leicester, sent photocopies of the book's incriminated parts to all Muslim organizations in Britain, as well as to the London embassies and High Commissioners of the states belonging to the Saudi-dominated Organization of Islamic Conference (OIC). After participating in a Union of Muslim Organizations meeting in London, Sher Azam, president of the Bradford Council of Mosques, carried the campaign down to the local level. The ritual burning of the *Satanic Verses* on 14

January 1989 in Bradford's central square, under the approving eyes of some of the city's Muslim notables, was the event that created the 'Rushdie affair' as a matter of domestic politics.[68]

Khomeini's infamous *fatwa*, issued in February 1989, catapulted the conflict back from domestic to international politics. Having first travelled from South Asia to Britain, the Rushdie affair now gravitated toward the Middle East, where Iran and Saudi Arabia were competing for leadership of the Islamic world. Before the *fatwa*, the British anti-Rushdie campaign was Saudi-dominated, consisting of discreet lobbying of publisher and government; after the *fatwa*, Iran was in charge, and the young Muslim protesters shouting in the streets of London that 'Rushdie must be chopped up' held up pictures of the Ayatollah. This was a significant coup: so far organized Islam in Britain had been supported by Saudi Arabia, which had poured some £50 million into the building of mosques and Islamic centres between 1980 and 1990 alone (Samad, 1992: 509). It was also an unlikely coup, because only 10 per cent of British Muslims belonged to the Iran-centred Shi'ite sect. The pro-Saudi Muslim bodies in Britain, such as the Union of Muslim Organizations, the Islamic Foundation, and the Muslim College, did not support the *fatwa*, and some moderate Islamic jurists pointed out that Islamic law applied only to Muslim citizens in pure Islamic states, but not in non-Islamic states (Malik, 1993). However, the strident defence of the Prophet had popular resonance. A Harris poll in September 1989 showed that about 80 per cent of those questioned favoured action against Rushdie; of these 35 per cent endorsed the death sentence, with the share rising to 45 per cent among young respondents (aged sixteen to twenty years) (Hiro, 1992: 187). The UK Action Committee on Islamic Affairs (UKACIA), formed in October 1988 by moderate Muslim leaders to lobby the government to ban the *Satanic Verses*, took an ambivalent position. Yes, the death penalty was jurisdictionally correct, because apostasy and blasphemy constituted a capital offence according to Islamic law; no, the sentence was not applicable outside the jurisdiction of Islamic law. That meant neither compromising nor condemning the *fatwa*: 'It is certainly not for the individual or Muslim leaders to lift the sentence, as it is not within their jurisdiction and it was not they who issued the *fatwa* in the first place' (Ahsan and Kidwai, 1993: 58).[69]

Whereas the *foulard* affair had united the French political and intellectual élites behind the defence of secularism (*laicité*) and Republican assimilation, the Rushdie affair divided the British élite, which reflects the entrenchment of multiculturalism in Britain. Parts of the Labour

Party, especially those dependent on the Muslim vote, sided with the anti-Rushdie campaign. Labour deputy-leader Roy Hattersley, from the predominantly Muslim district of Birmingham Sparkbrook, denounced the *Satanic Verses* as 'intentional blasphemy' and called 'racist' the proposition that Muslims should 'stop behaving like Muslims'.[70] Jack Straw, Labour's education spokesman, used the occasion to commit his party to the controversial Muslim demands for single-sex education and state-financed Muslim schools. Max Madden, Labour MP for Bradford West, urged his party to console the Muslims: 'We understand, we know that you've been hurt.'[71] So did the Church of England, which supported the Muslim campaign for an amended Blasphemy Law that protected not only the Christian faith. Some Conservatives, like Foreign Secretary Geoffrey Howe, disliked the parts of the *Satanic Verses* deemed offensive to British society, and sided at least indirectly with the Muslims: 'The book is extremely critical and rude about us and compares Britain to Hitler's Germany. We resent that, and don't like it any more than the people of the Muslim faith like the attacks on their faith contained in the *Satanic Verses*.'[72] This motley coalition of Muslim sympathizers was united by a Burkean distaste for defending abstract principles, such as 'free speech', over historically reached accords and understandings.

On the other hand, the Rushdie affair led to an unprecedented questioning of multiculturalism, even by those who had helped to create the latter. Roy Jenkins, hero of the liberal hour, now found some 'assumptions of the Sixties' retroactively invalidated, even wishing that 'we might have been more cautious about allowing the creation in the 1950s of substantial Muslim communities here'.[73] The chairman of the Commission for Racial Equality (CRE) ritually invoked that 'British society must learn how to give space and value to other cultures', but added a caveat not heard from these quarters before: 'that does not mean abandoning its [British society's] own beliefs and traditions' (Day, 1990: 109). In fact, the Rushdie affair induced a reflection on the British 'beliefs and traditions' that every minority group had to respect. In an Open Letter to British Muslims, the Home Office Minister of State, John Patten, laid down the government position of 'What it means to be British', particularly what it means to be a 'British Muslim'.[74] The Home Office minister reassured the Muslims that no one expected them to 'lay aside their faith, traditions or heritage'. But he emphasized the necessity of a shared link to keep a pluriethnic society together. According to the government, this shared link consisted of two principles: freedom of speech and the rule of law. Far from repudiating multiculturalism, this moderate response by a Conservative government sought to reconcile multiculturalism with a minimal sense of Britishness: 'At the heart of our thinking is a Britain where Christians, Muslims, Jews, Hindus, Sikhs and others can all work and live together, each retaining proudly their own faith and identity, but each sharing in common the bond of being by birth or choice, British.'[75]

In the wake of the Rushdie affair, three Muslim demands crystallized at the national level: extending the Blasphemy Law to other religions, including Islam; outlawing religious discrimination, analogous to already outlawed race discrimination; and supporting Muslim schools with state funds. All three demands were rebuffed by the government. Regarding the law of blasphemy, the government faced the odd demand to reactivate and extend a law that had been applied only six times in the last 120 years, and that the Law Commission had recommended to abolish in 1985. In the Home Office's Open Letter to Muslims, the government refused to amend the Blasphemy Law, citing the difficulty of defining which faith qualified for protection and the rush of 'divisive' and 'damaging' litigation expected in case of an amendment (UKACIA, 1989: 9).[76] Regarding the introduction of religious anti-discrimination law, Muslims have pointed to the laws against religious hatred and discrimination already in place in Northern Ireland.[77] By the same token, reference to the exceptional situation of Northern Ireland has allowed the government to refuse similar emergency legislation on the more tranquil British mainland.

By far the most delicate has been the long-standing Muslim demand for state-supported Muslim schools. One-third of all state-maintained schools in Britain have 'voluntary-aided' status, according to which schools are subject to private or denominational (instead of Local Educational Authority) control but nevertheless receive government funding. Why has this status been granted to Catholic or Jewish, but not to Muslim schools? The government has repeatedly stressed that it has no objection in principle to grant voluntary-aided status to Muslim schools, pointing instead to surplus places in existing schools due to a declining birth rate since 1970.[78] But it is an open secret that the government had set itself firmly against supporting separate Muslim schools, using existing vacancies, even allegedly ill-suited buildings, only as pretexts.[79] Why? Will Kymlicka (1992), who is not suspicious of anti-Muslim sentiment, cited the British Muslim campaign for separate schools as part of a larger attempt to establish a millet-like system of group rights that is repressive of individual liberties (p. 39). This is not far-fetched. Note that Muslim leaders have rejected the multicultural Swann Report for its secularism and relativistic perspective on religion, which would allow the Muslim child to take a critical attitude to Islam. According to the London-based Islamic Academy, the Swann Committee was guilty of '[imposing] on Muslim children what it considers of educational value—such as autonomy and a critical approach to their own faith and culture . . . The Muslim community cannot accept the secular philosophical basis of the report' (quoted in Kepel, 1997: 120). Similarly, the Muslim Parliament's White Paper on Muslim Education in Great Britain (1992) has criticized the multicultural curriculum for its 'dilution if not disintegration of traditional faith-based identity' (p. 13), presenting its quest for voluntary-aided status as one for an 'Islamic system of education' that was to '[insulate Muslim children] from the harmful effects of secularity and the sexual permissiveness it often encourages' (p. 30). There is no easy solution to dealing with an illiberal group in a liberal state. Granting voluntary-aided status would certainly fuel the separatist thrust of British Muslims, which is why the government has stubbornly denied this request. But it would also make the National Curriculum (passed in the 1988 Education Act) mandatory for Muslim schools, and thus enable the government to better control the latter.

State intransigence in the Rushdie affair and world political events have further isolated and radicalized British Muslims. The Gulf War in 1991, which saw Western troops trampling on the holy land of *Hijaz*,[80] fuelled the confrontation between Islam and the West, subjecting British Muslims to a loyalty conflict. After the Allied bombing of a bunker in Baghdad that killed close to 300 civilians, the Bradford Council of Mosques professed its 'deep outrage': 'These deaths must . . . be avenged in accordance with Islamic law in due course.'[81] Bradford Muslims obviously sided with Iraq rather than the British troops that were part of the Allied forces.[82] The Bosnian crisis shortly thereafter created a sense of Muslims 'as the world's persecuted people'.[83] Even Zaki Badawi, a respected British Muslim intellectual and a voice of moderation in the Rushdie affair, gave in to a conspiratorial view of the West hounding Islam: 'The West is back to its old tricks and has no qualms about Muslims being massacred . . . There is now a tremendous feeling across Europe that Muslim lives are devalued, that to be a Muslim is dangerous, and an apprehension that we will be hounded out of Europe.'[84] The chain of events from Rushdie to Gulf War to Bosnia made British Muslims discover their Muslimness. A young female Muslim academic, who refused to wear the headscarf and had been pro-Rushdie, expresses her experience: 'After Rushdie, the Gulf War, and now Bosnia, I have been forced to describe myself in terms of my religion.'[85]

A demographic characteristic of British Muslims is their young age. In 1991, 42.5 per cent of Pakistanis and 47.3 per cent of Bangladeshis were under sixteen years old (as against 19.3 per cent of white Britons) (see Joly 1995: 6). As recent studies have shown (Knott and Khokher, 1993; Jacobson, 1997), young Muslims are prone to develop a Muslim identity that is purged of ethnic or national-origins components. Estranged from a country of origin most of them have never seen, young Muslims seek membership in a world-wide *umma* that compensates for their marginal existence in Britain. Characteristic for many, a young Muslim interviewed by Jacobson (1997: 245) describes herself: '[I would identify myself] hopefully as a Muslim! That's how I'd like to be recognised—not as a Pakistani—or a British person or anything. As a Muslim.' Interestingly, the non-ethnic Muslim identities among youngsters are adopted more by peer than by parental pressure, and they are often a deliberate stance against the traditional ways of the older generation. In London's Tower Hamlets, a stronghold of Bengali Muslims, there is a youth culture of wearing the headscarf (referred to by the Arabic word *hijab* rather than the Bengali *burka*), of opposing arranged marriage because in Islam (as opposed to Bengali culture) women have the right to choose their partners, and of taking self-defence classes (something young Muslims have picked up from anti-racists). From this viewpoint, the parents' world is 'doing things for appearances', from which true Islam offers a rescue.[86]

The disposition for a non-ethnic Islam is articulated by new political groups. Already the Muslim Parliament, created in 1992 by the former Guardian journalist Kalim Siddiqui as the 'next best thing' to a territorial Islamic state in Britain,[87] was dominated by 'new' intellectuals apart from the traditional *ulama* (clergy).[88] It gave a prominent place to women, and conducted its affairs in English to bridge ethnic differences. Siddiqui's strange mimicking of British parliamentary traditions would be anathema to the more militant *Hizb ut Tahrir* (Islamic Liberation Party), which now dominates the Muslim student societies at London colleges and universities. For *Hizb ut Tahrir*, 'there is no such thing as a British Muslim. There are only Muslims.'[89] Linked to Middle East terrorist groups like the Palestinian Hamas or the Algerian FIS and opposing the Iranian Shi'ite regime, *Hizb ut Tahrir* advocates a global Islamic state (Caliphate) to unite all Sunni Muslims in the world.[90]

London is now the headquarters of the world's Islamic movements, which are competing for the allegiance of young British Muslims. Traditional Islamic organizations are trying hard to win back the disaffected young, often at the cost of giving in to fundamentalist chic. The 1995 International Islamic Conference in London, held one week before *Hizb ut Tahrir* was scheduled to rally in Trafalgar Square, lined up fundamentalists from Sudan, the United States, and Bangladesh.[91] British Muslim leaders realize that the extreme fragmentation of British Islam, divided into some 1,400 Islamic organizations and 1,000 mosques, has allowed the media-amplified, radical groups to prosper. But the attempt to create, in co-ordination with the Home Office, a Board of British Muslims (modelled on the Board of Deputies of British Jews) has so far been unsuccessful, because of the opposition from entrenched mosque committees and traditional clergymen. A member of the Bradford Council of Mosques explains the difficulty: 'Such a body would be impossible to set up. We all come from different countries and different sects.'[92]

A Nation against Europe

There is a new genre in the British race-relations literature: travel notes from Europe. A Muslim activist attending a Council of Europe conference on Women and Migration felt like a 'time-traveller beamed backwards': 'I realised that however bad things were in Britain for Muslims, they were much, much worse in Europe . . . I returned to Britain, happy to be home, and happy to be British.'[93] The negative attitude toward Europe is a good indicator of successful immigrant integration in Britain. If confronted with the lesser tolerance for minority identities and the weaker anti-discrimination provisions in the other member states of the European Union, even hardened race activists switch to a triumphalist reading of the British race-relations framework. Herman Ouseley, the former anti-racist from Brent and current chair of the CRE, is proud of 'the best anti-discrimination legislation in Europe', and he salutes the black and Asian people who 'fly the Union flag with pride to positively demonstrate their Britishness'.[94]

Against Europe the British nation stands united, the immigrant minorities included. Strikingly, when Conservative Home Secretary Michael Howard rejected new plans for harmonized anti-discrimination laws at the European level in reference to the 'effective legislation' already in place in Britain, the CRE was on his side, fearing a possible downgrading (Favell, 1998: 329).[95] When confronted with immigrant activists on the Continent, the Britishness of race-relations activists is thrown into sharp relief. Catherine Neveu (1994) reports the odd wish of a group of British race-relations activists to 'meet Black people' in France, not knowing that to their Algerian immigrant hosts the distinction between *immigrés* and French was more relevant than one in terms of race. In such encounters one sees, flash-like, the unwitting nationalization of immigrants across Europe.

Consider the lukewarm British reception of the Migrants Forum, set up by the European Commission in 1989 as a sounding-board for the problems of Europe's immigrant populations. The Migrants Forum seeks to strengthen the position of third-state nationals in the European Union—clearly not a problem for British immigrants who always had citizenship status. Accordingly, the CRE helped set up a rival organization in Brussels, the Standing Conference on Racial Equality in Europe (SCORE), to concentrate on free movement for European citizens marked by non-white skin. This is a very British perspective, and one that turns its back on the more pressing problems of asylum-seekers, the stateless, and new non-citizen migrants in Europe. Britain's postcolonial immigrants are national egoists no less than the Europhobic political élite. 'Multiculturalism in one nation' (Favell, 1998: 342) has made immigrants Britons, after all.

This chapter discussed the peculiar problem of integrating (nominal) co-nationals, whose major distinguishing mark was race. To accomplish this, Britain counterpointed its restrictive immigration policy with a liberal race-relations policy. It stood in a tension between Marshallian citizenship universalism and racial-group particularism, moving toward the latter over time. While race-relations policy stopped short of affirmative action, it practised multiculturalism *avant la lettre*. A statist race-relations consensus bred the tendency to be outflanked by a militant 'anti-racist' Left and a nationalist 'anti-antiracist' Right. I have shown this in the tempestuous course of local race politics in the 1980s. A second, more recent challenge to the British race-relations consensus has been raised by Muslims, who emerged as a separate claimant in the Rushdie affair. Their demand for religious recognition shows the limits of an integration approach that has extolled race at the cost of other group markers. Perhaps more importantly still, Muslim demands for separate Islamic schools and book-banning show the limits of multiculturalism in a liberal state.

8

Conclusion: Resilient Nation-States

Nation-states may be looked at in two different ways. In a particularizing view, a nation-state is a thing with a name that does not happen twice in the world. In this view, nation-states, each with its distinct history and identity, are bedrocks of particularism in a world that is undergoing economic and cultural homogenization—which is, perhaps, why people cling so desperately to this antiquated thing. In a generalizing view, nation-states are the same everywhere, characterized by 'structural isomorphism' despite differences in resources and traditions (Meyer *et al.*, 1997). In this view, the world is divided into like units, nation-states, each characterized by the same structural features, such as sovereignty and citizenship, and legitimized by the same narratives of progress and rational action.

Depending on the view taken, this book can be summarized in two ways. From a particularizing view, it has revealed sharply distinct immigration experiences, conditioned by the particular nation-state undergoing immigration. In this view, the nation-state figured as independent variable, with particular nationhood conceptions and nation-state problematiques channelling immigration in distinct ways.

The United States, under the impact of the domestic civil-rights revolution that outlawed racial discrimination, reopened itself to the outside world as a universal 'nation of immigrants' that welcomed newcomers not just from Europe, but from all parts of the world equally. As I have pointed out, this has not been the only concept of American nationhood, but the one that has come to prevail since the 1960s. America's self-description as a nation of immigrants, which is now shared across the political élite spectrum, has allowed it to remain expansive toward immigrants even in times of economic contraction and domestic backlash. So powerful is the hold of this national self-description that even the political movement to restrict immigration has generally not dared question it—its mainstream, represented by the 1990s Federal Commission on Immigration Reform, opposes only specific categories or aspects of immigration, such as illegal immigration or legal immigrants' access to welfare benefits, but not immigration per se.

Germany and Britain offer sharp contrasts to the American immigration experience. (West) Germany, an incomplete nation-state until 1990, prolonged its legacy of ethnic nationhood under the mantle of defining itself as homeland state of all Germans who were dispersed by the consequences of World War II and suffered reprisal under communist regimes. It is no small irony that Germany, the perpetrator, and Israel, the victim, emerged after World War II as the two countries with the most pronounced systems of ethnic-priority immigration. As long as Germany was divided, and the free western part defined itself as the homeland of all Germans who were unfree to determine their own fate—a definition enshrined in the Preamble of the Basic Law, Germany could tolerate immigrants only as 'guestworkers', who were expected to stay out of the nation's own unfinished business. After unification and the demise of communism, the dual approach of excluding guestworkers and including ethnic Germans has lost its rationale. Accordingly, less than a decade after this historical caesura, ethnic-priority immigration has been phased out, guestworkers and their offspring are encouraged to enter the citizenry, and the ritual formula that Germany is 'not a country of immigration' has receded from political discourse.

If Germany's particular nation-state problematique channelling postwar immigration was that political boundaries were smaller than the cultural boundaries of nationhood, imperial Britain's reverse problematique was that political boundaries were larger than those of the nation. As a result, Britain had immigration from its former colonies, unimpeded at first, and its gradual containment coincided with the devolution of empire and evolution into a nation-state proper, in which political overlap with cultural boundaries. Such postcolonial immigration had little in common with either guestworker immigration, German-style, or wanted-settler immigration, US-style. It was politically processed within a dual, strangely contradictory, approach of closing down essentially unwanted immigration, in which immigration policy from the start was a control policy aiming at zero-immigration, and of providing full, substantive citizenship rights to those who had entered with formal membership rights at hand, within an exceptionally liberal regime of multiculturalism *avant la lettre*.

In this particularizing reading, this book has tried to differentiate more clearly than previous studies have done between the different logics of guestworker, postcolonial, and wanted-settler immigration, in the context of the particular nationhood constellations in which they occurred. These three logics encompass a good part of the immigration that Western states underwent after World War II. Juxtaposing them, one sees more clearly than before a major difference between the United States and Europe combined: German guestworker and British postcolonial immigration have come to an end; by contrast, American wanted-settler immigration is an ongoing process. In Germany and Britain, the closing of legal immigration has shifted the focus of immigration policy to containing mass asylum-seeking and, increasingly, illegal immigration, and this within the new parameters of the emergent European Union that has removed all immigration barriers for member-state nationals and now sees itself confronted with controlling the entry and stay of third-state nationals. Accordingly, an entirely new, as yet protean and unchartered, immigration problematique is opening up in Germany and Britain as members of the European Union, which could be touched upon here only in passing. By contrast, America is likely to experience more of the same, described in some detail in this book—client politics over the size and nature of legal immigration quotas, renewed, and probably inconclusive, attempts to contain illegal immigration, and (more muted perhaps than in the past) racial claims-making in education, employment, and politics.

From a generalizing view, this book comes to a different set of conclusions. This view turns the nation-state from independent to dependent variable, looking at immigration as a challenge to some of the nation-state's generic features, such as sovereignty and citizenship.[1] From this angle, this book can be summarized in two propositions. First, there is no sign that the sovereignty of liberal states to admit or reject aliens is waning. Constraints on sovereignty are self-imposed, rather than externally inflicted, and they stem from the domestic logic of client politics, the autonomy of the legal process in liberal states, and (particularly in Europe) moral obligations toward particular immigrant groups. Secondly, there is little evidence that the postnational membership schemes established in some (continental European) states in response to postwar immigration have rendered national citizenship less important. As especially the German case made clear, citizenship for immigrants matters. At the same time, such citizenship comes without the expectation of assimilation, at least in the states considered here.[2] It is multicultural citizenship, in which immigrants are allowed, even encouraged, to maintain their ethnic identities, as long as these do not clash with the basic procedural rules of liberal states.

Whatever view is taken, particularizing or generalizing, this study found nation-states resilient in the face of immigration. This is a trivial outcome if one takes the nation-state as an independent variable, which precludes consideration of its possible transformation in response to immigration. It is a non-trivial outcome if immigration is seen as impacting on the nation-state as a dependent variable. In the second view, the diagnosis of resilient sovereignty and citizenship sets a counterpoint to popular diagnoses, more often journalistic than scholarly, that the nation-state is in decline. In the following, I seek to refute a more serious version of the nation-state-in-decline hypothesis, which argues that states are globally impaired to control immigration effectively and that postnational membership has devalued, perhaps even rendered obsolete, national citizenship. I close with an outlook of the immigration challenges in that part of the world where the decline of the nation-state seems to be most obvious: the emergent European Union.

Self-Limited Sovereignty

A basic image in recent writings on immigration and refugee policies is this: sovereign states have an interest in keeping out foreign migrants; but they meet foreign migrants protected by universal human-rights norms and regimes; and if states accept unwanted immigrants, then it is because they give in to externally imposed obligations. This is a view of the state as externally constrained by global human-rights precepts (e.g. Jacobson, 1996; Soysal, 1994). It is sometimes combined with a political economy argument, according to which state attempts to control the movement of people in a world of global factor mobility are futile—if money, goods, and ideas flow effortlessly around the globe, people will have to follow eventually (Sassen, 1998).

The opposition of an external human-rights regime and sovereign states may be justified in the case of illiberal states or fledgling democracies (see Sikkink, 1993; Risse and Sikkink, 1997). It is misleading in the case of liberal states, in which the protection of human rights is embedded in domestic law and traditions. This changes the basic image: sovereignty and human rights are still conflicting principles, but they are located under the roof of liberal states. If liberal states accept unwanted immigrants, then it is because of self-limited, rather than globally limited, sovereigny (see Joppke, 1998*b*). The typical conflict in immigration control is not a monolithic, sovereign state pitted against, and presumably dodging, external human-rights obligations, but a restrictionist executive pitted against independent courts who defend the family or resident rights of immigrants on the basis of domestic law.[3]

The diagnosis of globally limited sovereignty may be countered in two ways. First, its premiss of an golden age of state sovereignty, which is said to have come to an end in the age of globalization, is false. The Westphalian state, understood as a form of political rule based on territory and immunity from outside interference, has always been compromised, voluntarily by conventions and contracts or involuntarily by coercion and imposition: 'Compromising the Westphalian model is always available as a policy option because there is no authority structure to prevent it' (Krasner, 1995*a*: 117). Human-rights considerations, in particular, have been one form of compromising sovereignty since the inception of the modern state system. International human-rights regimes are no invention of the postwar era. The first such regime was the Peace of Westphalia, which mandated religious toleration from its signing princes and monarchs; other examples are the abolition of the slave trade under British leadership or the Wilsonian minority protections after World War I, which were forcibly imposed on the successor states of the Habsburg and Ottoman empires (Krasner, 1995*b*). The universal human-rights regime set up after World War II is only the latest attempt to discipline states from the outside, and one of the less effective at that.

Political scientists have long grappled with the paradox that sovereign states set up international regimes only to curtail their range of action (see Krasner, 1983). Realists, for whom inter-state relations are zero-sum games between strong and weak states, argue that strong states set up international regimes to further their interests, to the detriment of weak states. A liberal co-operation perspective argues that international regimes are a response to market failure, allowing states to overcome the prisoners' dilemma and to make all better off, the weak included. Steven Krasner (1995*b*: 140 f.) showed that international human-rights regimes, while dear to liberals, cannot be understood from a liberal perspective: if all states were committed to the same principles of human rights, there would be no need for an international regime. Instead, international human-rights regimes are devised to make some states behave in ways they would not otherwise behave. Human-rights regimes thus require a realist explanation: 'Only when powerful states enforced principles and norms were international human rights regimes consequential' (ibid. 141).

How does the universal human-rights regime established by the United Nations after World War II fare on this account? If its strength depends on the will of powerful states to implement its norms and principles, it would be absurd to assume that the United States, the world's hegemon, would use it against itself, or against the Western allies that had helped to set it up. There is also no need for liberal states to turn to an international human-rights regime for settling their internal affairs because this regime has only externalized the norms and principles that these states have always adhered to internally. But even against illiberal offenders of international regime norms the range of intervention has been limited, and human-rights concerns have generally been subordinated to the principle of non-interference. An exception is intervention against newly set-up states with non-democratic regimes, outside the communist hemisphere. The strongest injection of human-rights norms into inter-state relations is the protection under international law not of sovereignty as such, but of popular sovereignty (Reisman, 1990). Article 1 of the UN Charter establishes as one of its purposes friendly relations between states, 'based on respect for the principles of equal rights and self-determination of peoples' (p. 867). Accordingly, the major legitimation for US-led, Western interference in the domestic affairs of other states has been the violation of the popular sovereignty norm by autocratic regimes, such as in Grenada, Panama, or Haiti.

Regarding immigration, the universal human-rights regime has put two major limits on state discretion: the right of asylum and the principle of racial non-discrimination. Both have matured into customary international law that is binding on states. Refugee and asylum law, particularly its non-refoulement principle, is the strongest limit on state discretion, reflecting the original impetus of the UN regime, the protection of individuals qua individuals from criminal states. But note that international asylum law leaves state sovereignty fully intact, because it makes asylum a right of the state to grant asylum, not a right of the individual to enjoy asylum. Accordingly, the restrictive asylum laws passed by most Western states in response to post-1980s mass asylum-seeking revoked self-imposed, generous asylum rules and practices that had exceeded these states' international obligations (see Joppke, 1997: 262 f.). A second limit on state discretion is the principle not to discriminate against people on racial grounds. The non-discrimination principle is fully realized by source-country universalism in immigration policy. The United States made a beginning in abolishing its national-origins quota in 1965. However reluctantly, European states have followed, Britain phasing out its patrial scheme in the Nationality Act of 1981, and Germany its *Aussiedler* scheme in the *Kriegsfolgenbereinigungsgesetz* of 1992. If one excepts the special case of removing immigration restrictions for nationals of other member states in the European Union, and special transition rules for living patrials and ethnic Germans, there are no longer any ethnically or racially motivated double standards in European states' admission practices. Like all international law, the asylum and non-discrimination precepts are not enforceable against offenders. But the lack of sanctions does not render them ineffective. Most states follow their international obligations most of the time, if only to qualify as 'member[s] of good standing' in an increasingly interdependent world (Chayes and Chayes, 1995: 28).

Internationally guaranteed asylum and non-discrimination rights are only a small fraction of foreign-migrant rights. A second objection to the diagnosis of globally limited sovereignty is that crucial migrant rights, such as residence and family rights, have domestic, not international, roots. The United States, the hegemon of most international regimes set up after World War II, has notoriously ignored international human-rights conventions and treaties, refusing to incorporate the latter in domestic law. As we saw, the successive empowerment of legal permanent residents, illegal immigrants, and asylum-seekers draws upon a constitution that protects individuals qua persons rather than quacitizens. The recent slashing of the welfare rights of legal immigrants, however, demonstrates that this empowerment is reversible, if the federal government, backed by the plenary power doctrine, so decides (see Schuck, 1998).

Even in Europe, endowed with the highest density of international human-rights norms anywhere in the world, most migrant rights are grounded in domestic law. Only 2.5 per cent of the decisions of the European Court of Human Rights involve foreigner rights, and all were issued in the last ten years—after essential residence and family rights had already been established at the domestic level (Guiraudon, 1997: 14 f.). France, for instance, ratified the European Convention on Human Rights (ECHR) only in 1974, allowed individual petition under Article 25 in 1981, and gave full effect to Article 8 (which protects family life) as late as 1991. But the crucial decision by the Conseil d'Etat against government restrictions on foreign-family reunion occurred already in 1978, and its reference was the preamble of the domestic constitution that protects family rights (see Tomuschat, 1979). As Richard Plender (1988: 366) points out, a plethora of international and regional provisions notwithstanding, there is '[no] evidence of a right to family reunification in general international law'. One of the European Court's major family unification decisions, *Abdulaziz, Cabales and Balkandali* (1985), notably refused to deduce a right of family unification from Article 8 of the ECHR, while reaffirming that states have the right to prevent non-nationals from entering their territory. Family unification, a major source of legal immigration to Europe despite zero-immigration state policies, happened because of domestic, rather than international, legal constraints. And it is important to point out that even constitutionally protected family rights are not absolute, but weighed by courts against the equally legitimate interest of the state to curtail immigration. This is the spirit of the German Constitutional Court's 1987 decision in the Turkish and Yugoslav Case, which refused to deduce a right of entry for foreign spouses from the family clause of the Basic Law, but stipulated that the state's immigration policy had to be 'in proportion' to the family rights of settled foreigners.

Germany is still an extreme case of self-limited sovereignty. This is ironic, because Germany has readily incorporated all international human-rights treaties and conventions into domestic law, and (in Article 25 of the Basic Law) has even endowed the primacy of international over municipal law with constitutional dignity. But the extensive human-rights provisions in the Basic Law have rendered the resort to international law unnecessary, and accordingly few complaints have been filed against Germany before the European Court of Human Rights. Crucial protections of guestworkers from deportation, and residence and family rights have all been derived by domestic courts from a constitution that has gone further than any other constitution in the world to subject sovereign state powers to universal human rights. Judges helped make Germany a 'country of immigration', rendering obsolete the opposite state philosophy. Josef Isensee (1974) argued that the state's self-limitation *vis-à-vis* foreigners does not extend to the decision over first-time entry, which is discretionary. However, until the asylum reform of 1993, Germany's self-limitation even affected on-entry sovereignty, because its constitution granted asylum-seekers the unique right to have their cases examined by national courts.

Yasemin Soysal (1994) considers universal human rights less as a political regime than as global 'discourse', which shapes actors' identities—be they states, non-governmental organizations, or individuals: 'The notion of human rights . . . has become a pervasive element of world culture' (p. 7). To the degree that human rights are not legally or politically institutionalized, one could conceptualize them as moral constraints on states. However, a close look reveals that even such moral constraints do not meet states from the outside, as abstract human-rights precepts applied to indiscriminate migrants. Instead, moral human-rights considerations are always tied up with particular national responsibilities toward particular migrant groups. This is the case even in asylum debates, in which universal human-rights concerns are most prevalent. A study of parliamentary asylum debates in Switzerland, Germany, and Britain noted the absence of abstract moral argument, and the tendency of asylum advocates to present nationally bounded arguments in favour of generous asylum laws and practices (Steiner, 1997). This resonates with the findings presented in this book. German asylum advocates invoked a negative national history to derive special German responsibilities for asylum-seekers. The American liberalization of asylum law, which ran contrary to the parallel European developments, fed upon the positive founding myth of America as an 'asylum of nations' and the internal inconsistency of selecting refugees according to their country of origin, while (since 1965) immigrants could enter without national-origin restrictions.

The gradation of moral obligations toward particular immigrant groups is especially visible in Europe. In order to phase out postcolonial and guestworker immigration, European states developed a language of primary and secondary immigration that has no parallel in the United States. Moral obligations are strongest *vis-à-vis* primary immigrants, who have been actively recruited, and they become weaker *vis-à-vis* secondary immigrants, who have entered in recognition of the family rights of primary immigrants. Accordingly, Germany allowed its recruited guestworkers to bring in their spouses without restrictions, while imposing a waiting-period on the foreign spouses of second-generation immigrants. Similarly, Britain (until 1988) allowed its primary New Commonwealth immigrants to bring in their spouses freely, while subjecting the post-1973 generation to its tough marriage tests. Both countries thus concentrated their moral obligations on particular immigrant groups. This allowed them to cold-shoulder the rest. Immigration did not make European countries 'nations of immigrants'. Primary immigrants were simply subjected to the exigencies of nation-building as usual, while toward the outer layers of secondary (and tertiary) immigration the sense of moral obligation and the family rights of migrants became successively weaker. Without such gradations, primary immigration would have forever spun forward new immigration, which European states were not willing to accept.

As mentioned earlier, Britain does not fully fit the theory of self-limited sovereignty. But neither does it fit the opposite theory of globally limited sovereignty. Gary Freeman (1994: 297) even argues: 'The British experience demonstrates that it is possible to limit unwanted immigration.' Britain's exceptional efficacy of immigration control has been visible in its conflation of asylum with immigration policy, and the cold-hearted removal of the Immigration Act's Section 1(5), which had exempted primary immigrants from the marriage tests, once it came in the way of controlling secondary immigration. I attributed this efficacy to two factors, the weak sense of moral obligation toward immigration that has never been wanted, and the absence of an autonomous legal system keeping the executive in check. In Britain, Parliament is sovereign, and it may grant and take away individual rights as it sees fit. It is important to see that the lack of constitutional rights affects citizens and immigrants alike (even though this distinction is moot in the case of most postcolonial immigrants). Accordingly, the British fight against secondary immigration has pushed the family rights of all citizens below the European standard. There are signs that in the course of Europeanization British exceptionalism is coming to an end. In *M* v. *Home Office*, the Court of Appeal's unwillingness to grant 'crown immunity' to a high-handed executive violating elementary asylum rights ventured on continental-style judicial review, and the new Labour government has pledged to incorporate the European Convention on Human Rights into domestic law, which would introduce an equivalent to a written constitution.

Self-limited sovereignty has made liberal states broadly expansionist, rather than restrictionist, toward immigrants.[4] This is, for instance, expressed in the fact that after the general switch to zero-immigration policies in post-1973 Western Europe large-scale immigration continued, though at a reduced pace.[5] But it would be wrong to conclude from this that the sovereignty of liberal states to control immigration is in decline. The thesis of sovereignty in decline may be operationalized as two separate claims (see Freeman, 1998): first, that the locus of decision-making over immigration policy is shifting from nation-states to extranational, particularly supranational, actors; second, that the empirical capacity of states to implement immigration controls is waning. For both claims there is no empirical evidence. The emergent immigration and refugee regime of the European Union, the most extreme instance of an international, in important respects even supranational immigration regime, has strengthened the capacity of member states to control the entry of third-state nationals—otherwise the polemical notion of Fortress Europe would make no sense (see Bigo, 1997; Koslowski, 1998). Regarding the claim of declining empirical capacity, there is much evidence for the opposite claim that state capacity is growing over time. Modern technology has greatly increased the infrastructural power of the state, allowing the German state to screen its border to Poland with infrared devices, the British state to detect false family unification claims through genetic fingerprinting, and the Schengen states to beef-up their external borders through advanced information systems. In addition, legal niceties like visa schemes, carrier sanctions, and the creation of anomalous, extraterritorial zones at airports and other points of entry (for the latter, see Neuman, 1997) have allowed states to deflect unwanted entrants from their territory.

Dramatic scenarios of a pending 'migration crisis' in the West (e.g. Hollifield, 1994), which proliferated after the breakdown of communism, are exaggerated. Most people do not move. Of the 5 billion people making up the current world population only 120 million (2.5 per cent) live outside their country of origin or citizenship. Moreover, receiving states continue to be open only to particular migrant nationalities, which reflect historical migration legacies. Seventy per cent of the foreigners living in France in the early 1990s were EU nationals or originated in the former French colonies of North Africa, 50 per cent of new permanent settlers in Britain in 1991 stemmed from New Commonwealth countries or Pakistan, and the largest groups of asylum-seekers in Germany in 1995 were from Yugoslavia and Turkey, Germany's main guestworker countries (Messina, 1996: 143 f.).[6] Considering that the breakdown of communism, in combination with modern transport and information technologies, have driven to the extreme the core contradiction of the international migration system—free exit and restricted entry, Western states have proved remarkably resilient to new migration pressures. If 'poor people at the gate' was the alarmist cry in the early 1990s,[7] swift asylum reforms across Western states have rendered such fears baseless. As a result of asylum restrictions, the total numbers of asylum-seekers are down in most OECD countries (Freeman, 1998: 95), Germany being the extreme with a decline from over 400,000 new asylum-claimants in 1993 to just over 100,000 in 1997.[8] Certainly, closing one gate of entry will only open another one. In response to the quietening of the asylum front, illegal immigration, now propelled by organized human smuggling and transnationally operating crime cartels, has made new headways, especially in Europe. But, judged by past experience, states will respond quickly and effectively. Containing illegal immigration and combating transnational crime is already on top of the agenda of European interior ministers and driving further attempts at European harmonization.[9] Acting alone or in concert, nation-states are not likely to give in to perpetually new migration challenges.

Citizenship Matters

The postnational membership argument is closely linked with, in some respects implied by, the argument of globally limited sovereignty. It suffers from the same weaknesses: a hypostasized before and after, and a false projection of domestic state functions to the transnational level. Regarding the first, the postnational membership argument is premised on a colossus of 'national citizenship' that never was. Yasemin Soysal (1997: 6) thinks that in the old nation-states 'national belonging constitutes the source of rights and duties of individuals'. This is a fiction, building upon T. H. Marshall's flawed identification of individual rights with citizen rights. Contrary to Marshall's assumption that civil, political, and social rights in modern states are all citizen rights, civil and social rights have never been dependent on citizenship (see Ferrajoli, 1996). Instead, modern constitutions, since the French Declaration of the Rights of Man and Citizens of 1789, have conceived of civil and social rights as rights of the person residing in the territory of the state, irrespective of her citizenship status. Article 7 of Napoleon's Civil Code states that 'the exercise of civil rights is independent of citizenship status' (ibid. 4). These civil rights, which are invested in personhood rather than citizenship, include the right to freedom (of speech, opinion, and the press), the right to private autonomy (that is, to conclude contracts and act in law), and the right of ownership. Later on, when states took on welfare functions, civil rights were accompanied by social rights, which were likewise not premised on citizenship, but on residence and labour-market participation. Since their inception in Bismarckian Germany, social insurance schemes took territoriality as their reference point; after all, they had arisen only in response to industrial-age migrations and the incapability of local poor-relief provisions to cope with them (Zacher, 1993: 448). Accordingly, Paragraph 30 of the German Social Statute (*Sozialgesetzbuch*) states: 'The regulations of this statute are binding for all persons who are residents in the realm of its validity [*in seinem Geltungsbereich*]' (ibid. 445). The only class of rights reserved since 1789 to the citizen is the political right to take part in the formation of the general will and to hold public office.

As Luigi Ferrajoli (1996: 12) notes, in modern constitutions there are two civil rights generally *not* extended to persons, but reserved to citizens: residence and free movement in the state's territory. The dramatic moment in the evolution of migrant rights was the decoupling of resident and free-movement rights from citizenship. Only, this was not a postnational moment driven by abstract human-rights considerations. Instead, it was a crypto-national moment that equated long-term residency with *de facto* membership in the national community. This is especially visible in the German case. German legal scholars coined the notion of 'legal fate of dependency' (*Rechtsschicksal der Unentrinnbarkeit*) to justify the near-total approximation of non-citizen to citizen rights. Once the labour migrants had struck deep roots in German society, a return to the home country was no longer a realistic option, and they had become dependent on protection by the German state, this state could no longer withhold from them crucial residence and other rights usually reserved for citizens. The underlying motif is communitarian, not universalist: migrants are not conceived of as abstract holders of human rights, but as particular members of a community with historically derived entitlements to due consideration and protection.

This extension of residence rights to non-citizens is not unconditional: it applies only if the state had not clarified *ex ante* the ultimate termination of residence, and the foreign migrant had reason to plan her life in the new society. Accordingly, the German Constitutional Court argued in the Indian Case (1978) that the non-citizen plaintiff had a constitutionally protected 'reliance interest' (*Vertrauensschutz*) in a renewed residence permit only because the state had not originally prescribed its non-renewability. The German guestworker programme thus turned into *de facto* immigration not because of some general logic of postnational membership, but because the state had failed to be firm and explicit about the temporal limitation of its guestworker recruitment. Interestingly, the German state has learned from this experience. Its second-generation guestworker programmes, established since the early 1990s with Poland and other Eastern European countries, include strict termination clauses and legal safeguards to prevent permanent settlement (Rudolph, 1996). The obvious gradation of migrant rights cannot be captured within the postnational membership model, according to which all migrants alike are protected by the same rights of personhood.

The communitarian logic of investing (some, not all) labour migrants with permanent resident and free-movement rights casts doubt on Soysal's (1997: 8) blanket statement that 'rights acquire a more universalistic form and are divorced from national belonging'. Flawed is not only the implicit assumption of a comprehensive 'national citizenship', which never was. Flawed is also the assumed dualism between rights, transposed to the transnational level, and states. This is where the postnational membership argument meets the argument of globally impaired state sovereignty. Both invite the same objection: individual rights are not external to, but part and parcel of liberal states. Otherwise one could not explain why human-rights constraints are more urgently felt in the states of the West than, for instance, in the migrant-receiving states in the Middle East, which do not allow their foreign workers to acquire property or to bring in their families, and which routinely practise mass expulsions (see Weiner, 1995: 80–3).

The postnational membership model meets two further objections: it lacks spatial and temporal markers. Regarding space, Soysal (1994) derives her postnational model from the Western European experience, but claims that it is 'not exclusive to Europe' (p. 156). This is consistent with its globalizing thrust. But it is empirically questionable. As we saw, even within Europe the model does not apply to the British case, which moved in the opposite direction from non-national membership (as pre-national subjectship) to national citizenship. For a while at least, it applied to the German case, which used postnational membership to leave its ethnic citizenship regime intact. Postnational membership was (West) Germany's 'national model' of integrating immigrants. While postnational membership thus has a certain relevance for (some) European ethnic nation-states, it must be an awkward concept for American ears. The low entry thresholds into a non-ethnic, politically constituted immigrant nation have minimized the importance of second-tier membership. There are no 'postnational members' in the United States, only permanent resident aliens who have not yet naturalized. Most importantly, a civic-territorial citizenship regime guarantees that there will never be postnational members in the second generation.

Regarding time, postnational membership is seen as having a clear beginning—the postwar period, but as having no end. Its proponents hypostasize the historically specific adjustment to a finite immigration episode into a fundamental transformation of nation-states. Soysal (1994: 139) clearly delimits her postnational membership model from 'denizenship' models that treat second-tier membership as an anomaly subject to correction and that remain 'within the confines of the nation-state model'. She continues: 'As I see it, the incorporation of guestworkers is no mere expansion of the scope of national citizenship, nor is it an irregularity. Rather, it reveals a profound transformation in the institution of citizenship, both in its institutional logic and in the way it is legitimated' (ibid.). However, immigrant-receiving societies have treated a generations-spanning postnational membership of significant portions of their population as an intolerable anomaly. In Germany, there is no political actor today, the immigrants included, who does not consider the permanent exclusion of second- and third-generation foreigners from the citizenry as a serious deficit. For postnational membership advocates, the current movement, overwhelmingly supported by the moderate conservative to left-liberal spectrum, in favour of *jus soli* citizenship for third-generation immigrants must be utterly incomprehensible.[10] As a generations-spanning phenomenon, non-citizen membership is not celebrated; it is detested. Similarly, in the United States, the drastic cutting of welfare benefits for legal immigrants has demonstrated the inherent political vulnerabilities of non-citizens. The current urge by immigrants to naturalize,[11] which includes previous naturalization laggards like Hispanics, may be instrumentally motivated. But it suggests that citizenship matters, even in a country where it historically has not mattered much. Only if postnational membership advocates could show that such membership is a recurrent, transmittable, and positively valued status with its own institutional apparatus would it be a viable alternative to national citizenship.

While citizenship matters, it is increasingly decoupled from the expectation of cultural assimilation. This contradicts Rogers Brubaker's (1992) assumption of inert 'cultural idioms' of nationhood determining distinct citizenship laws, policies, and identities over the centuries. States with *jus soli* regimes, like the United States, have to routinely accept the decoupling of citizenship from cultural assimilation, because they have no means of withholding citizenship from second-generation immigrants. Perhaps for this reason, the United States still clings to an assimilation requirement, however minimal and ritual, in its naturalization procedure for first-generation immigrants. However, a dramatic transformation occurred in the German naturalization procedure, which shifted not only from a discretionary to an as-of-right mode (as in the United States), but was also decoupled from an individual assimilation test. This reflects a common trend in liberal states not to require the cultural assimilation of their immigrants, not even at the point of acquiring citizenship.[12] Irrespective of national variations, liberal states share an intransitive notion of immigrant integration, in which immigrants are free to pursue their own ways of life.

The multiculturalism of liberal states may be illustrated by three court rules, issued almost simultaneously in different parts of Europe on a touchy issue—the education of Muslim girls (see Albers, 1994). In November 1989, the French Conseil d'Etat decided that Muslim girls had the right to wear a veil in school, as long as this was the expression of their religious identity and they abstained from proselytizing. In June 1993, the Swiss Federal Court ruled that Muslim girls, even if they had not yet reached puberty, could be withdrawn by their parents from coeducational swimming lessons. The court argued: 'Non-nationals and members of other cultures must respect the legal order [of this country]. But they are not legally obliged to [abandon] their customs and ways of life' (ibid. 987). In August 1993, the German Federal Administrative Court ruled that young Muslim girls had the right to stay away from physical instruction in school, if the responsible *Land* administration had failed to offer separate classes for boys and girls. The court argued that the educational mandate of the state was outweighed in this case by constitutional parent rights and religious freedoms.

These are, admittedly, trivial cases. Physical is not physics instruction, and the same courts would have probably prohibited a religious abstention from natural science classes. Moreover, the courts simply followed the non-discrimination principle of modern law, which protects minority groups only indirectly, through guaranteeing individual rights of education and religious worship. This is less than group rights, in which designated minorities would be singled out for special protection and promotion. As trivial as the cases may be, the underlying issue of educating Muslim girls in a liberal state is not. It exposes the dilemma for liberal states to reconcile the conflicting principles of tolerance and autonomy. 'Tolerance' forces these states to be lenient toward cultural difference; 'autonomy' to enable their members (including female Muslims) to take a reflective attitude to any given

cultural tradition (see Kymlicka, 1995*b*: 15). This dilemma is irresolvable, and liberal states have tackled it in different ways. Britain, for
instance, tolerates private Muslim schools, but has refrained from supporting them with state funds. With the exception of the United States
(where third-world immigrants came to profit from the gains of black
Americans), liberal states have not granted special group rights to their
immigrants, sticking to passive non-discrimination instead. This may
meet the objection that even liberal states are not culturally neutral,
but one huge 'group right' arrangement for the majority culture. Such
is the nature of nation-states, even in the age of multiculturalism. As
the finest normative defence of multicultural citizenship concedes,
voluntary immigrants have 'waived' the right to recreate their homeland culture in the receiving society (Kymlicka, 1995*a*: ch. 5).
However, as not only the three court cases but our three-country
comparison of multicultural integration shows, the more moderate
'polyethnic rights' advocated by Kymlicka, which amount to a flexibility of law and policy to the religious and cultural needs of immigrants, are widely instituted and respected in liberal states.

Europe and Immigration

Germany and Great Britain no longer live in two separate immigration
worlds. Christmas 1997 gave a glimpse of a new, European immigration reality. Boatloads of Kurdish refugees had arrived on the southern coast of Italy, not on their own but with the help of the Turkish
mafia's lucrative human-smuggling branch. Italian authorities, well-
knowing that the refugees' destination was further north in a free border zone that stretched from Palermo to Rotterdam and Hamburg,
allowed them to enter and move around freely. In response, Austria
quickly reintroduced border controls with its southern neighbour,
and in Germany there was public outrage about Italy's lax border
enforcement. It suddenly became clear that after Italy's accession to
the Schengen Treaty in October 1997, her borders were also Austria
and Germany's borders. The Kurdish episode exposed the new as
injected with a heavy dose of old immigration realities. Italian negli-
gence tacitly counted on the force of established migration patterns,
with the large Kurdish diasporas in Germany and the Netherlands
attracting Kurdish newcomers, no matter where they first entered
Europe.[13] At the same time, the Kurds landing in Italy were no longer
'national' (would-be) immigrants in the sense guestworkers or post-

colonial immigrants had been 'German' or 'British' immigrants. Instead, the Kurds were perhaps the first 'European' immigrants, for whom no national government but an emergent European Union was responsible—in principle at least, if an effective European immigration and asylum regime had existed at this point.

There are two European migration regimes, with opposite purposes and in different stages of development (see Koslowski, 1998). An elaborate regime exists to ensure the free movement of member-state citizens in an 'area without internal frontiers', as stipulated in the 1987 amendment to the Treaty of Rome. This is not just an inter- but a supranational regime, withdrawn from the control of member states, and entrusted to the European Commission and the European Court of Justice. Outlawing discrimination on the basis of nationality, the intra-European migration regime has incapacitated the member states to reject the entry and stay of citizens of other member states. This is a remarkable novelty in the history of the international state system. But its impact on migration has been negligible. Despite the accession of less-developed member states like Spain, Portugal, and Greece, the size of the resident alien population from EU member states increased only minimally, from 4.5 million in 1987 to 4.9 million in 1992 (ibid. 165). National economic development entailed by membership in the EU seems to have greatly diminished intra-European migration pressure.

If the humanitarian aids commissioner of the European Commission took the Kurdish refugee episode to deplore the lack of a 'European immigration policy', her reference point was the considerably less developed inter-European migration regime.[14] It is only an 'intergovernmental' arrangement, in which the sovereignty of member states over the entry and stay of third-state nationals reigns supreme. Long neglected at the European level, the control of Europe's external borders became an issue once the effort to erase its internal borders switched to high gear in the mid-1980s. The geopolitical context of a crumbling Soviet empire and the civil war in the Balkans, which produced population movements of historical magnitude, made 'internal security' the guiding principle of the emergent inter-European migration regime. This is expressed in the polemical notion of Fortress Europe. The fortress was forged in a plethora of secretive forums composed of national interior ministry and police officials, acting outside European Union institutions. But there is a strong pull of EU institutions on these intergovernmental forums. The Maastricht Treaty first formalized the latter in the so-called Third Pillar, in which the member states were called upon to co-operate more closely in the combat against illegal immigration, drug-trafficking, and international terrorism. The Amsterdam Treaty of 1997 even shifted the entire asylum and immigration complex from the intergovernmental Third into the supranational First Pillar—with the safety valve of requiring unanimous voting by the (member-state dominated) Council of Ministers for another five years. As a legal observer put it, 'every step taken in direction of supranational structures [is balanced] by some intergovernmental elements in order to guarantee each government's control of this sensitive policy area' (Bank, 1998: 20). While the trend is toward diminished member-state sovereignty also in the control of third-state nationals, this does not make the member states less effective in restricting immigration. On the contrary, the whole point of European harmonization is to make them more effective. The best example is asylum policy, in which the reference to European harmonization has allowed France and Germany to curtail their constitutional asylum rights (see Lavenex, 1998). Intergovernmental or supranational, the inter-European migration regime will remain a regime to contain, rather than to solicit, immigration. It could not be otherwise because no state in Europe has been recruiting immigrants in the last thirty years.[15]

Germany and Britain have taken radically opposite stances toward the European migration regimes. These stances reflect their larger attitudes toward Europe (see Risse, 1997), but also the differential impact of these migration regimes on domestic policy. Germany, forever embracing Europe as an alternative to the nation-state, has championed the drive to harmonize and supranationalize immigration and refugee policies. This was not only a matter of identity but of interest, because it allowed Germany to farm out the control of her multiple, vulnerable land borders. In addition, it allowed her to remove domestic obstacles to effective immigration control, as in the asylum reform of 1993. Britain, by contrast, the notorious Euro-pessimist, has fiercely resisted the transfer of authority to European Union institutions. Accordingly, Britain has championed intergovernmental immigration control forums like the Trevi Group, while insisting that they remain just that, or 'opting out' in case they took on supranational features. As in the German case, this stance is conditioned as much by identity as by interest. If Germany stands only to win from Europeanization, Britain faces considerable transition costs. The free-movement regime forces Britain to abandon its island logic of controlling ports of entry in favour of the continental logic of controlling domestic society, a process now well underway. Moreover, the importation of human-rights constraints and judicial control of the executive are undermining the guiding principle of British immigration and refugee policy—unhindered state discretion.

Whereas the Europeanization of immigration control is clearly marked, the Europeanization of immigrant integration is much less so. Most visible so far has been the long-standing campaign, led by the European Commission itself, to endow third-country nationals legally residing in a member state with free movement, residence, and employment rights in other member states. It was a political decision, dictated by populist pressure on member states in the mid-1980s, to exclude the legal immigrant population from the intra-European free-movement regime. This regime's central constitutional clause, Article 8(a) of the Single European Act, speaks of 'persons', and thus allows the inclusion of non-EU nationals also.[16] Accordingly, the European Commission rightly finds that the free movement of persons 'logically implies the free movement of all legally resident third-country nationals for the purpose of engaging in economic activities' (in Papademetriou, 1996: 90). Judged by expansive denizen rights at the member-state level, the exclusion of legal immigrants from free-movement rights in an enlarged European polity is difficult to defend.[17]

One may still question if Europe is the adequate level at which to integrate immigrants. First, building a European integration regime appears quixotic, considering that Europe does not want new immigrants and that the old immigrants are already incorporated at the nation-state level. Secondly, the unclear meaning of Europe raises the question what immigrants are supposed to become integrated into. If Europe itself is a 'multi-cultural and multi-ethnic entity',[18] no further effort seems necessary to integrate immigrants into this liberal thing. The supposed necessity of European immigrant integration snubs the old nation-state model, but remains under its spell. However, even nation-states, as we have seen, have long adhered to an intransitive mode of integration, which leaves the identity of immigrants intact. There is no added value of a European integration. Not to mention that immigrants in Europe still meet nationally bounded education, employment, welfare, and political systems. In absence of a structured Euro-society, the range of European immigrant integration seems rather limited.

Does the emergent European Union mark the decline of the nation-state? First, a look at Europe's own south-eastern backyard shows that, in the global picture, the old nation-state is disturbingly vital. In John Meyer's (1997) interesting thought-experiment, an unknown island society suddenly 'discovered' would quickly take on all the insignia of nation-states, including passports, census, and a science ministry. Secondly, the debate about the European Union itself has moved beyond the earlier dispute if the EU is the supranational successor to, or the rescuer of, the nation-state. Here a unique, multi-tiered polity with fractured sovereignty and multiple allegiances is in the making, still best captured in Hedley Bull's metaphor of 'new medievalism'. In a continent destroyed by exalted nationalisms, a peculiar fatigue of the national principle has provided an opening for a unique reconfiguration of political space. It is unlikely to be emulated elsewhere: NAFTA is not the European Union.[19] By the same token, even a United States of Europe (an unlikely outcome by any chance) will not resemble the United States of America in at least one respect. Europe's constitutive units are nation-states, not individuals leaving nation-states. Immigration will alway be the periphery, never the core, of the European experience.

Notes

CHAPTER 1

1. Hedley Bull (1977: 146) realized the incompatibility of the state system and universal justice: 'Carried to its logical extreme, the doctrine of human rights and duties under international law is subversive of the whole principle that mankind should be organized as a society of sovereign states. For, if the rights of each man can be asserted on the world political stage over and against the claims of his state, and his duties proclaimed irrespective of his position as a servant or a citizen of that state, then the position of the state as a body sovereign over its citizens, and entitled to command their obedience, has been subject to challenge, and the structure of the society of sovereign states has been placed in jeopardy.'
2. See my review essay (Joppke, 1995).
3. A similar view is presented by Jacobson (1996).
4. I follow Jürgen Habermas (1994): 'The two ideas of popular sovereignty and human rights have shaped the normative self-understanding of constitutional states up to the present day. With the first idea we postulate that members of a democratic community are governed by themselves collectively; with the second, that they are governed by law and not by man' (p. 1).
5. See the masterful study of absolutism by Perry Anderson (1974).
6. Sophisticated discussions of modern 'territoriality' can be found in Kratochwil (1986), Ruggie (1993), and Spruyt (1994).
7. Absolute sovereignty is a fiction: if states could exclude their own nationals, they could no longer exclude aliens—because no state would be required to take them. The acceptance of nationals was first an exigency of the interdependency of states, but later turned into a right on part of the individual (see Plender, 1988: ch. 2).
8. See the frightening survey by Paul J. Smith, 'Anti-Immigrant Xenophobia Around the World', *International Herald Tribune*, 14 Feb. 1996, 8. See also the instructive comparison of Persian Gulf and Western European policies on labour migrants by Myron Weiner (1995: 80–3).
9. One should not forget, however, that about one-third of US immigrants during the peak period between 1880 and 1920 remigrated to their countries of origin (see Piore, 1979). The novelty seems to be the technologically conditioned obsolescence of a final choice of place, and the diasporic loss of a sense of having departed at all.
10. Next to Brubaker (1992), an outstanding example of in-depth 'small-N' comparison remains Gary Freeman's (1979) now classic comparison of immigration policies and politics in France and Britain.

INTRODUCTION TO PART I

1. See Joseph Carens's (1987) normative case for a policy of open borders.

2. Even in the United States, where the gulf between (national interest) principle and (special interest) reality in immigration policy has been the widest of all. Tellingly, the influential 1980 report of the Select Commission on Immigration and Refugee Policy is entitled *US Immigration Policy and the National Interest*. The first report of the 1990s US Commission on Immigration Reform (1995) also uses national-interest rhetoric: 'A properly regulated system of legal immigration is in the national interest' (p. i).

3. See the instructive comparison of family reunification in French and US immigration law by Guendelsberger (1988). Regarding the US, the author suggests the exemption of the nuclear family of permanent legal residents from quota restrictions. This restrictive feature of US family reunification rules, which falls short of the European standard, is neutralized by low hurdles to naturalization.

4. Asylum-seekers are 'unwanted' in the analytical sense of not being actively recruited, but admitted in response to an external, unsolicited claim.

5. This line of reasoning has been most clearly developed by Isensee (1974).

CHAPTER 2

1. The Asia-Pacific triangle provision set a quota of 100 for each country in this region. It inherited the racial logic of oriental exclusion, because a person of oriental ancestry could enter the United States only under the quota of her ancestors' country, even if she was a French or British citizen.

2. The numbers are quoted in *New York Times*, 24 July 1963, 12.

3. Among the major advocates for abolishing the quota system were the AFL-CIO, National Council of Churches, American Committee for Italian Migration, National Council of Jewish Women, National Catholic Welfare Conference, and the Japanese-American Citizen League (Reimers, 1985: 70).

4. Aristide Zolberg, *Again a Nation of Immigrants: The US Faces a New Wave* (lecture at the European University Institute, Florence, 12 Dec. 1995).

5. 'Quota Immigration Backed at Hearing', *New York Times*, 21 May 1965, 68.

6. These are the words of Italo-American Peter Rodino, a major Congressional player in immigration reform during the last 30 years (quoted in Cose, 1992: 109).

7. Until 1976, Western hemisphere countries were exempted from the preference system and country ceilings.

8. 'Flow of 3d World Immigrants Alters Weave of US Society', *New York Times*, 30 June 1980, 1.

9. 'Some Hard Choices Emerge in Debate on Illegal Aliens', *New York Times*, 16 Aug. 1982, A12.

10. See Hispanic leader Antonia Hernandez (MALDEF), who indicted an earlier version of IRCA as 'contradictory, ineffective and anti-Hispanic' (quoted in *Congressional Record-Senate*, Nov. 1982, 29423).

11. The total level of immigration during the 1980s is estimated between 6.7 and 8.7 million persons, thus exceeding the levels of all previous decades except the first decade of the twentieth century (Bean and Fix, 1992: 41 f.).

12. Interview with Jim Dorcy (FAIR), 24 Mar. 1994, Washington.

13. 'O'Neill Says Bill on Illegal Aliens is Dead for 1983', *New York Times*, 5 Oct. 1983, 1.

14. For instance, Joaquin G. Avila (MALDEF), 'Immigrant Non-Bill', *New York Times*, 17 Dec. 1982, 39.

15. Interview with Rick Swartz (National Immigration Forum), 26 Mar. 1994, Washington, DC.

16. William Saffire, 'The Computer Tattoo', *New York Times*, 9 Sept. 1982, A27.
17. Congressman Bill Richardson, quoted in 'Aliens Bill Nears Reality', *New York Times*, 18 June 1984, 1.
18. 'Amid Charges, Immigration Bill Dies', *New York Times*, 12 Oct. 1984, 16.
19. 'Message of Immigration Bill is Disputed', *New York Times*, 12 Oct. 1984, 17.
20. A Gallup poll in Nov. of 1984 found that only 35 per cent of Americans supported the amnesty (Fuchs, 1990).
21. Congressman Charles Schumer, quoted in 'Immigration Bill: How "Corpse" Came Back to Life', *New York Times*, 13 Oct. 1986.
22. Interview with Rick Swartz, 26 Mar. 1994, Washington.
23. '1986 Amnesty Law is Seen as Failing to Slow Alien Tide', *New York Times*, 18 June 1989, 1. Good assessments of the impact of IRCA on illegal flows are Bean, Edmonston, and Passel (1990) and Espenshade (1992).
24. The persistence of illegal immigration is not only due to the laxity of sanctions, but to legalization itself, which provided attractive fixpoints for new flows. For instance, since 1986 the proportion of women among illegal immigrants has been rising, because wives were joining their legalized husbands (Bean, Edmonston, and Passel, 1990: 263).
25. Quoted in 'Looking for Skills and Good English', *New York Times*, 10 Apr. 1988, IV, 5.
26. Interview with Demetrios Papademetriou (Carnegie Endowment for International Peace), 20 Apr. 1994, Washington.
27. From the testimony of Daniel Stein (FAIR), in *Immigration Act of 1989 (Part 1): Hearings before the Subcommittee on Immigration, Refugees, and International Law*. Washington: US Government Printing Office, Serial No.21, 1989, 571.
28. Quoted in *Immigration Act of 1989 (Part 3): Joint Hearings Before the Subcommittee on Immigration, Refugees, and International Law*. Washington: US Government Printing Office, Serial No.21, 1990, 661.
29. Cecilia Munoz (National Council of La Raza), in *Immigration Act of 1989 (Part 1)*, 203.
30. 'Key Senators Back Immigration Shift', *New York Times*, 14 Feb. 1988.
31. Quoted in 'Senate Back Bill on Aliens that Emphasizes Job Skills', *New York Times*, 16 Mar. 1988, A14.
32. Kennedy's chief immigration counsellor recounts a meeting between Kennedy and House Judiciary Committee chair Peter Rodino in 1988: 'Kennedy was really mad at Rodino, who would defend the Fifth Preference. "Peter, why do you think this is such an important thing: Fifth Preference for Italians, it's gonna be 25, 30 years [of waiting time], it would take a mortician to bring them in when their petition becomes relevant." Rodino mentioned a bishop in Newark feeling strongly about this. Kennedy banged the table and said: "You tell me that bishop's name, and I call that bishop!" Well, the bill died. Rodino wouldn't let it come to the floor' (Interview with Jerry Tinker, US Senate Subcommittee on Immigration and Refugee Affairs, 30 Mar. 1994, Washington).
33. 'Senate Debates Overhauling the Laws Governing Legal Immigration', *New York Times*, 13 July 1989.
34. Reverend Joseph Cogo, quoted in *Immigration Act of 1989 (Part 1)*, 254.
35. Donald Martin, quoted in *Immigration Act of 1989 (Part 1)*, 218.
36. Cecilia Munoz, quoted in *Immigration Act of 1989 (Part 1)*, 216.
37. Daryl Buffenstein, quoted in *Immigration Act of 1989 (Part 1)*, 432.
38. See the statement by Warren Leiden (American Immigration Lawyers Association), in *Immigration Act of 1989 (Part 1)*, 487–9.

39. Gary Rubin (American Jewish Committee), in *Immigration Act of 1989 (Part 1)*, 273.
40. 'Immigration Bill Debated in House', *New York Times* 3 Oct. 1990.
41. Interview with Demetrios Papademetriou, 20 Apr. 1994, Washington.
42. 'Two Reasons to Rejoice on Immigration', *New York Times*, 29 Oct. 1990, 20.
43. Interview with Demetrios Papademetriou, 20 Apr. 1994, Washington.
44. See also Anon., 'Developments in the Law' (1983).
45. 'Developments in the Law'.
46. Ibid. 1292.
47. Exceptions are the right to vote, to serve on juries, and to run for high elective office or federal appointment, all of which are reserved for US citizens. In addition, LPRs have lesser rights to sponsor family immigration, and they are theoretically (but almost never practically) subject to deportation. See Schuck (1995*b*: 18–27).
48. The court quotes are from 'Developments in the Law', 1403.
49. However, the legal empowerment of permanent resident aliens has remained limited to the state level. At the federal level, the plenary power doctrine has stood in the way of restricting the government's power to classify aliens. See Rosberg (1978).
50. In *Plyler* v. *Doe*, the Supreme Court interpreted the word *jurisdiction* in a 'predominantly geographic sense.' In a critique of *Plyler*, Schuck and Smith (1985: 103) have suggested a 'political, consensualist understanding' of the jurisdiction requirement. The authors conclude that birthright citizenship for the children of illegal aliens is not commanded by the constitution.
51. Quoted from Justice Brennan's majority opinion, excerpts of which are reprinted in *New York Times*, 16 June 1982, D22.
52. However, for three reasons such an expansive reading may be misleading. First, the Texas law barring the children of illegal immigrants from public education amounted to an immigration policy measure, which is a federal prerogative and thus subject to the principle of federal pre-emption. Since the Court ruled against a state statute, plenary power was never in question; in fact, the Court indicated that in case of an explicit, countervailing policy choice by Congress it might have arrived at a different conclusion. Second, the Court distinguished education as separate from and superior to other welfare benefits, elevating the state school to 'a most vital civic institution' indispensable for democratic government and the transmission of values. Accordingly, the Court ruled out an expansion of substantial benefits for illegal aliens to other welfare areas. Finally, the Court limited its generosity to the children of illegal immigrants, who were 'innocent' and should not be punished for the misdeeds of their parents: 'Legislation directing the onus of a parent's misconduct against his children does not comport with fundamental conceptions of justice' (Justice Brennan, quoted in 'Justices Rule States Must Pay to Educate Illegal Alien Pupils', *New York Times*, 16 June 1982, D22). Given this specific emphasis on education and the needs of children in the Court's reasoning, an extension of *Plyler* to either illegal alien adults or other welfare functions appears unlikely indeed.
53. Quoted in 'Developments in the Law', 1309.
54. The era of general parole had lasted from 1954, the closing of the Ellis Island detention centre in New York, to 1981, when the new Reagan policy of detaining undocumented entrants was instituted. During this period, detention was limited to aliens who were likely to abscond or who posed a threat to national security. See Scott (1985: 1123, n. 104).

55. The Knauff–Mezei doctrine, established in two Supreme Court cases in the early 1950s, grants unlimited exclusion powers to the government by positioning the entering alien as a 'non-person' outside the Constitution. It consists of two elements: conceiving of alien admission as a privilege, not a right; and the legal fiction that the entering alien is not on US territory, so that constitutional protection does not apply. The Knauff–Mezei doctrine draws a capricious line between 'excludable' and 'deportable' aliens. Deportable aliens, even those who have entered illegally, are considered on US territory, so that constitutional protection via personhood applies. By contrast, excludable aliens are effectively treated as non-persons.

56. See the discussion of the Supreme Court's *Jean* v. *Nelson* decision by Motomura (1990).

57. 'Fixing Immigration', *New York Times*, 8 June 1993, B2.

58. Teitelbaum (1984: 85 f.) realized this very clearly.

59. Elliott Abrams, 'Diluting Compassion', *New York Times*, 5 Aug. 1983, I, 23.

60. See the *New York Times* editorial 'Why Poles but Not Salvadorians?', 31 May 1983, I, 20. Salvadorians were eventually granted 'extended voluntary departure' status as part of the 1990 Legal Immigration Act.

61. By late 1986, the number of detained or imprisoned Marielitos awaiting deportation was at 7,600 ('US Laws Put Imprisoned Cubans in Legal Limbo With Few Rights', *New York Times*, 24 Nov. 1986, 1).

62. Jose Fuentes, 'Immigration: Is US Policy On Cubans Just?', *New York Times*, 2 Oct. 1983, XI, 30.

63. '1980 Cuban Refugees Gain on Citizenship Claim', *New York Times*, 21 Oct. 1984, I, 23. The 1986 Immigration Act finally allowed the Haitians to convert to immigrant status.

64. This was the line taken by the liberal Ninth Circuit court, responsible for the majority of asylum cases in the American Southwest. Other courts did not follow. See Porter (1992: 251 f.).

65. See the symposium in *Cornell International Law Journal*, 26 (1993), 495–818.

66. Still in 1989, 94 per cent of the 95,505 refugees approved for admission came from communist countries ('Study Asks New Safeguards For Refugees Asking Asylum', *New York Times*, 16 Mar. 1990).

67. Quoted in 'US to Make it Easier to Gain Asylum', *New York Times*, 1 July 1990.

68. 'US Adopts New Policy for Hearings On Political Asylum for Some Aliens', *New York Times*, 20 Dec. 1990, B18.

69. Since 1980, the government had denied 97 per cent of applications for political asylum by Salvadorians and 99 per cent of those by Guatemalans, while approving 76 per cent of Soviet and 64 per cent of Chinese applications (ibid.).

70. 'Aid to Aliens Said to Spur Illegal Immigration', *New York Times*, 23 Dec. 1985, 1.

71. By 1995, the proportion of foreign-born in the US rose to 8.7 per cent, which is the highest level since World War II. Between 1990 and 1994 alone, 4.5 million new immigrants entered the USA, almost as many as during the entire decade of the 1970s. As a result, about 20 per cent of the 22.6 million foreigners living in the USA in 1995 had entered in the previous five years. 'That's much higher than numbers we've had historically, going back 20, 30, 40, 100 years,' says Jeffrey Passel of the Urban Institute ('Surprising Rise In Immigration Stirs Up Debate', *New York Times*, 30 Aug. 1995).

72. These numbers are reported in *Roll Call*, 15 July 1993, 8.

73. Reported in Freeman (1996: 6 f.).

74. Lamar Smith, Republican from Texas, had introduced his sweeping House bill dealing jointly with legal and illegal immigration as 'put[ting] the interests of America first'. 'House G.O.P. Moves to Cut Immigration', *New York Times*, 22 June 1995.
75. See the detailed reviews of Brimelow's *Alien Nation* by Miles (1995) and Schuck (1996).
76. See the survey on the fiscal impacts of US immigration by Rothman and Espenshade (1992), especially 389–91.
77. Roger Waldinger, 'The Jobs Immigrants Take', *New York Times*, 11 Mar. 1996. However, Waldinger's case is not for closing immigration, but for improved job training and employer pressure to hire more blacks.
78. All these lawsuits were eventually dismissed.
79. Pete Wilson, 'Piety, but No Help, On Illegal Aliens', *New York Times*, 11 July 1996.
80. 'California Immigration Measure Faces Rocky Legal Path', *New York Times*, 11 Nov. 1994.
81. 'California Immigration Law is Ruled to be Partly Illegal', *New York Times*, 21 Nov. 1995.
82. In fact, the same political leaders who jumped aboard the anti-immigrant bandwagon had helped produce California's immigration crisis. Diane Feinstein, now a Democratic Senator for California advocating a $1 border toll to raise money for stronger border enforcement, had been lax toward illegal immigrants as a mayor of San Francisco, when she supported the 'sanctuary' movement and even prevented local police and city officials from enforcing federal immigration law. More interestingly still, the converted immigrant foe Pete Wilson had pushed as a Senator for a loosely administered, fraud-riddled Special Agricultural Worker (SAW) programme in the context of IRCA, which became a major magnet for illegal immigration to California. See the instructive report by Joel Brinkley, 'California's Woes on Aliens Appear Largely Self-Inflicted', *New York Times* 15 Oct. 1994, 1.
83. Composed of four Democratic and four Republican appointees, the Commission members included Lawrence Fuchs, the executive director of the 1981 commission on immigration reform, Warren Leiden, executive director of the American Immigration Lawyers Association, and Bruce Morrison, the House broker of the 1990 Immigration Act. As the Commission's chairwoman Barbara Jordan said, 'among Commission members, immigration is seen as having more of a positive impact than negative' ('Panel May Hold Key to Consensus on Immigration', *Los Angeles Times*, 11 July 1994, A3).
84. Most importantly Secretary of Labor, Robert Reich.
85. 'The United States can no longer be an "immigrant country" ' (Brimelow, 1995: 205); 'The United States is not a nation of immigrants, and never has been' (Lind, 1995: 286).
86. Barbara Jordan, 'The Americanization Ideal', *New York Times*, 11 Sept. 1995.
87. 'The Strange Politics of Immigration', *New York Times*, 31 Dec. 1995.
88. 'Unlikely Allies Battle Congress Over Anti-Immigration Plans', *New York Times*, 11 Oct. 1995.
89. 'Congress Plans Stiff New Curb on Immigration', *New York Times*, 25 Sept. 1995.
90. Roy Beck, 'The Pro-Immigration Lobby', *New York Times*, 30 Apr. 1996.
91. 'House Panel Approves Plan to Register Immigration Status', *New York Times*, 22 Nov. 1995.

92. 'Author of Immigration Measure in Senate Drops Most Provisions on Foreign Workers', *New York Times*, 8 Mar. 1996.
93. *Migration News*, Oct. 1996.
94. 'Bill to Limit Immigration Faces a Setback in Senate', *New York Times*, 14 Mar. 1996.
95. Quoted in 'Senate Votes Bill to Reduce Influx of Illegal Aliens', *New York Times*, 3 May 1996.
96. A study of the General Accounting Office (GAO) found that 25 per cent of the recipients of SSI (which supports old-age pensions) had been the parents of legal immigrants, who had been too short in the US to claim pensions on the basis of own contributions.

CHAPTER 3

1. See, for instance, Thomas Faist's (1994: 51) denouncing of the 'not a country of immigration' maxim as 'counterfactual ideology'. His question: 'How did a *de facto* country of immigration manage to espouse a counterfactual ideology in the 1980s and early 1990s?' denies the normative, self-definitional quality of the 'not a country of immigration' maxim. As a normative statement, this 'ideology' is necessarily 'counterfactual'. Rogers Brubaker (1992: 174) has seen this: 'The *kein Einwanderungsland* claim articulates not a social or demographic fact but a political-cultural norm, an element of national self-understanding'.
2. Ulrich Herbert (1990: 201), for instance, identifies a 'break in historical perception' between the Nazi regime's forced deployment of 7 million 'foreign workers' (*Fremdarbeiter*) and West Germany's 'guestworker' (*Gastarbeiter*) recruitment since the 1950s. The break of memory is evident in the different wording. In France too there has been a break of memory *vis-à-vis* prewar immigration (see Noiriel, 1996: ch. 1).
3. 'The Federal Republic of Germany is not a country of immigration. West Germany is a country in which foreigners reside for varying lengths of time before they decide on their own accord to return to their home country' (*Vorschläge der Bund-Länder-Kommission zur Fortentwicklung einer umfassenden Konzeption der Ausländerbeschäftigungspolitik*, Feb. 1977, quoted in Katzenstein, 1987: 239).
4. Quoted in 'Manchem Gastarbeiter bangt vor der Zukunft', *Frankfurter Allgemeine Zeitung*, 9 Nov. 1974.
5. Interior Minister Gerhard Baum (FDP), quoted in: *Das Parlament*, 32/9, 1982.
6. In German parlance, first-generation foreigners are the directly recruited guestworkers. Second-generation foreigners are either born in Germany or born abroad and admitted as children through family reunification. Third-generation foreigners are born in Germany as children of the second generation.
7. After praising its 'liberal and cosmopolitan' foreigner policy, the government points out that such a policy was contingent upon 'the possibility to realize state interests against foreign nationals, and especially to protect effectively the own citizens from harm' (quoted in Hailbronner, 1984: 4).
8. By 1992, 46.5 per cent of the foreigners residing in the Federal Republic held either an unrestricted residence permit or a residence entitlement. If one adds the 25.8 per cent of EU nationals exempted from a residence permit requirement, 74.3 per cent of all foreigners had a secure residence status. See Federal Ministry of the Interior (1993: 23 f.).
9. Initially, this residence right was given only to the foreign wives of German

husbands, but withheld from the foreign husbands of German wives, who were assumed to follow their husbands into their country of origin. In response to the first foreigner-related grassroots mobilization in the Federal Republic, by the *Interessengemeinschaft der mit Ausländern verheirateten deutschen Frauen*, the federal government revoked this obvious case of sex discrimination in 1975.

10. Foreign minister Klaus Kinkel, quoted in *Migration News* 3/7, July 1996.
11. This constitutional aspect of German 'semi-sovereignty' is omitted by Katzenstein (1987), who stresses instead federalism and neocorporatism.
12. David Currie (1990: 363) characterized Article 2(1) as 'the heart of substantive due process in Germany'.
13. An expansive interpretation of Article 2(1) as a 'super constitutional right' is not uncontested in the legal literature (see Hailbronner, 1983: 2113).
14. For the latter, see Hailbronner (1992).
15. Note that Isensee (1974: 72) denied the existence of a constitutional right of permanent residence: 'The discretion of the state to limit temporally or revoke a residence permit is not cancelled out by the constitutionally required status security.'
16. *Decision of 18 July 1973* (1 BvR 23, 155/73); henceforth quoted as the 'Arab Case'.
17. Since one of the plaintiffs was married to a German national, the Court also argued that in this case Article 6(1) of the Basic Law (which protects marriage and the family) had been violated.
18. *Decision of 26 Sept. 1978* (1 BvR 525/77); henceforth referred to as the 'Indian Case'.
19. The Court added, however, that a strict indication of the temporal limitation of a residence permit could preclude the emergence of a reliance interest: 'If the residence permit had been first issued with the explicit indication of its non-renewability (after the original purpose had been realized), the plaintiff could not have counted on its renewal.' By implication: a guestworker system based on strict rotation is constitutionally possible, but only if the intention to rotate is unmistakably stated from the start—which was obviously not the case in the German guestworker programme. This reasoning underlies Schwerdtfeger (1980: A131): 'After the political branches [of government] have allowed the "guestworker wave" to happen, the automatism of constitutional law steps in.'
20. Still in the early 1970s, Manfred Zuleeg attacked a 'divided legal state' (Zuleeg 1974) that treated foreigners like 'second class human beings' (Zuleeg 1973). After the Arab and Indian decisions of the Constitutional Court, Zuleeg (1982: 120) reconsidered his earlier indictments: 'One can no longer talk about a divided legal state [*vis-à-vis* foreigners].'
21. *Decision of 12 May 1987* (2 BvR 1226/83, 101, 313/84), in the following referred to as the 'Turkish and Yugoslav Case'.
22. Accordingly, the Turkish and Yugoslav decision has been heavily criticized by some legal scholars. Huber (1988: 609) attacks the 'reduction of constitutional rights in favour of an encompassing primacy of the state's foreigner policy'; Zuleeg (1988: 587) even finds that the decision 'leaves behind a constitutional ruin' (*verfassungsrechtlichen Trümmerhaufen*).
23. I owe this insight to recent work by Ted Perlmutter (1996*a*,*b*).
24. For the latter, see Eckart Schiffer's (1990: 51) characterization of the reformed Foreigner Law of 1990 as a 'fair compromise' between foreigners and Germans in Germany.
25. The principle of *Karenzzwang* was practised during the German Empire, when seasonal Polish *Wanderarbeiter* were forced to return home after the year's agricultural season had ended (see Herbert, 1986: ch. 1).

26. In September 1976, 27 per cent of surveyed companies employing 41 per cent of the total workforce in West Germany expected a lack of needed workers because of the recruitment stop (Dohse, 1981: 314 f.).
27. These numbers are quoted in the Constitutional Court rule in the Turkish and Yugoslav Case (1988: 33).
28. The latter numbers are quoted in 'Neue Einsichten in der Ausländer-Frage', *Frankfurter Allgemeine Zeitung*, 7 Dec. 1981.
29. The survey is summarized in 'Ausländerfeindlichkeit: Exodus erwünscht', *Der Spiegel*, 18, 1982, 37–44.
30. An SPD member of parliament, quoted in 'Ausländer: "Schmerzhafte Grenze gezogen" ', *Der Spiegel*, 50, 1981, 26.
31. Günther Gillessen, 'Die Orientalisierung Europas', *Frankfurter Allgemeine Zeitung* 2 Apr. 1980, 1.
32. The last two quotes are from the same cabinet paper, in: 'Integrieren, nicht "Eindeutschen" ', *Frankfurter Allgemeine Zeitung*, 28 Oct. 1981, 12.
33. This is how the Constitutional Court summarized the position of the federal government (Turkish and Yugoslav Case, 1988: 33 f.).
34. This and the following quotes are from the CDU/CSU parliamentary *Entschliessungsantrag zur Ausländerpolitik* of November 1981, in: 'CDU/CSU will die Bundesrepublik nicht als Vielvölkerstaat', *Frankfurter Rundschau*, 2 Dec. 1981.
35. This and the following quotes are from the parliamentary debate of 4 Feb. 1982, in: *Das Parlament*, 32/9, 6 Mar. 1982.
36. The arrival of Asians and Africans was expected in the case of 'increasing xenophobia in Great Britain' (A. Dregger).
37. 'We don't want to Germanize anyone', said Alfred Dregger.
38. Interview with Jürgen Haberland (Federal Ministry of the Interior), 23 Feb. 1994, Bonn.
39. This crusade was interestingly presented as an integration measure. A survey done in Baden-Württemberg showed that 80 per cent of foreign children who entered primary school at age six reached at least a lower High School degree (*Hauptschulabschluss*). For those who entered school at a more advanced age the chances of reaching a degree decreased considerably (see Haberland, 1983: 58).
40. Both quotes are from 'Nimm deine Prämie und hau ab', *Der Spiegel*, 34, 1983, 31.
41. Quoted in 'Nachzugsregelung bleibt Reizthema der Koalition', *Die Welt*, 2 Oct. 1984.
42. In 1982 and 1983, the migration balance was negative. This was grist to the mill of those who argued that a more restrictive Foreigner Law was currently not necessary (see 'Von drohender Überfremdung kann nicht die Rede sein', *Süddeutsche Zeitung*, 25 Jan. 1984).
43. Quoted in 'Zuwanderungen von Ausländern abwehren', *Der Spiegel*, 18 Apr. 1988, 23.
44. A position paper of the CDU's Employee Section is entitled 'From the Rejection of Threats to Partnership—For a New Paradigm of Foreigner Policy', quoted in 'Beim Ausländerrecht langsam voran', *Frankfurter Allgemeine Zeitung*, 7 Apr. 1988.
45. In a meeting at the Evangelical Academy in Tutzing, even Johannes Gerster, speaker for Home Affairs of the CDU parliamentary faction, distanced himself from Zimmermann: 'It will be difficult for the Interior Minister to find a qualified majority for his draft law, because the majority of the qualified opposes the latter' (quoted in 'Ein politischer Irrgarten wird angelegt', *Süddeutsche Zeitung*, 2/3 July 1988).

46. Quoted in 'Bis an die Grenzen', *Der Spiegel*, 28 Nov. 1988, 36.
47. These are the words of Wolfgang Wieland, chair of the leftist Republican Lawyers Association. See his (still critical) evaluation of Schäuble's draft law, 'Trotz schöner Verpackung schleppt der Entwurf sämtliche Mängel mit', *Frankfurter Rundschau*, 16 Nov. 1989.
48. See the critique of the new Foreigner Law by a leader of the Turkish lobby, Hakki Keskin, 'Ausländer sind zum Arbeiten grade recht . . .', *Frankfurter Rundschau*, 20 Feb. 1990.
49. The Federal Constitutional Court decided in Oct. 1975: 'The constitutional right of asylum . . . guarantees to a person seeking refuge from persecution . . . not to be rejected at the border of the state obliged to grant asylum . . .' This court rule became incorporated in Paragraph 9 of the Asylum Procedures Law, which states that rejection at the border may occur only if the asylum-seeker enjoys alternative protection from persecution. See Pfaff (1992: 131).
50. Asylum policy is only one example of the larger post-Nazi recovery of German state sovereignty at the European level. See the general accounts of the German uses of Europe by Garton Ash (1994) and Katzenstein (1996). But German Eurostealth may be coming to an end now (see 'Germany resolves to pursue its interests', *The Economist*, 13 July 1996, 25–6).
51. So Burkhard Hirsch (FDP), one of the main protagonists in the German asylum debate (quoted in Wolken, 1988: 105).
52. Heinrich Lummer (CDU), quoted in *Der Spiegel*, 12, 1986, 68 and 66, respectively.
53. In July 1990, Lebach, a town of 22,000, was 'overrolled' by the sudden arrival of 1,400 Gypsy refugees from Romania. Local outrage included the mayor barricading the town-hall and public swimming-pool, and business people closing their shops; a protest march to the refugee camp was narrowly averted. In response, the Minister President conceded: 'The law of asylum must be made acceptable to the population' ('Asylrecht: "Oskar quält sich" ', *Der Spiegel*, 32, 1990, 32).
54. Limiting territorial access through visa requirements, though practised since the mid-1970s, proved ineffective because of (West) Germany's open land borders.
55. Between 1973 and 1974, the number of new asylum claims jumped from 5,595 to 9,424 (Quaritsch, 1985: 41). In addition, the post-oil-crisis asylum-seekers came no longer from Eastern Europe but from Third World countries. The proportion of non-European asylum-seekers increased from 7 per cent in 1968 to 75 per cent in 1977 (Münch, 1992: 63). It should be mentioned that Germany too, not surprisingly perhaps for the front state in the Cold War confrontation, had a 'double standard' in accepting refugees: from 1966 to 1989, Eastern European refugees were generally not deported. Only, unlike in the United States, it never aroused much public attention, not to mention criticism.
56. 'Da sammelt sich ein ungeheurer Sprengstoff', *Der Spiegel*, 23, 1980, 17–18.
57. In one of the first parliamentary debates about *Scheinasylanten*, Eduard Spranger, a conservative hardliner from Bavaria, had this to say: 'It is the merit of the CDU/CSU faction in the Bundestag to discuss again today the unbearable conditions [*unerträglichen Zustände*], which a perpetually growing stream [*unaufhörlich wachsender Strom*] of asylum-seekers has brought for our country and for our people' (*Das Parlament*, 15, 12 Apr. 1980).
58. 'Die Spreu vom Weizen trennen', *Der Spiegel*, 40, 1986, 84–98. Because West Germany did not recognize communist East Germany as a sovereign state, transborder traffic was only perfunctorily controlled. By the mid-1980s, most new asylum-seekers from countries with visa requirements (which included Turkey,

Pakistan, Bangladesh, Iran, and India) would arrive by air in East Berlin Schönefeld, from where they slipped unnoticed via bus and metro connections into West Berlin. Pressured by Bonn, the East German regime agreed, in Sept. 1986, to allow entry only to holders of third-state visas. This abruptly closed the *Asyl-Schleuse*.

59. The President of the Federal Administrative Court reported that 'we have asylum applicants who have ended up four times at the Federal Administrative Court' (see his interview in 'Massenware, bei der nichts herauskommt', *Der Spiegel*, 17, 1982, 53).

60. Such lawyers often co-operated with *Schlepper* organizations; they have no resemblance with the high-minded public interest lawyers in the United States, who are largely unknown in Germany (see *Der Spiegel*, 40, 1986, 84–96).

61. 'Asyl—"Bis and die Grenze des Zulässigen" ', *Der Spiegel*, 31, 1986, 22–32.

62. According to the Geneva Convention on Refugees of 1951, a refugee is 'any person who is outside the country of his nationality . . . because he has or had a well-founded fear of persecution by reason of his race, religion, nationality, membership of a particular social group or political opinion . . .' The element of 'well-founded fear' entails a subjective refugee definition. By contrast, the Basic Law stipulates that 'politically persecuted enjoy the right of asylum.' The notion of 'politically persecuted' entails an objective refugee definition.

63. *Der Spiegel*, 31, 1986, 32.

64. The 'small asylum' is provided by Article 14 of the Foreigner Law: 'A foreigner must not be deported into a state in which his life or liberty is threatened because of his race, religion, nationality, membership of a particular social group, or his political opinion' (quoted in Hailbronner, 1984: 753). From a total of one million non-recognized or rejected asylum-seekers in 1992, about 500,000 were allowed to stay temporarily on the basis of 'small asylum'. 'Wer will Menschen das antun?', *Der Spiegel*, 46, 1992, 43.

65. Compiling the elements of the restrictive asylum policy in place by 1987, *Der Spiegel* (3 Aug. 1987, 24 f.) spoke of a 'catalogue of horror': visa obligations for most non-EU countries; no recognition of so-called 'post-flight asylum reasons' (which had allowed what Teitelbaum [(1984)] called 'bootstrapping', the post-factum creation of asylum causes), immediate departure in case of 'obviously unfounded' asylum claims; deportation also into countries of civil war (a speciality of Bavaria); forced encampment during the whole asylum procedures; a five-year work ban; and restrictive courts that did not automatically recognize asylum claims despite proved torture.

66. A first questioning of Article 16 had occurred during the first asylum crisis of 1980, when a few politicians (including Chancellor Helmut Schmidt and the Minister President of Schleswig-Holstein, Gerhard Stoltenberg) and constitutional lawyers (including the president of the Federal Administrative Court and legal experts Kay Hailbronner and Werner Kanein) called for the insertion into the Basic Law of a *Gesetzesvorbehalt* (legal condition) to neutralize Article 16 (see Quaritsch, 1985: 43). But these remained isolated voices.

67. Commenting on the failure of seven asylum reforms since 1978 to stop the new movement of asylum-seekers, Burkhart Hirsch (FDP) said: 'In the end nothing is achieved if after a final legal decision no consequent deportation follows' (*Der Spiegel*, 45, 1990, 44).

68. 'Wer will Menschen das antun?' *Der Spiegel*, 46, 1992, 54. The asylum-recognition rate for Gypsies, one of the biggest migrant groups in the early 1990s, was zero per cent.

69. 'Die Koalition spricht von drohendem Staatsnotstand', *Frankfurter Allgemeine Zeitung*, 2 Nov. 1992, 1.
70. Friedrich Karl Fromme, 'Aussiedler und Asylbewerber', *Frankfurter Allgemeine Zeitung*, 26 Oct. 1988, 1.
71. Interview with Klaus Wedemeier, Lord Mayor of Bremen, *Der Spiegel*, 32, 1991, 20.
72. 'Anklang an Weimar', *Der Spiegel*, 41, 1992, 18–29.
73. *Der Spiegel*, 46, 1992, 34.
74. The Minister President of Lower Saxony, Gerhard Schröder (SPD), in *Der Spiegel*, 11, 1992, 59.
75. Jürgen Habermas ('Die zweite Lebenslüge der Bundesrepublik', *Die Zeit*, 51, 18 Dec. 1992, 19) speaks of a *'Junktim* between the questions of political asylum and immigration'.
76. Lower Saxony's Minister for Refugee Affairs, Jürgen Trittin (Greens), in *Der Spiegel*, 37, 1992, 27 and 28 f.
77. The Interior Minister of Bavaria, Edmund Stoiber (CSU), in *Der Spiegel*, 45, 1990, 52.
78. Alfred Dregger (CDU) in the parliamentary debate over the change of Article 16, *Das Parlament*, 11 June 1993.
79. Discussions of Germany's 'Euro-solution' to its asylum crisis are in Kanstroom (1993) and Neuman (1993).
80. The German government has repeatedly tried to make its asylum law international standard practice. At a Geneva United Nations Conference in 1977, only one state voted unconditionally for the (West) German proposal to adopt its subjective right of asylum: the Vatican (Quaritsch, 1985: 18 f.).
81. For instance, in 1991 the German campaign failed to delegate national competences for a unified asylum law and procedure to the European Commission.
82. Wolfgang Schäuble, 'Asylrecht im europäischen Vergleich' (1992), in Bade (ed.) (1992).
83. The Bavarian CSU had even advocated legislation that would impose quotas on political refugee acceptance, in gross violation of non-refoulement obligations.
84. See 'Einmal Deutschland und zurück', *Die Zeit*, 22 Sept. 1995, 17.
85. Violent crimes motivated by xenophobia declined to 1,233 in the first eleven months of 1994, from 2,232 cases in 1993 and 2,630 in 1992 (figures provided by the Federal Office for the Protection of the Constitution, quoted in *International Herald Tribune*, 6 Apr. 1995, 6).
86. Ted Perlmutter's (1996b) good discussion of the German asylum debate, which attributes the resort to a non-incremental solution to the politicization of asylum by vote-seeking (conservative) parties, misses the objective grounding of the asylum crisis in impaired sovereignty.
87. See the new Preamble to the German Basic Law: 'The Germans . . . have completed the unity and freedom of Germany in free self-determination. This Basic Law is now valid for the entire German people.'
88. Johannes Gerster (CDU), quoted in *Das Parlament*, 25 Aug. 1989.
89. Erika Trenz (the Greens), quoted in *Das Parlament*, 25 Aug. 1989.
90. In a survey done at the peak of the influx of ethnic Germans, more than half of the respondents characterized the resettlers as 'economic refugees' (see 'Reden nix deutsch, kriegen aber alles', *Der Spiegel*, 8, 1989, 72). Among the odder ways of classifying *Aussiedler* was acknowledging the Nazi naturalizations of 'Germanizable' Poles, which allowed ethnic Poles to immigrate as ethnic Germans. The social benefits for *Aussiedler* included state-provided housing and

employment, interest-free credits, and old-age pensions equivalent to those of domestic citizens.

91. Before the 1993 law, the burden of proof had been the reverse: the German government had to disprove that an applicant had suffered from expulsion-type repression. However, exempting ethnic Germans from the former Soviet Union from this reversed burden of proof had great practical importance, because since the early 1990s the *Aussiedler* pressure originated almost exclusively from this region (see Ronge, 1995: 9).

92. Quoted from the text of the asylum compromise, which is reprinted in *Süddeutsche Zeitung*, 8 Dec. 1992, 5.

93. The quote is from Manfred Kanther, CDU chief of Hesse, 'Sesam, öffne dich', *Der Spiegel*, 17, 1992, 51.

94. See, for instance, the 'Manifesto of the Sixty', in which sixty renowned social scientists of all political leanings demanded 'comprehensive concepts for migration policy and immigration legislation' (Bade, 1994*b*).

95. *Entschliessung des Bundesfachausschusses Innenpolitik der CDU Deutschlands zur Forderung nach einem Einwanderungsgesetz* (Bonn, 15 Sept. 1993, press release).

96. 'Begrenzt oder unbegrenzt?' *Frankfurter Allgemeine Zeitung*, 11 July 1996, 2.

97. 'Germans Consider Immigration Policy', *Migration News*, 3/7, July 1996.

98. Heinrich Lummer (CDU), letter to the *Frankfurter Allgemeine Zeitung*, 4 Oct. 1995, 11.

99. Kay Hailbronner, 'Es bleibt nicht viel zu regeln übrig', *Frankfurter Allgemeine Zeitung*, 26 Apr. 1996, 14.

CHAPTER 4

1. Former Home Secretary Carr, quoted in Goodwin-Gill (1978: 92 f.).

2. See David Coleman (1994: 60 f.): 'Britain acquired its Commonwealth immigrant population in a fit of absence of mind. There was no plan to start the immigration and no intended purpose of it.'

3. There were, of course, some efforts at recruiting New Commonwealth immigrants, for instance, by the Ministry of Health and London Transport, but they did not add up to a concerted state policy.

4. Home Secretary Reginald Maudling during the 1971 immigration debate, in *Parliamentary Debates*, House of Commons, 8 Mar. 1971, v.813, c.44.

5. *Parliamentary Debates*, House of Commons, 7 July 1948, v.453, c.411.

6. Home Secretary Ede, ibid., c.394.

7. Sir Maxwell Fyfe, ibid., c.411.

8. Lord Altrincham, quoted in Evans (1983: 92).

9. Quintin Hogg (MP), in *Parliamentary Debates*, House of Commons, 27 Feb. 1968, v.759, c.1262.

10. Lord Chancellor Viscount Kilmuir in a May 1961 report to the Cabinet, quoted in *The Times*, 1 Jan. 1992, 5.

11. Labour Shadow Home Secretary Gordon Walker, in *Parliamentary Debates*, House of Commons, 16 Nov. 1961, v.649, c.714. Over 40 per cent of New Commonwealth immigrants had settled in London, and 30 per cent in the industrial cities of the West Midlands—and in rather small sections of those urban areas at that. This came on top of an acute housing shortage during the 1950s, aggravated by a reduction of council housing and relaxation of private-sector rent control under the Macmillan government, which produced severe racial clashes over scarce council housing (Carter *et al.*, 1993: 61–3).

12. Ibid., c.687 f.
13. Ibid., c.701.
14. Quoted in *The Times*, 1 Jan. 1992, 5.
15. *Parliamentary Debates*, House of Commons, 16 Nov. 1961, v.649, c.695.
16. The passport criterion, which would become the embattled subject of the Act's amendment in 1968, was introduced for sheer administrative convenience, because it helped avoid the verification of birth at the point of entry.
17. Ibid., c.792–803.
18. *Parliamentary Debates*, House of Commons, 27 Feb. 1968, v.759, c.1242.
19. Ibid., c.1255.
20. The Kenyan Independence Act of 1963 stated that its Asian residents—formally citizens of the United Kingdom and Colonies—had the option of either acquiring local citizenship or retaining UK citizenship, which entitled them to UK government passports. But the existence of a British government pledge to exempt the East African Asians from immigration control was questioned by some. For instance, Enoch Powell (1988: 42) argued that the right of entry was 'quite unintentionally' conferred upon the East African Asians, because after the abolition of the Colonial government only the local High Commissioner (i.e. the UK government) could issue British passports. Accordingly, 'a flaw in the drafting' (Powell) of the 1962 Act, and no intentional pledge, exempted the East African Asians from immigration control. During the second reading of the 1968 Commonwealth Immigrants Bill, the Under-Secretary of State for the Home Department, David Ennals, rejected this view: 'Those who did not automatically obtain Kenyan citizenship were given a right to claim a British passport and thus to be exempt from immigration control. It is disingenuous to suggest that those who were involved in the negotiations for Kenyan independence did not know the consequences of the decisions which were taken' (*Parliamentary Debates*, House of Commons, 27 Feb. 1968, v.759, c.1354).
21. Ibid., c.1345.
22. *Parliamentary Debates*, House of Commons, 27 Feb. 1968, v.759, c.1251.
23. Quintin Hogg, ibid., c.1265.
24. *East African Asians* v. *United Kingdom* (1973), 3 E.H.R.R. 76 (quote from p. 83).
25. *Parliamentary Debates*, House of Commons, 8 Mar. 1971, v.813, c.42.
26. Ibid., c.46.
27. BOCs are citizens in former colonies without local citizenship, most notably East African Asians still residing in Africa or who moved to India. BDTCs are citizens in existing colonies, most notably Hong Kong. The 1977 Green Paper estimated the pool of BOCs and BDTCs at 190,000 and 3.3 million, respectively (UK Home Office, 1977: 10).
28. Home Secretary William Whitelaw, *Parliamentary Debates*, House of Commons, 28 Jan. 1981, v.997, c.939.
29. Whitelaw, ibid., c.936.
30. 'From the humiliation of having no nation to which we distinctively belong, the people of the United Kingdom are now setting themselves free' (E. Powell, quoted in Dixon, 1983: 172).
31. Section 1(5) of the 1971 Immigration Act stipulated: 'The rules shall be so framed that Commonwealth citizens settled in the United Kingdom at the coming into force of this Act and their wives and children are not, by virtue of anything in the rules, any less free to come into and go from the United Kingdom than if this Act had not been passed.' It was removed in the 1988 Immigration Act.
32. David Coleman (1994: 60) used a 'hydraulic analogy' to visualize this policy,

'with constant repairs and additions being made to a basically sound structure in order to stop water slopping over the top or finding its way through new or previously undetected leaks'. Clumsy and cynical as the 'hydraulic analogy' may be, it catches the spirit of Britain's firm policy on secondary immigration.

33. The official 'pressure to emigrate' theory is documented in CRE (1985: 157).

34. Home Office Secretary of State Timothy Raisin, in *Parliamentary Debates*, House of Commons, 25 June 1982, v.26, no.140, c.691–2.

35. This is revealed in the CRE investigation on immigration control procedures on the Indian subcontinent, which had free access to secret instruction materials and interview protocols of British entry-clearance officers in Pakistan and Bangladesh (CRE, 1985).

36. This was denied by the government, which considered the existence of queues a matter of fact, not of policy. As Secretary of State David Waddington put it, 'The number of applicants [on the Indian subcontinent] seeking to settle in the United Kingdom exceeds the capacity of the resources available to deal with them without people having to wait in queues. This is a fact . . . There is therefore no deliberate policy of delay.' Quoted in the Joint Council for the Welfare of Immigrants statement to the 1978 Home Affairs Committee on Immigration from the Indian Sub-Continent (House of Commons, 1986*b*: 88).

37. Since 1975 there have been priority queues for newly married and young children. But they further lengthened the waiting times for the non-privileged rest. The system of differentiated queues was evermore refined over the years. In 1985, for instance, the British High Commission in Dhaka operated with five queues: 1. newly married wives (waiting-time to first interview: two weeks); 2. wives of UK passport-holders with a claim to right of abode (waiting-time: six months); 3. first and only wives with no children over the age of ten years, unaccompanied children under twelve (waiting-time: six months); 4. all other first time applicants, including husbands and male fiancés (waiting-time: 21 months); 5. repeat applications (waiting-time: 24 months). See House of Commons (1986*b*: 175).

38. There is the possibility of appealing a denied entry clearance, but only in Britain, on the basis of the interview protocols and generally in absence of the applicant. See the discussion about the rationale and fairness of this procedure in House of Commons (1986*b*: 146–8).

39. At the 1978 United Nations Conference on Racism and Racial Discrimination in Geneva, the UK delegation rejected the call for a right of family reunion: 'The United Kingdom Government cannot recognize family reunion as a fundamental right, owing to considerations of public policy and national security' (quoted in CRE, 1985: 28).

40. Statement during the 1978 election campaign, quoted in *Parliamentary Debates*, House of Commons, 25 June 1982, v.26, n.140, c.637.

41. Tony Marlow (MP), in *Parliamentary Debates*, House of Commons, 10 Dec. 1982, v.33, n.28, c.431.

42. Quoted in *Parliamentary Debates*, House of Commons, 25 June 1982, v.26, n.140, c.637.

43. The total number of new admissions for settlement dropped from 82,400 in 1975 to 53,000 in 1983. The decline of New Commonwealth settlement was especially steep, from 55,100 new admissions in 1976 to 27,500 in 1983, about two-thirds of whom were wives and children (CRE, 1985: pp. v and 6, respectively).

44. Quoted in 'New Immigration Rules Breach Convention, Lord Scarman Says', *The Times*, 18 Jan. 1980.

45. This had to be clear from the European Commission's verdict in *East African Asians* v. *United Kingdom*, where three cases of husbands prevented from joining their British wives were found in violation of Articles 14 and 8, which prohibit sexual discrimination and protect family life, respectively (see Evans, 1983: 97–100).

46. *Parliamentary Debates*, House of Commons, 10 Dec. 1982, v.33, n.28, c.360. The White Paper put it this way: 'The present rules were drafted at a time when British nationality law contained no satisfactory definition of persons with a close connection with this country. But the new status of British citizen introduced by the British Nationality Act 1981 provides such a definition and it is now appropriate to rely on that status to define those women who, because of their close connection with the United Kingdom, should be allowed to have their husbands or fiancés join them here, provided that the other conditions are met' (Home Office, 1982, p. iii).

47. When approached about the continued discrimination against settled immigrant women, the Minister of State pointed out that the Government was 'still concerned about the employment implication' ('Widespread Anger at Immigration Changes', *The Times*, 26 Oct. 1982). There was a second motive for withholding family rights from settled female immigrants: upgrading the newly created British citizenship. This was expressed by Lord Elton: 'Acquisition of British citizenship [was] an important step which demonstrated that a person had decided to throw in his or her lot with us. If a woman chose some other citizenship the Government saw no reason why she should be able to bring her husband here' ('Minister Defends New Rules', *The Times*, 22 Feb. 1983). Such employment and citizenship concerns pointed into a clear direction: no sex equality in family reunification without abolishing Section 1(5) of the 1971 Immigration Act.

48. 'Immigration Rule Change to Go Ahead', *The Times*, 12 July 1982.

49. Another, rather draconian, proposed safeguard was to increase to two years the probationary period for immigrant husbands, including immediate deportation in case of a marriage breakdown, whatever its reason. This safeguard was later dropped.

50. Quoted in 'Ministers Expect Immigrants Victory', *The Times*, 7 Dec. 1982.

51. See the statement by Secretary of State David Waddington before the second vote on the revised immigration rules, in *Parliamentary Debates*, House of Commons, 11 Feb. 1983, v.36, n.57, c.241: 'In the context of immigration as a whole the figures are small.'

52. European Court of Human Rights, *Case of Abdulaziz, Cabales and Balkandali*, Judgment of 28 May 1985, Series A, no.94, 38.

53. Rejecting the birth discrimination charge (which had earlier been accepted by the European Commission) sanctioned the 'substantive connection' and 'patriality' doctrines established in the 1968 Commonwealth Immigrants Act and the 1971 Immigration Act. However, the point was moot since the 1981 British Nationality Act had gone into effect and the 1980 immigration rules had been changed accordingly.

54. Ibid. 34.

55. *Parliamentary Debates*, House of Commons, 22 July 1985, v.83, n.160, cc.893–6.

56. Ibid., c.895.

57. Ibid., c.896.

58. Gerald Kaufman, ibid., c.901.

59. Either unaware of or shrewdly passing over his contradiction, Home Secretary Brittan pointed out himself that the extension of the marriage tests would require 'to introduce legislation', that is, the dropping of Section 1(5). See ibid., c.894.

60. Interestingly, Minister of State Timothy Renton sought to soften this break of commitment by pointing out that those who now profited from Section 1(5) had been infants in 1971: 'Those who are receiving the benefit of Section 1(5) are not those who were adult males at the time of the 1971 Act but the young children who had then just been born' (ibid., c.856).
61. 'Immigrants: Keep Out', *The Economist*, 14 Nov. 1987.
62. Ian Macdonald, 'Bits and Pieces that Don't Add Up', *Guardian*, 13 Nov. 1987.
63. *Parliamentary Debates*, House of Commons, 16 Nov. 1987, v.122, no.44, c.795–6. That 'most tawdry little measure', the 1988 Immigration Act, exemplifies the logic of loophole-closing underlying British immigration policy. Among its other provisions are the prevention of polygamous family reunions (which concerned only twenty-five cases per year) and the removal of appeal rights for someone claiming to be British citizen by descent. The last measure was in response to a concrete episode of some 1,500 foreign women and children claiming such appeal rights. As Home Secretary Hurd had to admit, there had been no such claims in the past year: 'But again, we need to close the loopholes' (ibid., c.792). The most serious provision was making overstaying a criminal offence without a meaningful right of appeal. This further increased the already considerable deportation powers of the government.
64. In practice, however, it remained much easier for wives and fiancées to pass the marriage tests than for husbands or male fiancés (Macdonald and Blake, 1991: 260).
65. Other secret instructions recommend taking into account 'the fact that it has been traditional in some countries for the wife to follow the husband to his home after marriage', which suggests that arranged marriages are immigration marriages; they provide hypothetical questions (e.g. 'If your fiancée did not live in the UK would you still marry her? If your family had asked you to marry a local girl, would you have done so?'), and suggest to take negative answers as indicators of an immigration marriage (however, not 'solely'); or they suggest more concretely that a man who intends to marry a divorced woman (shunned in Muslim culture) must have immigration as his primary purpose in marriage. Such 'hidden' immigration rules are outside the law, but primary purpose decisions came to be made on their basis (all quotes are from House of Commons, 1986*b*: 112–13).
66. It may be useful to cite the relevant passage in the Immigration Rules (version of 1990, HC 251): 'A passenger seeking admission to the United Kingdom as the spouse of a person who is present and settled in the United Kingdom . . . must hold a current entry clearance granted for that purpose. An entry clearance will be refused unless the entry clearance officer is satisfied: (a) that the marriage was not entered into primarily to obtain admission to the United Kingdom; and (b) that each of the parties has the intention of living permanently with the other as his or her spouse; and (c) that the parties to the marriage have met; and (d) that there will be adequate accommodation for the parties and their dependants without recourse to public funds in accomodation of their own or which they occupy themselves; and (e) that the parties will be able to maintain themselves and their dependants adequately without recourse to public funds' (quoted in Macdonald and Blake, 1991: 574 f.). Much of the conflict over primary purpose centred on the relationship between (a) and (b), the Home Office claiming that the genuineness of marriage (b) did not yet imply that the primary purpose was not immigration (a), immigrants and their legal advisers claiming that fulfilling (b) was conclusive evidence that also (a) was fulfilled.
67. *Parliamentary Debates*, House of Commons, 5 Mar. 1984, v.55, no.112, c.662.

68. See Marrington (1985); Macdonald and Blake (1991: 260–5); Scannell (1992); and Sachdeva (1993: ch. 4).
69. The quote is from the High Court opinion in *Regina* v. *Immigration Appeal Tribunal, Ex parte Bhatia*, which is summarized in *The Times*, 12 Apr. 1985.
70. To convey the flavour of later case-law, I quote from the Court of Appeal decision in *Sumeina Masood* (1991): 'The wife had the whip hand. She was the person who was saying quite firmly "I am a British citizen, . . . I am not going to live with you permanently unless you can" . . . The husband's intention to live with her . . . was itself contingent upon him obtaining an entry clearance certificate. Once the entry-clearance officer and the adjudicator both reached that stage . . . , it followed that it was but a short step to the conclusion that the marriage was entered into primarily to obtain admission to the United Kingdom' (in Scannell, 1992: 6).
71. There are numerous immigration rules devised to make life difficult for specific categories of family immigrants. For instance, the 'sole responsibility' rule keeps Caribbean single immigrant mothers apart from the children they had left behind, even though the father had never lived with the child and did not oppose the application (Macdonald and Blake, 1991: 272–4). Or take the classic catch-22 implicit in the rules on dependent relatives. They stipulated that the applicant had to have 'a standard of living substantially below that of their own country'. In the case of applicants from poorer countries (that is, the Caribbean or the Indian subcontinent), the fact of dependency on remittances from the UK had to elevate applicants above the minimum level, so that they no longer qualified (ibid. 285 f.). After a High Court rule on this 'manifestly unjust' and 'absurd' immigration ban, the 'standard of living' clause was withdrawn in 1986 (see 'Judge Rejects "Absurd" Immigration Ban', *Guardian*, 11 July 1986).
72. See Gillespie (1992) and Menski (1994). New immigration rules passed in 1994 make marriage-based immigration contingent upon 'adequate accommodation for the parties and any dependants without recourse to public funds in accommodation which they own or occupy *exclusively*' (in Menski, 1994: 115; emphasis supplied). The new 'exclusivity' test not only imposes new financial burdens, but also amounts to a deliberate challenge to the extended family life patterns of South Asians.
73. European Court of Justice, *Judgment on Surinder Singh*, 7 July 1992, C–370/90, pp. I–4288 ff.
74. In anticipation of *Singh*, Britain has softened its primary purpose rule by exempting marriages that have existed for at least five years or that involve children with the right of abode.
75. A *Times* editorial ('Tamil Fears', 29 May 1985) warns of the 'possibility that the disturbances in Sri Lanka (are) being used as a pretext for evasion of the strictness with which our immigration controls are habitually enforced, a strictness that is one of the props of good race relations within Britain'.
76. Douglas Hurd, 'Firm but Fair Control on Asylum Builds Harmony in Our Cities', *Independent*, 26 July 1989. Characteristically, the subtitle reads: 'Douglas Hurd defends the Government's much criticised immigration [*sic*] policy'.
77. Home Secretary Kenneth Clarke, *Parliamentary Debates*, House of Commons, 2 Nov. 1992, v.213, n.64, c.24.
78. The Immigration Rules of 1980 exempted asylum-seekers from the need to have an entry clearance or visa. But would-be entrants without proper documentation were still technically processed as 'illegal' entrants, who could appeal against a denial of entry (and asylum) only from overseas. Judicial review was available, but

ineffective because limited to the review of procedures (rather than substantive merit of a case).

79. *Regina* v. *Secretary of State for the Home Department, Ex parte Bugdaycay* (see *The Times* law-report, 'Refugee Status Questions are for Administrators not Judiciary', 12 Nov. 1985). This High Court rule was upheld by the House of Lords in 1987.

80. Interview with Ann Owers (formerly Joint Council for the Welfare of Immigrants), 18 July 1995, London.

81. As *The Economist* ('Back-door and Front-door', 1 June 1985) put it, '[the Home Office] cannot afford to treat the Tamils better than those to whom it is already denying established rights'.

82. Andrew Rawnsley, 'Brando Hurd has them Raving in the Gallery', *Guardian*, 19 Jan. 1989.

83. 'Britain Leads in Politics of Closed Door', *Sunday Times*, 22 Jan. 1989, B3.

84. The Sinhalese government made no attempt to arrest Mendis after his arrival, and Sri Lankans generally remained 'indifferent to his fate'. There he complained about his 'horrendous treatment in Britain', professing that 'my political struggle has been and continues to be focused upon opposition to racism and imperialism in Britain' ('Mendis "Wrong" on Threat to Life', *Guardian*, 28 Jan. 1989). In 1991, Mendis was eventually granted asylum—by Germany. In his balanced assessment of the Mendis case, Robin Cohen (1994: 155) admits that 'the high ground . . . was ultimately won by the frontier guards and not by the anti-deportation movement'.

85. 'Expelled Tamils Beaten in Sri Lanka', *Guardian*, 7 May 1989.

86. 'Hurd "Deported Tamils Illegally" ', *Guardian*, 17 Aug. 1989.

87. 'Baker Admits Bar on Kurds was Unlawful', *Guardian*, 25 Jan. 1991.

88. Quoted in 'Baker in Contempt of Court', *Guardian*, 28 July 1993, 1.

89. The five Tamils refouled in 1988 had argued that their denial of an in-country appeal possibility was in breach of the European Convention on Human Rights. Irony of ironies, the European Court of Human Rights decided that the convention had not been violated, and that a judicial review of procedures (rather than of merit and facts) was sufficient (see the *Guardian* law-report 'Expulsion of Tamils was Lawful', 6 Nov. 1991).

90. 'Asylum Bill Condemned as "Racist" Legislation', *Independent*, 12 Jan. 1993.

91. 'EC Rules May Return Genuine Refugees', *Guardian*, 1 Dec. 1992.

92. 'Britain "Barring More Refugees" ', *Guardian*, 1 Dec. 1994. The increase of the refusal rate has been at the cost of 'exceptional leave to remain' admissions, which have been down from 77 per cent in the first half of 1993 to 21 per cent in the first quarter of 1994 (National Council, 1995: 28).

93. See the *Guardian* ('Welcome to Britain', 8 June 1994) documentation of life in Campsfield House, called a 'first-class facility' by the Home Office.

94. 'Expulsion Row Grows', *Guardian*, 27 Dec. 1993, 1.

95. British asylum policy is still in flux, moving toward further restrictions. In Dec. 1995, a new Asylum and Immigration Bill was passed which would cut off welfare benefits from post-entry asylum seekers. A related new immigration rule was struck down by the Court of Appeal in June 1996 in unusually fervent language ('Troublesome Foreigners', *The Economist*, 29 June 1996, 39).

96. The 'Bangemann-wave' is named after single market commissioner Martin Bangemann, who had worked out this compromise with Home Secretary Kenneth Clarke shortly before the coming into force of Europe's internal market in Jan. 1993. The British government quickly withdrew the compromise.

97. 'No Land is an Island', *The Economist*, 1 Aug. 1992, 49.
98. Quoted in 'Treaty Under Fire Over Immigration', *Guardian*, 29 Jan. 1993.
99. Most importantly the fourth protocol of the European Convention on Human Rights. When asked in 1968 why it had not signed it while all other European governments had, the British government wistfully responded that no other country 'has quite the same difficulties as we have over immigration' (Macdonald and Blake, 1991: 321).
100. On the bill of rights, see most prominently *The Economist*, 'Why Britain Needs a Bill of Rights', 21 Oct. 1995. See also Lester (1994) and Storey (1994). On judicial review, see Sterett (1994).

INTRODUCTION TO PART II

1. Among the more sophisticated articulations of this concern is Ward (1991).

CHAPTER 5

1. Among the few exceptions are refugee settlement programmes, policies designed to promote English language acquisition (discussed below), and the anti-discrimination provisions in IRCA (see Ch. 2). Until the changes in welfare and immigration law in 1996, the eligibility of legal immigrants for most mainstream social programmes has amounted to *'de facto* immigrant policy' (Fix and Zimmermann, 1994).
2. A good overview on cultural pluralism is Higham (1975: ch. 10).
3. See Richard Alba (1990: 290), who observed 'a paradoxical divergence, between the long-run and seemingly irreversible decline of objective ethnic differences—in education and work, family and community—and the continuing subjective importance of ethnic origins to many white Amercans.' Alba's data reconfirm the 'symbolic ethnicity' hypothesis. However, his further claim of an emergent new group of 'European Americans', defined by 'a history of immigration and mobility' (ibid. 314), is added on rather than genuinely derived from his data.
4. '. . . that what the son wishes to forget the grandson wishes to remember' (Hansen, 1952: 495).
5. Waters's (1990: 35) popularity ranking of ethnicities had 'Italian' at the top, followed by English, Irish, German, and—at the very bottom—Scottish. This is an astonishing reversal of the public attitude toward Italian immigrants, who were once characterized as 'the most vicious, ignorant, degraded, and filthy paupers, with something more of an admixture of the criminal element', or simply as 'dago ditchdiggers' (quoted in Portes and Bach, 1985: 35).
6. The most extreme case is perhaps the Cuban exile community in Miami, which accomplished what Portes and Stepick (1993) called 'acculturation in reverse', the importation of foreign customs, institutions, and language into the native population. In the American Southwest, the massive arrival of immigrants from contiguous Mexico is sometimes dubbed *La Reconquista*, the recovery of territory that had once been Mexican. George Borjas even sees a 'Chicano Quebec' in the making, 'as a group emerges with strong cultural cohesiveness and sufficient economic and political strength to insist on changes in the overall society's ways of organizing itself and conducting its affairs' ('The Reconquista', *Atlantic Monthly*, Nov. 1996, 68).
7. Accordingly, national-origins restrictionism rejected even the assimilationist

melting-pot model, and thus is located entirely outside of the usual melting-pot versus cultural-pluralism contest (see Higham, 1955: ch. 11).

8. 'The racial dimension [is] present . . . in *every* identity, institution and social practice in the United States' (Omi and Winant, 1986: 68).

9. Senator Hubert Humphrey put the rejection of quotas in folksier terms: 'If . . . in Title VII . . . any language [can be found] which provides that an employer will have to hire on the basis of per centage or quota related to color, . . . I will start eating the pages [of the bill] one after another' (in Petersen, 1987: 200).

10. 'You do not take a person who for years has been hobbled by chains and liberate him, bring him to the starting-line and then say, "You are free to compete with all the others" . . . We seek not just freedom but opportunity, not just equality as a right and a theory but equality as a fact and as a result' (President Johnson, in Graham, 1990: 6).

11. The only systematic documentation thus far available of how and why the federal government has recognized minority status is about the Small Business Administration's (SBA) selection of minority groups entitled to 'set asides'. George LaNoue and John Sullivan's (1994) fascinating analysis of the selection process reveals that the SBA employed a 'hodgepodge of rationales' that appear largely to be pretexts for its erratic decisions (p. 461).

12. The dilemma is clear: majority minority districts increase the number of minority representatives in the polity, but weaken the strength of the Democratic Party that has traditionally represented minority interests. For instance, as a result of creating black-majority districts after the 1990 census, the number of blacks elected to Congress from the southern states jumped in 1992 from 5 to 17, the highest number since Reconstruction. In the 1994 Congressional elections, however, Republicans took 15 previously Democratic seats across the South, which had been 'whitened' by colour-conscious redistricting ('For Very Strange Bedfellows, Try Redistricting', *New York Times*, 23 July 1995).

13. In its 1990 decision *Metro Broadcasting, Inc.* v. *Federal Communications Commission*, the Supreme Court applied the diversity rationale outside higher education, affirming the constitutionality of the FCC's preferential allocation of broadcast licences to minorities: this was in the interest of 'promot(ing) programming diversity' (in Foster, 1993: 118).

14. 'Census Sees a Profound Ethnic Shift in US', *New York Times*, 14 Mar. 1996, A16.

15. As Roger Waldinger (1996: ch. 7) described in the case of New York City, blacks have succeeded the Irish in monopolizing public-sector employment. In 1990, blacks constituted 25 per cent of the city's population, but made up 36 per cent of the city's work force (p. 227). This created conflicts with Hispanics, who held only one-third as many municipal jobs as blacks despite being equally big in numbers (p. 249). Waldinger concludes: 'African-American New Yorkers now occupy an ordinary ethnic role in New York's segmented system, as just another, albeit important, self-interested player in the same old game of splitting up the pie' (p. 253). While Waldinger does not explicitly discuss affirmative action, his analysis suggests that it fulfills the functions of the old political machine (for the latter, see Erie, 1988).

16. Quoted in Kamasaki and Yzaguirre (1991: 7). The quote refers to the assimilationist thrust of pre-civil rights era Hispanic politics, in which Mexican-Americans successfully asked to be considered 'white' for the census and other government purposes.

17. Interview with Charles Kamasaki (National Council of La Raza), 1 Apr. 1994, Washington.

18. 'A Black-Hispanic Struggle Over Florida Redistricting', *New York Times*, 30 May 1992, 6.
19. Ibid.
20. This is the result of Paul Sniderman and Thomas Piazza's (1993) sophisticated survey analysis of white American attitudes toward blacks.
21. This view has been influentially advanced by legal scholar Owen Fiss (1976).
22. Quoted in *New York Times*, 13 June 1995, D24.
23. Ibid.
24. Ibid.
25. Quoted in 'US Issues New, Strict Tests for Affirmative Action Plans', *New York Times*, 29 June 1995, A16.
26. 'Not Over Till It's Over', *The Economist*, 16 Nov. 1996.
27. David Hollinger (1995: ch. 2) has introduced the (polemical) notion of an ethno-racial pentagon to denote the official races that make up US society: whites, blacks, Hispanics, Asians, and American Indians.
28. 'More Than Identity Rides On a New Racial Category', *New York Times*, 6 July 1996, 1.
29. This is no mere abstraction. In *Malone* v. *Haley* (1989), the Supreme Judicial Court of Massachusetts had to deal with fair-haired and light-skinned twin brothers claiming to be black in order to catch jobs in the Boston fire department. All they could produce was a questionable and inconclusive photograph of an allegedly black woman they claimed was their great-grandmother. The court rejected their claim. However, had the depicted woman indeed been black and ancestrally related to the Malones, the twins would be entitled to call themselves 'black', according to the curious 'one drop of blood' determination of blackness in the United States (formulated in *Plessy* v. *Fergusson* but never officially rescinded). For a history of the 'one drop of blood' rule, see Davis (1991).
30. For instance, the EEO–1 form that employers are required to file according to Title VII of the Civil Rights Act adds Hispanic to the racial categories of black, white, Asian, and American Indian, making them mutually exclusive entries. According to the census, however, Hispanics can be of any race, resulting in over-lapping entries.
31. This polemical thrust is visible in the titles of some of the few (more or less) read-able accounts of American multiculturalism: 'Dictatorship of Virtue' (Bernstein, 1995); 'Twilight of Common Dreams' (Gitlin, 1996); 'The Disuniting of America' (Schlesinger, 1992); or 'Postethnic America: Beyond Multiculturalism' (Hollinger, 1995).
32. 'Bilingual education' proper (1) requires the teaching of all school subjects in the native language for several years, so that the students learn the subject mattter while making, with the help of gradually increased English lessons, the transition from the native language to English. Among the alternatives to bilingual educa-tion are the traditional sink-or-swim method of 'structural immersion' (2), in which no attempt is made to teach in the native language, and 'English as a Second Language' (3), in which the lack of English proficiency is countered with what seems most logical: additional English lessons. For an insider view of how (1) pre-vailed over (2) and (3), see Porter (1990).
33. Public schools in the United States are mostly funded by local and state taxes, with federal funding amounting to about 10 per cent of their revenues. Title VI of the 1964 Civil Rights Act allows federal officials to withdraw these funds from schools that violate anti-discrimination laws and regulations. This became the

inroad for federally mandated bilingual education programmes. See Ravitch (1983: 268).

34. 'Schools Are Likely to Stop Automatic English Testing', *New York Times*, 27 Feb. 1996, B3.
35. Ada Jiminez, 'Trapped in the Bilingual Classroom', *New York Times*, 3 Feb. 1996.
36. James Crawford, '37 States Consider "English Only" Bills', *Education Week*, 17 June 1987, 14.
37. California's official English referendum, Proposition 63, was approved by 73 per cent of the voters in Nov. 1986; two years later, a similar campaign in Florida succeeded with 84 per cent of the vote. A Jan. 1991 Gallup survey of 995 registered voters found 78 per cent in favour of 'making English the official language of government in the United States'.
38. At the grassroots, as in Florida's heavily Cuban Dade County, nativist rhetoric is certainly never far from the surface: 'The United States is not a mongrel nation. We have a common language, it's English and we're damn proud of it . . . And when I see the Cuban flag flying all over our town, flown as high and as lofty as the American flag, I don't know about you, but I get angry as hell!' (Terry Robbins, *Bilingualism*, Dade Americans United to Protect the English Language: Miami, 8 Oct. 1987, flyer).
39. Stanley Diamond, *Proposition 63—English Language Initiative* (California English Campaign: San Francisco, undated flyer, c. Nov. 1987).
40. On the other hand, the Federation of Americans for Immigration Reform (FAIR), eager to take a liberal-centrist stance, has separated its case for restricting immigration from any argument about the cultural integration of immigrants. In reality, of course, FAIR and US English are closely intertwined organizations, with overlapping funding and personnel (Crawford, 1992: ch. 6).
41. This is the title of US English's full-page advertising campaign in America's major news magazines, such as *Time* and *Newsweek*, in the early 1990s. Why a Hispanic heads US English is answered as follows: 'I am proud of my heritage. Yet when I emigrated to the United States from Chile in 1965 to study architecture at Columbia University, I knew that to succeed I would have to adopt the language of my new home . . .'
42. The author remembers the not-so-subtle pressure by his former department chairman to have his (and his colleagues') sociology courses meet a new university-wide 'diversity' requirement, which would increase enrolment—and revenues for the department. This was at a southern Californian university once ridiculed as a bastion of conservatism.
43. Interview with Angela Oh, 25 July 1994, Los Angeles.
44. Both quotes are from Porter (1990: 162).
45. Thomas Sobol, 'Understanding Diversity' (letter to the Board of Regents of the New York State Education Department, Albany, New York, 12 July 1991, 1). On file by author.
46. Ibid. 12.
47. New York State Social Studies Review (1991: 20 and 21, respectively).
48. By contrast, New York (like 21 other states) allows individual school districts to use which textbooks they like.
49. Quoted in Robert Reinhold, 'Class Struggle', *New York Times Magazine*, 29 Sept. 1991, 26.
50. Ibid. 46.
51. Ibid. 27.
52. Ibid. 47.

53. The Oakland school district recently acquired notoriety for its attempt to declare black English a separate language, 'Ebonics'.
54. 'A City's Determination To Rewrite History Puts Its Classrooms in Chaos', *New York Times*, 18 Sept. 1991, A17.
55. A core tenet of Afrocentrism is the belief that ancient Greece pirated its philosophy and mathematics from a presumably 'black' Egypt: accordingly, the roots of Western civilization are in Africa.
56. 'Look Who's Saying Separate is Equal', *New York Times*, 1 Oct. 1995, 1.
57. This is the questionable argument made by D'Souza (1995) about American blacks.
58. In response to the tragic killing in 1982 of Vincent Chin, a Chinese-American who was mistaken by his two white killers for a Japanese. Asian-American civil-rights groups have tried to unravel a societal groundswell of anti-Asian violence, and they have lobbied for a 'Hate-Crime Statistics Act'. See Espiritu (1992: ch. 6).
59. A repeated exercise in Asian-American scholarship is to destroy the 'insidious "model minority" stereotype' (Wei, 1992: 49). This is usually done in two ways: pointing at the huge gap in income and education between, say, recent Hmong refugees and fourth-generation Japanese immigrants; and rendering visible the 'glass ceiling' that is said to prevent the Asian élite from acquiring top positions in the corporate world. After the ritual rejection of the 'model minority' image, Bill Ong Hing (1994: 11) mentions some countervailing facts: in 1990, Asians constituted 19 per cent of the freshman cohort at Harvard, 20 per cent at MIT, and 25 per cent at Berkeley (while their population share is only 2.9 per cent); and the 1990 median annual income of $42.250 for Asian-American households exceeded that of $36.920 for the white population.
60. For a history of the Chicano movement, see Munoz (1989).
61. Interview with Mario Moreno (MALDEF), 28 Mar. 1994, Washington.
62. 'The affirmative-action logic pervading America's political culture means that steadily increasing numbers of Mexican immigrants translate into demands for steadily increasing quotas for Latino employees and Latino-majority electoral districts' (Peter Skerry, 'Why Some of L.A.'s Latino Leaders Take a Walk on Immigration', *Los Angeles Times*, 22 Aug. 1993, M6).
63. For brief histories of MALDEF, see O'Connor and Epstein (1984) and MALDEF (1988).
64. According to the *1993 National Roster of Hispanic Elected Officials*, there were 5,170 Hispanics holding publicly-elected offices throughout the United States. This is still a small proportion of the nation's 504,404 elected officials that year, but also a 41.3 per cent increase since 1984 (Pachon and Alegre, 1993: p. viii, x). The great majority of such elected offices are local school-board and city council seats.
65. The National Council of La Raza, today the perhaps most influential Hispanic public policy group in the United States, was set up in 1969 with the help of a Ford Foundation grant, quite like MALDEF. However, in contrast to MALDEF, La Raza is constituency-based, and it functions as an umbrella for over 140 affiliated Hispanic community organizations throughout the United States (see National Council of La Raza, 1992).
66. Interview with Mario Moreno (MALDEF), 28 Mar. 1994, Washington.
67. 'What's the Problem with "Hispanic"? Just ask a "Latino" ', *New York Times*, 15 Nov. 1993, 6. The survey is summarized in Garza *et al.* (1992).
68. 'Hispanic Pragmatism Seen in Survey', *New York Times*, 15 Dec. 1992, 20.

69. In Waters's (1994) sample of second-generation West Indians and Haitian Americans in New York City, 42 per cent of respondents opted for a 'black' and 30 per cent for an 'ethnic' identity. The remaining 28 per cent remained neutral to American race and ethnic classifications, and self-identified as 'immigrants'.
70. Applying Raymond Breton's (1964: 194) terms, ethnic enclaves are characterized by 'institutional completeness', which exists 'whenever the ethnic community could perform all the services required by its members'.
71. Examples of the 'transnational' migration paradigm are Glick Schiller *et al.* (1992), Goldring (1996), or Rouse (1991).
72. This conclusion is confirmed by Maxine Margolis's (1994: ch. 9) observation of lacking community ties among recent Brazilian immigrants in New York City. Margolis attributes this lack of community to the illegal status and the return-orientation of the observed immigrants.

CHAPTER 6

1. 'Germans Planning to Make it Easier for Some to Become Citizens', *New York Times*, 25 Jan. 1993, A4.
2. In its decision on the constitutionality of the Basic Treaty (*Grundlagenvertrag*) with communist East Germany, the Constitutional Court concluded from the Preamble's unity mandate 'that the institutions of the state have to abstain from all measures that are legal obstacles to reunification or render the latter factually impossible' (quoted in Münch, 1981: 9). The creators of the Basic Law evaded the obvious question which of the conflicting goals—national reunification or European unity—should have priority. Of course, the collapse of communism rendered this question obsolete.
3. In an interesting interpretation of German citizenship law, Albert Bleckmann (1990) distinguishes between 'material' and 'formal' citizenship (*Staatsangehörigkeit*), the former being the condition for receiving the latter. From this he concludes that once 'material citizenship'—in the sense of membership in the German cultural nation (*Kulturnation*)—has been achieved through assimilation, the foreign applicant has a right to formal citizenship. This is unorthodox reasoning, because it uses the logic of ethnocultural nationhood to strengthen the legal position of (some) foreign applicants for German citizenship.
4. Albert Bleckmann (1980: 698) concludes from the Basic Law's universal liberty and equality guarantees that the former 'does not try to impose its values on other states and their population groups'. Accordingly, 'the Basic Law demands a balanced policy between assimilating the foreigner to the German population and an integration policy that protects the cultural particularity of the foreigners' (p. 697).
5. Hakki Kestin, 'Die Deutschen fühlen sich den Ausländern gegenüber als Herren', *Frankfurter Rundschau*, 22 July 1987.
6. 'Per Moneta', *Der Spiegel*, 41, 1964, 44.
7. Article 20(1) of the Basic Law says: 'The Federal Republic of Germany is a democratic and social federal state.' The second characterization is commonly referred to as the 'welfare state principle' (*Sozialstaatsprinzip*) of the Basic Law.
8. For instance, the German government must finance the education of a daughter of an Italian guestworker at an Italian university, according to the *Bundesausbildungsförderungsgesetz*; child-rearing abroad must be included in the calculation of German old-age pensions, even though in the country of origin no pension entitlements arise from child-rearing; and a claim to *Kindergeld* (child

allowance) for an EU migrant arises also from her unemployed child living abroad. To be sure, the comprehensive equality of EU nationals is not unconditional, but tied to their labour-market participation. As the European Court of Justice decided, there is no right to free movement only to reap social benefits in another member-state. See Hailbronner (1992: 90–3).

9. A more detailed elaboration can be found in Joppke (1996: 465–76).

10. The chief adviser to the Federal Commissioner for Foreigners admits: 'We don't use the concept of nation-state here, we don't think in these terms' (Interview with Bernd Geiss, 23 Feb. 1994, Bonn).

11. According to one of its proponents, intercultural education 'would acknowledge the immigrant cultures as equal and prepare the children for a life in a multi-national society' (Jürgen Zimmer, 'Integration—aber wie?', *Die Zeit*, 21 Nov. 1980, 34).

12. See the documentation of the 1992 anti-discrimination law symposium at the Evangelical Academy in Tutzing (Foreigner Commissioner of Berlin, 1993), and Rittstieg and Rowe (1992). Outlawing discrimination on the basis of nationality reflects the German reality of foreigner-related discriminations; yet it meets the formal difficulty that unequal treatment on the basis of nationality is a common and legitimate practice in the state system. Accordingly, advocates of an anti-discrimination law construct foreigner-related discrimination as a form of (internationally outlawed) ethnic or race discrimination. On these difficulties, see Mager (1992).

13. But see Bleckmann (1980: 698), who finds 'elements of real minority group protection' in the Basic Law's guarantees of religious freedoms, private schools, and parent rights.

14. Minority rights for Danes and Frisians were guaranteed by the subfederal constitution of Schleswig-Holstein.

15. See Dieter Oberndörfer, 'Völkisches Denken', *Die Zeit*, 10 June 1994, 12.

16. 'Aussen vor', *Der Spiegel*, 1–2, 1981.

17. 'Kleine Bresche', *Der Spiegel*, 6 Feb. 1989.

18. See 'Bohrung und Durchstich', *Der Spiegel*, 41, 1989, 97–101.

19. There is a huge legal literature about the German alien suffrage debate. For its advocates, see Zuleeg (1980; 1987); for its opponents, see Birkenheier (1976), Quaritsch (1983), Bleckmann (1988), and Stöcker (1989; 1991). An excellent summary of the arguments on both sides is Neuman (1992).

20. Accordingly, Josef Isensee derives his opposition to alien suffrage from the 'principle of democracy': 'Alien suffrage would be anti-democratic alien rule [*demokratiewidrige Fremdbestimmung*]' (Isensee, 1987: 304).

21. Quoted in 'Wer ist das Volk?', *Die Zeit*, 29 June 1990, 8.

22. As Josef Isensee (1987: 304) paraphrased the logic of the open republic: 'All state authority derives from the residents of the state [*Wohnbevölkerung*].'

23. Article 28(1) of the Basic Law says: 'In the states, districts [*Kreise*] and municipalities [*Gemeinden*] the people must have a representation that results from general, immediate, free, equal, and secret elections.'

24. Isensee (1987: 306) pointed out that the state-embeddedness of local government was implied in the Basic Law itself. If local government were a part of society, its principles would have to be laid out in the first part of the Basic Law, dealing with individual rights; instead, the Basic Law lays out these principles in the later part on state organization.

25. Presented in 1979 by the first Federal Commissioner for Foreigner Affairs, Heinz Kühn, the Kühn Memorandum had demanded far-reaching measures for integrating immigrants, especially of the second generation.

26. 'Gleich vor Gott', *Der Spiegel*, 30, 1987, 26–8.
27. Federal Constitutional Court, *Judgment of 31 Oct. 1990* (2 BvF2, 6/89), 52.
28. In conjunction with the low birth-rate of the domestic population, the non-citizenship status of most immigrants in Germany means that one of five babies are now born to non-Germans ('Who is a German', *The Economist*, 5 Apr. 1997, 29 f.).
29. Barbara John, 'Wer ist ein Deutscher?', *Zitty* (Berlin), 10 Jan. 1991.
30. Article 116(1) says: 'A German according to the Basic Law is someone who . . . owns German citizenship or who as refugee or expelled of German origin [*deutscher Volkszugehörigkeit*] . . . has been admitted to the territory of the German Reich as it existed on 31 Dec. 1937.' Accordingly, the definition of citizenship is presupposed, rather than prescribed by the Basic Law. But to be 'German' is obviously broader than German citizenship, including also the so-called 'status [or, ethnic] Germans'. This indirectly prescribes a descent-based citizenship regime.
31. The Naturalization Rules are reprinted in Hailbronner and Renner (1991); here, p. 626.
32. Ibid.
33. Ibid. 628.
34. See the excellent documentation 'Wir wollen Deutsche werden', *Zeit-Magazin*, 21 Sept. 1979, 7–16, 70. Unsurprisingly, Bavaria went the extra mile to test assimilation, asking its applicants for the 'first verse of the Bavarian national anthem', how to 'recognize a German *Volkszugehöriger*', or to 'name the German territories lost after the Second World War'. Helmut Quaritsch (1981) is liberal enough not to require enthusiasm for *Erbsensuppe*, *Volkswandern*, or *Büttenreden*. But he still would like prospective Germans to adopt 'industrial virtues' and a 'German attitude to work', and a 'positive attitude to the state', implying not to defraud taxes (p. 78). One wonders how many Germans would have to be expatriated for not following these principles.
35. An excellent overview of ever more inclusive stances toward citizenship policy across the entire political party spectrum is Murray (1994). According to Murray, the party debates over citizenship policy in the 1980s 'effectively demonstrate the fluidity of ideas of national membership, and the way in which national identity may be influenced and shaped by the changing composition of domestic society' (p. 51).
36. The response of the Interior Ministry is reprinted in *Frankfurter Rundschau*, 11 Sept. 1984, 10.
37. For first-generation immigrants, this offer was limited until 31 December 1995; for later-generation immigrants, it was unlimited.
38. See Schmidt Hornstein (1995), which is an instructive portrait of three Turkish residents and their difficult decision to naturalize.
39. Quoted from *Information Sheet of CDU/CSU Bundestagsfraktion*, 10/93, 30 Apr. 1993, 9.
40. Of the twenty-six members of the Council of Europe, only Germany, Austria, and Luxembourg stick to the principle of avoiding multiple citizenship ('In Europa weitgehend akzeptiert', *Frankfurter Allgemeine Zeitung*, 20 Feb. 1993).
41. 'Die erleichterte Einbürgerung', *Frankfurter Allgemeine Zeitung*, 1 July 1993, 4.
42. 'Schiefe Bahn', *Der Spiegel*, 1, 1995, 25.
43. 'Einbürgern, Ausbürgern, Einbürgern', *Die Zeit*, 28 Mar. 1997, 69.
44. Ibid.
45. 'Justizministerin erwartet Gesetzentwurf zur Staatsbürgerschaft bald', *Frankfurter Rundschau*, 3 June 1993, 4.

46. Horst Eylmann, 'Der Mythos der unteilbaren Staatsangehörigkeit', *Frankfurter Allgemeine Zeitung*, 25 Apr. 1997, 18.
47. Johannes Gerster, *Doppelte Staatsbürgerschaft—sachliche Lösung statt Scheindebatte*, CDU–CSU Fraktion im Deutschen Bundestag, DUD, 9, 4 June 1993, 4. Recall the opposite view in the Naturalization Rules, according to which an applicant for citizenship 'must accept economic disadvantages in the state of origin (for instance, limitations on the right to inherit or the requirement to sell property)' (in Hailbronner and Renner, 1991: 634).
48. 'Offensive gegen Gewalt und Fremdenfeindlichkeit', *Das Parlament*, 25 June 1993, 2.
49. Spiros Simitis, 'Zwei Pässe-warum nicht?', *Die Zeit*, 20 Jan. 1995, 4.
50. 'Scholz warnt die FDP vor "wechselnden Mehrheiten" ', *Frankfurter Allgemeine Zeitung*, 19 Dec. 1994, 3.
51. 'Gerster schlägt neues Modell für Staatsbürgerschaft vor', *Frankfurter Allgemeine Zeitung*, 19 Dec. 1994, 1.
52. 'Streit über Staatsbürgerschaft', *Frankfurter Allgemeine Zeitung*, 9 May 1997, 2.
53. 'Schiefe Bahn', *Der Spiegel*, 1, 1995, 25.
54. Horst Eylmann, 'Es gibt keine nationale Blutgruppe', *Die Zeit*, 18 Apr. 1997, 8.
55. 'Unter Blutsbrüdern', *Die Zeit*, 28 June 1996, 4.
56. Interview with Herbert Leuninger (Pro Asyl), 10 Feb. 1994, Hofheim im Taunus.
57. 'Ethnicization is a many-sided variant of discrimination' (Hinnekamp, 1990: 45).
58. Interview with Herbert Leuninger.
59. 'Different Cultures, Equal Rights' was the slogan of the church-organized 'Day of the Foreign Co-Citizen' in 1980 (*Frankfurter Rundschau*, 25 Sept. 1980, 10).
60. The federal and *Länder* governments paid the charity organizations for about two-thirds of their foreigner-related expenses.
61. Thomas Schwarz's (1992: 255) informative study of foreigner-related social policy in Berlin concludes on a sceptical note: '. . . The situation of the clientele has not significantly improved because of this social policy.' The Berlin Senate could venture its experiment in supporting the self-help sector because of the lesser structural influence of subsidiary charity organizations in Berlin.
62. The most detailed study of Turkish self-organizations in Germany is Özcan (1989). A general introduction to the life of Turks in Germany is Sen and Goldberg (1994).
63. The word 'Westberlin' betrayed FIDEF as Moscow-oriented. The Western label was 'West-Berlin'.
64. Interview with Ülkü Schneider-Gürkan (FIDEF), 23 Feb. 1994, Frankfurt am Main.
65. Turkish law proscribed the duplication of Turkish parties abroad. The latter therefore had to operate under different names, as camouflage organizations.
66. As a student of the Turks in Germany observed, the relationship between Turks and Germans is 'complicated by the . . . ethos of both nationalities', which is 'strongly ethno-centrist' (Ashkenasi, 1990: 289 and 306, respectively).
67. A 1981/2 survey of German opinion toward various foreigner groups found the Turks right at the top of an 'antipathy scale'. Eighty-four per cent of Germans found the Turks 'little sympathetic' (even though 71 per cent indicated they had little or no contact to foreigners). See Petra Kappert's informative essay, 'Was bleibt den Türken in der Fremde', *Frankfurter Allgemeine Zeitung*, 25 Sept. 1982.
68. The approximately 300,000 Alevites in Germany belong to the Shi'a branch of Islam. They mix elements of mysticism and folk religion, but hold to less rigid practices than Sunni Muslims: they do not visit mosques or send their children to

Quran schools, and they tend to be politically more liberal. See the instructive portrait of Turkish Alevi and Sunni migrants in Berlin by Wilpert (1988).
69. Kappert, 'Was bleibt den Türken in der Fremde?'.
70. By far the most informative and best-balanced study of organized Turkish Islam in Germany is Binswanger and Sipahioglu (1988). A critical Turkish insider view is Gür (1993).
71. 'Our programme has much in common with the Greens, it is critical of society, really critical, that is, beyond industrialism' (Interview with three members of Milli Görüs, 16 June 1994, Frankfurt am Main).
72. 'Der Islam ist der Weg', *Spiegel*, 12 Feb. 1996, 44–9.
73. The Netherlands are an interesting contrast case, because here the early presence of Turkish state Islam has left no space for Islamic sects to flourish. Accordingly, Islamic institutions in the Netherlands have performed a 'bridge-like function' between Muslim immigrants and the receiving society, which was not the case in Germany (see Doomernik, 1995: 60).
74. This is the estimate of the Federal Office for the Protection of the Constitution (*Verfassungsschutz*), in 'Türkische Extremisten', *Frankfurter Allgemeine Zeitung*, 2 June 1993, 2.
75. 'Wenn die Muftis kommen, gibt's Zoff im Pütt', *Der Spiegel*, 15, 1983, 92.
76. 'Offensive gegen Gewalt und Fremdenfeindlichkeit', *Das Parlament*, 25 June 1993, 2.
77. 'Drinnen vor der Tür', *Die Zeit*, 11 June 1993, 11–13.
78. But this income was earned by, and distributed over, the relatively large average household size of 4.1 persons (see Sen and Goldberg, 1994: 28). For accounts of the new Turkish middle class, see also Goldberg (1992) and Goldberg and Sen (1993).
79. An advertisement 'Proclamation to German Politicians!', published in the *Süddeutsche Zeitung* after the Solingen murders (18/19 July 1994), was signed mostly by this new type of business and professional association: Turkish Academics of Bochum; Turkish–German Physicians' Society (Cologne); Association of Turkish Engineers (Aachen), Association of Turkish Engineers and Architects (Frankfurt), Association of Turkish Engineers, Natural Scientists, and Architects (Munich), Association of Turkish Dentists in Germany (Essen), and the Association of German–Turkish Employers (Cologne).
80. Interview with Ertugrul Uzun (EATA), 13 June 1994, Berlin.
81. Ibid.
82. Ibid. *Deutschländer* is the word homeland Turks use for the young Turks who grew up in Germany.
83. Interview with Zafer Senocak, 13 June 1994, Berlin.
84. Ibid.
85. 'Das Bild von Türken korrigieren', *Frankfurter Allgemeine Zeitung*, 14 Nov. 1995, 4.
86. See Slavenka Drakulic's (1993: 51) reflections on being 'pinned to the wall of nationhood'.
87. See the excellent documentation 'Die Freundschaft zersplittert', *Die Zeit*, 31 Mar. 1995, 17–19.
88. 'Türken, Kurden, Sunniten, Alewiten, Laizisten und Islamisten?', *Frankfurter Allgemeine Zeitung*, 1 Dec. 1996, 6. This charge was not all wrong. Keskin had successfully lobbied the Turkish government for a less restrictive citizenship policy, thus removing all homeland-based legal hurdles for Turkish immigrants to acquire German citizenship. The Turkish Community's first campaign 'We Want

to Become German Citizens' envisages making half of the two million Turkish immigrants German citizens by the year 2000 ('Einbürgern, Ausbürgern, Einbürgern', *Die Zeit*, 28 Mar. 1997, 69).

89. Illegal since Nov. 1993, the German branch of PKK is believed to consist of 5,000 activists and 40,000 sympathizers, which is about 10 per cent of the 450,000 Kurds living in Germany. Their secure residence status has made it impossible to resolve the problem by means of deportation ('Des Innenministers stumpfe Waffe', *Die Zeit*, 4 Aug. 1995, 2).

90. 'Zeitbomben in den Vorstädten', *Der Spiegel*, 16, 1997, 78–93.

91. See 'Jeder Deutsche ein Nazi', *Spiegel*, 47, 1990, 157–74.

92. 'So ein Gefühl der Befreiung', *Der Spiegel*, 46, 1990, 54.

93. Interview with members of the 36-er and Ghetto Sisters streetgangs, in: *Der Spiegel*, 47, 1990, 160.

94. Ibid. 166.

95. Ibid. 170.

96. 'Türksun = Du bist Türke', *Die Zeit*, 12 Jan. 1996, 65.

97. Ibid.

98. Interview with Ertugrul Uzun.

99. Abdullah (1993: ch. 1) claims that only 12 per cent of Turks between 10 and 15 years stick to the religious traditions of their parents; that 58 per cent have abandoned Islam; and that 22 per cent practice Islam only because their parents want it. Unfortunately, he does not indicate the origins of these numbers.

CHAPTER 7

1. These are the four targeted areas of immigrant integration in the 1965 White Paper. In their interesting comparison of the empirical meanings of citizenship in the UK and the United States, Conover *et al.* (1991) found that ordinary Britons espouse 'communal' views of citizenship, with a stress on social rights (whereas Americans hold 'contractual' views of citizenship, with an emphasis on civil rights).

2. *Parliamentary Debates*, House of Commons, 3 May 1965, v.711, c.942.

3. Ibid., c.942. See also the retrospective characterization of race-relations policy by Mark Bonham-Carter, chairman of the Race Relations Board during the mid-1960s 'liberal hour' of British race relations: 'Race-relations policy should seek to convince the public that a policy of equal treatment irrespective of race is in the interests of the whole of society, and that it is not designed for the benefits of particular groups' (Bonham-Carter, 1987: 3).

4. In this most famous speech by a British politician in the postwar era, Enoch Powell depicted a gloomy scenario of US-style violent race conflict in Britain: 'Like the Roman, I seem to see "the River Tiber foaming with much blood". That tragic and intractable phenomenon which we watch with horror on the other side of the Atlantic but which there is interwoven with the history and existence of the State itself, is coming upon us here by our own volition and our own neglect' (Powell, 1992: 169).

5. *Parliamentary Debates*, House of Commons, 12 Mar. 1979, v.964, c.56.

6. The 'positive discrimination' charge has been the most serious in this list. This is evident in its vehement denial by the bill's defenders. For the Home Office Minister of State, Brynmor John, the bill 'gives the lie to those who have alleged that it involves a form of positive discrimination—if by that they mean giving advantage to people who are already on equal terms. It is merely bringing to a position of equality those who are disadvantaged' (ibid. c.166).

7. *Parliamentary Debates*, House of Commons, 3 May 1965, vol.711, c.943.
8. The 1967 PEP report was based on 'situation tests' in six British towns, in which a coloured West Indian immigrant, a Hungarian immigrant, and a white Englishman applied for various opportunities in fields of employment, housing, and commercial service, each claiming equal occupational qualifications or housing requirements. The results displayed systematic discrimination against coloured immigrants. Regarding housing, out of 60 personal applications to landlords West Indians were refused or asked a higher rent in 45 cases, whereas Hungarians underwent similar discrimination on only 3 occasions; regarding employment, only one of 40 firms offered the West Indian a job, whereas the English and Hungarian testers reaped 15 and 10 offers, respectively; and regarding insurance, the West Indian was refused cover in 6 of 20 applications for motor insurance, and was quoted a higher premium on 11 occasions (Lester and Bindman, 1972: 80 f.).
9. Home Secretary Roy Jenkins, quoted in Lester and Bindman (1972: 84).
10. *Parliamentary Debates*, House of Commons, 23 Apr. 1968, vol.763, c.53–4.
11. Ibid., c.55.
12. Regarding employment, small employers, private households, employment abroad, and ships and aircraft were exempted from the 1968 Act, as were small premises and private transactions in the field of housing. In addition, commercial vessels were still free to racially segregate their passengers. For a more complete list of exemptions, see Lester and Bindman (1972: ch. 4).
13. *Parliamentary Debates*, House of Commons, 23 Apr. 1968, vol.763, c.63.
14. The new PEP study showed that even after the 1968 Act a coloured unskilled worker had a one in two chance of being discriminated against when applying for a job; a coloured skilled worker had a one in five chance, and a coloured white-collar worker a one in three chance of being discriminated against (see Macdonald, 1977: ch. 1).
15. Roy Jenkins, in his second spell as Labour Home Secretary, had picked up the concept of indirect discrimination when visiting the United States in 1974 (see Sooben, 1990: 1).
16. Quoted sections are from the 1976 Race Relations Act (see Macdonald, 1977: 517). A third form of discrimination under the 1976 Act is 'victimization' of those who bring proceedings under the Act. The criterion of 'nationality' was deliberately inserted after a House of Lords rule had interpreted it as outside the 1968 Act (see Lester 1987: 24 f.).
17. *Parliamentary Debates*, House of Commons, vol. 906, no. 62, 4 Mar. 1976, c.1552.
18. In American parlance, 'equal opportunity' figured as the colour-blind alternative to the colour-conscious 'equal result' principle in civil-rights law and practice; in British parlance, 'equal opportunity' became a code-word for pushing toward the 'equal result' principle, that is, affirmative action.
19. The Brixton riots lasted three days, with 226 people injured (including 150 policemen) and 200 people arrested. There was extensive property damage, including 26 buildings and 20 cars burnt by rioters. Soon thereafter, similar riots occurred in Toxteth near Liverpool (see Layton-Henry, 1986: 87).
20. In Jan. 1983, the Home Office instituted new Section 11 rules that corresponded to some recommendations of the Home Affairs Select Committee's *Racial Disadvantage* report (1981), such as relaxing the conditions on the size and length of residence of the respective local beneficiary group. However, the government was not prepared to extend provision to non-Commonwealth immigrants over a wider range of needs (as stipulated in the original Ethnic Groups bill). See FitzGerald (1986: 267).

21. Interview with Joe Charlesworth, Commission for Racial Equality, 17 Aug. 1994, London.
22. CRE, *Annual Report 1989*, 9.
23. Having refused to respond to the CRE's first review of the Race Relations Act in the late 1980s, the Tory government finally responded to the second review, two years after its publication, and negatively. All CRE proposals, including strengthening the commission's investigative powers and tightening the screw of anti-discrimination and equal opportunity measures, were rejected as too expensive, impractical, or inappropriate. Defending this affront to the CRE, Home Secretary Michael Howard reiterated the non-legal, conciliatory approach of British race relations: 'Good race relations is not just about legislation to penalize those who transgress. It is as much about promotion, advice, information, help and education. Measures that build confidence, trust, and mutual understanding' ('Fast-Track Route to Tackle Racism', *Independent*, 5 July 1994, 2).
24. 'Domicile', which is unaffected by citizenship, denotes an individual's 'real home' or 'permanent base', as indicated by her 'intention' to live there permanently (Poulter, 1990: 3).
25. English law refuses to acknowledge only overseas 'bare *talaqs*', which occur without notice, delay, or administrative involvement (as practised in India and Saudi Arabia); it recognizes the more formalized and state-supervised *talaq* in Pakistan (Poulter, 1990: 46 f.). *Talaqs* within Britain are outlawed by the Domicile and Matrimonial Proceedings Act of 1973.
26. The Law Lords did not follow the headmaster's defence of minimizing the external differences of pupils from different classes and races and maintaining the Christian character of his school.
27. The Code of Practice does not have the force of law. But courts and tribunals have taken its violation as presumption of unlawful discrimination.
28. Select Committee on Race Relations and Immigration, Session 1972–3, *Education*, i. London: HMSO.
29. Quoted in the preface to the Runnymede Research Report (1985), *'Education For All': A Summary of the Swann Report on the Education of Ethnic Minority Children*. Runnymede Trust: London.
30. The 1981 interim report of the Select Committee under Anthony Rampton, a dedicated race activist from the Lambeth Community Relations Council, had been a sweeping indictment of teachers' 'racism, both intentional and unintentional', having 'a direct and important bearing on the performance of West Indian children in our schools' (quoted in Swann, 1985: 9). The newly installed Tory government found such reasoning unacceptable, and it replaced Rampton by Lord Swann, a 'neutral respected establishment figure' (Rex, 1989: 21). Swann redrafted the chapter on the causes of 'black underachievement', stressing socio-economic factors rather than racism as the cause of black underachievement. In angry response, two distinguished Select Committee members, Ann Dummett and Father M. Hollings, resigned (see 'Swann's Way', *Searchlight*, May 1985, 119, 18). Lord Swann's personal 'guide' to *Education for All* (Swann, 1985b) makes no mention of racism. However, the final report's chapter on 'racism' still makes ample use of the word.
31. See the Swann report's discussion of the principle of 'permeation' (p. 21 in the abbreviated Runnymede version).
32. See also Messina (1989) for a similar, but updated interpretation. Bulpitt (1986) sees 'racial buffering' as part of a general disposition of British élites to push political problems from the 'centre' to the 'periphery'.

33. Dipak Nandy, quoted in Hill and Issacharoff (1971: 30).
34. 'Community Relations Council' is the new word for the old voluntary liaison committees introduced by the second Race Relations Act in 1968; since 1990, they have been renamed again as 'Race Relations Council'.
35. Interview with Makhan Bajwa (IWA and Greenwich Racial Equality Council), 16 Aug. 1994, London.
36. This was one of the few 1981 Home Affairs Committee recommendations that was fully supported by the government: 'The Government agrees that it is essential that local authorities have regular and direct contact with ethnic minority communities in their areas to ensure that the authorities are fully aware of the particular needs and anxieties of these communities' (quoted in Prashar and Nicholas, 1986: 6).
37. Messina (1987: 199), referring to a personal interview with a CRE official.
38. Outside London, similar race initiatives were launched by Labour councils in Bradford, Leicester, Coventry, the West Midlands and Greater Manchester (Ouseley, 1984: 134).
39. Anne Sofer, 'Ken Livingstone's Pantomime Cow', *The Times*, 6 May 1983.
40. See the interview with Ken Livingstone, 'Champion of the People', in *Asian Times* (London), 6 May 1983, 11.
41. In force until the local Labour defeat in 1990, Brent's 'race spy' programme never took off because of bad management and ill-qualified execution ('Race "Spies" Branded Failure', *Guardian*, 15 May 1991).
42. Henry Porter, 'Big Brother is Watching You Down in Brent', *Sunday Times*, 7 Dec. 1986.
43. For a collection of anti-racist follies, see Lansley *et al.* (1989: ch. 7).
44. 'Die Laughing', *Sun*, 7 Sept. 1985.
45. 'Britannia to Rule Down Our Street', *Sun*, 19 Sept. 1985.
46. John Casey, 'One Nation: The Politics of Race', *Salisbury Review*, Autumn 1982, 23–8.
47. David Dale, 'The New Ideology of Race', *Salisbury Review*, Oct. 1985, 17–22. See also the comprehensive review of the British Commonwealth immigration history from such premises by E. J. Mishan, 'What Future for a Multi-Racial Britain?', pt. I and II, *Salisbury Review*, June 1988, 18–27, and Sept. 1988, 4–11.
48. 'Tories Play Loony Left Card', *Guardian*, 18 Nov. 1986.
49. Ironically, there were more cost-effective alternatives to abolishing the GLC and the other Metropolitan Councils. According to O'Leary (1997), Thatcher was driven to the extreme solution by her 'Nietzschean' style: 'Nietzschean policymaking is heroic, designed to transform values. Thatcher's Cabinet refusal to bend to cost-benefit analysis in GLC abolition, and its willingness to send ministers out to defend the indefensible were fascinating folly' (p. 214). Mrs Thatcher thus proved to be a worthy opponent to the anti-racists.
50. The strengthening of parental choice in education cut both ways, allowing radical Muslim groups to reinforce their quest for separate Islamic schools (see Muslim Parliament, 1992).
51. 'Race Equality Staff Ponder New Political Landscape', *The Times*, 10 Dec. 1990, 4.
52. Indians and Caribbeans are Britain's largest ethnic minority groups, with 840,000 and 500,000 members, respectively, in 1991.
53. Afro-Caribbeans combined, in contrast to American blacks, do not differ dramatically from whites regarding housing, employment, or residential segregation; and there is an exceptionally high proportion of mixed black and white

households. Peach (1996: 23) therefore characterizes British blacks as 'one of the most integrated groups'.

54. See the manifesto *Charter 90 for Asians* (hectographed: London, 1 July 1990), whose demands include protection from racial attacks, recognition of cultural identity, and a less restrictive immigration policy—all of them absent from the Afro-Caribbean/anti-racist agenda.

55. 'British Asians Protest at Being Called Black', *Sunday Times*, 26 June 1988, A5.

56. One may interpret this wide definition of racial group, which left out no one, as an ironical reflection of citizenship universalism or 'racial inexplicitness' (Kirp). When asked during the Second Reading of the 1965 Race Relations Bill what 'ethnic' added to the race criteria of 'colour, race, or ethnic or national orgins', Home Secretary Soskice underlined his intention to 'include every possible minority group in the country', including Germans or Cypriots. He added: 'We hope, by the use of the word "ethnic", to cover everybody who is neither of a particular national origin nor of a particular racial origin but who would be distinguished by colour' (*Parliamentary Debates*, House of Commons, 3 May 1965, vol.711, c.933). This was confused thinking, because it combined 'ethnic origins' with 'colour', which was already on the list. But it expresses the inclusive, rather than exclusive, intention of the lawmaker.

57. See Booth (1985), Bhrolchain (1990), Nanton (1992), Sillitoe and White (1992), and Coleman and Salt (1996).

58. Only 7 per cent of Asian respondents rejected the ethnic-group categories of the 1991 census; the 20 per cent of Afro-Caribbeans rejecting these categories must be seen against their overwhelming opposition to an ethnicity question ten years earlier (Bhrolchain, 1990: 560). An obvious shortcoming of the mutually exclusive, discrete ethnic group categories is their failure to capture the offspring from the large and growing number of mixed-race couples in Britain (see Nanton, 1992).

59. See *The All England Law Reports 1983* (1983). London: Butterworths, i. 1062–72.

60. Ibid. 1072.

61. See 'Law Report: Rastafarians Not an Ethnic Group', *Independent*, 16 Feb. 1993, 22. Michael Banton (1989) used Lord Templeman's 'more than' religious group criterion of defining ethnic groupness in *Mandla* to criticize an earlier rule of the Birmingham Industrial Tribunal that Rastafarians were an ethnic group. In contrast to Sikhs and Jews, some but not all of whom were religious, Rastafarians were by definition members of a religious sect—thus lacking the 'more than' religious criterion making them ethnic (p. 156).

62. Quoted in *EOR Discrimination Case Law Digest*, 2, Winter 1989, 4.

63. 'Muslims are Not Covered by Race Act, Tribunal Says', *Independent*, 27 July 1991.

64. The most intelligent comparison of the British Rushdie affair and the French *foulard* affair I have come across is in the pages of the *Financial Times* (Edward Mortimer, 'Liberté, Egalité, Laicité', 12 Dec. 1989).

65. Highlighting the fragmentation of minority groups, as against their politically required unity, is a taboo in the race-relations literature. For exceptions, see Ellis (1991) and Werbner (1991).

66. Because the census does not count the population by religion, there are only rough estimates of the size of the British Muslim population, derived indirectly from national-origins indicators. Wahhab (1989: 8) concluded from the 1981 census that there were about 940,000 Muslims in Britain, more than a third of them

from Pakistan; Anwar (1994: 23) concludes from the 1991 census that the Muslim population was about 1.5 million.

67. The preference for in-marriage persists. By the mid-1980s, only 7 per cent of Pakistani men and 2 per cent of Pakistani women were married to native Britons. For Bangladeshis the mixed marriage rate is even lower. See Joly (1995: 7).

68. It was no accident that the domestic campaign caught fire in Bradford. The majority of its Muslims are Barelvis, whose religious sentiments are centred around the cult of holy men (*pirs*) and the Prophet.

69. In practical terms, this meant '[opposing] the book, not the author' (Interview with Iqbal Sacranie, UK Action Committee on Islamic Affairs, 18 July 1995, London).

70. Roy Hattersley, 'The Racism of Asserting That "They" Must Behave Like "Us" ', *Independent*, 21 July 1989.

71. 'Labour on the Rack Over Rushdie', *Independent*, 22 July 1989.

72. 'Howe Says Rushdie Book is Offensive', *Guardian*, 3 Mar. 1989.

73. Roy Jenkins, 'On Race Relations and the Rushdie Affair', *Independent Magazine*, 4 Mar. 1989.

74. The 'unprecedented' letter was published in *The Times* of 5 July 1989. Along with the Muslim response, it is reprinted in UKACIA (1989).

75. Ibid. 9. Interestingly, some of the addressed Muslim leaders, especially in the UK Action Committee on Islamic Affairs, found fault with the government's reflex-like framing of the issue as one of 'race relations'. In their response to Patten, UKACIA found it 'most misleading to see the Muslim community as an ethnic community', and even advocated a colour-blind stance directly opposite to the race-relations mainstream: 'We look forward to the time when people in Britain will not be classified according to the colour of their skin or ethnic origin but according to their worth and contribution to the well-being of society' (UKACIA, 1989: 11). See also UKACIA (1993). This was certainly not the only stance taken by Muslim organizations (see the overview in Modood, 1993).

76. This government reasoning was supported in the court decision on *Regina* v. *Bow Street Magistrates Courts, Ex parte Choudhury* (1990): 'Their Lordships agreed that extending the law of blasphemy would pose insuperable problems and would be likely to do more harm than good' (quoted in Malik, 1993: 131).

77. So has the CRE in its *Second Review of the Race Relations Act* (1992), which recommends introduction of a law against incitement to religious hatred and giving 'further serious consideration' to a law against religious discrimination, stressing that the latter had to be located outside the race relations nexus (p. 77).

78. Rejecting the quest for voluntary-aided status by the well-equipped Islamia School in London's Brent borough, the Department of Education pointed to 1,500 surplus primary school places within a two mile radius of Islamia ('Muslim School Denied State Aid', *Independent*, 19 Aug. 1993). Because of the declining birth-rate, there were 400 fewer voluntary-aided schools in 1987 than in 1981 (Poulter, 1990: 83).

79. 'Muslims on the March', *Sunday Times*, 9 July 1989. Under the new Labour government of Tony Blair, the rejection of Muslim schools seems to be softening.

80. *Hijaz* refers to the 150,000 square miles of Saudi Arabia that encompass the holy cities of Mecca and Medina.

81. 'Crisis in the Gulf: Muslims Outraged by Attack on Shelter', *Independent*, 15 Feb. 1991.

82. Whereas the Rushdie affair had united British Muslims, the Gulf War divided them. Barelvis, who had always been at odds with the Saudi Arabian Wahabi

tradition of Islam, sided with Saddam for playing the anti-Saudi card. Some Deobandi Imams, the ideological brethren of the Wahabis but concerned about the integrity of the holy shrines, were summoned up by the Saudi government to cool their critique of the Saudi–US alliance. Pro-Iranian Muslim organizations, like the Muslim Parliament, refused to take sides because of the neutral position taken by Iran ('British Moslems Sharply Divided', *Financial Times*, 21 Jan. 1991).

83. Interview with Tariq Modood (Institute for Policy Studies), 19 July 1995, London.
84. Yasmin Alibhai-Brown, 'Made to Feel Like Trespassers on European Soil', *Independent*, 5 July 1993.
85. Ibid.
86. See the instructive portrait of Muslim youth culture in Tower Hamlets, 'Why They Can't Turn Their Backs on the Veil', *Independent*, 28 Apr. 1994.
87. See Kalim Siddiqui (14 July 1990), *Generating "Power" Without Politics*. London: The Muslim Institute, hectographed, 10.
88. See Eickelman and Piscatori (1996: 72).
89. 'Radical Time-Bomb Under British Islam', *Guardian*, 7 Feb. 1994, 6.
90. A *Hizb ut Tahrir* pamphlet says: 'Throw a stone, trigger a bomb, plant a mine, hijack a plane, do not ask how', and 'the believers fight the Jews and kill them.' Quoted in *Guardian*, 7 Feb. 1994, 6.
91. 'Muslim Extremists Challenged for Hearts of Youth', *Guardian*, 5 Aug. 1995.
92. 'The Tragedy is Salman Rushdie has Created More Muslim Leaders Here Than Anyone', *Guardian*, 13 June 1995.
93. Humera Khan, 'Muslims, Be Careful of Europe', *Q-News* (London), 14–20 July 1995, 6.
94. 'Introduction by the Chairman' (1993), *Annual Report*. London: CRE, 6.
95. The CRE's *Second Review of the Race Relations Act 1976* says: 'There is a real danger that one day a process of harmonisation of laws might lead, not to an improvement in protection from racial discrimination across Europe, but to a reduction to, as it were, the lowest common denominator' (CRE, 1992: 68). The rejection of intergovernmental harmonization is to be distinguished from the CRE's campaign for adding 'race' to the EU's Equal Treatment Directive, which as of now covers only sex discrimination. A first step toward this was achieved in a new anti-discrimination provision in the Amsterdam Treaty of 1997. However, the provision is worded so that it cannot have a direct effect at the national level (Elspeth Guild, 'After the Amsterdam Treaty', MERGER [Utrecht], 5/1, 1997, 8).

CHAPTER 8

1. I have spelled out this perspective in Joppke (1998*a*).
2. For *de facto* multiculturalism in philosophically assimilationist France, see Schain (forthcoming).
3. As I outlined in the introduction to Part I, self-limited sovereignty rests on the triple pillars of interest-group politics ('client politics', as Gary Freeman says), domestic legal constraints on the executive, and (particularly in Europe) moral élite constraints toward particular immigrant groups. In the following, I concentrate on legal and moral constraints only.
4. Interestingly, the thesis of pervasive restrictionism is often presented by the same people who see the state globally impaired to control immigration effectively (Sassen, 1996: ch. 3; Sassen 1998). See the rebuttal by Freeman (1998).

5. In the fifteen states that currently constitute the European Union, the size of the international migrant population increased at a yearly average of 3.7 per cent during 1965 and 1975, 2.1 per cent during 1975 to 1985, and 2.0 per cent during 1985 to 1990. In absolute numbers, the immigrant population in Europe grew from 10.9 million in 1965, 15.8 in 1975, 19.4 in 1985, to 21.5 in 1995. See Lahav (1997).

6. The continued relevance of historical migration legacies and networks even for asylum flows casts doubt on the often-heard view, shared by conservatives and liberals alike, that improvements in the sending countries could lower global migration pressures.

7. 'Poor People at the Gate', *The Economist*, 15 Mar. 1991.

8. The Office of European Statistics reported a decline in asylum requests by over 50 per cent between 1992 and 1995 (see Wolf, 1996: 229).

9. See Koslowski's (1998*b*) interesting observation that 'personal security' is increasingly legitimizing a further transfer of power to supranational European Union institutions.

10. Soysal would respond that the dual citizenship implied by territorial birthright citizenship would be yet another instance of postnational membership (see Soysal, 1997: 6 f.). There is a systematic ambiguity about the role of formal state membership in her model—witness that in her earlier study (Soysal, 1994) she speaks alternately of postnational 'citizenship' and 'membership', while its main thrust is to show that guestworkers had acquired full civil and social rights without having formal state membership (i.e. 'citizenship'). If dual citizenship also is postnational membership, the latter shrinks from an institution to an attitude. As throughout this book, I therefore use 'postnational membership' in its narrower, original meaning of non-citizen membership.

11. In 1996, 1.3 million naturalization petitions were filed, then the largest in history; in 1997, an estimated 1.8 million petitions were filed (Schuck, 1998: 195).

12. See Randall Hansen's (1998) instructive discussion of liberalized naturalization procedures in Europe, which states a convergence around granting second-generation immigrants a right to citizenship.

13. Note that only a few months earlier the Italian government had denied entry to boatloads of Albanian refugees, whose final destination was believed to be Italy.

14. See the interview with Emma Bonino, 'Europei, e colpa vostra', *La Repubblica*, 7 Jan. 1998, 2.

15. But there is conflict over the direction of European immigration policy between the 'progressive' European Commission and the more conservative member states. The Commission's 1994 *Communication to the Council and the European Parliament on Immigration and Asylum Policies* states that 'immigration has been a positive process', and that 'a complete halt to immigration [is] neither feasible nor desirable' (in Papademetriou, 1996: 85). The Justice and Home Affairs (JHA) Council, in charge of Third-Pillar issues, drily responded that 'no Member State (was) pursuing an active immigration policy . . . (but) on the contrary . . . (all had) curtailed the possibility of permanent legal immigration for economic, social, and thus political reasons' (ibid. 87). The JHA Council then adopted a resolution restricting the employment of non-EU legal residents in other member states.

16. Article 8(a), added to the Treaty of Rome by the Single European Act of 1987, defines the internal market to be created by late 1992 as 'an area without internal frontiers in which the free movement of goods, *persons*, services and capital is ensured . . .' (in Hailbronner and Polakiewicz, 1992: 52, emphasis supplied).

17. The Amsterdam Treaty requires the Commission to bring forward proposals to resolve the issue of free movement rights for third-country nationals. This suggests a liberal outcome (see Geddes, 1998: 26 f.).
18. Quoted from a European Commission proposal for a comprehensive control and integration policy, in Papademetriou (1996: 85).
19. The European experience in mind, the United States explicitly rejected relinquishing sovereignty to the institutions created to implement NAFTA (like the Free Trade Commission), or bestowing direct rights on individuals. Moreover, immigration questions were deliberately excluded from the ambit of NAFTA. During the treaty negotiations, the Bush administration stated that 'what we are negotiating here is a trade agreement not a social contract. We don't in NAFTA try to parallel the kinds of things which the EC, for instance, is engaged in with respect to political and social rights . . .' (quoted in Cassise, 1996: 1372).

Appendix: Interviews

United States

Angelo Ancheta, Coalition for Humane Immigrant Rights of Los Angeles, 7 July 1994, Los Angeles.

Diana Aviv, Council of Jewish Federations, 1 Apr. 1994, Washington.

Richard Dale, US Senate Judiciary Subcommittee on Immigration, 25 Mar. 1994, Washington.

Jim Dorcy, Federation of Americans for Immigration Reform (FAIR), 24 Mar. 1994, Washington.

Joe Hicks, Southern Christian Leadership Conference, 20 July 1994, Los Angeles.

Charles Kamasaki, National Council of La Raza, 1 Apr. 1994, Washington.

Stewart Kwoh, Asian Pacific American Legal Center, 6 July 1994, Los Angeles.

Daphne Kwok, Organization of Chinese Americans, 23 Mar. 1994, Washington.

Warren Leiden, American Immigration Lawyers Association, 5 Apr. 1994, Washington.

Ira Mehlman, Federation of Americans for Immigration Reform (FAIR), 18 July 1994, Los Angeles.

Mario Moreno, Mexican American Legal Defense and Educational Fund (MALDEF), 28 Mar. 1994, Washington.

Mauro Mujica, US English, 19 Apr. 1994, Washington.

Angela Oh, 25 July 1994, Los Angeles.

Harry Pachon, Tomas Rivera Center, 26 July 1994, Claremont, California.

Demetrios Papademetriou, Carnegie Endowment for International Peace, 20 Apr. 1994, Washington.

Gary Philips, Multi-Cultural Collaborative, 5 July 1994, Los Angeles.

Eugene Pugliese, House Subcommittee on International Law, Immigration, and Refugees, 7 Apr. 1994, Washington.

Irma Rodriguez, Mexican American Legal Defense and Educational Fund (MALDEF), 27 July 1994, Los Angeles.

Frank Sharry, National Immigration Forum, 25 Mar. 1994, Washington.

Rick Swartz, National Immigration Forum, 26 Mar. 1994, Washington.

Jerry Tinker, US Senate Subcommittee on Immigration and Refugee Affairs, 30 Mar. 1994, Washington.

Carlos Vaqcerano, Central American Resource Center, 22 July 1994, Los Angeles.

Charles Wheeler, National Immigration Law Center, 8 July 1994, Los Angeles.

Linda Wong, Rebuild L.A., 15 July 1994, Los Angeles.

Jerry Yu, Korean-American Coalition, 14 July 1994, Los Angeles.

Germany

Ozan Ceyhun (The Greens), Office for Immigrants and Refugees in the Hesse Ministry for Youth, Family, and Health, 24 Feb. 1994, Wiesbaden.

Daniel Cohn-Bendit, Office for Multicultural Affairs, 10 Feb. 1994, Frankfurt am Main.

Theodor Gavras, Foreigner Council Munich, 18 Feb. 1994, Munich.

Bernd Geiss, Office of the Federal Commissioner for Foreigner Affairs, 23 Feb. 1994, Bonn.

Jürgen Haberland, Federal Ministry of the Interior, 23 Feb. 1994, Bonn.

Helmut Huber, Referent for Foreigner Affairs in the Bavarian Ministry for Labour and Social Affairs, 9 Feb. 1994, Munich.

Chong-Sook Kang, Commissioner for Foreigner Affairs of the City of Munich, 22 Feb. 1994, Munich.

Huseyen Kurt, Turkish-Islamic Union and Member of the Communal Foreigner Parliament, 15 June 1994, Frankfurt am Main.

Reinhard Leicht, Referent for Foreigner Affairs in the Hesse Ministry for Women, Labour, and Social Affairs, 25 Feb. 1994, Wiesbaden.

Herbert Leuninger, Pro Asyl, 10 Feb. 1994, Hofheim im Taunus.

Bahman Nirumand, Office for Multicultural Affairs, 25 Feb. 1994, Frankfurt am Main.

Elke Pohl, Office of the Commissioner for Foreigner Affairs of the Berlin Senate, 13 June 1994, Berlin.

Klaus-Henning Rosen (SPD), Federal Ministry of the Interior, 22 June 1994, Bonn.

Semer Sargut, Turkish Community Rhein-Main, 24 Feb. 1994, Frankfurt am Main.

Ülku Schneider-Gürkan, Türkisches Volkshaus (FIDEF), 23 Feb. 1994, Frankfurt am Main.

Thomas Schwarz, Berliner Institut für vergleichende Sozialforschung, 13 June 1994, Berlin.

Zafer Senocak, 13 June 1994, Berlin.

Gulay Simsek and two other members of Milli Görüs, 16 June 1994, Frankfurt am Main.

Ertugrul Uzun, European Association of Turkish Academics, 13 June 1994, Berlin.

Rosi Wolf-Almanasreh, Office for Multicultural Affairs, 24 Feb. 1994, Frankfurt am Main.

Turgut Yüksel, Member of the Communal Foreigner Parliament, 15 June 1994, Frankfurt am Main.

Gregorios Zarkadas, Chair of the Communal Foreigner Parliament, 16 June 1994, Frankfurt am Main.

Great Britain

Yasmin Alibhai-Brown, writer on minority affairs, 17 July 1995, London.

Makhan Bajwa, Greenwich Racial Equality Council, 16 Aug. 1994, London.

Jenny Bourne, Institute of Race Relations, 9 Aug. 1994, London.

Joe Charlesworth, Commission for Racial Equality (CRE), 17 Aug. 1994, London.

Unmesh Desai, Newham Monitoring Project, 11 Aug. 1994, London.

Carol Dixon, 1990 Trust and National Black Caucus, 17 July 1995, London.

Ann Dummett, European Consultant of the Commission for Racial Equality (CRE), 19 July 1995, London.

Suresh Grover, Southall Monitoring Group, 17 Aug. 1994, Southall, Middlesex.

Raga Miah, Tower Hamlets Race Equality Council, 12 Aug. 1994, London.

Tariq Modood, Institute for Policy Studies, 19 July 1995, London.

Ann Owers, former Managing Director of Joint Council for the Welfare of Immigrants (JCWI), 18 July 1995, London.

Bhikhu Parekh, University of Hull, 11 Nov. 1994, Florence.

Rahul Patel, Anti-Nazi League, 8 Aug. 1994, London.

A.R. Rawsthorne, Home Office (Immigration and Nationality Department), 10 Aug. 1994, Croydon, London.

Jill Rutter, British Council of Refugees, 17 Aug. 1994, London.

Iqbal Sacranie, UK Action Committee on Islamic Affairs (UKACIA), 18 July 1995, London.

John Salt, University of London, 8 Aug. 1994, London.

Sarah Spencer, Institute for Public Policy Studies, 18 Aug. 1994, London.

Mark Wadsworth, Anti-Racist Alliance, 12 Aug. 1994, London.

Kalpana Wilson, Migrant Support Unit, 19 Aug. 1994, London.

References

Abdullah, Mohammad (1993), *Was will der Islam in Deutschland?* Gütersloh: Mohn.

Ahsan, M. M., and Kidwai, A. R. (1993) (eds.), *Sacrilege versus Civility*. Leicester: The Islamic Foundation.

Alba, Richard (1990), *Ethnic Identity*. New Haven: Yale University Press.

Albers, Hartmut (1994), 'Glaubensfreiheit und schulische Integration von Ausländerkindern', *Deutsches Verwaltungsblatt*, 1 Sept., 984–90.

Almaguer, Tomas (1996), *Racial Fault Lines: The Historical Origins of White Supremacy in California*. Berkeley and Los Angeles: University of California Press.

Amiraux, Valerie (1996), 'Turkish Islam in Germany', in W. A. R. Shadid and P. S. Van Koningsveld (eds.), *Political Participation and Identities of Muslims in Non-Muslim States*. Kampen: Kok Pharos Publishing House.

—— (1998), 'Transnationalism as a Resource for Turkish Islamic Associations in Germany'. Seminar paper, European Forum on International Migrations, Florence, 5 Mar..

Amnesty International (UK) (1991), 'United Kingdom: Deficient Policy and Practice for the Protection of Asylum Seekers'. London: mimeograph.

Anderson, Margo J. (1988), *The American Census*. New Haven: Yale University Press.

Anderson, Perry (1974), *Lineages of the Absolutist State*. London: Verso.

Anker, Deborah, and Blum, Carolyn Patty (1989), 'New Trends in Asylum Jurisprudence', *International Journal of Refugee Law*, 1/1: 67–82.

Anon., 'Developments in the Law: Immigration Policy and the Rights of Aliens', *Harvard Law Review*, 96 (1983), 1286–465.

Anwar, Muhammad (1994), *Young Muslims in Britain*. Leicester: The Islamic Foundation.

Arab Case (1974), *Decision of the German Federal Constitutional Court* (1 BvR23, 155/73).

Asante, Molefi Kete (1992), 'Multiculturalism: An Exchange', in Paul Berman (ed.), *Debating P.C.*

Ashkenasi, Abraham (1990), 'The Turkish Minority in Germany and Berlin', *Immigrants and Minorities*, 9/3: 303–16.

Auster, Lawrence (1990), *The Path to National Suicide*. Monterey, Va.: The American Immigration Control Foundation.

Bade, Klaus (1992) (ed.), *Ausländer, Aussiedler, Asyl in der Bundesrepublik Deutschland*. Hannover: Niedersächsische Landeszentrale für politische Bildung.

—— (1994*a*), *Ausländer, Aussiedler, Asyl*. Munich: Beck.

—— (1994*b*), *Das Manifest der 60*. Munich: Beck.

Bank, Roland (1998), 'The Emergent EU Policy on Asylum and Refugees'. Seminar paper, European Forum on International Migrations, Florence, 22 Jan..

Banton, Michael (1985), *Promoting Racial Harmony*. Cambridge: Cambridge University Press.

—— (1989), 'Are Rastafarians an Ethnic Group?', *New Community*, 16/1: 153–64.

Barker, Sir Ernest (1951), *The Ideas and Ideals of the British Empire* (2nd edn.). Cambridge: Cambridge University Press.

Barnett, Pamelia S. (1985), 'United States Political Asylum for Salvadoran Refugees', *Houston Journal of International Law*, 8: 131–54.

Bean, Frank D., and Fix, Michael (1992), 'The Significance of Recent Immigration Policy Reforms in the United States', in Gary Freeman and James Jupp (eds.), *Nations of Immigrants*. Melbourne: Oxford University Press.

Berman, Paul (1992) (ed.), *Debating P.C.* New York: Dell.

Bernstein, Richard (1995), *Dictatorship of Virtue*. New York: Vintage.

Bevan, Vaughan (1986), *The Development of British Immigration Law*. London: Croom Helm.

Bhrolchain, Maire Ni (1990), 'The Ethnicity Question for the 1991 Census', *Ethnic and Racial Studies*, 13/4: 542–67.

Bickel, Alexander (1975), *The Morality of Consent*. New Haven: Yale University Press.

Bigo, Didier (1997), 'Europe passoire et Europe forteresse: La Securisation/humanitarisation de l'immigration'. MS.

Birkenheier, Manfred (1976), *Wahlrecht für Ausländer*. Berlin: Duncker and Humblot.

Binswanger, Karl (1990), 'Ökonomische Basis der Fundamentalisten', in Bahman Nirumand (ed.), *Im Namen Allahs*. Cologne: Dreisam.

—— and Sipahioglu, Fethi (1988), *Türkisch-Islamische Vereine als Faktor Deutsch-Türkischer Koexistenz*. Benediktbeuern: Riess.

Blake, Charles (1982), 'Citizenship, Law and the State: The British Nationality Act 1981', *Modern Law Review*, 45: 179–97.

Blake, Nicholas (1988), 'The Road to Sivakumaran', *Immigration and Nationality Law and Practice*, Apr., 12–16.

—— (1990), 'Life after the Lords: Developments in the Case of Sivakumaran and Others', *Immigration and Nationality Law and Practice*, Jan., 7–11.

Blauner, Robert (1972), *Racial Oppression in America*. New York: Harper and Row.

Bleckmann, Albert (1980), 'Ausländerpolitik und Verfassung', *Deutsches Verwaltungsblatt*, 95/17/18: 693–701.

—— (1988), 'Das Nationalstaatsprinzip im Grundgesetz', *Die öffentliche Verwaltung*, 41/11: 437–44.

—— (1990), 'Anwartschaft auf die deutsche Staatsangehörigkeit?', *Neue Juristische Wochenschrift*, 22: 1397–401.

Blumenwitz, Dieter (1993), 'Territorialitätsprinzip und Mehrstaatigkeit', *Zeitschrift für Ausländerrecht und Ausländerpolitik*, 13/4: 151–6.

—— (1994), 'Abstammungsgrundsatz und Territorialitätsprinzip', *Zeitschrift für Politik (ZfP)*, 41/3: 246–60.

Bommes, Michael (1991), *Interessenvertretung durch Einfluss*. Osnabrück: Arbeitsgemeinschaft Kommunale Ausländervertretungen Niedersachsen.

Bonham-Carter, Mark (1987), 'The Liberal Hour and Race Relations Law', *New Community*, 14: 1 ff.

Booth, Heather (1985), 'Which "Ethnic Question"?', *Sociological Review*, 33/2: 254–74.

Borjas, George (1990), *Friends or Strangers: The Impact of Immigrants on the U.S. Economy*. New York: Basic Books.

Bourne, Randolph (1916), 'Trans–National America', *Atlantic Monthly* 118: 86–97.

BRC. See British Refugee Council.

Breton, Raymond (1964), 'Institutional Completeness of Ethnic Communities and the Personal Relations of Immigrants', *American Journal of Sociology*, 70/2: 193–205.

Briggs, Vernon M. (1992), *Mass Immigration and the National Interest*. Armonk, NY: Sharpe.

Brimelow, Peter (1995), *Alien Nation*. New York: Random House.

British Refugee Council (1992), 'UK Asylum Statistics 1982–1992'. London: mimeograph.

Brubaker, Rogers (1989) (ed.) , *Immigration and the Politics of Citizenship in Europe and North America*. Lanham: University Press of America.

—— (1992), *Citizenship and Nationhood in France and Germany*. Cambridge, Mass.: Harvard University Press.

—— (1995), 'Comments on "Modes of Immigration Politics in Liberal Democratic States" ', *International Migration Review*, 29/4: 903–8.

Bull, Hedley (1977), *The Anarchical Society*. London: Macmillan.

Bulpitt, Jim (1986), 'Continuity, Autonomy and Peripheralisation', in Zig Layton-Henry and Paul B. Rich (eds.), *Race, Government and Politics in Britain*. London: Macmillan.

Burgess, David (1991), 'Asylum by Ordeal', *New Law Journal*, 18 Jan., 50–2.

Calavita, Kitty (1994), 'U.S. Immigration and Policy Responses', in Cornelius, Martin, and Hollifield (eds.), *Controlling Immigration*.

Calderon, Jose (1992), ' "Hispanic" and "Latino": The Viability of Categories for Panethnic Unity', *Latin American Perspectives*, 19/4: 37–44.

California Senate Office of Research (1993), *Californians Together: Defining the State's Role in Immigration*. Sacramento: Senate Publications.

Carens, Joseph H. (1987), 'Aliens and Citizens: The Case for Open Borders', *Journal of Politics*, 49/2: 251–73.

Carter, Bob, Harris, Clive, and Joshi, Shirley (1993), 'The 1951–55 Conservative Government and the Racialization of Black Immigration', in Winston James and Clive Harris (eds.), *Inside Babylon*. London: Verso

Cassise, Christopher J. (1996), 'The European Union v. The United States under the NAFTA', *Syracuse Law Review*, 46: 1343–79.

Chavez, Linda (1991), *Out of the Barrio*. New York: Basic Books.

—— (1992), 'Hispanics, Affirmative Action, and Voting', *Annals of the American Academy of Political and Social Science*, 523: 75–87.

Chayes, Abram and Antonia Handler Chayes (1995), *The New Sovereignty*. Cambridge, Mass.: Harvard University Press.

Choldin, Harvey M. (1986), 'Statistics and Politics: The "Hispanic Issue" in the 1980 Census', *Demography*, 23/3: 403–18.

Citrin, Jack (1990), 'Language Politics and American Identity', *Public Interest*, 99: 96–109.

Cohen, Robin (1994), *Frontiers of Identity: The British and the Others*. London: Longman.

Coleman, David (1994), 'The United Kingdom and International Migration', in Heinz Fassmann and Rainer Münz (eds.), *European Migration in the Late Twentieth Century*. Aldershot: Elgar.

—— and Salt, John (1996), 'The Ethnic Group Question in the 1991 Census', in D. Coleman and J. Salt (eds.), *Ethnicity in the 1991 Census*, i. London: HMSO.

Colley, Linda (1992), *Britons*. New Haven: Yale University Press.

Commission for Racial Equality (1985), *Immigration Control Procedures*. London: CRE.

—— (1989), *Positive Action and Racial Equality in Housing*. London: CRE.

—— (1990), *Free Speech: Report of a Seminar*. London: CRE.

—— (1992), *Second Review of the Race Relations Act 1976*. London: CRE.

Cornelius, Wayne A., Martin, Philip L., and Hollifield, James F. (1994) (eds.), *Controlling Immigration*. Stanford: Stanford University Press.

Cose, Ellis (1992), *A Nation of Strangers*. New York: Morrow.

Crawford, James (1992), *Hold Your Tongue: Bilingualism and the Politics of "English Only"*. Reading, Mass.: Addison-Wesley.

CRE. See Commission for Racial Equality.

Currie, David P. (1990), 'Lochner Abroad: Substantive Due Process and Equal Protection in the Federal Republic of Germany', *1989 Supreme Court Review*, 333–72.

Cyrns, Manfred (1988), 'Rechtsstellung und politische Beteiligung von Ausländern', *Politische Bildung*, 19/1: 34–45.

D'Souza, Dinesh (1995), *The End of Racism*. New York: Free Press.

Davis, F. James (1991), *Who is Black?* University Park: Pennsylvania State University Press.

Day, Sir Michael (1990), 'The Salman Rushdie Affair: Implications for the CRE and Race Relations', in CRE, *Free Speech: Report of a Seminar.*

de Swaan, Abram (1988), *In Care of the State.* Cambridge: Polity Press.

Deakin, Nicholas (1968), 'The Politics of the Commonwealth Immigrants Bill', *Political Quarterly*, 39/1: 25–45.

Dean, D. W. (1987), 'The Labour Government and Black Communities in Great Britain 1945–51', *Immigrants and Minorities*, 6/3: 305–34.

Delfs, Silke (1993), 'Heimatvertriebene, Aussiedler, Spätaussiedler', *Aus Politik und Zeitgeschichte*, B48/92: 3–11.

Deutscher Juristentag (1980), *Verhandlungen des 53. Deutschen Juristentages*, ii. Munich: Beck.

Dinh, Viet D. (1994), 'Law and Asylum', in Nicolaus Mills (ed.), *Arguing Immigration.* New York: Touchstone.

Diversity Project (1991). *Final Report*, Institute for the Study of Social Change, University of California, Berkeley.

Divine, Robert A. (1957), *American Immigration Policy, 1924–1952.* New Haven: Yale University Press.

Dixon, David (1983), 'Thatcher's People: The British Nationality Act 1981', *Journal of Law and Society*, 10/2: 161–80.

Döhring, Karl (1979), 'Die Wiedervereinigung Deutschlands und die europäische Integration als Inhalte der Präambel des Grundgesetzes', *Deutsches Verwaltungsblatt*, 94/17/18: 633–9.

Dohse, Klaus (1981), *Ausländische Arbeiter und bürgerlicher Staat.* Königstein, Taunus: Hain.

Dong, Selena (1995), ' "Too Many Asians" ', *Stanford Law Review*, 47: 1027–57.

Doomernik, Jeroen (1995), 'The Institutionalization of Turkish Islam in Germany and The Netherlands', *Ethnic and Racial Studies*, 18/1: 46–63.

Drakulic, Slavenka (1993), *The Balkan Express.* New York: Norton.

Dummett, Ann, and Nicols, Andrew (1990), *Subjects, Citizens, Aliens and Others.* London: Weidenfeld and Nicolson.

Eastland, Terry (1996), *Ending Affirmative Action.* New York: Basic Books.

Edmonston, Barry, Passel, Jeffrey S., and Bean, Frank D. (1990), 'Perceptions and Estimates of Undocumented Migration to the United States', in F. Bean, B. Edmonston, and J. Passel (eds.), *Undocumented Migration to the United States: IRCA and the Experience of the 1980s.* Washington: Urban Institute.

Edwards, John (1987), *Positive Discrimination, Social Justice, and Social Policy.* London: Tavistock.

Eickelman, Dale F., and Piscatori, James (1996), *Muslim Politics.* Princeton: Princeton University Press.

Ellis, Jean (1991), 'Local Government and Community Needs: A Case Study of Muslims in Coventry', *New Community*, 17/3: 359–76.

Elwert, Georg (1982), 'Probleme der Ausländerintegration', *Kölner Zeitschrift für Soziologie und Sozialpsychologie*, 34: 696–716.

Erie, Steven P. (1988), *Rainbow's End*. Berkeley and Los Angeles: University of California Press.

Espenshade, Thomas J. (1992), 'Policy Influences on Undocumented Migration to the United States', *Proceedings of the American Philosophical Society*, 136/2: 188–207.

Espiritu, Yen Le (1992), *Asian American Panethnicity*. Philadelphia: Temple University Press.

Evans, A. C. (1983), 'United Kingdom Immigration Policy and the European Convention of Human Rights', *Public Law*, Spring 1983, 90–107.

Evans, J. M. (1983), *Immigration Law* (2nd edn.). London: Sweet and Maxwell.

Faist, Thomas (1994), 'How to Define a Foreigner?', *West European Politics*, 17/2: 50–71.

Fanon, Frantz (1963), *The Wretched of the Earth*. New York: Grove Press.

Favell, Adrian (1995), 'Philosophies of Integration: The Theory and Practice of Ethnic Minority Policies in France and Britain', Ph.D. thesis, European University Institute, Florence.

—— (1997), 'European Citizenship and the Incorporation of Migrants and Minorities in Europe'. Seminar paper, European Forum on International Migrations, Florence, 23 Oct.

—— (1998), 'Multicultural Race Relations in Britain', in Joppke (ed.), *Challenge to the Nation-State*.

Ferrajoli, Luigi (1996), 'From the Rights of the Citizen to Rights of the Person'. Seminar paper, European Forum on Citizenship, Florence, 1996.

Fisher, Maxine P. (1978), 'Creating Ethnic Identity: Asian Indians in the New York City Area', *Urban Anthropology*, 7/3: 271–85.

Fiss, Owen M. (1976), 'Groups and the Equal Protection Clause', *Philosophy and Public Affairs*, 5/2: 107–77.

FitzGerald, Marian (1986), 'Immigration and Race Relations: Political Aspects— No.15', *New Community*, 13/2: 265–71.

Fix, Michael, and Zimmermann, Wendy (1994), 'After Arrival: An Overview of Federal Immigrant Policy in the United States', in Barry Edmonston and Jeffrey S. Passel (eds.), *Immigration and Ethnicity*. Washington.: Urban Institute.

—— —— (1995), 'Immigrant Families and Public Policy: A Deepening Divide'. MS.

Ford, Christopher (1994), 'Administering Identity: The Determination of "Race" in Race-Conscious Law', *California Law Review*, 82: 1231–85.

Foreigner Commissioner of Berlin (1993) (ed.), *Schutzgesetze gegen ethnische Diskriminierung*. Berlin: Verwaltungsdruckerei.

Foster, Sheila (1993), 'Difference and Equality: A Critical Assessment of the Concept of "Diversity" ', *Wisconsin Law Review*, 105: 105–61.

Franke, Dietrich, and Hofmann, Rainer (1992), 'Nationale Minderheiten: ein Thema für das Grundgesetz?', *Europäische Grundrechts Zeitschrift*, 19/17: 401–9.

Franz, Fritz (1980), 'Einwanderer ohne Einwanderungsland', *Kursbuch*, 62: 159–71.

—— (1990), 'Der Gesetzentwurf der Bundesregierung zur Neuregelung des Ausländerrechts', *Zeitschrift für Ausländerrecht*, 1: 3–10.

Freeman, Gary P. (1979), *Immigrant Labor and Racial Conflict in Industrial Societies*. Princeton: Princeton University Press.

—— (1994), 'Britain, the Deviant Case', in Cornelius, Martin, and Hollifield, *Controlling Immigration*.

—— (1995a), 'Modes of Immigration Politics in Liberal Democratic States', *International Migration Review*, 29/4: 881–902.

—— (1995b), 'Rejoinder', *International Migration Review*, 29/4: 909–13.

—— (1996), 'Change or Continuity in American Immigration Policy?', *People and Place*, 4/1: 1–7.

—— (1998), 'The Decline of Sovereignty? Politics and Immigration Restriction in Liberal States', in Joppke (ed.) *Challenge to the Nation-State*.

Fuchs, Lawrence H. (1983), 'Immigration Reform in 1911 and 1981: The Role of Select Commissions', *Journal of American Ethnic History*, 3/1: 58–89.

—— (1990), 'The Corpse that Would not Die: The Immigration Reform and Control Act of 1986', *Revue européenne des migrations internationales*, 6/1: 111–26.

Gans, Herbert (1979), 'Symbolic Ethnicity: The Future of Ethnic Groups and Cultures in America', *Ethnic and Racial Studies*, 2/1: 1–20.

Garcia, Mario T. (1989), *Mexican Americans*. New Haven: Yale University Press.

Garton Ash, Timothy (1994), *In Europe's Name: Germany and the Divided Continent*. New York: Random House.

Garza, Rodolfo de la, De Sipio, Louis, Garcia, F. Chris, Garcia, John, and Falcon, Angelo, (1992), *Latino Voices*. Boulder, Colo.: Westview Press.

Geddes, Andrew (1998), *Breaching Fortress Europe? Migrant Interest Representation at the EU Level*. Seminar paper, European Forum on International Migrations, Florence, 5 Feb.

Gellner, Ernest (1983), *Nations and Nationalism*. Ithaca, NY: Cornell University Press.

German Interior Ministry (1993), 'Aufzeichnung zur Ausländerpolitik und zum Ausländerrecht in der Bundesrepublik Deutschland'. Bonn: hectographed.

Gilanshah, Bijan (1993), 'Multiracial Minorities', *Law and Inequality*, 12: 183–204.

Gillespie, Jim (1992), 'Maintenance and Accomodation and the Immigration Rules', *Immigration and Nationality Law and Practice*, 6/3: 97–100.

Gitlin, Todd (1996), *The Twilight of Common Dreams*. New York: Holt.

Gitmez, Ali, and Wilpert, Czarina (1987), 'Social Organization and Ethnicity Amongst Turkish Migrants in Berlin', in John Rex, Daniele Joly, and Czarina Wilpert (eds.), *Immigrant Associations in Europe*. Aldershot: Gower.

Glazer, Nathan (1954), 'Ethnic Groups in America', in Morroe Berger, Theodore Abel, and Charles H. Page (eds.), *Freedom and Control in Modern Society*. New York: Van Nostrand.

—— (1987), *Affirmative Discrimination*. Cambridge, Mass.: Harvard University Press.

—— (1988), *The New Immigration*. San Diego: San Diego State University Press.

—— (1991), 'In Defense of Multiculturalism', *New Republic*, 2 Sept.

—— (1995), 'Immigration and the American Future', *Public Interest*, Winter, 45–60.

—— (1997), *We Are All Multiculturalists Now*. Cambridge, Mass.: Harvard University Press.

GLC. See Greater London Council.

Gleason, Philip (1980), 'American Identity and Americanization', in Stephan Thernstrom (ed.), *Harvard Encyclopedia of American Ethnic Groups*. Cambridge, Mass.: Harvard University Press.

Glick Schiller, Nina, Basch, Linda, and Blanc-Szanton, Cristina (1992) (eds.), 'Towards a Transnational Perspective on Migration', *Annals of the New York Academy of Sciences*, 645.

Goering, John M. (1989), 'The "Explosiveness" of Chain Migration', *International Migration Review*, 23/4: 797–812.

Goldberg, Andreas (1992), 'Selbständigkeit als Integrationsfortschritt?', *Zeitschrift für Türkeistudien*, 75–92.

—— and Sen, Faruk (1993), 'Ein neuer Mittelstand?', *WSI Mitteilungen*, 3: 163–73.

Goldring, Luin (1996), 'Blurring Borders: Constructing Transnational Community in the Process of Mexico–U.S. Migration', *Research in Community Sociology*, 6: 69–104.

Goodwin-Gill, Guy (1978), *International Law and the Movement of Persons between States*. Oxford: Clarendon Press.

—— (1983), *The Refugee in International Law*. Oxford: Clarendon Press.

Gordon, Milton M. (1964), *Assimilation in American Life*. New York: Oxford University Press.

Goulbourne, Harry (1992), 'New Issues in Black British Politics', *Social Science Information*, 31/2: 355–73.

Graham, Hugh Davis (1990), *The Civil Rights Era*. New York: Oxford University Press.

Grant, Stefanie (1987), 'Family Rights in UK and EEC Immigration Law', *Immigration and Nationality Law and Practice*, July, 38–40.

Greater London Council (1983), 'The GLC's Work to Assist Ethnic Minorities'. London: hectographed.

Griffith, J. A. G. (1979), 'The Political Constitution', *Modern Law Review*, 42/1: 1–21.

Guendelsberger, John (1988), 'The Right to Family Unification in French and United States Immigration Law', *Cornell International Law Journal*, 21/1: 1–102.

Gür, Metin (1993), *Türkisch-islamische Vereinigungen in der Bundesrepublik Deutschland*. Frankfurt am Main: Brandes and Apsel.

Guiraudon, Virginie (1997), 'Sovereign After All? International Norms, Nation-States, and Aliens'. MS.

—— (1998), 'Citizenship Rights for Non-Citizens: France, Germany, and The Netherlands', in Joppke (ed.), *Challenge to the Nation-State*.

Gutierrez, David G. (1995), *Walls and Mirrors: Mexican Americans, Mexican Immigrants, and the Politics of Ethnicity*. Berkeley and Los Angeles: University of California Press.

Haberland, Jürgen (1983), 'Die Vorschläge der Kommission "Ausländer-politik"', *Zeitschrift für Ausländerrecht*, 2: 55 ff.

Habermas, Jürgen (1994), 'Human Rights and Popular Sovereignty', *Ratio Juris*, 7/1: 1–13.

Hahn, Richard F. (1982), 'Constitutional Limits on the Power to Exclude Aliens', *Columbia Law Review*, 82/5: 957–97.

Hailbronner, Kay (1980), 'Zur Reform des Ausländerrechts', *Zeitschrift für Rechtspolitik*, 9: 231–7.

—— (1983), 'Ausländerrecht und Verfassung', *Neue Juristische Wochen-schrift*, 36/38: 2105–13.

—— (1984), *Ausländerrecht. Ein Handbuch*. Heidelberg: C. F. Müller.

—— (1989), 'Citizenship and Nationhood in Germany', in Brubaker (ed.), *Immigration and the Politics of Citizenship*.

—— (1990), 'Der Gesetzentwurf der Bundesregierung zur Neuregelung des Ausländerrechts', *Zeitschrift für Ausländerrecht*, 2: 56–62.

—— (1992), 'Der Ausländer in der deutschen Sozialordnung', *Vierteljahres-schrift für Sozialrecht*, 2: 77–98.

—— and Renner, Günter (1991), *Staatsangehörigkeitsrecht: Kommentar*. Munich: Beck.

—— and Polakiewicz, Jörg (1992), 'Non-EC Nationals in the European Community', *Duke Journal of Comparative and International Law*, 3: 49–88.

Hammar, Tomas (1990), *Democracy and the Nation State*. Aldershot: Avebury.

Handlin, Oscar (1951), *The Uprooted*. Boston: Little, Brown and Company.

Hansen, M. L. (1952), 'The Third Generation in America', *Commentary*, 14: 492–500.

Hanson, Randall (1998), *Citizenship, Immigration and Nationality Law in the European Union*. Paper presented at the ERCOMER/European Forum on International Migrations Workshop on Migrants, Minorities and New Forms of Citizenship in the European Union, Florence, 6–7 Mar. 1998.

Harlow, Carol (1994), 'Accidental Loss of an Asylum Seeker', *Modern Law Review*, July, 620–6.

Hassan, Farooq (1983), 'The Doctrine of Incorporation', *Human Rights Quarterly*, 5: 68–86.

Heineman, Benjamin (1972), *The Politics of the Powerless*. London: Oxford University Press.

Heinrich, Herbert (1987), 'Einwanderung und Begrenzung des Ausländerzuzugs in der Rechtsprechung des Bundesverwaltungsgerichts', in Walther Fürst, Roman Herzog, Dieter C. Umbach (eds.), *Festschrift für Wolfgang Zeidler*. Berlin: de Gruyter.

Heinze, Rolf G., and Olk, Thomas (1981), 'Die Wohlfahrtsverbaende im System sozialer Dienstleistungsproduktion', *Kölner Zeitschrift für Soziologie und Sozialpsychologie*, 33: 94–114.

Heitmeyer, Wilhelm, Müller, Joachim, and Schrüder, Helmut (1997), *Verlockender Fundamentalismus*. Frankfurt am Main: Suhrkamp.

Heller, Thomas C. (1997), 'Modernity, Membership, and Multiculturalism', *Stanford Humanities Review*, 5/2: 2–69.

Herbert, Ulrich (1990), *A History of Foreign Labor in Germany, 1880–1980*. Ann Arbor: University of Michigan Press (German edn. (1986): *Geschichte der Ausländerbeschäftigung in Deutschland, 1880–1980*. Berlin: Dietz Verlag).

Higham, John (1955), *Strangers in the Land*. New Brunswick: Rutgers University Press.

—— (1984), *Send These To Me*. New York: Atheneum.

Hill, Michael J., and Issacharoff, Ruth M. (1971), *Community Action and Race Relations*. Oxford: Oxford University Press.

Hinnenkamp, Volker (1990), 'Ethnisierung: Eine vielseitige Variante der Diskriminierung', *Informationsdienst zur Ausländerarbeit*, 4: 39–45.

Hiro, Dilip (1992), *Black British, White British*. London: Paladin.

Hoffmann, Lutz (1994), 'Einwanderungspolitik und Volksverständnis', *Österreichische Zeitschrift für Politikwissenschaft*, 23/3: 253–66.

Hollifield, James (1994), 'The Migration Crisis in Western Europe', paper presented at the 1994 Annual Meeting of the American Political Science Association, New York.

Hollinger, David A. (1995), *Postethnic America*. New York: Basic Books.

Home Office (UK) (1977), *British Nationality Law: Discussion of Possible Changes*. London: HMSO.

—— (1982), *Proposals for Revision of the Immigration Rules*, Cmnd. 8683, London: HMSO.

Horwitz, Morton J. (1993), 'The Constitution of Change', *Harvard Law Review*, 107/1: 32–117.

House of Commons (1981), *Racial Disadvantage*, i: *5th Report from the Home Affairs Committee, Session 1980–81*, 20 July. London: HMSO.

—— (1986), *Immigration From the Indian Sub-Continent: Second Report from the Home Affairs Committee, Session 1985–86*, 2 vols. London: HMSO.

Huber, Bertold (1988), 'Zur Verfassungsmässigkeit der Beschränkungen des Ehegatten- und Familiennachzugs im Ausländerrecht', *Neue Juristische Wochenschrift*, 10: 609–11.

ILEA. See Inner London Education Authority.

Indian Case (1979), *Decision of the German Federal Constitutional Court* (1 BvR 525/77).

Inner London Education Authority (1983), 'Race, Sex and Class. (3) A Policy for Equality: Race'. London: hectographed.

Isensee, Josef (1974), 'Die staatsrechtliche Stellung der Ausländer in der Bundesrepublik Deutschland', *Veröffentlichungen der Vereinigung der Deutschen Staatsrechtslehrer*, 32. Berlin: de Gruyter.

—— (1987), 'Kommunalwahlrecht für Ausländer aus der Sicht der Landesverfassung Nordrhein-Westfalens und der Bundesverfassung', *Kritische Vierteljahresschrift für Gesetzgebung und Rechtswissenschaft*, 4: 300–21.

Jacobson, David (1996), *Rights Across Borders*. Baltimore: Johns Hopkins University Press.

Jacobson, Jessica (1997), 'Religion and Ethnicity: Dual and Alternative Sources of Identity among Young British Pakistanis', *Ethnic and Racial Studies*, 20/2: 238–56.

John, Barbara (1985), 'Ausländerpolitik für Inländer?' *Zeitschrift für Ausländerrecht*, 1: 3–7.

Johnston Conover, Pamela, Crewe, Ivor, and Searing, Donald (1991), 'The Nature of Citizenship in the United States and Great Britain', *Journal of Politics*, 53/3: 800–32.

Joly, Daniele (1995), *Britannia's Crescent: Making a Place for Muslims in British Society*. Aldershot: Avebury.

Jones, Catherine (1977), *Immigration and Social Policy in Britain*. London: Tavistock.

Jones, Trevor (1996), *Britain's Ethnic Minorities*. London: Policy Studies Institute.

Joppke, Christian (1995), 'Toward a New Sociology of the State', *Archives européennes de sociologie*, 36/1: 168–78.

—— (1996), 'Multiculturalism and Immigration', *Theory and Society*, 25/4: 449–500.

—— (1997), 'Asylum and State Sovereignty', *Comparative Political Studies*, 30/3: 259–98.

—— (1998a), 'Immigration Challenges the Nation-State', in Joppke (1998c).

—— (1998*b*), 'Why Liberal States Accept Unwanted Immigration', *World Politics*, 50/2: 266–93.

—— (1998*c*) (ed.), *Challenge to the Nation-State: Immigration in Western Europe and the United States*. Oxford: Oxford University Press.

Kallen, Horace M. (1915), 'Democracy Versus the Melting-Pot', in H. Kallen, *Culture and Democracy in the United States*. New York: Boni and Liveright, 1924.

Kamasaki, Charles, and Yzaguirre, Raul (1991), 'Black-Hispanic Tensions'. Paper presented at the 1991 Annual Meeting of the American Political Science Association, Washington.

Kanein, Werner (1973), 'Das Ausländergesetz im Meinungsstreit', *Neue Juristische Wochenschrift*, 26/17: 729–35.

Kanstrom, Daniel (1993), 'The Shining City and the Fortress', *Boston College International and Comparative Law Review*, 16/2: 201–43.

Katzenstein, Peter (1987), *Policy and Politics in West Germany*. Philadelphia: Temple University Press.

—— (1996), 'Tamed Power: Germany in Europe'. MS.

Katznelson, Ira (1973), *Black Men, White Cities*. New York: Oxford University Press.

Kaye, Ronald (1994), 'Defining the Agenda: British Refugee Policy and the Role of Parties', *Journal of Refugee Studies*, 7/2/3: 144–59.

Kennedy, John F. (1964), *A Nation of Immigrants*. New York: Harper and Row.

Kepel, Gilles (1997), *Allah in the West*. Cambridge: Polity Press.

Kibria, Nazli (1993), *Family Tightrope: The Changing Lives of Vietnamese Americans*. Princeton: Princeton University Press.

Kirp, David L. (1979), *Doing Good by Doing Little: Race and Schooling in Britain*. Berkeley: University of California Press.

Knott, Kim, and Khokher, Sajda (1993), 'Religious and Ethnic Identity among Young Muslim Women in Bradford', *New Community*, 19/4: 593–610.

Koslowski, Rey (1998*a*), 'European Union Migration Regimes, Established and Emergent', in Joppke (ed.), *Challenge to the Nation State*.

—— (1998*b*), *European Migration Regimes: Emerging, Enlarging and Deteriorating*. Paper presented at the ERCOMER/European Forum on International Migrations Workshop on Migrants, Minorities and New Forms of Citizenship in the European Union, Florence, 6–7 Mar.

Krasner, Stephen D. (1983) (ed.), *International Regimes*. Ithaca, NY: Cornell University Press.

—— (1995*a*), 'Compromising Westphalia', *International Security*, 20/3: 115–51.

—— (1995*b*), 'Sovereignty, Regimes, and Human Rights', in Volker Rittberger (ed.), *Regime Theory and International Relations*. Oxford: Clarendon Press.

Kratochwil, Friedrich (1986), 'Of Systems, Boundaries, and Territoriality', *World Politics*, 39: 27–52.

Kymlicka, Will (1992), 'Two Models of Pluralism and Tolerance', *Analyse und Kritik*, 13: 33–56.

—— (1995a), *Multicultural Citizenship*. Oxford: Oxford University Press.

—— (1995b), 'Introduction', in W. Kymlicka (ed.), *The Rights of Minority Cultures*. Oxford: Oxford University Press.

—— and Norman, W. J. (1994), 'Return of the Citizen', *Ethics*, 104/2: 352–81.

LaNoue, George R., and Sullivan, John C. (1994), 'The Small Business Administration's Decisions on Groups Entitled to Affirmative Action', *Journal of Policy History*, 6/4: 439–67.

Lahav, Gallya (1997), 'Devolution and Privatization of Migration Regulation'. Seminar paper, European Forum on International Migrations, Florence, 27 Nov.

Lansley, Stewart, Gross, Sue, and Wolmar, Christian (1989) (eds.), *Councils in Conflict: The Rise and Fall of the Municipal Left*. London: Macmillan.

Lavenex, Sandra (1998), 'Ironic Integration: The Europeanization of Asylum Policies in France and Germany'. Seminar paper, European Forum on International Migrations, Florence, 29 Jan..

Lawson, Miguel, and Grin, Marianne (1992), 'The Immigration Act of 1990', *Harvard International Law Journal*, 33: 255–76.

Layton-Henry, Zig (1986), 'Race and the Thatcher Government', in Z. Layton-Henry and Paul B. Rich (eds.), *Race, Government, and Politics in Britain*. London: Macmillan.

—— (1992), *The Politics of Immigration*. Oxford: Blackwell.

—— (1994), 'Britain: The Would-Be Zero Immigration Country', in Cornelius, Martin, and Hollifield (eds.), *Controlling Immigration*.

Legomsky, Stephen H. (1985), 'Immigration Law and the Principle of Plenary Congressional Power', *1984 Supreme Court Review*, 255–307.

—— (1995), 'Ten More Years of Plenary Power', *Hastings Constitutional Law Quarterly*, 22: 925–37.

Lester, Anthony (1987), 'Anti-Discrimination Legislation in Great Britain', *New Community*, 14/1/2: 21–31.

—— (1994), 'European Human Rights and the British Constitution', in J. Jowell and D. Oliver (eds.), *The Changing Constitution* (3rd edn.). Oxford: Clarendon Press.

—— and Bindman, Geoffrey (1972), *Race and Law*. London: Longman.

Leuninger, Herbert (1984), 'Ausländerfeindlichkeit', in Hartmut M. Griese (ed.), *Der gläserne Fremde*. Opladen: Leske and Buderich.

Lewis, Russell (1988), *Anti-Racism: A Mania Exposed*. London: Quartet Books.

Lewis, Philip (1994), *Islamic Britain*. London: Tauris.

Lind, Michael (1995), *The Next American Nation*. New York: Free Press.

Loescher, Gil and Scanlan, John A. (1986), *Calculated Kindness: Refugees and America's Half-Open Door.* New York: Free Press.

Lowry, Ira S. (1982), 'The Science and Politics of Ethnic Enumeration', in Winston A. Van Horne (ed.), *Ethnicity and Public Policy.* Madison: University of Wisconsin System, i.

Lustgarten, Laurence (1980), *Legal Control of Racial Discrimination.* London: Macmillan.

Macdonald, Ian A. (1977), *Race Relations: The New Law.* London: Butterworth.

—— (1983), *Immigration Law and Practice in the United Kingdom.* London: Butterworth.

—— and Blake, Nicholas J. (1991), *Immigration Law and Practice in the United Kingdom.* London: Butterworth.

Mager, Ute (1992), 'Schutz der Ausländer vor Diskriminierung durch Privatpersonen', in Foreigner Commissioner of Berlin (ed.), *Schutzgesetze gegen ethnische Diskriminierung.*

Mahler, Sarah J. (1995), *American Dreaming: Immigrant Life on the Margins.* Princeton: Princeton University Press.

MALDEF. See Mexican American Legal Defense and Educational Fund.

Malik, Akbar Ali (1993), *The Satanic Verses: Was it Worth All the Fuss?* London: Unique Books.

Margolis, Maxine (1994), *Little Brazil.* Princeton: Princeton University Press.

Marquand, David (1995), 'After Whig Imperialism: Can There Be a New British Identity?' *New Community*, 21/2: 183–93.

Marrington, Dave (1985), 'Legal Decisions Affecting Ethnic Minorities and Discrimination—No.24', *New Community*, 12/3: 536–45.

Marshall, T. S. (1992), *Citizenship and Social Class.* London: Pluto Press.

Martin, David A. (1983), 'Due Process and Membership in the National Community', *University of Pittsburgh Law Review*, 44: 165–235.

—— (1988), 'The New Asylum Seekers', in D. Martin (ed.), *The New Asylum Seekers.* Dordrecht: Nijhoff.

—— (1989), 'Effects of International Law on Migration Policy and Practice: The Uses of Hypocrisy', *International Migration Review*, 23/3: 547–78.

—— (1995), 'The Obstacles to Effective Internal Enforcement of the Immigration Laws in the United States'. MS.

Martineau, Robert J. (1983), 'Interpreting the Constitution: The Use of International Human Rights Norms', *Human Rights Quarterly*, 5: 87–107.

Marx, Reinhard (1992), 'The Criteria for Determining Refugee Status in the Federal Republic of Germany', *International Journal of Refugee Law*, 4/2: 151–70.

Massey, Douglas S. (1995), 'The New Immigration and Ethnicity in the United States', *Population and Development Review*, 21/3: 631–52.

Mehrländer, Ursula, Ascheberg, Carsten, and Ueltzhöffer, Jörg, (1996), *Situation der ausländischen Arbeitnehmer und ihrer Familienangehörigen in der Bundesrepublik Deutschland*. Bonn: Bundesministerium für Arbeit und Sozialordnung.

Meier-Braun, Karl-Heinz (1988), *Integration oder Rückkehr?*, Munich: Grünewald.

Meissner, Doris (1988), 'Reflections on the Refugee Act of 1980', in Martin (ed.), *The New Asylum Seekers*.

Menski, Werner (1994), 'Family Migration and the New Immigration Rules', *Immigration and Nationality Law and Practice*, 8/4: 112–24.

Messina, Anthony M. (1987), 'Mediating Race Relations: British Community Relations Councils Revisited', *Ethnic and Racial Studies*, 10/2: 186–202.

—— (1989), *Race and Party Competition in Britain*. Oxford: Clarendon Press.

—— (1996), 'The Not So Silent Revolution: Postwar Migration to Western Europe', *World Politics*, 49: 130–54.

Mexican American Legal Defense and Educational Fund (1988), 'The First Twenty Years, 1968–1988'. San Antonio, Texas: hectographed.

Meyer, John Boli, John Thomas, George M., and Ramirez, Francisco O. (1997), 'World Society and the Nation-State', *American Journal of Sociology*, 103/1: 144–81.

Miles, Jack (1995), 'The Coming Immigration Debate', *Atlantic Monthly*, 275/4: 130–40.

Miles, Robert, and Kay, Diana (1990), 'The TUC, Foreign Labour and the Labour Government 1945–1951', *Immigrants and Minorities*, 9/1: 85–108.

Mills, Nicolaus (1994) (ed.), *Debating Affirmative Action*. New York: Delta.

Milward, Alan (1992), *The European Rescue of the Nation-State*. London: Routledge.

Modood, Tariq (1990), 'British Asian Muslims and the Rushdie Affair', *Political Quarterly*, 61/2: 143–60.

—— (1993), 'Muslim Views on Religious Identity and Racial Equality', *New Community*, 19/3: 513–19.

—— (1994a), 'Political Blackness and British Asians', *Sociology*, 28/4: 859–76.

—— (1994b), 'Ethnic Difference and Racial Equality', in David Milliband (ed.), *Reinventing the Left*. Cambridge: Polity Press.

—— Beishon, Sharon, and Virdee, Satnam (1994), *Changing Ethnic Identities*. London: Policy Studies Institute.

—— and Berthoud, Richard (1997), *Ethnic Minorities in Britain*. London: Policy Studies Institute.

Mommsen, Wolfgang J (1990), *Nation und Geschichte*. Munich: Piper.

Motomura, Hiroshi (1990), 'Immigration Law After a Century of Plenary Power', *Yale Law Journal*, 100/3: 545–613.

—— (1995), 'Family Reunification in Immigration Law and Policy'. MS.

Münch, Ingo von (1981), *Grundgesetz-Kommentar*. Munich: Beck.

Münch, Ursula (1992), *Asylpolitik in der Bundesrepublik Deutschland*. Opladen: Leske and Budrich.

Muenz, Rainer, and Ulrich, Ralf (1995), 'Too Many Foreigners?' Center for German and European Studies, Georgetown University. Working paper.

Mufti, Rashid (1988), 'A Failure of Political Will: Report of a Review of Camden Council's Race Equality Policies and Strategies'. London: hectographed.

Muller, Thomas (1993), *Immigrants and the American City*. New York: New York University Press.

Munos, Carlos (1989), *Youth, Identity, Power: The Chicano Movement*. London: Verso.

Murray, Laura M. (1994), 'Explaining the Evolving Positions of German Political Parties on Citizenship Policy', *German Politics and Society*, 33: 23–56.

Muslim Parliament (1992), 'White Paper on Muslim Education in Great Britain'. London: hectographed.

Myrdal, Gunnar (1944), *An American Dilemma*. New York: Harper.

Nanton, Philip (1992), 'Official Statistics and Problems of Inappropriate Ethnic Categorisation', *Policy and Politics*, 20/4: 277–85.

Natapoff, Alexandra (1995), 'Trouble in Paradise: Equal Protection and the Dilemma of Interminority Group Conflict', *Stanford Law Review*, 47: 1059–96.

National Council for Civil Liberties (UK) (1995), 'The Last Resort: Violations of the Human Rights of Migrants, Refugees and Asylum Seekers'. London: mimeograph.

National Council of La Raza (1992), *State of Hispanic America 1991: An Overview*. NCLR: Washington.

Neuman, Gerald L. (1990), 'Immigration and Judicial Review in the Federal Republic of Germany', *New York University Journal of International Law*, 23: 35–85.

—— (1992), ' "We Are the People": Alien Suffrage in German and American Perspective', *Michigan Journal of International Law*, 13: 259–335.

—— (1993), 'Buffer Zones Against Refugees', *Virginia Journal of International Law*, 33: 503–26.

—— (1995), 'Nationality Law in the United States and the Federal Republic of Germany'. MS.

—— (1997), 'Anomalous Zones', *Stanford Law Review*, 48: 1197–234.

Neveu, Catherine (1994), 'Is "Black" an Exportable Category to Mainland Europe?' in J. Rex and B. Drury (eds.), *Ethnic Mobilization in a Multi-Cultural Europe*. Avebury: Aldershot.

New York State Social Studies Review (1991), 'One Nation, Many Peoples: A Declaration of Cultural Interdependence'. Albany, NY: hectographed.

Noiriel, Gerard (1996), *The French Melting-Pot*. Minneapolis: University of Minnesota Press.

O'Connor, Karen, and Epstein, Lee (1984), 'A Legal Voice for the Chicano Community', *Social Science Quarterly*, 65/2: 245–56.

O'Hare, William P. (1992), 'America's Minorities', *Population Bulletin* (Washington), Dec. 2–45.

O'Leary, Brendan (1987), 'Why Was the GLC Abolished?' *International Journal of Urban and Regional Research* 10: 193–217.

Oberndörfer, Dieter (1993), *Der Wahn des Nationalen*. Freiburg: Herder.

Özcan, Ertekin (1989), *Türkische Immigrantenorganisationen in der Bundesrepublik Deutschland*. Berlin: Hitit.

Omi, Michael, and Winant, Howard (1986), *Racial Formation in the United States*. New York: Routledge and Kegan Paul.

Ong Hing, Bill (1994), *Making and Remaking Asian Americans through Immigration Policy, 1850–1990*. Stanford, Calif.: Stanford University Press.

Ouseley, Herman (1984), 'Local Authority Race Initiatives', in Martin Boddy and Colin Fudge (eds.), *Local Socialism?* London: Macmillan.

—— (1990), 'Resisting Institutional Change', in Wendy Ball and John Solomos (eds.), *Race and Local Politics*. London: Macmillan.

Pachon, Harry P., and Alegre, Juan Carlos (1993), 'An Overview of Hispanic Elected Officials in 1993', *1993 National Roster of Hispanic Elected Officials*.

Padilla, Felix M. (1985), *Latino Ethnic Consciousness: The Case of Mexican Americans and Puerto Ricans in Chicago*. Notre Dame, Ind.: University of Notre Dame Press.

Papademetriou, Demetrios G. (1993), 'Illegal Mexican Migration in the United States and US Responses', *International Migration*, 31/2/3: 314–48.

—— (1996), *Coming Together or Pulling Apart? The European Union's Struggle With Immigration and Asylum*. Washington: Carnegie Endowment for International Peace.

Park, Robert E. (1950), *Race and Culture*. Glencoe, Ill.: Free Press.

Paul, Kathleen (1992), 'The Politics of Citizenship in Post-War Britain', *Contemporary Record*, 6/3: 452–73.

—— (1997), *Whitewashing Britain: Race and Citizenship in the Postwar Era*. Ithaca, NY: Cornell University Press.

Peach, C. (1996), 'Introduction', in C. Peach (ed.), *Ethnicity in the 1991 Census*, ii. London: HMSO.

Perlmutter, Ted (1996a), 'Bringing Parties Back In', *International Migration Review*, 30/1: 375–88.

—— (1996b), 'The Political Asylum Debates in Germany, 1978–1992'. MS.

Petersen, William (1987), 'Politics and the Measurement of Ethnicity', in William Alonso and Paul Starr (eds.), *The Politics of Numbers*. New York: Russell Sage Foundation.

Pfaff, Victor (1992), 'Flucht und Einwanderung', *Kritische Justiz*, 25: 129–46.

Pietzcker, Jost (1975), 'Die neuere Rechtsprechung des Bundesverfassungsgerichts zum vorläufigen Rechtschutz im Ausländerrecht', *Juristische Zeitschrift*, 14: 435–9.

Piore, Michael (1979), *Birds of Passage*. New York: Cambridge University Press.

Plender, Richard (1988), *International Migration Law* (2nd edn.). Dordrecht: Nijhoff.

Porter, Gregory (1992), 'Persecution Based on Political Opinion: Interpretation of the Refugee Act of 1980', *Cornell International Law Journal*, 25: 231–76.

Porter, Rosalie Pedalino (1990), *Forked Tongue: The Politics of Bilingual Education*. New York: Basic Books.

Portes, Alejandro, and Bach, Robert L. (1985), *Latin Journey: Cuban and Mexican Immigrants in the United States*. Berkeley and Los Angeles: University of California Press.

—— and Rumbaut, Ruben G. (1996), *Immigrant America*. 2nd edn. Berkeley and Los Angeles: University of California Press.

—— and Stepick, Alex (1993), *City on the Edge: The Transformation of Miami*. Berkeley and Los Angeles: University of California Press.

Poulter, Sebastian (1986), *English Law and Ethnic Minority Customs*. London: Butterworth.

—— (1987), 'Ethnic Minority Customs, English Law and Human Rights', *International and Comparative Law Quarterly*, 36: 589–615.

—— (1990), *Asian Traditions and English Law*. London: Trentham Books.

Powell, Enoch (1988), 'The UK and Immigration', *Salisbury Review*, Dec. 40–3.

—— (1992), *Reflections* (Selected Writings and Speeches, ed. Rex Collings). London: Bellew.

Prantl, Heribert (1994), *Deutschland—leicht entflammbar*. Munich: Hanser.

Prashar, Usha, and Nicholas, Shan (1986), *Routes or Roadblocks? Consulting Minority Communities in London Boroughs*. London: Runnymede Trust.

Preuss, Ulrich (1996), 'Two Challenges to Modern Citizenship'. MS.

Quaritsch, Helmut (1981), *Einwanderungsland Bundesrepublik Deutschland?* Munich: Carl Friedrich von Siemens Stiftung.

—— (1983), 'Staatsangehörigkeit und Wahlrecht', *Die öffentliche Verwaltung*, 36/1: 1–15.

—— (1985), *Recht auf Asyl*. Berlin: Duncker and Humblot.

Radtke, Frank-Olaf (1990), 'Multikulturell—Das Gesellschaftsdesign der 90er Jahre?', *Informationsdienst zur Ausländerarbeit*, 4: 27–34.

—— (1994), 'The Formation of Ethnic Minorities and the Transformation of Social into Ethnic Conflicts in a So-Called Multi-Cultural Society', in Rex and Drury (eds.), *Ethnic Mobilization in a Multi-Cultural Europe*.

Ramirez, Deborah (1995), 'Multicultural Empowerment', *Stanford Law Review*, 47: 957–92.

Randall, Chris (1994), 'An Asylum Policy for the UK', in Spencer (ed.), *Strangers and Citizens*.

Ravitch, Diane (1983), *The Troubled Crusade: American Education, 1945–1980*. New York: Basic Books.

—— (1992), 'Multiculturalism: E Pluribus Plures', in Berman (ed.), *Debating P.C.*

Reimers, David M. (1983), 'An Unintended Reform: The 1965 Immigration Act and Third World Immigration to the United States', *Journal of American Ethnic History*, 3/1: 9–28.

—— (1985), *Still the Golden Door: The Third World Comes to America*. New York: Columbia University Press.

Reisman, W. Michael (1990), 'Sovereignty and Human Rights in Contemporary International Law', *American Journal of International Law*, 84: 866–76.

Renner, Günter (1993), 'Asyl- und Ausländerrechtsreform 1993', *Zeitschrift für Ausländerrecht*, 3: 118–27.

—— (1994), 'Ausländerintegration, ius soli und Mehrstaatigkeit', *Familienrechtszeitschrift (FamRZ)*, 14: 865–72.

Rex, John (1989), 'Equality of Opportunity, Multiculturalism, Anti-racism and "Education for All" ', in Gajandra K. Verma (ed.), *Education for All: A Landmark in Pluralism*. London: Falmer.

Risse, Thomas (1997), 'Who Are We? A Europeanization of National Identities?'. MS.

—— and Sikkink, Kathryn (1997), 'The Socialization of Human Rights Norms into Domestic Practices'. MS.

Rittstieg, Helmut, and Rowe, Gerard C. (1992), *Einwanderung als gesellschaftliche Herausforderung*. Baden-Baden: Nomos.

Romig, Jeffrey L. (1985), 'Salvadoran Illegal Aliens', *University of Pittsburgh Law Review*, 47: 295–335.

Ronge, Volker (1995), 'Ethnic German Immigration and German Policy toward German Minorities in Eastern Europe and FSU'. MS.

Rosberg, Gerald M. (1978), 'The Protection of Aliens from Discriminatory Treatment by the National Government', *1977 Supreme Court Review*, 275–339.

Rose, E. J. B. (1969), *Colour and Citizenship*. Oxford: Oxford University Press.

Rothman, Eric S. and Espenshade, Thomas J. (1992), 'Fiscal Impacts of Immigration to the United States', *Population Index*, 58/3: 381–415.

Rottmann, Frank (1984), 'Das Asylrecht des Art.16 GG als liberal-rechtsstaatliches Abwehrrecht', *Der Staat*, 22/3: 337–68.

Rouse, Roger (1991), 'Mexican Migration and the Social Space of Postmodernism', *Diaspora*, 1: 8–23.

Rudolph, Hedwig (1996), 'The New *Gastarbeiter* System in Germany', *New Community*, 22/2: 287–300.

Ruff, Anne (1989), 'The Immigration (Carriers' Liability) Act 1987', *International Journal of Refugee Law*, 1/4: 481–501.

Ruggie, John (1993), 'Territoriality and Beyond', *International Organization*, 47/1: 139–74.

Sachdeva, Sanjiv (1993), *The Primary Purpose Rule in British Immigration Law*. London: Trentham Books.

Salyer, Lucy E. (1995), *Laws Harsh as Tigers: Chinese Immigrants and the Shaping of Modern Immigration Law*. Chapel Hill: University of North Carolina Press.

Samad, Yunas (1992), 'Book Burning and Race Relations: Political Mobilisation of Bradford Muslims', *New Community*, 18/4: 507–19.

San Miguel, Guadalupe (1984), 'Conflict and Controversy in the Evolution of Bilingual Education in the United States', *Social Science Quarterly*, 65/2: 505–18.

Sassen, Saskia (1996), *Losing Control?* New York: Columbia University Press.

—— (1998), 'The *de facto* Transnationalizing of Immigration Policy', in Joppke (ed.), *Challenge to the Nation-State*.

Scannell, Rick (1992), 'Primary Purpose: The End of Judicial Sympathy?', *Immigration and Nationality Law and Practice*, 6/1: 3–6.

Scarman, Lord (1981), *The Brixton Disorders, 10–12 Apr. 1981*. London: HMSO.

Schain, Martin (forthcoming), 'Minorities and Immigrant Incorporation in France: The State and the Dynamics of Multiculturalism', in C. Joppke and Steven Lukes (eds.), *Multicultural Questions*. Oxford: Oxford University Press.

Schiffer, Eckart (1990), 'Vor der Neuregelung des Ausländerrechts', *Zeitschrift für Ausländerrecht*, 2: 51–6.

—— (1992), 'Ausländerintegration und/oder multikulturelle Gesellschaft', *Politische Studien*, 43/321: 56–66.

Schlesinger, Arthur (1992), *The Disuniting of America*. New York: Norton.

Schmalz-Jacobsen, Cornelia *et al.* (1993), *Einwanderung—und dann?* Munich: Knaur.

Schmidt Hornstein, Caroline (1995), *Das Dilemma der Einbürgerung*. Opladen: Leske and Budrich.

Schmitt, Carl (1934), *Politische Theologie* (2nd edn.). Berlin: Duncker and Humblot.

Schmitter, Philippe (1991), 'The European Community as an Emergent and Novel Form of Political Domination'. Madrid: Juan March Institute, Working Paper no. 26.

Schnapper, Dominique (1992), *L'Europe des immigrés*. Paris: Éditions François Bourin.

—— (1994), 'The Debate on Immigration and the Crisis of National Identity', *West European Politics*, 17/2: 127–39.

Schuck, Peter (1984), 'The Transformation of Immigration Law', *Columbia Law Review*, 84/1: 1–90.

—— (1985), 'Immigration Law and the Problem of Community', in Nathan Glazer (ed.), *Clamor at the Gates*. San Francisco: Institute for Contemporary Studies.

—— (1989), 'Membership in the Liberal Polity: The Devaluation of American Citizenship', in Brubaker (ed.), *Immigration and the Politics of Citizenship*.

—— (1992), 'The Politics of Rapid Legal Change: Immigration Policy in the 1980s', *Studies in American Political Development*, 6: 37–92.

—— (1995*a*), 'The Message of 187', *American Prospect*, 21: 85–92.

—— (1995*b*), 'The Treatment of Aliens in the U.S.'. MS.

—— (1996), 'Alien Ruminations', *Yale Law Journal*, 105: 1963–2012.

—— (1998), 'The Re-Evaluation of American Citizenship', in Joppke (ed.), *Challenge to the Nation-State*.

—— and Smith, Rogers (1985), *Citizenship Without Consent*. New Haven: Yale University Press.

Schwarz, Thomas (1992), *Zuwanderer im Netz des Wohlfahrtsstaats*. Berlin: Edition Parabolis.

Schwerdtfeger, Gunther (1980), *Welche rechtlichen Vorkehrungen empfehlen sich, um die Rechtsstellung von Ausländern in der Bundesrepublik Deutschland angemessen zu gestalten?*, Gutachten A zum 53. Deutschen Juristentag Berlin 1980. Munich: Beck.

Scott, Margaret O'B. (1985), 'Significant Developments in the Immigration Laws of the United States 1983–1984', *San Diego Law Review*, 22: 1101–42.

Select Commission on Immigration and Refugee Policy (1981), *US Immigration Policy and the National Interest*. Washington: GPO.

Sen, Faruk, and Goldberg, Andreas (1994), *Türken in Deutschland*. Munich: Beck.

Senocak, Zafer (1993), 'Deutsche werden—Türken bleiben', in Claus Leggewie and Zafer Senocak (eds.), *Deutsche Türken*. Reinbek: Rowohlt.

Shaw, Alison (1994), 'The Pakistani Community in Oxford', in Roger Ballard (ed.), *Desh Pradat: The South Asian Presence in Britain*. London: Hurst.

Sikkink, Kathryn (1993), 'Human Rights, Principled Issue-Networks, and Sovereignty in Latin America', *International Organization*, 47/3: 411–41.

Sillitoe, K., and White, P. H. (1992), 'Ethnic Group and the British Census: The Search For a Question', *Journal of the Royal Statistical Society*, 155: 141–63.

Skerry, Peter (1989), 'Borders and Quotas', *Public Interest*, 96: 86–102.

—— (1992), 'The Census Wars', *Public Interest*, 106: 17–31.

—— (1993), *Mexican Americans*. New York: Free Press.

Skrentny, John (1996*a*), 'Cultural Analysis and the Administrative Origins of Affirmative Action'. Paper presented at the 1996 Annual Meeting of the American Sociological Association, New York.

—— (1996*b*), *The Ironies of Affirmative Action*. Chicago: University of Chicago Press.

Smith, Rogers M. (1993), 'Beyond Tocqueville, Myrdal, and Hartz: The Multiple Traditions in America', *American Political Science Review*, 87/3: 549–66.

Sniderman, Paul, and Piazza, Thomas (1993), *The Scar of Race*. Cambridge, Mass.: Harvard University Press.

Solomos, John, and Back, Les (1995), *Race, Politics and Social Change*. London: Routledge.

Sondhi, Ranjit (1987), *Divided Families: British Immigration Control in the Indian Subcontinent*. London: Runnymede Trust.

Sooben, Philip N. (1990), *The Origins of the Race Relations Act*. Centre for Research in Ethnic Relations, University of Warwick, Research Paper in Ethnic Relations, 12.

Soysal, Yasemin (1994), *Limits of Citizenship*. Chicago: University of Chicago Press.

—— (1997), 'Identity, Rights, and Claims-Making: Changing Dynamics of Citizenship in Postwar Europe'. MS.

Spencer, Sarah (1994) (ed.), *Strangers and Citizens*. London: IPPR/Rivers Oram Press.

Spruyt, Hendrik (1994), *The Sovereign State and its Competitors*. Princeton: Princeton University Press.

Steiner, Niklaus (1997), 'Interests, Humanitarianism and Refugee Debates in Switzerland, Germany, and Britain, 1970s–1990s'. MS.

Sterett, Susan (1994), 'Judicial Review in Britain', *Comparative Political Studies*, 26: 421–42.

Stöcker, Hans A. (1989), 'Nationales Selbstbestimmungsrecht und Ausländerwahlrecht', *Der Staat*, 28/1: 71–90.

—— (1991), 'Der Binnen– und der Aussenaspekt der Volkssouveränität', *Der Staat*, 30: 259–68.

Stoker, Gerry (1991), *The Politics of Local Government*. London: Macmillan.

Storey, Hugo (1994), 'International Law and Human Rights Obligations', in Spencer (ed.), *Strangers and Citizens*.

Stratmann, Friedrich (1984), 'Zwischen bürokratischem Eigeninteresse und Selbsthilfeanspruch', in Rudolf Bauer and Hartmut Diessenbacher (eds.), *Organisierte Nächstenliebe*. Opladen: Westdeutscher Verlag.

Studlar, Donley (1974), 'British Public Opinion, Colour Issues, and Enoch Powell', *British Journal of Political Science*, 4: 371–81.

—— (1980), 'Elite Responsiveness or Elite Autonomy: British Immigration Policy Reconsidered', *Ethnic and Racial Studies*, 3/2: 207–23.

Swann, Lord (1985*a*), *Education for All*. London: HMSO.

—— (1985*b*), *Education for All: A Brief Guide to the Main Issues of the Report*. London: HMSO.

Teague, Andy (1993), 'Ethnic Group: First Results From the 1991 Census', *Population Trends*, Summer, 12–17.

Teitelbaum, Michael S. (1984), 'Political Asylum in Theory and Practice', *Public Interest*, 76: 74–86.

The Greens (1990), *Die multikulturelle Gesellschaft*. Bonn: The Greens.

Thernstrom, Abigail M. (1980), 'E Pluribus Plura—Congress and Bilingual Education', *Public Interest*, 60: 3–22.

—— (1987), *Whose Votes Count? Affirmative Action and Minority Voting Rights*. Cambridge, Mass.: Harvard University Press.

Thomae-Venske, Hanns (1988), 'The Religious Life of Muslims in Berlin', in Tomas Gerholm and Yngve G. Lithman (eds.), *The New Islamic Presence in Western Europe*. London: Mansell.

Thomas, William I., and Znaniecki, Florian (1984), *The Polish Peasant in Europe and America* (ed. and abr. Eli Zaretsky). Urbana, Ill.: University of Illinois Press.

Thornberry, P. (1980), 'Seven Years On: East African Asians, Immigration Rules and Human Rights', *Liverpool Law Review*, 2: 136–50.

Thränhardt, Dietrich (1983), 'Ausländer im Dickicht der Verbände', *Neue Praxis* (special issue), 7: 62–78.

Tichonor, Daniel J. (1994), 'The Politics of Immigration Reform in the United States, 1981–1990', *Polity*, 26/3: 333–62.

Titmuss, Richard M. (1976), *Commitment to Welfare*. London: Allen and Unwin.

Todorov, T. (1993), *On Human Diversity*. Cambridge, Mass.: Harvard University Press.

Tomlinson, Sally (1986), 'Political Dilemmas in Multi-Racial Education', in Layton-Henry and Rich (eds.), *Race, Government and Politics in Britain*.

Tomuschat, Christian (1979), 'Das Recht auf Familieneinheit', *Europäische Grundrechte Zeitschrift*, 6: 191–8.

—— (1980), 'Zur Reform des Ausländerrechts', *Neue Juristische Wochenschrift*, 33/20: 1073–128.

Ture, Kwame (Stokely Carmichael), and Hamilton, Charles V. (1992; orig. 1967, *Black Power*. New York: Random House.

Turkish and Yugoslav Case (1988), *Decision of the German Federal Constitutional Court* (2 BvR 1226/83, 101, 313/84).

Ueda, Reed (1982), 'Naturalization and Citizenship', in Richard A. Easterlin *et al.*, *Immigration*. Cambridge, Mass.: Harvard University Press.

Uhlitz, Otto (1986), 'Deutsches Volk oder "Multikulturelle Gesellschaft" ', *Recht und Politik*, 22/3: 143–52.

UKACIA. See United Kingdom Action Committee on Islamic Affairs.

United Kingdom Action Committee on Islamic Affairs (1989), 'The British Muslim Response to Mr. Patten'. London: hectographed.

—— (1993), 'Muslims and the Law in Multi-Faith Britain'. London: hectographed.

US Commission on Immigration Reform (1995), *Legal Immigration: Setting Priorities*. Washington: GPO.

Uzun, Ertugrul (1993), 'Gastarbeiter-Immigranten-Minderheit', in Claus Leggewie and Zafer Senocak (eds.), *Deutsche Türken*. Reinbek: Rowohlt.

Wade, Sir William (1992), 'The Crown—Old Platitudes and New Heresies', *New Law Journal*, 18 Sept., 1275–6, 25 Sept., 1315–18.

Wahhab, Iqbal (1989), *Muslims in Britain*. London: Runnymede Trust.

Waldinger, Roger (1996), *Still the Promised City? African-Americans and New Immigrants in Postindustrial New York*. Cambridge, Mass.: Harvard University Press.

Walzer, Michael (1983), *Spheres of Justice*. New York: Basic Books.

—— (1990), 'What Does it Mean to Be an "American"?' *Social Research*, 57: 591–614.

Ward, Cynthia V. (1991), 'The Limits of "Liberal Republicanism": Why Group-Based Remedies and Republican Citizenship Don't Mix', *Columbia Law Review*, 91: 581–607.

Ward, Ian (1994), 'The Story of M: A Cautionary Tale from the United Kingdom', *International Journal of Refugee Law*, 6/2: 194–206.

Waters, Mary (1990), *Ethnic Options*. Berkeley and Los Angeles: University of California Press.

—— (1994), 'Ethnic and Racial Identities of Second-Generation Black Immigrants in New York City', *International Migration Review*, 28/4: 795–820.

Wei, William (1992), *The Asian American Movement*. Philadelphia, Pa.: Temple University Press.

Weides, Peter, and Zimmermann, Peter (1988), 'Verfassungsrechtliche Vorgaben für die Regelung des Familiennachzugs im Ausländerrecht', *Neue Juristische Wochenschrift*, 41/23: 1414–20.

Weil, Patrick, and Crowley, John (1994), 'Integration in Theory and Practice: A Comparison of France and Britain', *West European Politics*, 17/2: 110–26.

Weiler, Joseph H. H. (1995), *The State 'über alles': Demos, Telos and the German Maastricht Decision*. Florence: European University Institute, EUI Working Paper RSC, No.95/19.

Weiner, Myron (1995), *The Global Migration Crisis*. New York: HarperCollins.

Werbner, Pnina (1991), 'The Fiction of Unity in Ethnic Politics', in P. Werbner and Muhammad Anwar (eds.), *Black and Ethnic Leaderships in Britain*. London: Routledge.

White Paper (UK) (1965), *Immigration from the Commonwealth*. London: HMSO.

—— (1988), *1991 Census of Population*. London: HMSO.

White, R., and Hampson, F. J. (1982), 'The British Nationality Act 1981', *Public Law*, Spring 1982, 6–20.

Wilpert, Czarina (1988), 'Orientations, Perceptions and Strategies among Turkish Alevi and Sunni Migrants in Berlin', in Tomas Gerholm and Yngve G. Lithman (eds.), *The New Islamic Presence in Western Europe.* London: Mansell.

Wolf, Giovanna (1996), 'Efforts Toward "An Ever Closer" European Union Confront Immigration Barriers', *Indiana Journal of Global Legal Studies,* 4: 223–30.

Wolken, Simone (1988), *Das Grundrecht auf Asyl als Gegenstand der Innen- und Rechtspolitik in der Bundesrepublik Deutschland.* Frankfurt: Peter Lang.

Wollenschläger, Michael and Alexander Schraml (1994), 'Ius soli und Hinnahme von Mehrstaatigkeit', *Zeitschrift für Rechtspolitik,* 6: 225–9.

Wright, Lawrence (1994), 'One Drop of Blood', *New Yorker,* 25 July, 46–55.

Yancey, William L., Erickson, Eugene P., and Juliani, Richard N. (1976), 'Emergent Ethnicity', *American Sociological Review,* 41/3: 391–403.

Young, Ken (1983), 'Ethnic Pluralism and the Policy Agenda in Britain', in Nathan Glazer and K. Young (eds.), *Ethnic Pluralism and Public Policy.* Lexington, Mass.: Lexington Books.

Zacher, Hans F. (1993), 'Grundfragen des internationalen Sozialrechts', in H. F. Zacher, *Abhandlungen zum Sozialrecht.* Heidelberg: Müller.

Zolberg, Aristide R. (1978), 'International Migration Policies in a Changing World System', in William McNeill and Ruth Adams (eds.), *Human Migration.* Bloomington, Ind.: University of Indiana Press.

—— (1981), 'International Migrations in Political Perspective', in M. Kritz, C. Keely, and S. Tomasi (eds.), *Global Trends in Migration.* New York: Center for Migration Studies.

—— (1990), 'Reforming the Back Door', in Virginia Yans-McLaughlin (ed.), *Immigration Reconsidered.* New York: Oxford University Press.

—— (1992), 'Labour Migration and International Economic Regimes', in Mary Kritz, Lin Lean Lim, Hania Zlotnik (eds.), *International Migration Systems.* Oxford: Clarendon Press.

—— and Long, Litt Woon (1997), 'Why Islam is Like Spanish: Cultural Incorporation in Europe and the United States'. MS.

Zuleeg, Manfred (1973), 'Zur staatsrechtlichen Stellung der Ausländer in der Bundesrepublik Deutschland', *Die Öffentliche Verwaltung,* 26/11/12: 361–70.

—— (1974), 'Grundrechte für Ausländer', *Deutsches Verwaltungsblatt,* 15 Apr., 1 May, 341–9.

—— (1980), 'Einwanderungsland Bundesrepublik Deutschland', *Juristenzeitung,* 35/13: 425–31.

—— (1982), 'Stand und Entwicklung des Ausländerrechts in der Bundesrepublik Deutschland', *Zeitschrift für Ausländerrecht,* 3: 120–7.

—— (1987), 'Die Vereinbarkeit des Kommunalwahlrechts für Ausländer mit dem deutschen Verfassungsrecht', in M. Zuleeg (ed.), *Ausländerrecht und Ausländerpolitik in Europea*. Baden-Baden: Nomos.

—— (1988), 'Öffentliche Interessen gegen Familiennachzug', *Die öffentliche Verwaltung*, 14: 587–95.

—— (1989), 'Juristische Streitpunkte zum Kommunalwahlrecht für Ausländer', in Klaus Sieveking *et al.* (eds.), *Das Kommunalwahlrecht für Ausländer*. Baden-Baden: Nomos.

Index